W0050014

Springer
Berlin
Heidelberg
New York
Barcelona
Budapest
Hong Kong
London
Milano
Paris
Tokyo

CARDIAC ARRHYTHMIAS 1995

Edited by

Antonio Raviele

Proceedings of the
4th International Workshop
on Cardiac Arrhythmias

(Venice, 6-8 October 1995)

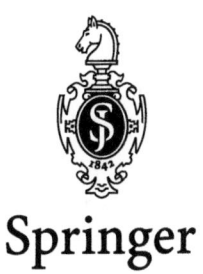

Springer

ANTONIO RAVIELE, MD
Divisione di Cardiologia
Ospedale Umberto I
Via Circonvallazione 50
I-30174 Venezia Mestre

ISBN-13: 978-3-540-75012-3   e-ISBN-13: 978-88-470-2223-2
DOI: 10.1007/978-88-470-2223-2

This work is subject to copyright. All rights are reserved, whether the whole or part of the material is concerned, specifically the rights of translation, reprinting, reuse of illustrations, recitation, broadcasting, reproduction on microfilm or in any other way, and storage in data banks. Duplications of this publication or parts thereof is permitted only under the provisions of the German Law of September 9, 1965, in its current version, and permission for use must always be obtained from Springer-Verlag. Violations are liable for prosecution under the German Copyright Law.

© Springer-Verlag Italia, Milano 1996

The use of general descriptive names, registered names, trademarks, etc, in this publication does not imply, even in the absence of a specific statement, that such names are exempt from the relevant protective laws and regulations and therefore free for general use.

Product liability: The publishers cannot guarantee the accuracy of any information about dosage and application contained in this book, in every individual case the user must check such information by consulting the relevant literature.

Table of Contents

SYNCOPE

CARDIAC PACING

SUPRAVENTRICULAR TACHYCARDIAS

SUDDEN DEATH AND VENTRICULAR ARRHYTHMIAS

Non-sustained Ventricular Tachycardia: Is It Possible to Identify the High-Risk Patients and How to Treat Them?

G. Turitto

Cardiac Electrophysiology Section, State University of New York,
Health Science Center at Brooklyn
Brooklyn, USA

Introduction

Identification of patients at high risk for sudden cardiac death, among those presenting with complex ventricular arrhythmias and spontaneous nonsustained ventricular tachycardia (NS-VT), is of paramount importance. This chapter reviews the role of risk stratification techniques, with particular emphasis on the signal-averaged electrocardiogram (ECG) and programmed ventricular stimulation (PVS), in the management of patients with NS-VT.

Complex ventricular arrhythmias are infrequent in the absence of organic heart disease and, in this setting, they are probably not associated with an adverse outcome. The prognostic role of frequent ventricular premature complexes (VPCs) and NS-VT in the presence of organic heart disease and left ventricular dysfunction is still under debate. The relationship between reduced ventricular function, complex ventricular arrhythmias, and sudden death has been analyzed mainly in two groups of patients: (1) survivors of myocardial infarction, and (2) patients with congestive heart failure secondary to ischemic or idiopathic dilated cardiomyopathy. In the 1980s, several studies suggested that frequent VPCs and NS-VT represent an independent risk factor for serious arrhythmic events, in postinfarction patients (1-4). On the other hand, the corollary demonstration that abolition of these arrhythmias prevents sudden death has not been achieved (5). The results of a large multicenter study sponsored by the National Institutes of Health, the Cardiac Arrhythmia Suppression Trial (CAST), exemplify this problem (6-8). CAST showed that the use of encainide, flecainide, or moricizine to treat asymptomatic or mildly symptomatic ventricular ectopy in patients with mild to moderate left ventricular dysfunction after myocardial infarction carries an excessive mortality risk. Thus, VPC suppression alone in this population is not an adequate indication that a drug can prolong survival. While the use of type I antiarrhythmic drugs has not been linked to increased survival in the CAST studies, preliminary data on the effect of amiodarone in postinfarction patients appeared to be more encouraging (9,10).

The prognostic value of complex ventricular arrhythmias in patients with dilated cardiomyopathy is controversial. Two recent reviews reached opposite conclusions regarding the predictive accuracy of frequent VPCs and NS-VT in this setting (11,12). Larsen et al. (11) stated that the identification of patients with dilated cardiomyopathy at risk for sudden death based on the presence of ventricular arrhythmias on the ambulatory ECG is difficult and unreliable. This may be partly related to the possibility that bradyarrhythmias are responsible for a significant number of sudden deaths in these patients. In contrast, Tamburro and Wilber (12) concluded that most evidence available in the literature confirms the prognostic significance of ambulatory arrhythmias in patients with dilated cardiomyopathy. However, data seemed insufficient to establish which criterion of spontaneous arrhythmia frequency or severity may provide the optimum indicator of risk.

Even if the CAST or subsequent studies could show that arrhythmia suppression significantly improves survival in postinfarction patients, a risk stratification strategy entailing other than the mere documentation of frequent VPCs or NS-VT on ambulatory ECG would be needed. In fact, these arrhythmias are low in sensitivity and specificity. Because of the low sensitivity, treatment may not be started in some patients at risk for sudden death, while, due to the low specificity, a large percentage of patients could be subjected to unnecessary long-term therapy. Based on these premises, the usefulness of PVS and the signal-averaged ECG for risk stratification of patients with NS-VT has received considerable interest.

Several studies and reviews have investigated the role of PVS in identifying subgroups of patients with NS-VT at high or low risk for serious arrhythmic events (13). The induction of sustained monomorphic VT in patients with spontaneous nonsustained runs may be interpreted as the demonstration of the ability of PVS to expose a fixed electrophysiologic substrate. Such abnormality may be implicated in the high risk of sudden death in this subgroup. Patients without sustained monomorphic VT induced by PVS may be at low risk for sudden death and may not warrant antiarrhythmic therapy. On the other hand, patients with induced VT may be at increased risk of sudden death. It is possible that, in these patients, antiarrhythmic therapy guided by the results of PVS may decrease the incidence of sudden death.

Only a fraction of patients with spontaneous NS-VT have induced sustained monomorphic VT during PVS; thus, several clinical, electrocardiographic and other noninvasive determinants of VT inducibility have been investigated as a means to screen patients for the invasive electrophysiologic procedure. The presence and type of heart disease, the extent of left ventricular dysfunction, as well as a history of syncope have been found to be significantly related to VT induction (13). The first prospective study of the value of the signal-averaged ECG as a predictor of the results of PVS in patients with NS-VT was published by Turitto et al. (14). This study used a stepwise discriminant function analysis which showed that the signal-averaged ECG was the single most accurate screening test for VT induction in a population of 105 patients with NS-VT (60 with coronary artery disease, 26 with idiopathic dilated cardiomyopathy, and 19 with apparently normal heart). The predictive accuracy of the signal-averaged ECG was 84% and was comparable in patients with coronary artery disease (85%) and dilated cardiomyopathy (81%). No combination between the signal-averaged ECG and other significant variables (left ventricular ejection fraction and history of syncope/presyncope) provided an improvement in predicting VT induction in comparison with the signal-averaged ECG alone.

The hypothesis that VT induction by PVS indicates patients at high risk for arrhythmic events has been tested by a number of investigators (13), discussed in a series of editorials (15-18), and is the basis for several ongoing multicenter trials enrolling patients with coronary artery disease and spontaneous NS-VT (18,19). Available reports on the prognostic significance carried by ventricular tachyarrhythmias during PVS in patients with NS-VT are characterized by one or more of the following shortcomings: (a) small sample size; (b) retrospective data collection; (c) lack of standardization of the stimulation protocol and its endpoints; or (d) lack of uniform therapeutic approach. The indications for antiarrhythmic therapy varied in different studies. Some authors only treated patients with induced sustained monomorphic VT, while others treated patients with induced ventricular fibrillation or induced NS-VT. Therapy was evaluated by means of repeat PVS in a small number of studies, while in others this was not the case. Guidelines for management of patients without induced tachyarrhythmias were also disparate; in some instances, these subjects did not receive any antiarrhythmic treatment, whereas in other studies there were subgroups followed on or off antiarrhythmic drugs. In none of the published studies was treatment randomized.

Most studies reported a low rate of serious arrhythmic events in patients with spontaneous NS-VT and no induced VT. The risk of sudden death was equally low in patients with induced NS-VT in at least two relatively large studies (20,21). In the series from

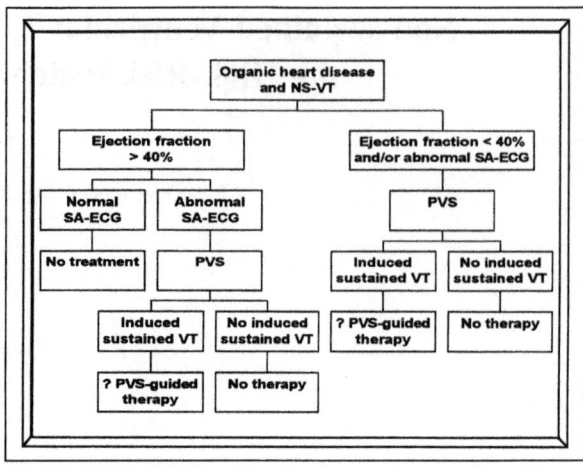

Fig. 1. Management algorithm for patients with organic heart disease and spontaneous non-sustained ventricular tachycardia. NS-VT, nonsustained ventricular tachycardia; PVS, programmed ventricular stimulation; SA-ECG, signal-averaged electrocardiogram

Turitto et al. (20), the 3-year sudden death rate was 9% in 56 patients with no induced sustained monomorphic VT followed off antiarrhythmic therapy. It seems reasonable to conclude that patients with spontaneous NS-VT and no induced sustained VT may be managed safely without the use of antiarrhythmic drugs. Conversely, VT induction seems to carry a poor prognosis, even if few studies failed to find a correlation between arrhythmia inducibility and increased risk of sudden cardiac death. In one study from Buxton et al. (22), sudden death occurred in 27% of patients with induced sustained VT, 5% of those with induced NS-VT, and 13% of those without induced VT, during a follow-up of 33 months. Sudden death occurred only in patients with left ventricular ejection fraction under 40%. Using multivariate analysis, patients with one poor prognostic marker (induced sustained VT or low ejection fraction) had a threefold increased risk of sudden death, whereas patients with both markers had a sevenfold increased risk.

The literature on the effects of antiarrhythmic therapy in patients with spontaneous NS-VT and induced VT is inconclusive. Some of the reported studies failed to document that therapy guided by PVS improved survival or was superior to empiric therapy. One caveat is that most of the early studies used large doses of type I antiarrhythmic drugs for VT therapy. On the other hand, a study by Buxton et al. that only used historical controls suggested that therapy guided by PVS was associated with a lower rate of sudden death compared to empiric therapy (23). A similar conclusion was reached by Wilber et al. (21) and Kadish et al. (17). The ability of drugs and devices to improve survival in patients with coronary artery disease, spontaneous NS-VT, and induced sustained VT is being evaluated in several prospective, randomized multicenter studies (18,19); most of them will include a control group of inducible patients who will not receive any antiarrhythmic intervention, in order to definitely prove the adverse prognostic significance of arrhythmias induced by PVS, as well as groups assigned to drug or device treatment.

An optimal protocol for risk stratification and

management of patients with organic heart disease and spontaneous NS-VT should be based on the results of the signal-averaged ECG, left ventricular function studies, and PVS, as follows (Fig. 1) (13, 20):

1. Patients with normal signal-averaged ECG and left ventricular ejection fraction ≥40% do not require PVS or long-term antiarrhythmic therapy, since the incidence of induced sustained monomorphic VT and sudden death are low in this subgroup.

2. Patients with normal signal-averaged ECG but ejection fraction <40%, as well as patients with abnormal signal-averaged ECG should be recommended for electrophysiologic evaluation, since the incidence of induced sustained monomorphic VT is high in these subgroups. Based on the results of PVS, patients with no induced sustained monomorphic VT may be followed off antiarrhythmic therapy. If VT is induced, however, these patients should be enrolled in one of the ongoing randomized studies to assess the value of antiarrhythmic therapy in preventing sudden death. If this is not feasible, inducible patients should probably receive antiarrhythmic therapy (possibly with type III drugs), with the understanding that the value of antiarrhythmic therapy has yet to be definitely established.

References

1. Bigger JT Jr, Fleiss JL, Kleiger R, Miller JP, Rolnitzky LM, the Multicenter Post-Infarction Research Group (1984) The relationships among ventricular arrhythmias, left ventricular dysfunction, and mortality in the 2 years after myocardial infarction. Circulation 69:250
2. Mukharji J, Rude E, Poole WK et al (1984) Risk factors for sudden death after acute myocardial infarction: two-year follow-up. Am J Cardiol 54:31
3. Maisel AS, Scott N, Gilpin E et al (1985) Complex ventricular arrhythmias in patients with Q wave versus non-Q wave myocardial infarction. Circulation 72:963
4. Bigger JT Jr, Weld FM, Rolnitzky LM (1981) Prevalence, characteristics and significance of ventricular tachycardia (three or more complexes) detected with ambulatory electrocardiographic recording in the late phase of acute myocardial infarction. Am J Cardiol 48:815
5. Yusuf S, Venkatesh G, Teo KK (1993) Critical review of the approaches to the prevention of sudden death. Am J Cardiol 72:51F
6. Cardiac Arrhythmia Suppression Trial (CAST) (1989) Preliminary report: effect of encainide and flecainide on mortality in a randomized trial of arrhythmia suppression after myocardial infarction. N Engl J Med 321:406
7. Echt DS, Liebson PR, Mitchell LB et al (1991) Mortality and morbidity in patients receiving encainide, flecainide, or placebo. The Cardiac Arrhythmia Suppression Trial. N Engl J Med 324:781
8. Cardiac Arrhythmia Suppression Trial II (1992) Effect of the antiarrhythmic agent moricizine on survival after myocardial infarction. N Engl J Med 327:227
9. Burkart F, Pfisterer M, Kiowski W, Follath F, Burckhardt D (1990) Effect of antiarrhythmic therapy on mortality in survivors of myocardial infarction with asymptomatic complex ventricular arrhythmias: Basel antiarrhythmic study of infarct survival (BASIS). J Am Coll Cardiol 16:1711
10. Ceremuzynski L, Kleczar E, Krzeminska-Pakula M et al (1992) The effect of amiodarone on mortality after myocardial infarction: a double-blind, placebo controlled, pilot study. J Am Coll Cardiol 20:1056
11. Larsen L, Markham J, Haffajee CL (1993) Sudden death in idiopathic dilated cardiomyopathy: role of ventricular arrhythmias. PACE 16:1051
12. Tamburro P, Wilber D (1992) Sudden death in idiopathic dilated cardiomyopathy. Am Heart J 124:1035
13. El-Sherif N, Turitto G (1995) Ventricular premature complex: risk stratification and management. In: Mandel WJ (ed) Cardiac arrhyhthmias. Their mechanisms, diagnosis and management. Lippincott, Philadelphia, pp 605-625
14. Turitto G, Fontaine JM, Ursell SN, Caref EB, Henkin R, El-Sherif N (1988) Value of the signal-averaged electrocardiogram as a predictor of the results of programmed stimulation in non-sustained ventricular tachycardia. Am J Cardiol 61:1272
15. Wiener I, Stevenson W, Weiss J, Nademanee K (1990) Are electrophysiologic studies indicated in nonsustained ventricular tachycardia? Am J Cardiol 66:642
16. Kowey PR, Taylor JE, Marinchak RA, Rials SJ (1992) Does programmed stimulation really help in the evaluation of patients with nonsustained ventricular tachycardia? Results of a meta-analysis. Am Heart J 123:481
17. Kadish A, Schmaltz S, Calkins H, Morady F (1993) Management of nonsustained ventricular tachycardia guided by electrophysiological testing. PACE 16:1037
18. Pires LA, Huang SKS (1993) Nonsustained ventricular tachycardia: identification and management of high-risk patients. Am Heart J 126:189
19. Buxton AE, Fisher JD, Josephson ME et al (1993) Prevention of sudden death in patients with coronary artery disease: the multicenter unsustained tachycardia trial (MUSTT). Prog Cardiovasc Dis 36:215
20. Turitto G, Fontaine JM, Ursell S, Caref EB, Bekheit S, El-Sherif N (1990) Risk stratification and management of patients with organic heart disease and non-sustained ventricular tachycardia: role of programmed stimulation, left ventricular ejection fraction and the signal averaged electrocardiogram. Am J Med 88(1):35N
21. Wilber DJ, Olshansky B, Moran JF, Scanlon PJ (1990) Electrophysiological testing and nonsustained ventricular tachycardia: use and limitations in patients with coronary artery disease and impaired left ventricular function. Circulation 82:350
22. Buxton AE, Marchlinski FE, Waxman HL, Flores BT, Cassidy DM, Josephson ME (1984) Prognostic factors in nonsustained ventricular tachycardia. Am J Cardiol 53:1275
23. Buxton AE, Marchlinski FE, Waxman HL et al (1987) Nonsustained ventricular tachycardia in patients with coronary artery disease: role of electrophysiology study. Circulation 75:1178

QT Prolongation in Postinfarction Patients and Sudden Death: Which Relationship?

X. Viñolas Prat and A. Bayés de Luna

Cardiology Department, Hospital de Sant Pau,
Barcelona, Spain

Prognosis of Postinfarction Patients: A Multifactorial Problem

The prognosis of postmyocardial infarction (post-MI) patients depends in particular upon the interaction between ischemia, left ventricular dysfunction, and electrical instability. The risk can be found in the center of an imaginary triangle formed by these three factors. These factors interact bidirectionally (Fig. 1), so that any of the apices affects the next directly or indirectly, and the modification of any one of these factors consequently alters the other two. Ischemia, therefore, affects left ventricular dysfunction either directly or indirectly through the electrical instability pathway and the sames happens with other two factors. We should also emphasize that the three angles of the triangle, electrical instability, left ventricular dysfunction, and ischemia, include different parameters as we can see in Fig 2. In Tables 1-3 we summarize the most important relationships between these three parameters.

First, we will briefly discuss the interaction between these three factors and then address the role of specific parameters such as QT prolongation in the risk stratification of postinfarction patients.

As we can see all parameters are interrelated, so

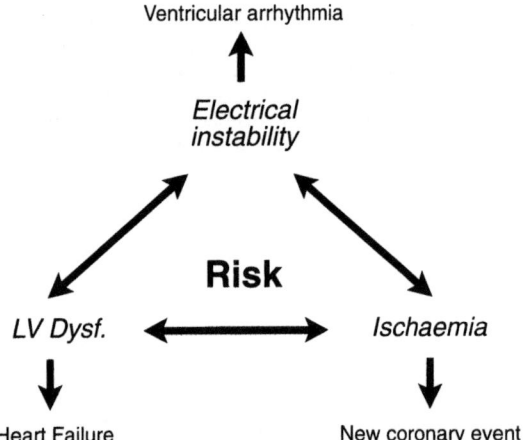

Fig. 1. Prognosis of postinfarction patients is related to three main factors: left ventricular dysfunction, ischemia and electrical instability, leading respectively to progressive heart failure, a new coronary event, or a malignant ventricular arrhytmia. But each of them interacts with the other two bidirectionally, so the modification of one of them always alters the others

Table 1. Interactions between electrical instability and ischemia

Ischemia - electrical instability
    Slowing of conduction,
    prolonged recovery of excitability
    Changes in refractoriness (shorter than in normal myocytes)
    Refractoriness dispersion allowing reentry
    Automatic and triggered activity

Electrical Instability - Ischemia
    Decreased blood flow in rapid heart rates

Table 2. Interactions between left ventricular dysfunction and electrical instability

Left ventricular dysfunction → electrical instability
    Neurohumoral factors
    Electrolytic disturbances
    Proarrhythmic effects of drugs
    Morphofunctional factors
        Anatomical block allowing reentry
        Functional block
        Triggered activity

Electrical instability - left ventricular dysfunction
    Hemodynamic disturbances in rapid heart rates
    Loss of atrial activity

Table 3. Interaction between left ventricular dysfunction and ischemia

Left ventricular dysfunction → ischemia
    Increased diastolic ventricular pressure produces
    reduced subendocardial coronary blood flow
    Low cardiac output
    Increased ischemia during exercise
    Increased wall tension (Laplace law) leads to an
    increase oxygen demand

Ischemia - left ventricular dysfunction
    Hibernating myocardium
    Stunned myocardium

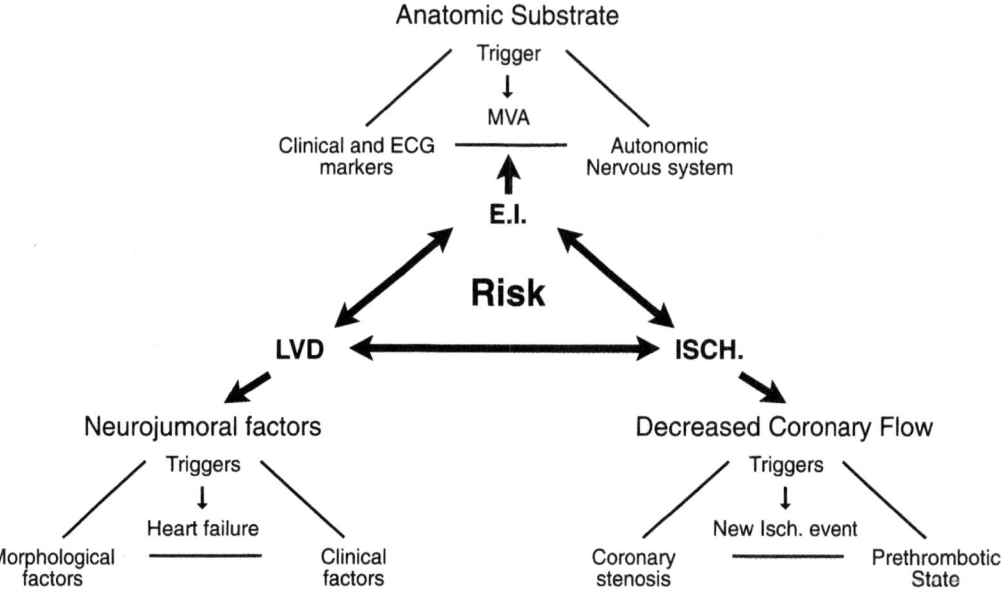

Fig. 2. Electrical instability (*E.I.*) also depends on other interrelated factors. The analysis of QT interval is one of the parameters used to analyze the status of autonomic nervous system. As is shown, other factors are important in the evaluation of electrical instability that can be assessed with other techniques. *MVA*, malignant ventricular arrhythmias; *LVD*, left ventricular dysfunction; *ISCH.*, ischemia

the best approach for post-MI risk stratification is probably also a multifactorial approach using several parameters. The most important parameters for risk stratification of post-MI patients are related to the three factors previously discussed (see Table 4).

Table 4. Parameters and techniques used to stratify risk in postmyocardial infarction patients (see Fig. 2)

	Parameters	Techniques
Electrical instability	Ventricular arrhythmias	Holter PES
	Autonomic nervous system	Holter
	Heart rate variability	
	QT interval	
	Anatomic substrate	Late potentials (conventional or Holter techniques)
Ischemia	Coronary flow	Exercise testing
		Holter Imaging techniques
	Coronary stenosis	Coronary angiography MRI
	Prethrombotic state	Blood test
Left ventricular dysfunction	Diastolic function	Echo-Doppler
	Systolic function	Echocardiography, angiography, and isotopic techniques
	State of RAA axis	Blood test

PES, Programmed electrical stimulation; MRI, magnetic resonance imaging; RAA, renin-angiotensin

There seems to be no doubt that exercise testing is the best technique to study residual ischemia, Holter technology to detect different abnormalities in the parameters related to electrical instability, and imaging techniques the most useful to detect left ventricular dysfunction and morphological alterations. As we can see in Table 4, electrical instability can be evaluated by Holter recordings, programmed ventricular stimulation and ventricular late potentials analysis. Signal-averaged electrocardiogram (ECG) allows us to noninvasively analyze the presence of ventricular late potentials indicating an arrhythmogenic substrate. It is a simple, cheap, noninvasive technique and which is available in all hospitals, and for these reasons its value for risk assessment in postinfarction patients has been extensively analyzed. It is not the aim of this paper to review this subject extensively.

QT analysis is another noninvasive parameter of electrical instability. Furthermore, as we will see in this chapter QT also allows the evaluation of the autonomic nervous system, thus complementing other variables such as heart rate variability.

QT Prolongation and Sudden Death in Post-MI Patients

From a practical point of view, electrical instability depends upon various factors which are also interrelated, as we show in Fig. 2, and can be evaluated accordingly. But QT analysis is only one method of evaluating the autonomic nervous system. We must keep these limitations in mind: QT mainly evaluates arrhythmic death after myocardial infarction and mainly analyzes autonomic nervous system function.

The relationship between the duration of the QT interval and the presence of malignant ventricular arrhythmias and its maximum expression in the presence of congenital long QT syndrome are known. Interest in the QT interval also derives from observations that excessive prolongation of the QT interval with group I drugs is associated in some cases with proarrhythmia. But, in contrast, prolongation of the QT interval by amiodarone, within limits that have not been well established, is considered a good parameter of the drug's effectiveness. All these findings have awakened interest in the relation ship between QT and ventricular arrhythmias or sudden cardiac death in post-MI patients.

The QT interval is a simple measurement on the surface ECG so the possibility of finding a relation between this measurement and the presence of malignant ventricular arrhythmias could be very important. However, measurement of the QT interval always has limitations. It is a simple measurement of cardiac repolarization, which is an extremely complex process that is influenced by many factors: presence or absence of underlying organic heart disease, the autonomic nervous system, circulating catecholamines, electrolytes, drugs (cardiac and noncardiac), and others. Moreover, the QT interval varies with heart rate, being shorter in shorter cycles, an effect that usually is corrected by the Bazett formula (1), which somewhat distorts the results. This distortion of results occurs primarily at the upper and lower limits of heart rate.

QT Interval in Surface ECG and Prognosis

As we have already mentioned, it would be very interesting to find a relation between the value of QT (and/or QTc) on the surface ECG and the risk of sudden death or ventricular arrhythmias. Some studies have been conducted (2-9) but the results are discordant. Some of them found that a QT prolongation is an independent factor of prognosis and others did not find this relation.

For instance, in some cases these discordant results can be due to the important limitations of a single 12-lead surface ECG in evaluating QT interval. First of all a single measure of QTc simply reflects the state of the autonomic nervous system at a precise moment, and, as we will see later, QT and QTc show a dynamic behavior with changes over 24 h. Thus a patient with a borderline QT at a moment during the day can show prolongation some hours later. Another factor to be kept in mind is that QT varies with heart rate, and for this reason we must make some kind of correction using different formulas, none of which are exact.

Furthermore, heart rate is not the only factor that changes QT; for instance, at the same heart rate isoproterenol infusion shortens the QT interval. Likewise, in patients with VVI pacemakers with a fixed heart rate, the QT interval becomes shorter with exercise. This indicates that the QT interval is influenced by a number of factors, many of them dependent on the autonomic nervous system. Therefore, the study of the dynamic behavior and circadian rhythm of the QT interval seems to be more important than a single measurement of QT because it reflects this multiple interaction. Another important aspect of the study of the dynamics of QT prolongation is that the circadian variations in the QT interval examined in relation to the circadian rhythm of malignant ventricular arrhythmias or sudden death may clarify some of the triggering mechanisms of sudden death.

QT Variations in Postinfarction Patients With and Without Ventricular Arrhytmias

In order to test the possible value of dynamic QT behavior in post-MI patients, we first analyzed the value of QT variations in the Holter tapes of postinfarction patients with and without malignant ventricular arrhythmias. A manual measurement was made (10) of the QT intervals on the Holter tape and then an algorithm developed for automatic measurement of the QT interval. Manual measurement of the QTc intervals was done by selecting several beats per hour. These measurements do not provide information on subtle and transitory changes in the QT-QTc interval. We found no differences in mean QTc value between postinfarction patents with and without malignant ventricular arrhythmias. However, patients with malignant ventricular arrhythmias during follow-up had QTc peaks >500 ms more frequently than patients without these arrhythmic complications. Manual measurement is very time consuming and therefore not applicable to large series of patients. Another limitation is that manual measurement, as we have already mentioned, does not provide information about the transient changes of QT because it only analyzes some beats per hour.

Automatic Measurement of the QT Interval

Using the automatic algorithm we studied two groups of postinfarction patients (10). Group I consisted of 14 consecutive postinfarction patients admitted to the coronary unit of our hospital for ventricular tachycardia (eight patients) or after an aborted sudden death episode (six patients). Arrhythmia secondary to an acute ischemic episode was excluded in all patients. In seven patients, ventricular arrhythmias occurred between the subacute phase and the second month postinfarction and in the rest of the patients it occurred after 2 months. The clinical characteristics are summarized in Table 5. The second group included 28 postinfarction patients matched by clinical data, ejection fraction, and infarction site who did not have malignant ventricular arrhythmias in a similar period of time. There were no significant differences in the clinical characteristics of the two groups of patients. Holter

Table 5. Clinical characteristics of postmyocardial infarction patients with and without life-threatening arrhythmias

	Group I (n=14)	Group II (n=28)	p value
Sex (M/F)	12/2	25/3	NS
Age (years)	59±13	57±10	NS
Anterior MI	9 (64%)	16 (57%)	NS
LV ejection fraction (%)	40±6	44±8	NS
LV ejection fraction <40%	6 (42%)	13 (46%)	NS
Angina	3 (21%)	7 (25%)	NS
Diabetes mellitus	3 (21%)	8 (28%)	NS
Hypertension	8 (57%)	15 (53%)	NS

Group I, Postmyocardial infarction patients with secondary life-threatening arrhythmia; group II, postmyocardial infarction patients without life-threatening arrhythmias. MI, myocardial infarction; NS, not significant.

Table 6. Automatic QTC analysis in the three studied groups

	Group I (n=14)	Group II (n=28)	Group III (n=10)	p value I vs II	p value I vs III
Total beats automatically analyzed	682,960	1,276,498	563,910	–	–
Global QTc	425±15	408±19	402±20	<0.005	<0.001
Total number of peaks of QTc >500 ms	11,114 (1.62%)	823 (0.06%)	0 (0%)	<0.005	<0.005
Patients with peaks of QTc >500 ms	7 (50%)	2 (7%)	None	<0.005	<0.03
Patients with clusters of peaks of QTc >500 ms	4 (28%)	None	None	<0.02	<0.02

Group I, Postmyocardial infarction patients who presented with a secondary life-threatening arrhythmia; group II, postmyocardial infarction patients who did not present with life-threatening arrhythmias; group III, healthy subjects.

recordings were made routinely in all patients as a control before hospital release after MI or as a routine "screening" method during follow-up. At most, the Holter recording preceded the arrhythmic episode by 1 year. A 3-channel Holter recorder was used in every case. The QT interval was analyzed on the channel that had the best signal-to-noise ratio.

The mathematical algorithm for automatic measurement of the QT interval has been described in detail elsewhere (11). It is important to emphasize that we analyzed the results based on a QT interval reaching the end of the T wave. Other authors use a QT interval ending at the peak of the T wave (peak QT) because it is considered simpler and more stable. However, with use of peak QT values part of the information gets lost because QT may be prolonged exclusively at the expense of the terminal parts of the T wave. Later, the QT interval was corrected using the Bazett formula (1), which is simple and widely used in spite of its limitations. Other formulas could have been used but none of these is accepted universally and all have limitations so we used the most widely accepted correction method. Data from the various QTc intervals could be represented as a trend that allowed exact assessment of the behavior of the QTc interval throughout the day in a practical form.

The next step was to validate the algorithm. This was done by comparing the results obtained from manual measurements by two cardiologists on recordings printed at 25 mm/s with the results obtained by automatic analysis (11). An analysis was made of 650 beats on 18 different tapes. The mean error between the manual and automatic measurements was 2.4±17 ms and 2±14 ms and the difference between the manual measurements by the two experts was 1.9±10 ms. Therefore, the differences between automatic and manual measurements were similar to those of manual measurements by two experts. This validated the use of this method for analysis of larger patient groups and, above all, the analysis of all QT values, which cannot be done manually. Automatic measurement is the only valid means of evaluating transitory changes in the value of QT intervals, and thus analyzing "peaks" of QT.

We analyzed mean QTc value, "peaks" of QTc (QTc values above a certain value), and clusters (groups of peak QT values lasting more that 1 min). The mean QTc interval was longer in patients with malignant ventricular arrhythmias than in patients with-

out these arrhythmias: 425±20 ms versus 408±19 ms (Table 6).

The behavior of the QT interval in relation to time of day is shown in Fig. 3. The data in Fig. 3 confirm the tendency toward longer QTc values from 11 p.m. to 11 a.m. than from 11 a.m. to 11 p.m. (430±18 ms versus 425±19 ms). These differences were not statistically significant, perhaps because of the small sample size, but they suggested a trend and concurred with findings in healthy subjects.

QT Peaks. QT peaks were analyzed for different cut-off points: >440, >460, >480, and >500 ms. Statistically significant differences were found only when the group of patients with QT interval values above 500 ms were analyzed (Table 7). Fifty percent of the postinfarction patients who had malignant ventricular arrhythmias had QT values over 500 ms as compared with only 7% (2 of 28) of postinfarction patients who did not have malignant ventricular arrhythmias. None of the healthy subjects analyzed had peak QTc over 500 ms. When we examined the presence of clusters, we found that none of the postinfarction patients without malignant ventricular arrhythmias had clusters but 28% of the postinfarction patients with malignant ventricular arrhythmias did (Table 6). When the number of beats with QTc >500 ms was analyzed, postinfarction patients with malignant ventricular arrhythmias had long QTc in 1.62% of beats compared with only 0.06% of beats in postinfarction patients without malignant

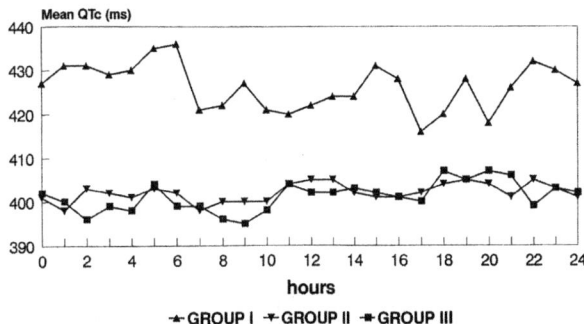

Fig. 3. Plot of the mean hourly QTc interval of the postmyocardial infarction patients with (Group I, ▲) and without (Group II, ▼) life-threatening ventricular arrhythmias and healthy subjects (Group III, ■). Note that patients who developed life-threatening ventricular arrhythmias presented a longer QTc over 24 h than postmyocardial infarction patients who did not present with life-threatening arrhythmias

9

Table 7. Patients with peaks of QTC lengthening measured automatically in Holter recordings according to a determined cut-off of QTc value

Peaks of QTc interval (ms)	Group I (n=14)		Group II (n=28)		p value
	n	%	n	%	
>440	14	100	20	71	NS
>460	10	71	14	50	NS
>480	7	50	8	28	NS
>500	7	50	2	7	<0.005

Group I, Postmyocardial infarction patients who presented with a secondary life-threatening arrhythmia; group II, postmyocardial infarction patient who did not present with life-threatening arrhythmias.

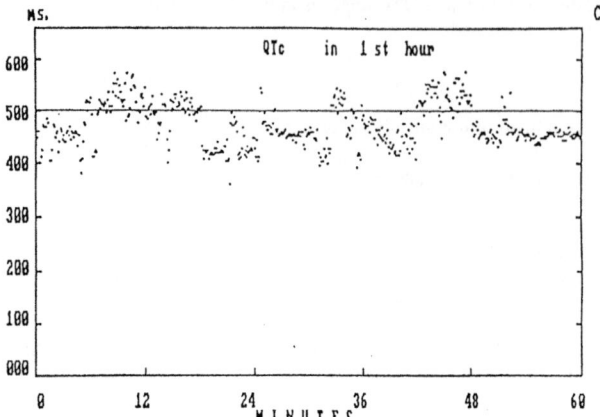

Fig. 4. Trend of QT in a patient showing transient prolongation of QT > 500 ms

ventricular arrhythmia. Figure 4 shows the graphic representation of postinfarction patients who had peak QTc >500 ms. It is important to note that these peaks sometimes occurred in groups and did not correspond to artifacts of automatic analysis. The trend in QTc intervals can also be seen in Fig. 4.

Circadian Rhythm of Peaks. QTc peaks >500 ms exhibited a circadian rhythm, the percentage of QT peaks per hour being higher between 11 p.m. and 11 a.m. than during the rest of the day. The most relevant results are summarized in Table 8. This finding coincides with hourly mean QTc values, which were longer during the same hours of the day. The QTc clusters also demonstrated circadian behavior, with a higher incidence between 11 p.m. and 11 a.m. If we analyze the total duration of QTc clusters, which also occurred at a period that coincided with the periods in which patients are at "higher risk," QTc duration was longer in the same hours. The mean duration of clusters from 11 p.m. to 11 a.m. was 10.60±9.64 min and from 11 a.m. to 11 p.m. it was 2.85±1.95 (Table 8). However, this behavior does not indicate whether the QT interval was a triggering factor in malignant ventricular arrhythmias or only an accompanying event.

The behavior of the QT/QTc interval varied throughout the day in postinfarction patients with malignant ventricular arrhythmias: there was a longer mean QTc/h, a larger number of QTc values >500 ms in absolute terms and as a percentage of beats, and more frequent and prolonged QTc clusters in the period between 11 p.m. and 11 a.m.

Algra et al. (12) recently published the report of a study in which QTc interval was analyzed automatically on Holter tapes. Here, prolongation of the QTc interval to more than 440 ms doubled the patients' risk of sudden death. Moreover, the presence of a short QTc interval (<400 ms) was also predictive of arrhythmic complications during follow-up. However, Algra's study is not entirely comparable to ours because only 50% of their very heterogeneous group of patients were postinfarction patients and many of them were taking drugs that can modify QT interval.

As already mentioned, the rate of occurrence of sudden death and malignant ventricular arrhythmias is greater between 6 a.m. and noon. Although this fact may show a link between these two factors, it does not demonstrate a cause-effect relationship. Prolongation of the QT interval may only be a marker of malignant ventricular arrhythmias but not a trigger. Although some isolated cases have been described, we have been unable to confirm in our review, that a sudden prolongation of QTc is the triggering mechanism of sudden death and not only a manifestation of an underlying mechanism.

As noted, the QT interval is influenced by sympathetic/parasympathetic tone. The QT and the RR interval also varies with sympathetic or parasympathetic stimulation. Variations in the QT interval may coincide with disturbances in the autonomic nervous system that may trigger malignant ventricular arrhythmias.

Conclusions

As we have seen, the presence of malignant ventricular arrhythmias and sudden cardiac death demonstrates a

Table 8. Circadian rhythm of the peaks and clusters of QTC lengthening over 500 ms in postmyocardial infarction patients wih malignant ventricular arrhythmias (group I)

	24 h of Holter	11 a.m.-11 p.m.	11 p.m.-11 a.m.	p value
Number of peaks of QTc > 500 ms/h	463±315	336±176	590±375	<0.05
Percentage of peaks of QTc > 500 ms/h	4.17±2.83	3.02±1.58	5.31±3.37	<0.05
Number of grouped peaks (clusters) with QTc lengthening > 500 ms/h	1.29±1.1.27	0.84±0.83	1.75±1.48	NS
Mean duration (min) of the grouped peaks per hour	7.41±8.31	2.85±1.95	10.60±9.64	<0.04

Results represent the mean±standard deviation taken from hourly Holter monitoring within the period of time indicated. The *p* value expresses the differences between time from 11 a.m. to 11 p.m. versus from 11 p.m. to 11 a.m.

circadian rhythm. Most of the actually known possible "triggers" such as ischemia, ventricular premature beats, etc. also show this circadian patttern. In the past years a good deal of attention has been focused on the important role of the autonomic nervous system as a triggering mechanism of malignant arrhythmias. Although we have not reviewed all the repolarization parameters of the sympathetic-parasympathetic balance, some of them, such as the heart rate variability, also show this circadian rhythm. QT and QTc interval is another important parameter for autonomic nervous system analysis, although it is also influenced by other factors (such as circulating catecolamines, drugs, etc.). In our study as in Algra's study (12), a QT prolongation during Holter recording is more frequently present in patients with arrhythmic events after MI. In postinfarction patients with malignant ventricular arrhythmias during follow-up this circadian pattern remains but sudden prolongation of QTc values ("peaks") appears, usually grouped in cluster form. The circadian rhythm of these peaks is quite similar to the circadian pattern of sudden death, although this is not a demonstration or evidence that QTc prolongation is the triggering factor of sudden death. This QTc prolongation may only be the manifestation of an underlying process such as a sudden imbalance of the autonomic nervous system. Circadian pattern factors offer a new avenue in the study of the mechanisms of sudden death. Many mechanisms, triggers, modulators, etc. are still unknown and why an arrhythmia develops at a given moment in the follow-up sometimes remains a mystery. There are still many questions that are open: does the circadian pattern of these parameters have any clinical relevance; is it only an external manifestation of an underlying mechanism or is it the actual triggering mechanism; does the lack of the circadian pattern represent a worse prognosis factor in postinfarction patients? Without any doubt the technological improvements in Holter equipment in the future, with the possibility of studying not only circadian variations of heart rate variability but also other repolarization parameters such as QT interval, T wave alternans, etc., and its modification before an arrhythmic episode (using Holter recordings of AICD devices) will increase our knowledge of sudden death mechanisms.

References

1. Bazett HC (1920) An analysis of the time-relation of the electrocardiogram. Heart 7:353-370
2. Schwartz PJ, Wolf S (1978) QT interval prolongation as predictor of sudden death in patients with myocardial infarction. Circulation 57:1074-1077
3. Haynes RE, Hallstrom AP, Cobb LA (1978) Repolarisation abnormalities in survivors of out-of-hospital ventricular fibrillation. Circulation 57:654-658
4. Anhve S, Gilpin E, Madsen EB, Froelicher V, Henning H, Ross J Jr (1984) Prognostic importance of QTc interval at discharge after acute myocardial infarction: a multicenter study of 865 patients. Am Heart J 108:395-400
5. Algra A, Tijsen JGP, Roeland J, Pool J, Lubsen J (1991) QTc prolongation measured by standard 12-lead electrocardiography is an independent risk factor for sudden death due to cardiac arrest. Circulation 83:1888-1894
6. Moller M (1981) QT interval in relation to ventricular arrhythmias and sudden cardiac death in post-myocardial infarction patients. Acta Med Scand 220:73-77
7. Wheelam K, Mukharji J, Rude RE (1986) Sudden death and its relation to QT prolongation after acute myocardial infarction: 2 year follow-up. Am J Cardiol 57:745-750
8. Boudoulas H, Sohn YH, O'Neill WM, Brown R, Weissler AM (1982) The QT<QS2 syndrome: a new mortality indicator in coronary artery disease. Am J Cardiol 50:1229-1235
9. Pohjola-Sintonen S, Siltanen P, Haapakosi J (1986) The QTc interval on the discharge electrocardiogram for predicting survival after acute myocardial infarction. Am J Cardiol 57:1066-1068
10. Martí V, Guindo J, Homs E, Viñolas X, Bayés de Luna A (1992) Peaks of QTc lengthening in Holter recordings as a marker of life-threatening arrhythmias in postmyocardial infarction patients. Am Heart J 124:234-235
11. Laguna P, Thakor NV, Caminal P, Jané R, Bayés de Luna A, Marti V, Guindo J (1990) New algorithm for QT interval analysis in 24-hour Holter ECG: performance and applications. Med Biol Eng Comput 28:67-73
12. Algra A, Tijssen JGP, Roetlandt JRTC, Pool J, Lubsen J (1993) QT interval variables from 24 hour electrocardiography and the two year risk of sudden death. Br Heart J 70:43-48

T wave Alternans. A Marker of Vulnerability to Ventricular Tachyarrhythmias

N. El-Sherif

Cardiology Division, State University of New York,
Health Science Center and Veterans Affairs Medical Center,
Brooklyn, USA

Introduction

Alternation of the configuration and/or duration of the repolarization wave of the electrocardiogram (ECG) – usually referred to as T wave alternans, and occasionally as ST alternans, U wave, or TU wave alternans – is seen under diverse experimental and clinical conditions (1,2). Interest in repolarization alternans is attributed to the hypothesis that it may reflect underlying dispersion of repolarization in the ventricle, a well-recognized electrophysiolgic substrate for reentrant ventricular tachyarrhythmias (3-6). Although overt T wave alternans in the ECG are not common, in recent years digital signal-processing techniques capable of detecting subtle degrees of T wave alternans have suggested that the phenomonem may be more prevalent than recognized and could represent an important marker of vulnerability to ventricular tachyarrhythmias (7-9). This report provides a brief review of the experimental and clinical conditions associated with T wave alternans and the electrophysiologic basis that links the phenomenon to ventricular vulnerability. Preliminary observations on a recently developed noninvasive technique to detect subtle T wave alternans will also be discussed (10).

Experimental T Wave Alternans

Tachycardia-Dependent Alternans of Normal Cardiac Fibers

Alternans of the action potential duration (APD) of normal Purkinje and ventricular muscle fibers under physiologic conditions can consistently be induced by a critical short cycle length. In Purkinje fibers, alternans induced by a decrease in cycle length always declined progressively and disappeared before the APD reached the new steady state. In ventricular muscle fibers, the magnitude of alternans induced by a decrease in cycle length also tended to decrease progressively because of declining memory effect. However, at very rapid rates, alternans of action potential shape in ventricular muscle fibers could continue indefinitely without a change in diastolic interval (11).

Alternation of APD of Purkinje fibers is explained by the differences in the recovery of membrane currents generated by the preceding action potential (12,13). The two recovery processes that could be curtailed by a reduction of the interval between successive action potentials are the recovery of the slow inward calcium current (I_{ca}) from inactivation and the difference in magnitude of the decaying time dependent outward current(I_k) (12,13). Although the same factors may also influence the alternation of APD of muscle fibers, the latter seem to have an independent mechanism for action potential alternans associated with tension alternans. The alternans in muscle fibers may be related to differences in the concentration and/or handling of intracellular calcium (11). Action potential alternans of muscle fibers can be limited to alternation of the configuration of the plateau without changes in APD or diastolic intervals (11). It is important to emphasize the differences between the mechanisms of alternans in Purkinje and muscle fibers because the relative contribution of both type of fibers to the configuration of the endocardial monophasic action potential (MAP) is still largely unknown.

Myocardial Ischemia and Alternans

Myocardial ischemia may create electrical alternans resulting from electrophysiologic nonhomogeneities within the ischemic myocardium as well as between the ischemic and nonischemic myocardium. The mechanism of electrical alternans at the cellular level during experimental myocardial ischemia has been studied in intact and isolated hearts (1,5,14,15). Acute ischemia shortened the APD and decreased action potential amplitude, velocity of depolarization, and resting membrane potential. Alternans of action potential amplitude was associated with alternation of baseline and ST segment level, and alternans of upstroke velocity of action potential was associated with alternating depolarization morphology in the extracellular signals (14). At a later stage of ischemia, postrepolarization refrac-

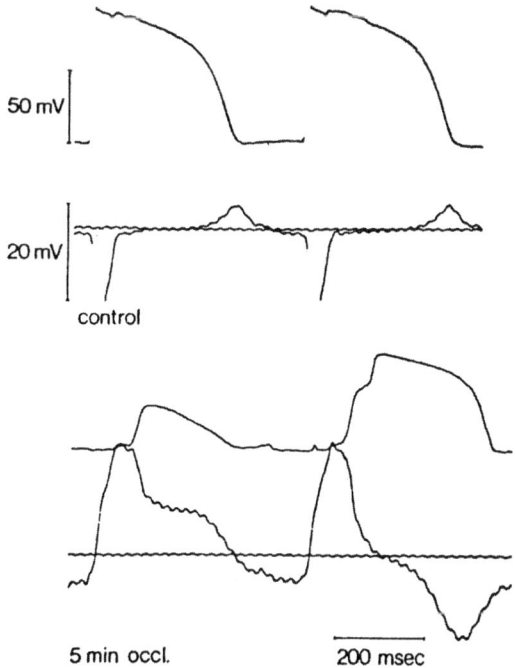

Fig. 1. Transmembrane action potential and local electrogram before (*top*) and 5 min after (*bottom*) coronary occlusion (*occl.*) in a pig heart. Two complexes occur during alternans. Note that delayed repolarization in the ischemic area results in a negative T wave in the electrogram. From Kleber et al. (14)

toriness resulted in progressive delay of recovery that eventually caused encroachment of the stimulated complex on the next stimulus, thus producing alternans of APD and refractoriness (Fig. 1). It has been suggested that the differences in action potential amplitude and resting membrane potential during alternans create the substrate for spontaneous reexcitation, contributing to ventricular tachyarrhythmias during ischemia (5,14,16).

Alternans caused by asynchrony of depolarization is not the only mechanism of ST segment alternans during acute ischemia because ST and T wave alternans have been recorded in association with alternating amplitude and duration of MAP without activation delay (16). The risk of ventricular fibrillation increases with increasing magnitude of ST alternans, particularly when the ST segment alternans is discordant (that is, the ST changes in the adjacent leads are out of phase) (17).

In addition to manifest alternans in the ECG, subtle forms of T wave alternans that could be detected by spectral analytical methods have been shown to be temporarily associated with occurrence of ventricular fibrillation in dogs following ligation of the left anterior coronary artery (8).

The ionic basis of repolarization alternans during acute ischemia is not well defined. It has been suggested that changes in electrical restitution that coincide with repolarization alternans may reflect a disturbance in ionic conductances related to either accumulation of extracellular potassium or impaired intracellular cycling of calcium (13). Antzelevitch and colleagues (18) have proposed that alternans of the ST segment and T wave may be due to loss of action potential dome on alternate beats during ischemia. They recorded action potentials from endocardial and epicardial myocytes

dissociated from canine left ventricle. When the tissue was superfused for 30 min with ischemic solution, there was a suppression of dome on alternate beats in the epicardial tissue but no effect on endocardial tissue. The simulated ECG obtained by differential recording of the endocardial and epicardial traces revealed an alternation pattern. It was postulated that these morphology changes leading to alternans could set the stage for dispersion of refractoriness and vulnerability to ventricular arrhythmias.

TU Alternans in Experimental Models of Long QTU Syndrome

El-Sherif et al. (19) suggested that TU alternans in the long QTU syndrome may be due to alternate propagation of early afterdepolarization (EAD). This was shown in an experimental model of bradycardia-dependent long QTU and torsade de pointes (TDP) ventricular tachyarrhythmia in the dog induced by anthopleurin A. The drug results in marked lengthening of APD by delaying inactivation of the sodium current and produces EADs preferentially in Purkinje fibers. El-Sherif et al. (19) studied the propagation of EAD in a Purkinje-muscle preparation exposed to anthopleurin-A and showed that conduction of EAD from Purkinje to muscle fibers was relatively slow and suggested that the conduction delay occurred predominantly at the Purkinje muscle junction. Tachycardia-dependent alternation of a deflection on the endocardial MAP in the same experimental model was interpreted to represent alternate conduction block of an EAD (Fig. 2).

However, the hypothesis that 2:1 propagation of EAD can explain TU alternans in the long QTU syndrome is based only on analysis of MAP repolarization recordings. The validity of the hypothesis depends on whether these deflections on the endocardial MAP actually represent EAD. The nature of the endocardial MAP in the in vivo heart is not well defined. The MAP recording may reflect activity generated in Purkinje fibers and in subendocardial muscle fibers. In a preliminary study from our laboratory, we have shown that, in vitro, mere differences in repolarization between Purkinje and adjacent muscle can produce MAP deflections similar to phase 3 EAD in normal endocardial preparations (20). The late phase 3 repolarization of the Purkinje fiber appeared as a late phase 3 EAD in the MAP. Thus it is possible that what has been interpreted as 2:1 occurrence of EAD on phase 3 of the endocardial MAP may have represented a greater degree of alternation of APD of Purkinje fibers compared to adjacent muscle fibers.

Clinical T Wave Alternans

Acute Ischemia and T Wave Alternans

Manifest T wave or ST alternans in the ECG have been frequently reported in clinical situations associated with acute myocardial ischemia such as Prinzmetal's angina (21,22), angioplasty (23), bypass graft occlusion (24), the postexercise period (25), and myocardial in-

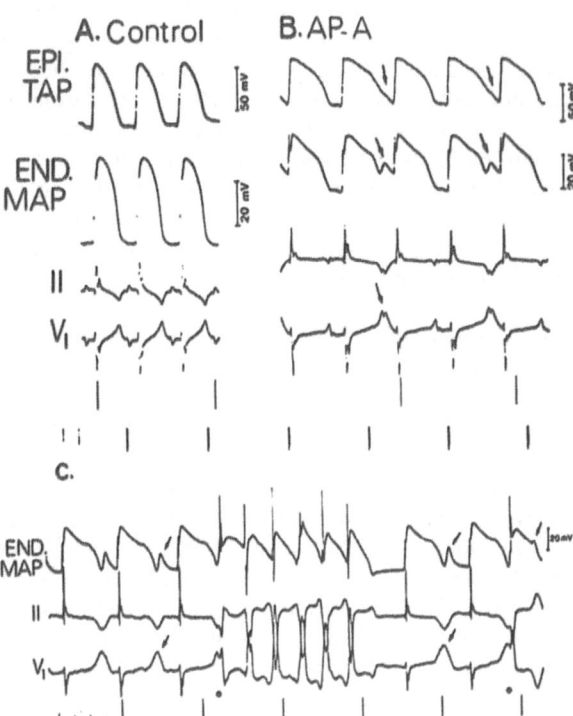

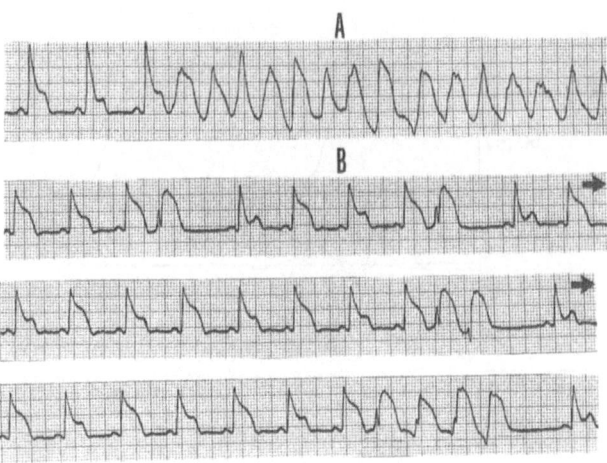

Fig. 3A,B. ECG recording of lead II from a patient during Prinzmetal's angina showing ST alternans and runs of ventricular tachycardia

Fig. 2. Recordings from a canine experiment of epicardial (*EPI*) transmembrane action potential (*TAP*), endocardial (*END*) monophasic action potential (*MAP*), and surface ECG showing QTU alternans. **A** Control recordings. **B** Recordings obtained 14 min after the administration of anthopleurin-A (*AP-A*) (4 µg/kg) showing QTU alternans due to 2:1 alternation of an early after depolarization EAD (marked by *arrows*) that was more prominent in the endocardial MAP. Cardiac cycle during the alternans was 450 ms. **C** Cardiac cycle length was increased to 700-750 ms by vagal stimulation. Epicardial TAP could not be maintained. There was further prolongation of the endocardial MAP and QTU segment with disappearance of the QTU alternans. Every action potential was followed by an EAD with an increased amplitude. A short run of ventricular tachycardia occurred and the first ectopic action potential arose from the peak of the EAD. Arrhythmia terminated by full repolarization of the last action potential, which did not show an EAD. From El-Sherif et al. (19)

farction (26,27). In patients with acute ischemia, ST alternans usually consists of alternating levels of ST elevation in the standard or anterior precordial leads, or both, displaying an acute injury pattern with an anteriorly or inferiorly directed ST vector. ST alternans during acute ischemia have been associated with the appearance or aggravation of ventricular tachyarrhythmia. For example, in a study by Turitto and El-Sherif (22) the incidence of ventricular arrhythmias was significantly higher in patients with Prinzmetal's angina and visible ST segment alternans (78%) than those without ST alternans (32% - $p<0.05$) (Fig. 3). The statistical correlation between alternans and arrhythmogenesis pertained only to the occlusion and not the reperfusion phase. The frequency of ischemic attacks accompanied by angina, the magnitude of ST segment elevation at the peak of the ischemic attack, and the duration of the attack, were all significantly greater in patients with visible ST alternans. However, it has been noted that the frequent occurrence of ventricular tachyarrhythmias and sudden cardiac death during coronary artery spasm in the absence of ST alternans makes it difficult to assess the specificity of this association (1).

T or TU Wave Alternans in Patients with Congenital or Acquired Long QTU and TDP

T or TU alternans are relatively common in patients with congenital or idiopathic long QTU and TDP as well as in those patients in whom the syndrome is related to electrolyte abnormality, including hypokalemia, hypomagnesemia, and hypocalcemia (28-31). In contrast, T or TU alternans are rare in patients with the acquired long QTU and TDP (31).

The acquired drug-induced long QTU and TDP is characteristically bradycardia dependent. On the other hand, bradycardia is not a requirement for the development of long QTU and TDP in patients with congenital or idiopathic long QTU syndrome as well as when the syndrome is associated with electrolyte abnormality.

On the contrary, patients with congenital or idiopathic long QTU syndrome characteristically develop TDP during periods of increased adrenergic activity (29) usually associated with relative increase of the heart rate, i.e., tachycardia dependent. It is in this group of patients that tachycardia dependent TU alternans is commonly observed and is associated with the onset of TDP (Fig. 4). It has been suggested that an abnormal adjustment of APD to shortening of the cardiac cycle length may play an important role in the mechanism of TDP in those patients (32). This can also easily explain the common occurrence of TU alternans on sudden increase of the heart rate. These observations raise the role of dispersion of repolarization versus EAD in the initiation and perpetuation of TDP in general and in this group of patients in particular (31).

There is strong experimental and clinical evidence that the initiating beat of TDP represents an action potential triggered by EAD arising from the Purkinje network. However, the electrophysiologic mechanism(s) of subsequent beats is less certain. These beats could result from a succession of triggered action potentials arising from EAD, from circus movement reentry due to dispersion of repolarization, or from a combination of more than one mechanism (33).

However, it is possible that the congenital/idiopathic and the acquired long QTU syndromes have

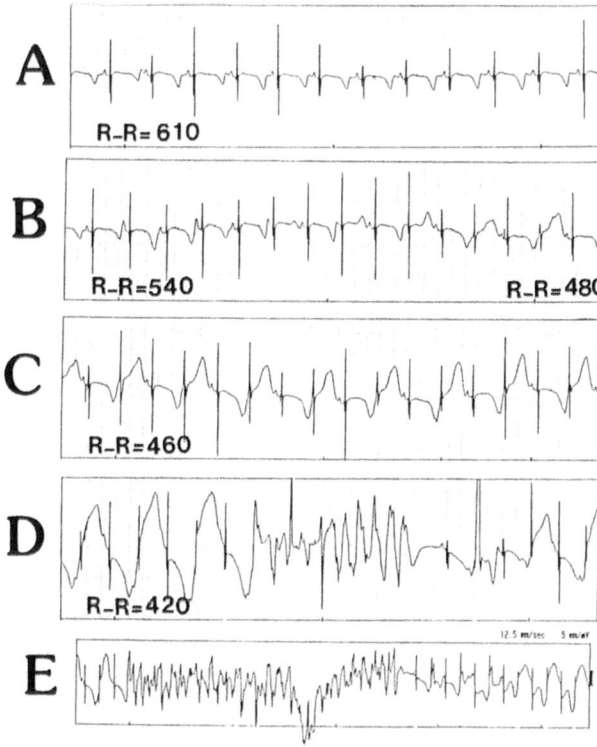

Fig. 4A-E. Representative ECG recordings from a newborn baby boy with congenital long QTU syndrome showing tachycardia-dependent TU alternans and torsade de pointes tachyarrhythmia. R-R cycle lengths are in milliseconds. From Habbab and El-Sherif (31)

similar electrophysiologic mechanisms but differ in the degree of the abnormality and/or the relative contribution of each mechanism. A recent report showing subtle T wave alternans in the ECG associated with alternans of the endocardial MAP recordings from a patient with procainamide-related long QTU and TDP (Figs. 5, 6) raises the possibility that subtle degrees of T wave alternans may be detected in patients with acquired long QTU and TDP if recent digital signal processing techniques are utilized.

Subtle T Wave Alternans and Vulnerability to Ventricular Tachyarrhythmias

T wave alternans in vivo may be so subtle as to preclude visual detection, yet be statistically significant and easily measurable with digital signal-processing techniques (7). In a recent study signal-processing techniques to measure electrical alternans at a microvolt level were utilized to establish the prognostic importance of electrical alternans in a group of 83 patients referred for diagnostic electrophysiologic testing (9). Irrespective of left ventricular mechanical function, subtle alternation of the ST segment or T wave was an independent marker of vulnerability to inducible ventricular arrhythmias and clinical arrhythmic events. The maximum level of T wave alternans recorded in this study was only 116 mV, indicating the need for sensitive signal-processing techniques and explaining why alternans is not commonly recognized on standard ECG tracings. In this study, however, alternans was measured during atrial pacing in order to eliminate any possible influence of heart rate or beat-to-beat

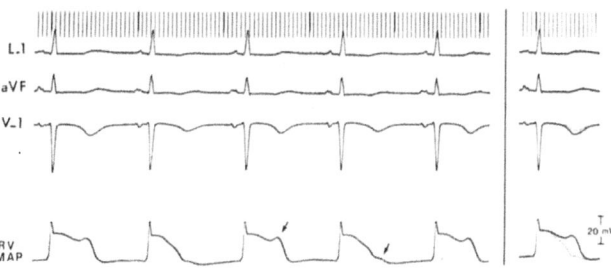

Fig. 5. Recordings from a patient with procainamide-related acquired long QTU and torsade de pointes tachyarrhythmia. Electrocardiographic leads L₁, aVF, and V₁ are shown. The endocardial monophasic action potential (*MAP*) recording from the right ventricle (*RV*) shows alternation of the configuration and duration of MAP associated with subtle but definite alternation of the TU wave at a constant cycle length of 1140 ms. The *right panel* illustrates a superimposed recording of two consecutive beats. The *arrows* point to deflections consistent with early afterdepolarization. From Habbab and El-Sherif (31)

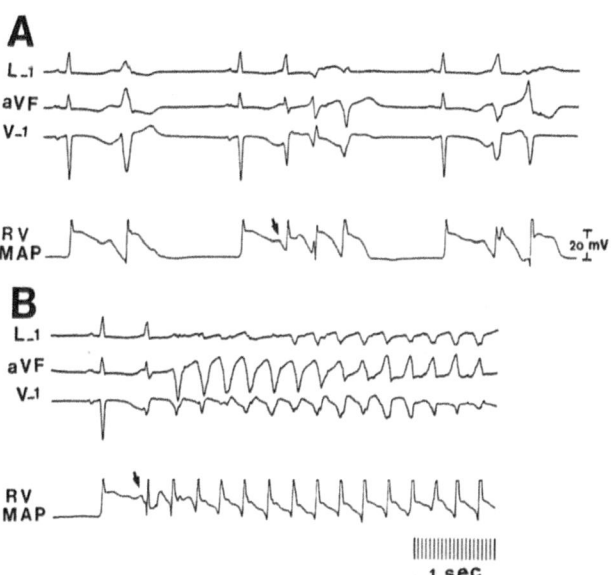

Fig. 6A,B. Recordings from the same patient in Fig. 5 showing the occurrence of torsade de pointes tachyarrhythmia. The *arrows* point to deflections on the endocardial monophasic action potential (*MAP*) recording from the right ventricle (*RV*) that are consistent with early afterdepolarizations (EAD). Electrocardiographic leads L₁, aVF, and V₁ are shown. Note that the first ectopic action potential seems to arise from the descending limb of the EAD and before complete repolarization of the sinus beat action potential. From Habbab and El-Sherif (31)

variability in heart rate on measured T wave alternans.

To make the measurement of repolarization alternans a suitable test for ambulatory patients, improvements in the algorithm are required to compensate for the fluctuations in heart rate associated with sinus rhythm. Recent technical improvements allow the detection of microvolt T wave alternans during sinus rhythm with the heart rate moderately elevated to >90 beats/min using bicycle exercise (Fig. 7). In a preliminary multicenter study (10) alternans voltage > 1.0 mV at rest or >1.9 mV during exercise and alternans ratio >3 were required for a positive alternans test. Arrhythmia vulnerability was defined by clinical or induced sustained ventricular tachycardia or fibrillation. The positive and negative predictive values of T wave alternans in this group of patients were 85% and 100%, respectively. Further studies will be required to evaluate

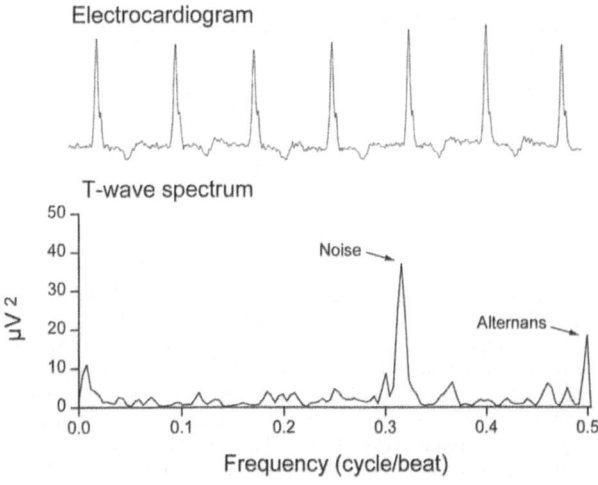

Electrocardiogram

T-wave spectrum

Fig. 7. Surface ECG lead and T wave power spectrum from a patient with resuscitated cardiac arrest and inducible fast ventricular tachyarrhythmia who later received an implantable cardioverter defibrillator. The ECG and T wave spectrum were obtained during bicycle exercise that increased the heart rate to approximately 100 beats/min. The spectrum shows a large noise peak at 0.33 cycle per beat reflecting the noise artifact associated with bicycling. A second peak at 0.5 cycle per beat illustrates the presence of T wave alternans. Note the absence of any visible beat-to-beat alternation of T wave in the surface ECG lead

the test as a noninvasive index of vulnerability to ventricular tachyarrhythmias and to compare the sensitivity and specificity to other indices of sudden cardiac electrical death.

References

1. Surawicz B, Fisch C (1992) Cardiac alternans. Diverse mechanisms and clinical manifestations. J Am Coll Cardiol 20:483-499
2. Verrier RL, Nearing BD (1994) Electrophysiologic basis for T wave alternans as an index of vulnerability to ventricular fibrillation. J Cardiovasc Electrophys 5:445-461
3. Han J, Moe GK (1964) Nonuniform recovery of excitability in ventricular muscle. Circ Res 14:44-60
4. Cinca J, Figueras J, Senador G et al (1984) Transmural DC electrograms after coronary artery occlusion and latex embolization in pigs. Am J Physiol 246:H475-H482
5. Dilly SG, Lab M (1988) Electrophysiological alternans and restitution during acute regional ischemia in myocardium of anesthetized pig. J Physiol (Lond) 402:315-333
6. Janse MJ, Wit AL (1989) Electrophysiological mechanism of ventricular arrhythmias resulting from myocardial ischemia and infarction. Physiol Rev 69:1049-1169
7. Smith JM, Clancy EA, Valeri CR et al (1988) Electrical alternans and cardiac electrical instability. Circulation 77:110-21
8. Nearing BD, Huang AH, Verrier RL (1991) Dynamic tracking of cardiac vulnerability by complex demodulation of the T wave. Science 252:437-440
9. Rosenbaum DS, Jackson LE, Smith JM et al (1994) Electrical alternans and vulnerability to ventricular arrhythmias. N Engl J Med 330:235-241
10. Eastes MNA, Zipes DP, El-Sherif N et al (1995) The value of T-wave alternans and signal-averaged electrocardiogram as predictors of arrhythmia vulnerability. Pace 18:796 (Abstract)
11. Saitoh H, Bailey JC, Surawicz B (1989) Action potential duration alternans in dog Purkinje and ventricular muscle fibers. Further evidence in support of two different mechanisms. Circulation 80:1421-1431
12. Hauswirth O, Noble D, Tsien RW (1972) The dependence of plateau currents in cardiac Purkinje fibers on the interval between action potentials. J Physiol (Lond) 222:27-49
13. Boyett MR, Jewell BR (1978) A study of the factors responsible for rate-dependent shortening of the action potential in mammalian ventricular muscle. J Physiol (Lond) 285:359-380
14. Kleber AG, Janse MJ, van Capelle FJL et al (1978) Mechanism and time course of S-T and T-Q segment changes during acute regional myocardial ischemia in the pig heart determined by extacellular and intracellular recordings. Circ Res 42:603-613
15. Downar E, Janse MJ, Durrer D (1977) The effect of acute coronary artery occlusion on subepicardial transmembrane potentials in the intact porcine heart. Circulation 56:217-224
16. Russel DC, Smith HJ, Oliver MD (1979) Transmembrane potential changes and ventricular fibrillation during repetitive myocardial ischaemia in the dog. Br Heart J 42:88-96.
17. Konta T, Ikeda K, Yamaki M et al (1990) Significance of discordant ST alternans in ventricular fibrillation. Circulation 82:2185-2189
18. Antzelevitch C, Siccouri S, Litovsky S et al (1991) Heterogeneity within the ventricular wall: electrophysiology and pharmacology of epicardial, endocardial, and M cells. Circ Res 69:1427-1449
19. El-Sherif N, Zeiler RN, Craelius W et al (1988) QTU prolongation and polymorphic ventricular tachyarrhythmias due to bradycardia-dependent early afterdepolarizations. Circ Res 63:286-305
20. Gough WB, Henkin R (1989) The early afterdepolarization as recorded by the monophasic action potential technique: fact or artifact. Circulation 80:II-130 (Abstr)
21. Kleinfeld MJ, Rozanski JJ (1977) Alternans of the ST segment in Prinzmetal's angina. Circulation 55:574-577
22. Turitto G, El-Sherif N (1988) Alternans of the ST segment in variant angina. Chest 93:587-591
23. Gilchrist IC (1991) Prevalence and significance of ST segment alternans during coronary angioplasty. Am J Cardiol 68:1534-1535
24. Sutton PMI, Taggart P, Lab M et al (1991) Alternans of epicardial repolarization as a localized phenomenon in man. Eur Heart J 12:70-78
25. Wayne VS, Bishop RL, Spodick DH (1983) Exercise-induced ST segment alternans. Chest 83:824-825
26. Puletti M, Curione M, Righetti G et al (1980) Alternans of the ST segment and T wave in acute myocardial infarction. J Electrocardiol 13:297-300
27. Salerno JA, Previtali M, Panciroli C et al (1988) Ventricular arrhythmias during acute myocardial ischaemia in man. The role and significance of R-ST-T alternans and the prevention of ischaemic sudden death by medical treatment. Eur Heart J 7:63-75
28. Schwartz PJ, Maliani A (1975) Electrical alternation of the T wave: clinical and experimental evidence of its relationship with the sympathetic nervous system and with the long Q-T syndrome. Am Heart J 89:45-50
29. Jackman WM, Clark M, Friday KJ et al (1984) Ventricular tachyarrhythmias in the long QT syndrome. Med Clin North Am 68:1079-1104
30. Reddy CVR, Riok JP, Khan RG et al (1984) Repolarization alternans associated with alcoholism and hypomagnesemia. Am J Cardiol 53:390-391
31. Habbab MA, El-Sherif N: (1992) TU alternans, long QTU, and torsade de pointes: clinical and experimental observations. PACE 15:916-931
32. Attwell D, Lee JA (1988) A cellular basis for the primary long QT syndromes. Lancet 1:1136-1139
33. El-Sherif N, Craeius W, Boutjdir M et al (1990) Early afterdepolarizations and arrhythmogenesis. J Cardiovasc Electrophysiol 1:145-160.

Idiopathic Ventricular Fibrillation: Which Prognosis and Treatment?

S.G. Priori and V. Paganini

on behalf of the Steering Committee of UCARE

Istituto di Clinica Medica Generale e Terapia Medica, Università di Milano,
Milan, Italy

Introduction

Ventricular fibrillation (VF) in the presence of is-chemic heart disease is the leading cause of sudden cardiac death (1). Other less common cardiac diseases are also associated to VF, among them the cardiomy-opathies, myocarditis, the long QT syndrome, infiltra-tive diseases such as amiloidosis, and valvular defects. However, in a small subset of patients who develop VF, no structural heart disease can be identified de-spite intensive examination. These patients are defined as having "idiopathic ventricular fibrillation" (IVF; 2-6).

Knowledge about IVF is very limited and this complicates the management of these patients. It is not known whether they are in an early stage of an undetectable structural heart disease, yet which is ca-pable of reducing cardiac electrical stability. The fre-quency of recurrence of lethal ventricular tach-yarrhythmias is also unknown and whether therapy is necessary or useful in modifying prognosis. The lack of conclusive answers to these very basic questions makes IVF a very difficult clinical condition to man-age and relegates clinical decision to an empirical process rather than a logical procedure soundly based on medical knowledge.

Historical Perspective

In 1992 we reviewed (5) the data published in the inter-national literature on IVF during the last 35 years. We identified only case reports or small cohorts of patients, with a total of 125 cases of IVF. Sixty-eight percent of patients were males, their age ranged from 9 to 79 years, and the follow-up period varied from 2 months to 14 years. Electrophysiologic studies were performed in 95 patients: nonsustained ventricular tachycardia (VT) was induced in 9% of patients, sustained VT in 26%, and VF in 12%. The therapies used in this group of patients were extremely varied and included class I antiarrhythmic drugs, amiodarone, ß-blockers, a combi-nation of the above, and implantable cardioverter de-fibrillators (ICDs). The need for therapy in patients with ventricular arrhythmias has to be weighed against the risk of proarrhythmic events, and the assessment of the risk-benefit ratio obviously depends on the risk of recurrence. Unfortunately, at this time, this risk cannot be quantified in patients with IVF.

Viskin and Belhassen (2) reported in their cohort of 45 patients a recurrence rate of 11%. In our own analysis, out of 100 patients, 12 died suddenly or were defibrillated by ICD and another nine experienced re-currence of nonsustained VT or syncopal episodes: the overall number of recurrence of arrhythmic events was therefore 21%. If this figure were confirmed in a clinical study one would conclude that IVF patients are at high risk of recurrence. Recently, Wever and coworkers (3) reported the first large series of IVF pa-tients studied prospectively at the same institution with an extensive evaluation of cardiac function and a relatively long follow-up (43 months, range 5-85 months). The results of this study are particularly im-portant for estimating the risk of recurrence. Major arrhythmic events occurred in 7/19 (37%) patients. Two patients were treated with antiarrhythmic drugs and experienced a recurrence of cardiac arrest: one died suddenly, and the other was successfully resusci-tated. In the remaining five patients termination of syncopal episodes occurred by ICD shock. None of the 19 patients included in the study developed signs of cardiac disease at follow-up. The authors concluded that IVF is a truly idiopathic disease which carries a high risk of recurrence of cardiac arrest and therefore suggested that implantation of ICD is recommended in survivors from IVF.

Mechanisms for Arrhythmias in IVF

The mechanisms for arrhythmogenesis in IVF can only be speculated upon. The presence of an anatomical substrate to initiate reentry is unlikely as no structural abnormality is, by definition, present in these patients. Indeed, the low rate of inducibility of monomorphic VT in IVF patients supports the concept of the absence of a structural abnormality. However, even if an anatomical pathway for reentry does not exist, reentry may still be the mechanism for arrhythmias when functional reentry (7) is initiated by a premature beat. As an alternative hypothesis focal arrhythmias originating from different foci may be the mechanism for polymorphic VT which may degenerate into VF (8). The two hypotheses may even coexist, as triggered or automatic beats may initiate the arrhythmias and a functional reentry may allow perpetuation of the VT and degeneration into VF.

Finally, recent knowledge about genetic abnormalities in ionic channels obtained in long QT syndrome (LQTS; 9,10) have raised the possibility that primary electrical disorders (of which LQTS may be considered one form characterized by prolongation of repolarization) may indeed be the consequence of congenital "channelopathies", i.e., primary abnormalities of ionic channels function that result in an increased susceptibility to ventricular arrhythmias.

A Prospective Registry for IVF

The implementation of an extensive international IVF data base has been advocated by several investigators (2,4) as the only approach that could lead to the collection of a large patient population. Such an international registry could provide not only epidemiological data on the gross incidence and outcome of IVF, but would also make it possible to evaluate the effectiveness of therapy.

It is very important that in such a study patients are monitored for at least 10-15 years in order to establish whether any structural heart disease might develop over time, thus suggesting that the cardiac arrest might have been the first and only symptom of the preclinical phase of an organic disease.

Previous experience with an international registry has proven successful in the understanding of another rare and lethal disease: the idiopathic LQTS (11,12). The international LQTS registry was initiated by A.J. Moss, R.S. Crampton, and P.J. Schwartz. As of today, after 16 years of activity, data are available for 7900 patients and family members and have provided a major contribution to the understanding of the disease.

In 1992 the Working Group on Cardiac Arrhythmias of the European Society of Cardiology officially endorsed the international IVF registry UCARE (Unexplained Cardiac Arrest Registry of Europe). Given the need for international collaboration for the success of this project the European Economic Community and the European Society of Cardiology have provided a research grant that will help to support UCARE and to increase awareness of IVF among clinicians.

The primary objective of UCARE is to collect information about individuals who survived a documented episode of IVF (Fig. 1) and to follow them for at least 10 years with yearly visits to acquire information on (1) recurrence of malignant arrhythmias or cardiac arrest, (2) development of a previously nonobvious organic heart disease, and (3) the difference in outcome in patients treated with different drugs or devices.

UCARE is a registry open to any physician worldwide willing to collaborate by providing cases of IVF for enrollment. UCARE is not a clinical trial, therefore there are no protocols to be followed and physicians are free to decide whether any treatment is required and, if so, which medication or device is the most appropriate in their judgment.

Since IVF is mainly a diagnosis of exclusion, it is difficult to define how and when it is possible to exclude, with a high degree of accuracy, the presence of structural heart disease. In fact, it may happen that an abnormality responsible for arrhythmic development is missed because a test is not performed, is incorrectly interpreted, or is simply not sensitive enough to detect disease at an early stage. The use of endomyocardial biopsy has been advocated by several investigators (13-16) as a procedure that may identify occult heart disease in patients with unexplained ventricular tachyarrhythmias. In our experience, myocardial biopsy in patients with IVF is likely to reveal normal specimens or "aspecific alterations" that might also be present in normal individuals. The interpretation of these findings remains difficult until a control group constituted by individuals with normal hearts and no arrhythmia is available in which the prevalence of the so-called aspecific alterations in the normal population is estimated. In the UCARE registry endomyocardial biopsy was performed in 49/127 patients (39%). In 39/49 (80%) no alterations were identified, while in the remaining ten

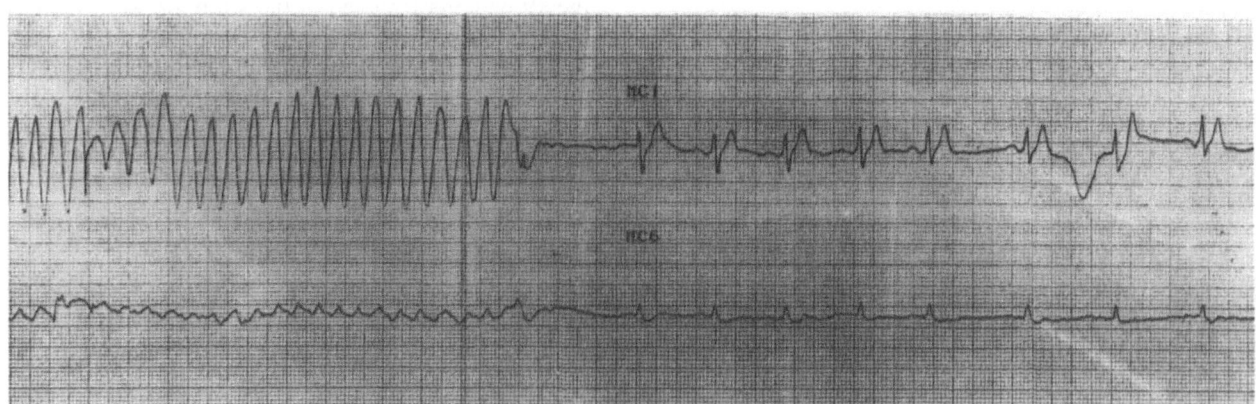

Fig. 1. Self-terminating ventricular fibrillation in a patient (L.E., female, 52 years old) without structural heart disease. (Courtesy of Dr. C. Menozzi and Dr. N. Bottoni)

patients mild fibrosis was observed in six, mild cellular hypertrophy in two, and mild disarray of fibers in other two: all these observations were defined as "nonspecific" for a diagnosis of structural heart disease.

We believe that the long follow-up planned for the UCARE patients will allow us to put these data into perspective since if they really represent an early marker of a structural disease in the preclinical stage, a full-blown disease will eventually develop and will be identified at follow-up.

Criteria and guidelines to exclude the presence of a structural heart disease have been prepared by the Steering Committee of the UCARE registry (Table 1) by taking into consideration the major diagnoses that need to be excluded (Table 2). However, no matter how carefully a patient is studied, a few clinical conditions potentially responsible for ventricular tachyarrhythmias such as coronary artery spasm or malformations, subclinical or focal myocarditis, sporadic LQTS, or LQTS with normal QT interval remain particularly difficult to identify: a follow-up over a prolonged period of time may in these cases be the only way to secure a correct diagnosis.

Table 1. Members of the Steering Committee of UCARE

Martin Borggrefe	Silvia G. Priori
A. John Camm	Peter J. Schwartz
Richard N.W. Hauer	Paul Touboul
Helmut Klein	Hein J.J. Wellens
Karl-Heinz Kuck	

Table 2. Clinical conditions to be excluded in the diagnosis of idiopathic ventricular fibrillation

Coronary artery disease
  Congenital malformation
  Atherosclerosis
  Spasm

Cardiomyopathies
  Hypertrophic
  Dilated
  Right ventricular dysplasia

Long QT syndrome

Ventricular pre-excitation

Iatrogenic arrhythmias
  Cocaine
  Digitalis
  Agents known to induce torsade de pointes (antiarrhythmic agents that prolong repolarization, antidepressants, macrolide antibiotics, antifungals of the "onazoles" group, antihistaminic drugs)

Electrolyte abnormalities
  Hypomagnesemia
  Hypokalemia

Infiltrative and inflammatory disorders
  Sarcoidosis
  Amyloidosis
  Postinflammatory fibrosis
  Myocarditis

Before enrolling a patient in UCARE it is recommended that a careful history is taken in order to identify a family history of sudden death, and that noninvasive as well as invasive procedures be performed (Table 3) such as standard ECG, signal-averaged ECG for the detection of late potentials, echocardiogram, Holter

Table 3. Diagnostic procedures performed in idiopathic ventricular fibrillation in patients

Test	Patients	Percentage
Echocardiogram	126	99
Holter	108	85
Exercise stress test	114	90
Coronary angiography	115	91
Electrophysiologic study	121	95

recording, exercise stress test, electrophysiologic study for the exclusion of pre-excitation and for the evaluation of inducibility of ventricular tachyarrhythmias, angiography, myocardial biopsy, heart rate variability, baroreflex sensitivity, and magnetic resonance imaging. Every year at the follow-up visit it is important to obtain information on recurrences of ventricular tachyarrhythmias and to repeat the noninvasive tests to exclude the presence of signs or symptoms suggestive of organic heart disease development.

As of 30 April 1995, 127 patients have been enrolled in UCARE: 92 males and 35 females. The mean age at the time of the first episode of cardiac arrest was 38±16 years. The analysis of factors associated to development of VF such as type of activity or the location in the minutes preceding the arrest has not offered relevant information that could help in identifying risk predictors for these individuals (Fig. 2). In 26 patients (20%) cardiac arrest occurred during physical exertion and in 11 (9%) it occurred after intense stress or emotion (Fig. 3). Overall, adrenergic activation was

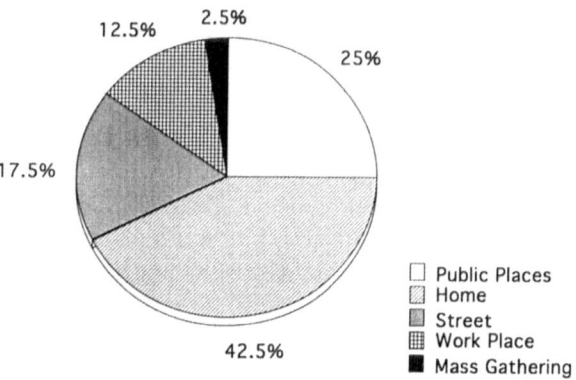

Fig. 2. Location of critical event

- □ Public Places
- ▨ Home
- ▦ Street
- ▤ Work Place
- ■ Mass Gathering

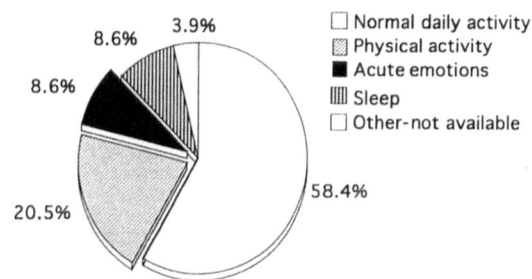

- □ Normal daily activity
- ▨ Physical activity
- ■ Acute emotions
- ▥ Sleep
- □ Other-not available

Fig. 3. Factors associated with the critical event

19

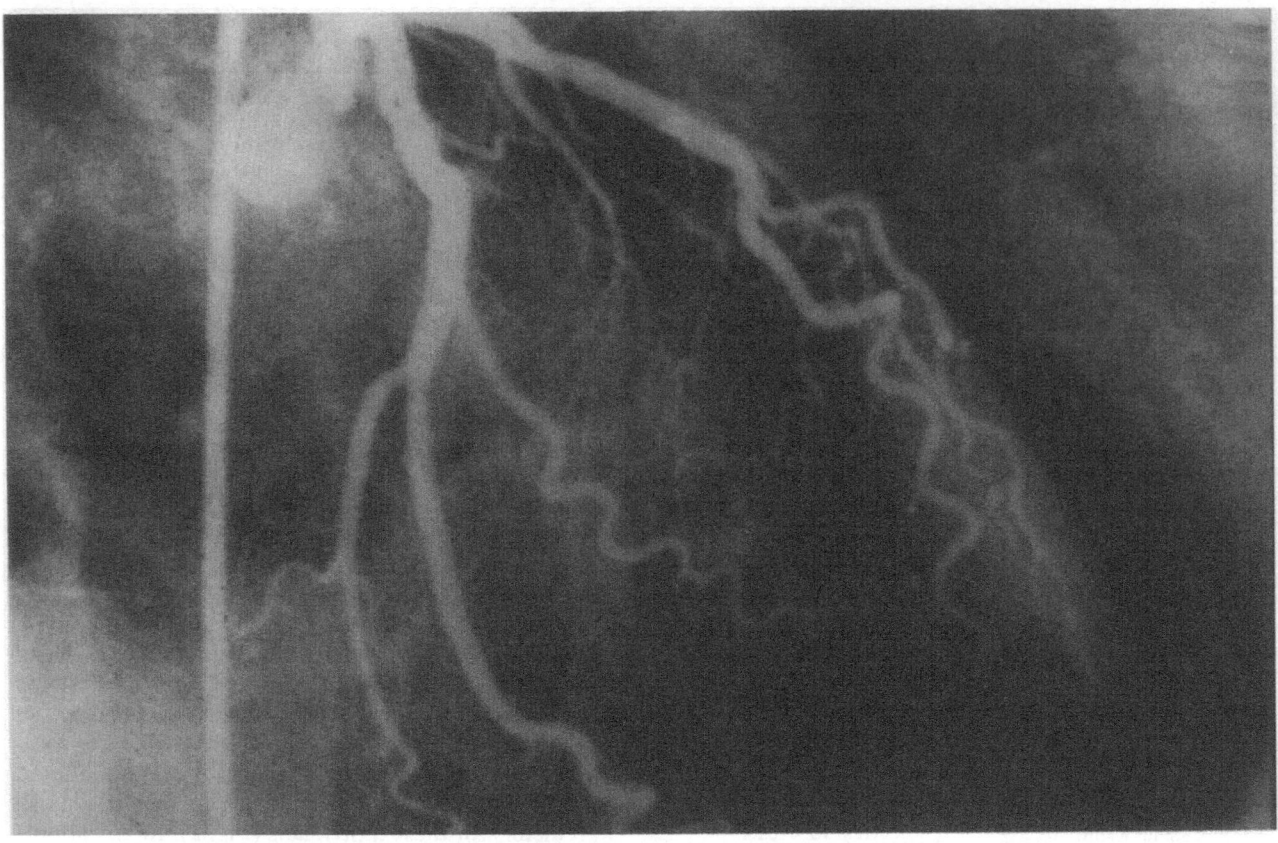

Fig. 4. Intact coronary arteries in a female patient 69 years old. (Courtesy of Dr. A. Saino)

present at the time of arrest in 29% of patients: these subjects may belong to a subgroup of individuals with catecholamine-dependent arrhythmias and otherwise normal heart (17). Forty patients (31.5%) had a history of syncopal episodes before the index event and none of these events required resuscitation.

Only 46% of patients (56/121) were inducible at baseline electrophysiologic study. Overall, sustained monomorphic VT occurred in a minority of inducible subjects (*n* = 3) while polymorphic VT and ventricular flutter/fibrillation occurred in 17 and 30 subjects, respectively; nonsustained VT occurred in the remaining six patients. Since monomorphic VT is largely attributed to the presence of an anatomical substrate that perpetuates a reentrant pattern of excitation, it appears logical that in IVF patients, in whom a lack of organic substrate is postulated,

monomorphic VT should be difficult to induce.

Coronary artery anatomy was evaluated by means of angiography in 115 (91%) patients and in no case stenoses >50% were identified. The use of the ergonovine test has been recently advocated (18) to assess the propensity of coronary arteries to develop vasospasms. This test was performed in 34 subjects and only in two cases it was positive; these patients have been excluded from the analysis (Fig. 4).

Recently, Brugada and Brugada (19) reported the existence of a new syndrome characterized by episodes of VF in subjects with no structural heart disease with a typical ECG pattern consisting of right bundle block and persistent ST segment elevation in V1-V3. This syndrome is described as a variant of IVF. Three patients in the population enrolled in UCARE presented with the electrocardiographic features described by

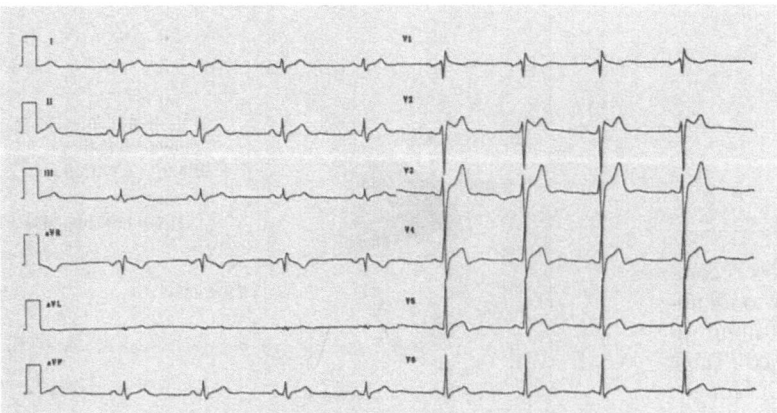

Fig. 5. ECG tracing showing the pattern described by Brugada and Brugada (19). (Courtesy of Dr. M. Fromer)

Brugada and Brugada (Fig. 5). In the series reported by Brugada and Brugada these patients experienced a high rate of recurrences, since out of the eight patients included in the study one experienced several episodes of polymorphic VT associated with circulatory arrest, one died suddenly, and one was successfully defibrillated by the ICD, while the remaining five subjects remained asymptomatic. No criteria were identified to differentiate patients who experienced recurrences from those who remained asymptomatic.

Therapy

The subgroup of patients with IVF has been previously considered at low risk of recurrence of cardiac arrest because they have often been grouped with patients with idiopathic ventricular tachycardia (IVT). However, there are no data to support the concept that the patients showing greater electrical instability of the heart which allows the development of VF share the same risk of recurrence as the subgroup of patients that only develops VT. Since it is well established that patients with IVT have a benign prognosis (20-24), it is rather obvious that in grouping the smaller population with IVF together with the larger group with IVT one will end up with an overall lower risk of recurrence to be attributed to both subgroups. Similarly, when a risk/benefit ratio is calculated to assess the need for therapy in IVT patients one might challenge the idea of life-long therapy versus the low risk of experiencing recurrence of VT. On the other hand, the evaluation of the need of treatment should be entirely different in a young and otherwise healthy patient resuscitated from a documented episode of VF in whom a recurrence may be fatal.

In the UCARE patient population pharmacological therapy was started in 58 patients (Table 4). Most patients (22/58) received ß-blockers on the assumption that adrenergic activation may be the most important trigger for the development of tachyarrhythmias in normal individuals. It is interesting to note that 13 subjects received therapy with sodium channnel blockers; however, they were all treated before 1990. This is likely to reflect a "post-CAST" attitude based more on emotional than on rational evidence. The CAST study (25) enrolled postmyocardial infarction subjects with frequent arrhythmias, and data obtained in this population cannot be directly extrapolated to the group of patients with IVF. Viskin and Belhassen (2) in their analysis of previously published reports of IVF suggested that sodium channel blockers prevent arrhythmia inducibility in several patients and are therefore likely to represent an effective therapy for IVF patients.

In the group of patients enrolled in UCARE, pharmacological therapy did not show any benefit in preventing arrhythmia recurrence. As a matter of fact five of seven patients (71%) treated with amiodarone, four of eight (50%) treated with class I agents, one of two (50%) treated with calcium antagonists, and three of 20 (15%) receiving ß-blockers experienced recurrence of arrhythmia.

It should be noted that these data refer to empirical therapy and not to pharmacological therapy guided by results of programmed electrical stimulation (PES). This is due to the fact that during PES only about half of the subjects who experienced IVF developed sustained arrhythmias and most of them VT, i.e., not the arrhythmia responsible for their cardiac arrest. Therefore it cannot be excluded that the drug proven to be effective at PES may offer better protection from arrhythmic recurrences.

It is remarkable to observe that in eight patients no therapy or devices were considered appropriate; in other words, the physicians of these subjects felt that chances of recurrences were so low that the risk/benefit ratio of any therapy was in favor of leaving the patients untreated. As a matter of fact, after a mean follow-up of 29 months none of these subjects experienced recurrence of major arrhythmic events.

The role of the ICD needs to be carefully evaluated in IVF. These patients, in fact, represent a subgroup of the survivors of out-of-hospital cardiac arrest at high risk of dying of an arrhythmic episode but with an otherwise long life expectancy. These characteristics reflect the profile of the ideal candidate for ICD implantation as outlined by the Working Group on Arrhythmias of the European Society of Cardiology (26).

As of today, 74 patients (57%) were implanted with the ICD; follow-up data are available for 49 patients implanted with a defibrillator and in this group 14 (29%) subjects experienced recurrence of VF, while four (8%) patients had inappropriate discharges of the defibrillator. Therefore if we wish to evaluate the cost/effectiveness of the ICD in IVF we should certainly acknowledge that while approximately 30% of patients are likely to be saved by the device, still 70% of subjects may have no benefit from the ICD. If we take into consideration the high cost of an ICD and how it affects the quality of life of the patients, it appears straightforward that the identification of risk factors predictive for recurrence may help in identifying those individuals that would benefit most from the device. Unfortunately, multivariate analysis of the potential prognostic parameters is not helpful in identifying patients at higher risk of recurrence (Table 5).

Table 4. Therapy at hospital discharge

Therapy	Patients	Percentage
Single AA agent	46	36
Two or more AA agents	12	10
ICD	57	45
ICD + AA agent	8	6
No therapy	4	3

AA, antiarrythmic agent; ICD, implantable cardioverter defibrillator

Table 5. Risk stratification

	Relative risk	95% C.I.
Age < 40 years	1.95	0.91 - 4.10
History of syncope	1.80	0.90 - 3.60
Positive LP	1.05	0.30 - 3.30
EPS inducibility	0.97	0.52 - 1.80
Arrhythmias at exercise	0.82	0.32 - 2.12
Arrhythmias at Holter	0.58	0.26 - 1.32

LP, late potentials; EPS, electrophysiologic study; C.I., confidence interval

Ninety patients out of the total of 127 (71%) have been clinically evaluated to define whether, after a mean period of 4±2.8 years, evidence of a structural heart disease has developed. Only three patients (3%) presented with evidence or were suspected of having structural heart disease (in two cases with positive results of the ergonovine test and in one case for thoracic chest pain during physical activity). These data support the hypothesis that IVF truly represents an electrical disorder unrelated to a structural heart disease.

Conclusions

Based on the current evidence it appears that IVF carries a high risk of recurrence of cardiac arrest and syncopal episodes (24%); empirical pharmacological therapy is associated with a high risk of recurrence of ventricular tachyarrhythmias (12 patients of 37 receiving drugs, i.e., 33% had a recurrence) and of death (four of 37 patients receiving pharmacological therapy i.e., 9%, died suddenly).

For these reasons the implantation of an ICD appears to be an appropriate therapeutic approach to IVF. However, in order to improve the quality of life of patients and to limit the number of shocks delivered, all efforts should be made to identify a pharmacological agent that could reduce the number of arrhythmic events; more specifically the role of programmed electrical stimulation-guided therapy should be defined in IVF patients with arrhythmias inducible in the electrophysiology laboratory.

Acknowledgment. UCARE is partially supported by educational grants from the European Society of Cardiology and Medtronic International, and the international coordination of the project is funded through a BIOMED 1 grant from the European Economic Commission.

References

1. Roberts WC (1986) Sudden cardiac death: definitions and causes. Am J Cardiol 57: 1410-1413
2. Viskin S, Belhassen B (1990) Idiopathic ventricular fibrillation. Am Heart J 120: 661-671
3. Wever EFD, Hauer RNW, Oomen A, Peters RHJ, Bakker PFA, Robles de Medina EO (1993) Unfavorable outcome in patients with primary electrical disease who survived an episode of ventricular fibrillation. Circulation 88: 1021-1029
4. Wellens HJJ, Lemery R, Smeets JL, Brugada P, Gorgels AP, Cheriex EC, de Zwaan C (1992) Sudden arrhythmic death without overt heart disease. Circulation 85 [Suppl 1]: I-92-I-97
5. Priori SG, Borggrefe M, Camm AJ, Hauer NWR, Klein H, Kuck K-H, Schwartz PJ, Touboul P, Wellens HJJ (1992) Unexplained cardiac arrest. The need of a prospective registry. Eur Heart J 13: 1445-1446
6. Proclemer A, Facchin D, Miani D, Feruglio GA (1994) Tachicardia e fibrillazione ventricolare idiopatiche. Inquadramento, diagnosi, terapia e prognosi. G Ital Cardiol 24: 1027-1041
7. Allessie MA, Schalij MJ, Kirchhof CJHJ, Boermsa L, Huyberts M, Hollen J (1989) Experimental electrophysiology and arrhythmogenicity. Anisotropy and ventricular tachycardia. Eur Heart J 10: E 8-14
8. Priori SG, Diehl L, Schwartz PJ (1995) Torsade de pointes. In: Podrid PJ, Kowey PR (eds) Cardiac arrhythmia: mechanisms, diagnosis and management. William and Wilkins, Baltimore, pp 951-963
9. Curran ME, Splawski I, Timothy KW, Vincent GM, Green ED, Keating MT (1995) A Molecular basis for cardiac arrhythmia: HERG mutations cause long QT syndrome. Cell 80: 795-803
10. Wang Q, Shen J, Splawski I, Atkinson D, Li Z, Robinson JL, Moss AJ, Towbin JA, Keating MT (1995) SCN5A mutations associated with an inherited cardiac arrhythmia, long QT syndrome. Cell 80: 805-811
11. Moss AJ, Schwartz PJ, Crampton RS, Locati E, Carleen E (1985) The long QT syndrome: a prospective international study. Circulation 71: 17-21
12. Moss AJ, Schwartz PJ, Crampton RS, Tzivoni D, Locati EH, MacCluer J, Hall WJ, Weitkamp L, Vincent GM, Garson A Jr, Robinson JL, Benhorin J, Choi S (1991) The long QT syndrome. Prospective longitudinal study of 328 families. Circulation 84: 1136-1144
13. Stran JE, Grose RM, Factor SM, Fisher JD (1983) Results of endomyocardial biopsy in patients with spontaneous ventricular tachycardia but without apparent structural heart disease. Circulation 68: 1171-1181
14. Sugrue DD, Holmes DR, Gersh BJ, Edwards WD, McLaren CJ, Wood DL, Osborn MJ, Hammill SC (1984) Cardiac histologic findings in patients with life-threatening ventricular arrhythmias of unknown origin. J Am Coll Cardiol 4: 952-957
15. Crijns H, Tuininga Y, Schoots C, Van Dijk R, Wiesfeld A, Lie K (1991) Value of target-directed endomyocardial biopsy in idiopathic right ventricular tachycardia. J Am Coll Cardiol 17: 97A
16. Martini B, Nava A, Thiene G, Buja GF, Canciani B et al (1989) Ventricular fibrillation without apparent heart disease: description of six cases. Am Heart J 118: 1203-1209
17. Lucet V, Grau F, Denjov I, Do Ngoc D, Geiger K, Ghisla R, Mselati JC, Leenhardt A, Coumel P (1994) Devenir à long terme des tachycardies ventriculaires polymorphes catécholergiques de l'enfant. A propos de 20 cas suivis pendant 8 ans. Arch Pediatr 1: 26-32
18. Myerburg RJ, Kessler KM, Mallon SM, Cox MM, de Marchena E, Interian A Jr, Castellanos A (1992) Life-threatening ventricular arrhythmias in patient with silent myocardial ischemia due to coronary artery spasm. N Engl J Med 326: 1451-1455
19. Brugada P, Brugada J (1992) Right bundle branch block, persistent ST segment elevation and sudden cardiac death. A distinct clinical and electrocardiographic syndrome. J Am Coll Cardiol 20: 1391-1396
20. Brooks R, Burgess JH (1988) Idiopathic ventricular tachycardia: a review. Medicine 67: 271-294
21. Pedersen DH, Zipes DP, Foster PR, Troup PJ (1979) Ventricular tachycardia and ventricular fibrillation in a young population. Circulation 60: 988-997
22. Kennedy HL, Whitlock JA, Sprague MK, Kennedy LJ, Buckingham TA, Goldberg RJ (1985) Long-term follow up of asymptomatic healthy subjects with frequent and complex ventricular ectopy. N Engl J Med 312: 193-197
23. Deal BJ, Miller SM, Scagliotti D, Prechel D, Gallastegui JL, Hariman RJ (1986) Ventricular tachycardia in a young population without overt heart disease. Circulation 73: 1111-1118
24. Lemery R, Brugada P, Della Bella P, Dugernier T, Wellens HJJ (1989) Ventricular fibrillation in six adults without overt heart disease. J Am Coll Cardiol 13: 911-916
25. The Cardiac Arrhythmia Suppression Trial "CAST" (1989) Preliminary report: effect of encainide and flecainide on mortality in a randomized trial of arrhythmia suppression after myocardial infarction. N Engl J Med 321: 406-412
26. A Task Force of Working Group of Arrhythmias and Cardiac Pacing of the European Society of Cardiology: Breithardt G, Camm AJ, Campbell RWF, Coumel P, Janse MJ, Kappenberg L, Klein H, Kuck KH, Luderitz B, Rehnqvist N, Schwartz PJ, Touboul P (1992) Guidelines for the use of implantable cardioverter defibrillators. Eur Heart J 13: 1304-1310

Beta Blockers, Sotalol, or Amiodarone for the Treatment of Malignant Ventricular Arrhythmias?

A. Proclemer, D. Facchin, D. Miani, D. Vanuzzo, and G.A. Feruglio

Divisione di Cardiologia, Ospedale S. Maria della Misericordia, Udine, Italy

In patients with malignant ventricular tachyarrhythmias the impact of drug therapy on total mortality has been difficult to evaluate with certainty because placebo-controlled studies could not be performed for ethical reasons. However, current clinical data indicate a need for a greater use of drugs that prolong repolarization, such as amiodarone and sotalol (class III of antiarrhythmics), than agents that delay conduction, such as sodium channel blockers (class I) (1-5). There is also increasing evidence that sympathetic inhibition represents a fundamental feature in the treatment of patients with ventricular tachycardia (VT) and ventricular fibrillation (VF) (4).

Beta Blockers

In patients who have survived acute myocardial infarction, beta blockers have short and long-term beneficial effects. A meta-analysis by Teo et al. (6) showed a significantly decreased mortality in patients who were treated with different β-adrenergic blockers compared with placebo-treated controls (1464 deaths out of 26973 patients in the first group versus 1727 out of 26294 in the control group, $p < 0.0001$, relative risk, 0.81). Several factors, such as antiarrhythmic activity, low incidence of proarrhythmic effects, increase of fibrillation threshold, anti-ischemic properties, and interaction with the autonomic nervous system may account for the prophylactic efficacy of these drugs. More specifically, the treatment with lipophilic beta blockers such as propranolol (7) and metoprolol (8, 9) was associated with a lower rate of VF, of sudden death, and of electrically treated VT compared to placebo. Lipophilicity allows a high penetration of these drugs into the brain, and the combining effect with $β_1$-adrenergic receptors causes an increase of vagal activity and of fibrillation threshold (10)

In patients with sustained ventricular arrhythmias, beta blockers are considered the first-choice treatment only in exercise-induced VT, catecholamine-sensitive VT, idiopathic VT, and "torsades de pointes" VT in the long QT syndrome. However, the role of these drugs is still controversial in patients with underlying heart disease who have suffered from sustained episodes of VT or VF. The rationale for using beta blockers in this category of patients is the low incidence of proarrhythmic phenomena and the relevant increase in the cardiac sympathetic activity. Recently, Meredith et al. (11) demonstrated a significant increase in the production of total and cardiac norepinephrine in patients with sustained VT or VF as a consequence of the left ventricular function reduction.

Clinical Studies in Patients with Sustained Ventricular Tachycardia or Ventricular Fibrillation

By using electrophysiologic studies, Duff et al. (12) evaluated the efficacy of propranolol in 28 patients with inducible sustained VT and observed a positive response to the parenteral administration of this drug in 21% of the cases. No significant differences have been noticed between the response to low doses (beta blocking effect) and high doses, and no relevant changes in ventricular refractoriness were demonstrated. In the follow-up, oral administration of propranolol was effective in four out of five of those patients who were considered responders in the acute phase. This study demonstrated that propranolol can suppress inducible VT in very few cases and that the efficacy of this drug is mainly due to its beta-blocking effect, rather than to traditional electrophysiologic effects.

Brodsky et al. (13) assessed the effectiveness of solitary beta blocker treatment in 30 nonconsecutive patients with sustained ventricular arrhythmias. Metoprolol, propranolol, atenolol, pindolol, acebutolol and nadolol were used. Episodes of VT were demonstrated in 57% of the patients during basic Holter monitoring; they were also provoked with exercise testing in 50% of the patients and induced by programmed electrical stimulation in 69% of the cases (86% with isoproterenol). The use of beta blockers determined arrhythmia suppression in 54% of cases on electrocardiogram (ECG) monitoring, in 83% during exercise, and prevented inducible VT in 37% during programmed electrical stimulation. A total of 24 patients underwent long-term treatment with beta blockers: six suffered from VT recurrence (25%), and in two the treatment, was interrupted because of side effects. No deaths were reported. Factors such as an ejection fraction greater than 45%, absence of coronary disease, and age below 60 years were predictive of effectiveness of the beta blocking therapy, whereas noninvasive investigations and electrophysiologic study were not. This study showed favorable effects of beta blockers, but has the obvious limitations of lack of randomization and of selection bias.

In an observational and noncontrolled study, Hallstrom et al. (14) evaluated the efficacy of empirical administration of beta blockers and class I antiarrhythmic drugs in 941 consecutive patients who had been resuscitated from an out-of-hospital cardiac arrest between 1970 and 1985. Beta blockers were administered in 28% of the cases, quinidine in 18.7%, and procainamide in 17.5%. No antiarrhythmic therapy was administered in 39.4% of the patients. During an average 9-year follow-up, the use of beta blockers has been associated with a better survival, whereas the use of quinidine and of procainamide has been associated with a worse prognosis (survival after 2 years, 75%, 55%, and 30%, respectively, $p < 0.0001$). The difference between groups was not significant after adjustment for baseline risk factors ($p = 0.08$). The authors concluded that the use of beta blockers should be considered in survivors of out-of-hospital VF, in spite of the limitations of a retrospective analysis.

The efficacy of empirical metoprolol treatment in patients with malignant ventricular arrhythmias was compared with conventional antiarrhythmic therapy guided by electrophysiologic testing in a prospective, randomized trial (15). This series included 85 patients with VT, 41 with cardiac arrest due to documented VF, and 36 with syncope and ventricular arrhythmias. A total of 55 patients whose arrhythmia was not initially inducible (mean ejection fraction, 53%) were empirically treated with metoprolol. Patients whose arrhythmia was inducible were randomized to guided treatment (61 patients; mean ejection fraction, 42%) or to metoprolol (54 patients; mean ejection fraction, 43%). Serial testing was performed at random with propafenone, flecainide, disopyramide, sotalol, and amiodarone. During a mean follow-up period of 23 months, the incidence of sudden death and arrhythmia recurrence was the same in the two randomized groups (guided therapy, 46%, metoprolol therapy, 48%). In patients treated with metoprolol, baseline noninducibility identifies a group with an incidence of fatal and nonfatal arrhythmia recurrence lower than that of inducible patients (29% versus 52%, respectively, $p = 0.009$). In conclusion, the empirical use of metoprolol was associated with a favorable prognosis in patients at low risk (baseline noninducibility, preserved left ventricular function) and a rather high rate of arrhythmia recurrence in inducible patients. Moreover, the recurrence rate was similar to that observed in patients who received electropharmacologically guided treatment.

Additional information on the use of beta blockers in malignant ventricular arrhythmias will be obtained from the CASH trial (Cardiac Arrest Study Hamburg), involving 400 patients who survived cardiac arrest and who were randomized to treatment with metoprolol, amiodarone, propafenone, or implantable cardioverter defibrillators (ICD). Preliminary results of this study (16) have shown no significant differences in the incidence of sudden death and total mortality between patients treated with metoprolol and amiodarone and patients treated with the ICD. A significantly higher incidence of events was observed in patients treated with propafenone, which led to an early interruption of this treatment.

Several studies reported a high efficacy of the association of beta blockers with antiarrhythmics in patients with recurrent episodes of VT and impaired left ventricular function (17-19). Recently, Leclercq et al. (20) retrospectively evaluated the role of nonrandomized association of nadolol or acebutolol to conventional antiarrhythmic therapy in 240 patients with ischemic heart disease or dilated cardiomyopathy. Multivariate analysis showed that low ejection fraction, advanced age, and absence of beta blocker therapy were independent predictors of cardiac and sudden deaths. The 5-year cardiac mortality was 48% in patients without beta blockers versus 20% in those receiving this treatment.

In conclusion, beta blockers should be considered as a first-line therapy for patients with idiopathic VT, especially if induced by physical activity or a hyperadrenergic state. These indications can be extended to patients with underlying heart disease and preserved or slightly depressed left ventricular function, especially in the absence of baseline inducibility. In patients with a more compromised ventricular function, empirical therapy with beta blockers is associated with a significant incidence of sudden death and arrhythmic recurrences (15). Retrospective studies showed more favorable results when beta blockers were combined with other antiarrhythmic drugs, mainly amiodarone (20). Electrophysiologic studies appear to be of limited clinical value for evaluating the efficacy of beta blockers. Finally, in survivors of cardiac arrest beta blockers appeared to be more effective than class I drugs. Ongoing studies are comparing these drugs with amiodarone and ICD (16).

Sotalol

Sotalol is an antagonist of β-adrenergic receptors devoid of membrane-stabilizing effects, local anesthetic activities, intrinsic sympathomimetic actions, or cardioselectivity (21). In addition to its beta blocking effect (class II), sotalol increases the action potential duration and prolongs the repolarization phase both in the atrium and in the ventricle, properties belonging to class III agents. Due to its pharmacologic actions, this drug has been widely used in the recent years.

Several studies reported the use of sotalol in patients with sustained VT or VF (Table 1). Most patients were refractory to class I drugs and were treated with sotalol on the basis of electrophysiologic testing. In these nonrandomized trials (22-34), noninducibility after sotalol was found in 20%-89% of the patients. This wide range can be explained by many factors such as patient selection, different daily dosage, nonstan-

Table 1. Studies including patients with ventricular tachycardia or ventricular fibrillation treated with sotalol

Reference	Patients	Daily dose (mg)	Noninducibility after sotalol		Average follow-up (months)	Patients under long-term sotalol alone		Arrhythmia recurrence		Deaths	
	(n)		(n)	(%)		(n)	(%)	(n)	(%)	(n)	(%)
(22)	18	320–480	12	67	16	9	50	1	11	0	0
(23)	37	160–480	15	42	9	16	43	0	0		
(24)	39	160–480	17	45	13	22	56	6	27	0	0
(25)	9	480–900	8	89	23	8	88	2	25	1	12
(26)	16	320–960	7	50	19	14	88	3	21	1	7
(27)	50	—	10	22	20	24	88	4	17	2	8
(28)	65	80–480	8	20	10	22	34	1	5	1	5
(29)	26	160–320	13	62	13	15	58	2	13	0	0
(30)	42	160–320	10	24	8	12	29	2	17	0	0
(31)	64	480–720	59	92	20	53	82	5	12	0	0
(32)	68	320	34	50	41	68	100	10	15	1	1
(33)	22	160–560	10	45	23	8	36	0	0	0	0
(34)	28	320–640	15	53	10	15	53	0	0	0	0

dardized stimulation protocols, and variable definitions of success or failure. During the follow-up period noninducible patients showed a very low death rate and a favorable reduction in arrhythmia recurrence (Table 1). However, patients at high risk due to persistent inducibility were excluded in most trials from the long term administration of sotalol. Similar results were obtained from a single centre in a nonrandomized prospective study of 171 patients with VT or VF (35). At a mean daily dosage ranging from 240 to 640 mg, the incidence of sudden death and VT recurrence was 4% in responders (52% of the patients), but 44% in patients whose arrhythmia was still inducible after sotalol (48%). Significant side effects were noted in 5% of the patients.

In a recent study, Young et al. (34) evaluated the efficacy of sotalol by programmed electrical stimulation in sustained VT or VF secondary to coronary heart disease. Sotalol revealed greater success in suppressing sustained arrhythmias in patients with VF (eight of nine, 89%) than in those with VT (seven of 19, 37%, $p < 0.01$). Patients without a history of myocardial infarction showed a high rate of suppression compared with patients with previous infarction (88% versus 40%, $p<0.05$). The baseline VT cycle length of the suppressed group was also significantly shorter than that of the nonsuppressed group (218 ms versus 270 ms, $p < 0.05$). Patients with fast VT or VF have a shorter reentry circuit and a shorter excitable gap; in these patients sotalol may have more effectively decreased the excitable window by prolonging refractoriness.

Sotalol was compared with amiodarone in an open-label, randomized multicenter study which included 59 patients with sustained VT or VF refractory or intolerant to class I drugs (36). Patients received either a maintenance dose of amiodarone of 400 mg/day or increasing doses of sotalol up to 640 mg/day. Over a 12-month period, therapy was discontinued in half of the patients in each group due to arrhythmia recurrence, adverse drug reactions, or protocol violation. By intention to treat analysis, there was no significant difference in either antiarrhythmic efficacy or the incidence of severe side effects. An increase in the left ventricular ejection fraction was also observed during the follow-up period in the group of patients treated

with sotalol: 37.9% versus a mean baseline value of 32.8%. Based on these data, sotalol appears to be an attractive alternative to amiodarone in patients with VT or VF who can tolerate β-adrenergic blockade. However, the impact of this study is limited by the the small number of patients and the brief follow-up period.

The ESVEM trial (37) compared the effectiveness of sotalol with that of imipramine, mexiletine, pirmenol, procainamide, and quinidine in patients with sustained VT or VF. This study was initiated in 1985, more than 2000 patients were screened, and ultimately only 486 patients enrolled. They received long-term treatment with the first antiarrhythmic drug that was predicted to be effective on the basis of the drug testing assigned (electrophysiologic study or electrocardiographic monitoring). Patients with a very low ejection fraction, congestive heart failure, and hypotension were not considered eligible to receive sotalol. In the electrophysiologic study group, the percentage of patients with drug efficacy was higher after sotalol than after therapy with antiarrhythmics of class I (35% versus 16%, $p < 0.001$), while there was no significant difference among the seven drugs in the Holter monitoring group. During a mean follow-up period of 6.2 years, the probability of arrhythmia recurrence after a prediction of drug efficacy by either drug testing was lower with sotalol than with other drugs (risk ratio 0.43; $p < 0.001$). The risk of death from any cause (risk ratio, 0.50; $p = 0.004$), of death from cardiac causes (0.50, $p = 0.02$), and of arrhythmic death (risk ratio, 0.50; $p < 0.04$) were also lower on sotalol than on other drugs. More specifically, in patients on sotalol, the 1- and 3-year actuarial incidence of arrhythmia recurrence, cardiac death, and arrhythmic death were 20% and 25%, 7% and 18%, and 6% and 15%, respectively. After 1 year sotalol is predicted to show complete efficacy in 33% of patients in the Holter group, but only in 23% in the electropharmacologic arm. The rate of adverse effects among patients receiving sotalol was 16% during titration and 7% during the follow-up period. These values were significantly better than in patients treated with class I drugs ($p < 0.001$). Torsades de pointes were recorded in 1.7% of patients treated with sotalol during titration and in 3.5% during long-term therapy, but no patients died as a consequence of this proarrhythmia. Although sotalol gave more favorable results, several limitations were observed in the ESVEM trial that reduce its clinical impact (38): (a) the entry requirement of the study restricted the conclusions to a specific group of patients with VT or VF; (b) the stimulation protocol used during drug evaluation was limited to the same protocol that induced the baseline arrhythmias, possibly resulting in a greater number of subsequent drug failures; (c) the exercise test was included in the drug-assesment only in the Holter monitoring arm, favoring a greater prediction of drug efficacy by this method; (d) the definition of arrhythmia recurrence was very wide, including nonsustained VT and syncope of unknown origin; (e) amiodarone was not used, most likely because its long half-time would have prevented other drugs from being tested and because of its frequent inability to demonstrate suppression of VT/VF induction.

In a double-blind parallel design multicenter study, the electrophysiologic and antiarrhythmic effects of intravenous and oral sotalol and procainamide were compared in 110 patients with a history of sustained and inducible VT (39). Sotalol produced a greater effect on lenghtening the ventricular effective refractory period and prevented the inducibility of VT in 30% of patients compared to 20% for procainamide (p = not significant, NS). Patients with a baseline VT cycle of less than 270 ms were more likely to effectively respond to sotalol than the other patients. A ventricular refractory period of more than 300 ms after sotalol was also determinant for the prevention of VT inducibility. After a 12-month period of follow-up, lifetable analysis showed a trend in favor of sotalol. According to ESVEM results, this study confirmed that sotalol is more effective than class I agents in preventing VT and VF when beta blockade is not contraindicated.

Some conflicting data about the prognostic value of programmed ventricular stimulation in patients treated with sotalol were obtained in two recent studies. In the trial by Haverkamp et al. (40), including 210 patients treated with a mean daily dose of 435 mg, persistent inducibility of VT predicted VT recurrence, but not sudden death. In contrast, in the series investigated by Kühlkamp et al. (41), 37 responders to sotalol (mean daily dose of 330 mg) had a VT/VF recurrence rate similar to 23 nonresponders treated with ICD who continued to receive sotalol (16% versus 22%, mean follow-up 16 months).

Sotalol was also effective at a daily dose of 320 – 640 mg/day in a group of patients with arrhythmogenic right ventricular disease (42). The overall efficacy in terms of arrhythmia prevention was 68.4% in patients with baseline inducible VT and 82.8% in patients evaluated by Holter monitoring and exercise testing for baseline noninducibility. Side effects severe enough to discontinue therapy were rare (5%) and occurred mainly within the first few days of treatment.

To evaluate whether the benefical effects of sotalol are due to a beta-blocking action, to a class III antiarrhythmic activity, or to a combination of both, Antz et al. (43) prospectively compared the use of metoprolol and sotalol in 34 patients with sustained VT, mainly associated with coronary heart disease.

Compared with metoprolol, sotalol significantly reduced the inducibility of sustained VT by ventricular stimulation (56% versus 14%). During an average 2-year follow-up the incidence of arrhythmia recurrence was not significantly different in the two groups (6% with metoprolol versus 27% with sotalol, p=NS), whereas the appearance of side effects was higher in the metoprolol group than in the sotalol group (31% versus 11%). Persistent inducibility of sustained VT did not predict arrhythmia recurrence in either group. The conclusion of this pilot study is that pure beta blocker metoprolol is as efficacious as sotalol in the treatment of patients with sustained VT. Moreover, these data emphasize the beta-blocking properties of sotalol, which can reduce the possible proarrhythmic effects of class III activity.

The safety of sotalol was evaluated in 3257 patients treated for cardiac arrhythmias in clinical trials that supported the drug approval in the United States (44). The overall incidence of adverse events was 73%, but therapy was discontinued in only 18% of patients. The main reasons for discontinuing the drug were fatigue (4%), dyspnea (3%), and bradycardia (3%). No evidence of extracardiac organ toxicity was found. New appearance or worsening of heart failure occurred in 4.6% of patients with VT or VF, but treatment was continued in more than half of the patients. There was no change in the ejection fraction even in patients with baseline values of < 40%. The negative inotropic effect of beta blockade may be attenuated by the positive effect of prolonged repolarization on contractility. The overall rate of proarrhythmia in patients with sustained VT or VF was 6.5%, and the rate of torsades de pointes was 4.1%. This arrhythmia occurred early during treatment and more frequently in patients with congestive heart failure and a low ejection fraction. Its occurrence was also related to a daily dose greater than 320 mg. With the exception of torsades de pointes, the adverse effects of sotalol are consistent with the beta-blocking action.

Amiodarone

Important data on amiodarone in the treatment of patients with ventricular tachyarrhythmias refractory to class I drugs come from studies done in the 1970s and in the 1980s (45-54). From these noncontrolled and nonrandomized studies the following conclusions can be drawn:
• When amiodarone was empirically administered, a cardiac death rate of 25%-30%, a sudden death rate of 8%-10% and an incidence of nonfatal arrhythmic recurrence of 15%-20%could be expected after 1 year.
• When amiodarone treatment was based on electrophysiologic studies, there was a further reduction of the incidence of sudden death and arrhythmic recurrence rates after 1 year: 2.5% and 2.0% in responders (20-30% of the cases) versus 11% and 27% in nonresponders, respectively. A feature peculiar to amiodarone is the high percentage of patients who remained asymptomatic in spite of persistent inducibility. Moreover, induction of slower and well-tolerated VT during amiodarone treatment in comparison to

baseline study identifies a group of patients with an intermediate risk of arrhythmia recurrence, but with low mortality (48). The induction of fast VT or VF on amiodarone seems to be related to a high incidence of sudden death.

• When amiodarone therapy was based on Holter monitoring, the suppression of ventricular premature complexes (VPC) was 70%-80% in 90% of patients and close to 100% in the case of nonsustained VT. In the majority of studies (55-57), the incidence of nonfatal arrhythmic recurrences after 1 year was about 20% in responders and 48% in nonresponders. In other studies (58, 59), a significant reduction in ventricular ectopic activity by amiodarone was of limited prognostic value in patients with inducible VT.

• During a follow-up period of 8-24 months, the overall rate of side effects was between 30% and 93%. A total of 9%-26% of patients were withdrawn from amiodarone treatment. Drug-related adverse events were associated with both dosage and length of the treatment.

Additional information on the effectiveness and tolerability of amiodarone therapy in patients refractory to class I agents comes from two large retrospective trials (60-61).

Herre et al. (60) followed 427 patients affected by different underlying heart disease (coronary heart disease in 77% of cases), who were empirically treated with amiodarone after an average of 2.6 class I antiarrhythmic drugs proved to be ineffective. The mean left ventricular ejection fraction was 36%. The sudden cardiac death rate after 1, 3, and 5 years of follow-up was 9%, 15%, and 21%, respectively, while the total death rate was 24%, 43% and 62% (Tables 2, 3). By multivariate analysis, survival time to sudden death was significantly decreased in elderly patients, in patients with an ejection fraction of less than 40% and with a history of cardiac arrest. Withdrawal from therapy due to side effects was necessary in 14%, 26%, and 37% after 1, 3, and 5 years, respectively. More specifically, the drug was discontinued due to lung toxicity in 11% of the patients, to neurologic toxicity in 5%, to gastrointestinal and hepatic toxicity in 2.6%, to ocular toxicity in 2.5%, and to hypothyroidism and hyperthyroidism in 0.5%. These data are in agreement with the results obtained by Weinberg et al. (61), who evaluated 469 patients with ventricular tachyarrhythmia during an average follow-up of almost 3 years. In 36% of the cases, amiodarone was initially combined with other antiarrhythmic drugs. The sudden death rate at 1 year was 9% and increased thereafter by 3% every year. The combined incidence of sudden death and sustained VT or VF recurrence was 19% at 1 year and 38% at 5 years (Table 2, 3). An insufficient dosage of amiodarone did not seem to justify such events. By years 2 and 5, the total death rate was 13% and 46% and the incidence of side effects necessitating discontinuation of amiodarone was 10% and 18%, respectively. Pulmonary toxicity was observed in 3.5% of patients at 1 year and in 9.1% at 5 years. A higher functional class appeared to be the best predictor of sudden death and treatment failure.

We evaluated the benefits of amiodarone as a first-choice antiarrhythmic drug in a nonrandomized study which included 128 consecutive patients with

Table 2. Clinical results of empirical amiodarone treatment: sudden death (SD), and nonfatal arrhythmia recurrences (AR) rates (%)

Reference	Patients (n)	1-year		3-year		5-year	
		SD	AR	SD	AR	SD	AR
(60)	427	9	19	15	33	21	43
(61)	469	9	19	16	30	22	38
(62)	128	9	5	16	15	20	25
(54)	52	9	15	22	24	22	43

Table 3. Clinical results of empirical amiodarone treatment: cardiac (CM) and total mortality (TM) rates (%)

Reference	Patients (n)	1-year		3-year		5-year	
		CM	TM	CM	TM	CM	TM
(60)	427	0	24	0	43	0	62
(61)	469	11	13	26	33	37	46
(62)	128	18	21	28	34	37	42
(54)	52	11	0	31	0	31	0

sustained VT or VF (62). The average age was 62 years, and the mean ejection fraction 36%. A total of 81% of patients had coronary artery disease. After 1, 3 and 5 years, the sudden death rate was 9%, 16% and 20%, the total cardiac death rate was 18%, 28% and 37%, and the nonfatal VT recurrence rate was 5%, 15%, and 25% respectively. These results are similar to those observed in studies in which amiodarone was considered to be a second- or third-choice drug (Tables 2, 3). Side effects occurred in 22.6% of patients and 8.6% of patients were withdrawn from therapy. Functional class III or IV and an ejection fraction of less than 35% proved to be risk factors for sudden and total cardiac deaths, whereas a history of cardiac arrest appeared to be predictive only of cardiac death. The conclusions of these retrospective and nonrandomized studies (60-62) are that amiodarone can be used safely and successfully after 5 years in approximately half of the patients with VT or VF and that the incidence of sudden death is relatively low after the first year (3% per year). Finally, few clinical and laboratory parameters can identify patients at high risk.

The superiority of amiodarone treatment in comparison to class I agents was demonstrated by CASCADE (Cardiac Arrest in Seattle: Conventional versus Amiodarone drug evaluation), a prospective study which included 228 survivors of cardiac arrest: 113 were randomized to empirical administration of amiodarone, and 115 to an electrophysiologically guided conventional treatment (quinidine and procainamide in most cases) (63, 64). The two groups did not differ in their basic clinical and laboratory characteristics or in the percentage of the patients simultaneously treated with ICD (46% and 47%, respectively). By years 2, 4, and 6, survival was significantly higher for patients on amiodarone treatment than for those receiving conventional treatment: 82%, 66%, and 53% versus 69%, 52%, and 40%, respectively ($p = 0.07$). Considering only the patients with ICD, 2-year survival free of all shocks and of syncopal shocks was also lower for amiodarone therapy: 77% versus 42% ($p = 0.014$), and 98% versus 81% ($p = 0.01$). Drug-related adverse events did not differ between the two groups at 6 months, although after 1 year more patients randomized to amiodarone had to discontinue their therapy.

In a retrospective case control investigation, Newmann et al. (65) compared the empirical use of amiodarone (120 patients) and ICD (60 patients). There was no difference between the groups in terms of age, ejection fraction, underlying heart disease, arrhythmia at presentation, and follow-up length. During a mean follow-up of 18 and 23 months, sudden death rate was lower in ICD recipients than in controls (5% versus 10%, $p < 0.01$). Actuarial survival after 1 and 3 years was also better in patients treated with ICD than with amiodarone (89% and 65% versus 72% and 49%, respectively $p < 0.05$), but after the fourth year the survival curves of the two groups overlapped. However, in patients treated with ICD, nonsudden cardiac death was less frequent (17% versus 39%), possibly because ICD patients were less sick. Therefore, clinical differences between groups may at least in part explain the favorable results observed in ICD group. Finally, another important confounding factor is the high percentage of ICD recipients maintained on amiodarone.

Three large trials are now in progress in order to evaluate prospectively the effectiveness of amiodarone treatment in comparison to sotalol, beta blockers, and ICD: the Cardiac Arrest Study of Hamburg (CASH) (16), the Canadian Implantable Defibrillator Study (CIDS) (66), and the Antiarrhythmics Versus Implantable Defibrillators investigation (AVID) (67). About 2000 patients will be enrolled in these three trials and preliminary data are now available. The CASH study (16) randomized the patients in four groups of nonguided treatment: propafenone, metoprolol, amiodarone, and ICD. The propafenone arm was stopped due to high mortality, but there were no significant differences in total mortality among the other groups. CIDS randomized patients between amiodarone and ICD and has extended the completion date to 1 January, 1997 (66). A preliminary report shows that addition of amiodarone to ICD occurred in 18% of cases, while crossover from amiodarone to ICD is to date only 9% (68). The AVID study randomized more than 350 patients to empirical treatment with amiodarone or ICD, while only a small number of cases received electrophysiologically guided therapy with sotalol (67). To date, the number of crossover between the two main treatments have been equal. With regard to total mortality reduction, preliminary data from these three prospective trials seem to confirm that amiodarone and ICD are equally effective.

Conclusions

Beta blockers. These should be considered the drugs of choice in patients with idiopathic VT. Their usefulness in patients with aborted sudden death or with sustained VT and relevant underlying heart disease is still debatable. Prospective trials on patients with a back up ICD may shed some light on the appropriateness of this treatment. Guided therapy with beta blockers seems to be of limited value, while an empirical administration may be an acceptable approach. Finally, these drugs are very useful in combination with other antiarrhythmic agents, especially with amiodarone.

Sotalol. This drug yields favorable short- and long-term results when therapy is guided by Holter monitoring or programmed ventricular stimulation. Randomized studies showed that guided treatment with sotalol is more effective than with class I agents. However, responders account for less than 50% of tested cases. The effectiveness of sotalol is explained by a combination of beta-blocking activity and of class III properties. There is also a low rate of long-term side effects but in patients with sustained VT or VF the treatment should be started under monitoring due to the possibility of early proarrhythmia, mainly torsades de pointes. There are no conclusive data on comparative effects of sotalol, amiodarone, and ICD.

Amiodarone. This drug has proven effective both in patients with VT or VF refractory to conventional treatment and when compared with other antiarrhythmic agents. The outcome is less favorable in high-risk patients, such as those with a history of cardiac arrest, a very low ejection fraction, and persistent inducibility of ill-tolerated sustained ventricular arrhythmias. Randomized prospective trials are needed to assess the role of amiodarone compared to ICD in this high-risk population. Available evidence indicates that the overall long-term prognosis is no different between patients treated with amiodarone and those treated with ICD. However, ICD-treated patients seem to have a lower sudden death rate in the first few years of follow-up, but many patients continue to take amiodarone as well. Finally, the high incidence of side effects mandates close monitoring and careful tailoring of treatment.

References

1. Josephson ME (1993) Evaluation of antiarrhythmic agents. In: Josephson ME (ed) Clinical cardiac electrophysiology. Lea and Febiger , Philadelphia, pp 630-682
2. Knilans TK, Prystowsky EN (1992) Antiarrhythmic drug therapy in the management of cardiac arrest survivors. Circulation 85 [Suppl I]: I 118-I124
3. Camm AJ, Katritsis D (1992) How to prescribe and manage antiarrhythmic drug therapy. Eur Heart J 13 [Suppl F]: 44-52
4. Singh BN (1993) Choice and chance in drug therapy of cardiac arrhythmias: technique versus drug-specific responses in evaluation of efficacy. Am J Cardiol 72: 114F-124F
5. Proclemer A, Facchin D, Miani D, Vanuzzo D, Feruglio GA (1994) Opzioni terapeutiche nel trattamento delle aritmie ventricolari maligne: farmaci antiaritmici. In: Rovelli F, De Vita C, Moreo A (eds) Cardiologia. Scientific Press, Florence, pp 366-389
6. Teo KK, Yusuf S, Furberg CD (1993) Effects of prophylactic antiarrhythmic drug theraphy in acute myocardial infarction. JAMA 270: 1589-1595
7. Beta-Blocker Heart Attack Trial Research Group (1982) A randomized trial of propranolol in patients with acute myocardial infarction: I. Mortality results. JAMA 247: 1707-1714
8. The Göteborg Metoprolol Trial in Acute Myocardial Infarction (1984) Am J Cardiol 53 (13) 1-50D
9. Rydén L, Ariniego R, Arnman K et al (1983) A double blind-trial of metoprolol in acute myocardial infarction. Effects on ventricular tachyarrhythmias. N Engl J Med 308: 614-618
10. Hjalmarson Å (1994) Empiric therapy with beta-blockers. PACE 17: 460-466
11. Meredith IT, Broughton A, Jennings GL, Esler MD (1991) Evidence of a selective increase in cardiac sympathetic activity in patients with sustained ventricular arrhythmias. N Engl J Med 325:618-624

12. Duff HJ, Mitchell B, Wyse G (1986) Antiarrhythmic efficacy of propranolol: comparison of low and high serum concentrations. J Am Coll Cardiol 8: 959-965

13. Brodsky MA, Allen BJ, Luckett CR, Capparelli EV, Wolff LJ, Henry WL (1989) Antiarrhythmic efficacy of solitary beta-adrenergic blockade for patients with sustained ventricular tachyarrhythmias. Am Heart J 272-280

14. Hallstrom AP, Cobb LA, Yu BH, Weaver WD, Fahrenbruch CE (1991) An antiarrhythmic drug experience in 941 patients resuscitated from an initial cardiac arrest between 1970 and 1985. Am J Cardiol 68:1025-1031

15. Steinbeck G, Andresen D, Bach P, Haberl R, Oeff M, Hofmann E, von Leitner E-R (1992) A comparison of electrophysiologically guided antiarhythmic drug therapy with beta-blocker therapy in patients with symptomatic sustained ventricular tachyarrhythmias. N Engl J Med 327:987-992

16. Siebels J, Cappato R, Rüppel R, Schneider MAE, Kuck KH and the CASH investigators (1993) Preliminary results of the Cardiac Arrest Study Hamburg. Am J Cardiol 72: 109F-113F

17. Hirsowitz G, Podrid PJ, Lampert S, Stein J, Lown B (1986) The role of beta-blocking agents as adjunct therapy to membrane stabilizing drugs in malignant ventricular arrhythmia. Am Heart J 11: 852- 860

18. Tonet J, Frank R, Fontaine G, Grosgogeat Y (1988). Efficacy and safety of low doses of beta-blocker agents combined with amiodarone in refractory ventricular tachycardia. PACE 11: 1984-1987

19. Brodsky MA, Allen BJ, Bessen M, Luckett CR, Siddiqi R, Henry WL (1988) Beta-blocker therapy in patients with ventricular tachyarrhythmias in the setting of left ventricular dysfunction. Am Heart J 115: 799-808

20. Leclercq JF, Chastang CL, Coumel PH (1995) Beta-blocking therapy: a main prognostic factor of survival in patients with sustained monomorphic ventricular tachycardia due to left ventricular disease. PACE 18: 810 (abstr)

21. Claudel JP, Touboul P (1995) Sotalol: from "just another beta-blocker" to "the prototype of class III antidysrhythmic compound". Pace 18: I: 451-467

22. Senges J, Lengfelder W, Jauernig R et al (1984) Electrophysiologic testing in assessment of therapy with sotalol for sustained ventricular tachycardia. Circulation 69: 577-584

23. Nademanee K, Singh BN (1990) Effects of sotalol on ventricular tachycardia and fibrillation produced by programmed electrical stimulation: comparison with other antiarrhythmic agents. Am J Cardiol 65: 53A-57A

24. Steinbeck G, Bach P, Haberl R (1986) Electrophysiologic and antiarrhythmic efficacy of oral sotalol for sustained ventricular tachyarrhythmias: evaluation by programmed stimulation and ambulatoy electrocardiogram. J Am Coll Cardiol 8: 949-958

25. Kienzle MG, Martins JB, Wendt DJ et al (1988) Enhanced efficacy of oral sotalol for sustained ventricular tachycardia refractory to type I antiarrhythmic drugs. Am J Cardiol 16: 1012-1017

26. Singh SN, Cohen A, Chen YW et al (1988) Sotalol for refractory sustained ventricular tachycardia and nonfatal cardiac arrest. Am J Cardiol 62: 399-402

27. Gonzales R, Scheinman MM, Herre JM et al (1988) Usefulness of sotalol for drug-refractory malignant ventricular arrhythmias. J Am Coll Cardiol 12: 1568-1572

28. Ruder MA, Ellis T, Lebsack C et al (1989) Clinical experience with sotalol in patients with drug-refractory ventricular arrhythmias. J Am Coll Cardiol 13: 145-152

29. Jordaens LJ, Palmer A, Clement DL (1989) Low-dose oral sotalol for monomorphic ventricular tachycardia: effects during programmed electrical stimulation and follow-up. Eur Heart J 10: 218-226

30. Kuchar DL, Garan H, Venditti FJ et al (1989) Usefulness of sotalol in suppressing ventricular tachycardia or ventricular fibrillation in patients with healed myocardial infarcts. Am J Cardiol 64: 33-36

31. Obel IW, Jardine R, Haitus B et al (1990) Efficacy of sotalol in reentrant ventricular tachycardia. Cardiovasc Drugs Ther 41 [Suppl 3]: 613-618

32. Trappe HJ, Klein H, Lichtlen P (1990) Sotalol in patients with life-threatening ventricular tachyarrhythmias. Cardiovasc Drug Ther 4: 1425-1432

33. Kus T, Campa MA, Nadeau R et al (1992) Efficacy and electrophysiologic effects of oral sotalol in patients with sustained ventricular tachycardia caused by coronary artery disease. Am Heart J 123: 82-89

34. Young GD, Kerr CR, Mohama R, Boone J, Yeung-Lai-Wah JA (1994) Efficacy of sotalol guided by programmed electrical stimulation for sustained ventricular arrhythmias secondary to coronary artery disease. Am J Cardiol 73: 677-682

35. Martinez-Rubio A, Chen X, Hief C, Büscher M, Borggrefe G, Breithardt G (1990) Acute and long-term efficacy of sotalol in patients with ventricular tachyarrhythmias. Eur Heart J 11: 242 (Abstr)

36. Amiodarone vs. Sotalol Study Group (1989) Multicentre randomized trial of sotalol vs amiodarone for chronic malignant ventricular tachyarrhythmias. Eur Heart J 10: 685-694

37. Mason JW, for the Electrophysiologic Study versus Electrocardiographic Monitoring Investigators (1993) A comparison of seven antiarrhythmic drugs in patients with ventricular tachyarrhythmias. N Engl J Med 329: 452-458

38. Gettes LS (1995) ESVEM and the hazards of clinical trials. Circulation 91: 1908-1909

39. Singh BN, Kehoe R, Woosley RL, Scheinman M, Quart B, and the Sotalol Multicenter Study Group (1995) Multicenter trial of sotalol compared with procainamide in the suppression of inducible ventricular tachycardia: a double-blind, randomized parallel evaluation. Am Heart J 129: 87-97

40. Haverkamp W, Lammers A, Möhlenkamp S, Witcher T, Borggrefe M (1994) Characteristics of patients developing either recurrences of ventricular tachycardia or sudden cardiac death on long-term oral sotalol. Circulation 90: I-544

41. Kühlkamp V, Mermi J, Mewis C, Braun U, Seipel L (1994) Does programmed electrical stimulation predict long term efficacy of d/l sotalol? Circulation 90: I -545

42. Wichter T, Borggrefe M, HaverkampW, Chen X, Breithardt G (1992) Efficacy of antiarrhythmic drugs in patients with arrhythmogenic right ventricular disease: results in patients with inducible and noninducible ventricular tachycardia. Circulation 86: 29-37

43. Antz M, Cappato R, Kuck KH (1995) Metoprolol versus sotalol in the treatment of sustained ventricular tachycardia. (in press)

44. MacNeil DJ, Davies RO, Deitchman D (1993) Clinical safety of sotalol in the treatment of arrhythmias. Am J Cardiol 72: 44A-50A

45. Morady F, Sauve MJ, Malone P et al (1983) Long-term efficacy and toxicity of high-dose amiodarone therapy for ventricular tachycardia or ventricular fibrillation. Am J Cardiol 52: 975-979

46. Heger JJ, Prystowsky EN, Zipes DP (1983) Clinical efficacy of amiodarone in treatment of recurrent ventricular tachycardia and ventricular fibrillation. Am Heart J 106: 887-894

47. Di Carlo LA, Morady F, Sauve MJ et al (1985) Cardiac arrest and sudden death in patients treated with amiodarone for sustained ventricular tachycardia or ventricular fibrillation: risk stratification based on clinical variables. Am J Cardiol 55: 372-374

48. Horowitz LN, Greenspan AM, Spielman SR et al (1985) Usefulness of electrophysiologic testing in evaluation of amiodarone therapy for sustained ventricular tachyarrhythmias associated with coronary heart disease. Am J Cardiol 55: 367-371

49. Manolis AS, Uricchio F, Estes M (1989) Prognostic value of early electrophysiologic studies for ventricular tachycardia recurrence in patients with coronary artery disease treated with amiodarone. Am J Cardiol 63: 1052-1057

50. Hamer AW, Finerman WB, Peter T, Mandel WJ (1981) Disparity between the clinical and electrophysiologic effects of amiodarone in the treatment of recurrent ventricular tachyarrhythmias. Am Heart J 102: 992-1000

51. Waxman HL, Groh WC, Marchilinski FE et al (1982) Amiodarone for control of sustained ventricular tachyarrhythmia: clinical and electrophysiologic effects in 51 patients. Am J Cardiol 50: 1066-104

52. Nademanee K, Singh BN, Cannon DS, Weiss J, Feld G, Stevenson WG (1983) Control of sudden recurrent arrhythmic deaths: role of amiodarone. Am Heart J 106:895-901

53. Proclemer A, Facchin D, Vanuzzo D, Feruglio GA (1993) Risk stratification and prognosis of patients treated with amiodarone for malignant ventricular tachyarrhythmias after myocardial infarction. Cardiovasc Drugs Ther 7: 683-689

54. Di Pede F, Raviele A, Gasparini G et al (1990) Trattamento

empirico con amiodarone in pazienti con tachiaritmie ventricolari sostenute. G Ital Cardiol 20: 819-827

55. Veltri EP, Griffith LSC, Platia E, Guarnieri T, Reid PR (1986) The use of ambulatory monitoring in the prognostic evaluation of patients with sustained ventricular tachycardia treated with amiodarone. Circulation 74: 1054-1060

56. Kim SG, Felder SD, Fifura I, Johnston DR, Waspe LE, Fisher JD (1987) Value of Holter monitoring in predicting long term efficacy and inefficacy of amiodarone used alone and in combination with class IA in antiarrhythmic agents in patients with ventricular tachycardia. J Am Coll Cardiol 9 :169-174

57. Marchlinsky FE, Buxton AE, Flores BT, Doherty JU, Waxman HL, Josephson ME (1985) Value of Holter monitoring in identifying risk for sustained ventricular arrhythmias recurrence on amiodarone. J Am Coll Cardiol 55: 709-712

58. Morady F, Scheinman M, Hess D (1983) Amiodarone in the management of patients with ventricular tachycardia and ventricular fibrillation. PACE 6: 609

59. Nasir N, Doyle TK, Wheeler SH, Pacifico A (1994) Usefulness of Holter monitoring in predicting efficacy of amiodarone therapy for sustained ventricular tachycardia associated with coronary artery disease. Am J Cardiol 73: 554-558

60. Herre JM, Sauve MJ, Malone P et al (1989) Long-term results of amiodarone theraphy in patients with recurrent sustained ventricular tachycardia or ventricular fibrillation. J Am Coll Cardiol 13: 442-449

61. Weinberg BA, Miles WM, Klein LS et al (1993) Five years follow-up of 589 patients treated with amiodarone Am Heart J 125: 109-120

62. Proclemer A, Facchin D, Vanuzzo D, Feruglio GA (1993) Risk stratification in patients treated with amiodarone for ventricular tachycardia or ventricular fibrillation of different etiology. PACE 16: 1212 (Abstr)

63. The CASCADE Investigators (1993) Randomized antiarrhythmic drug therapy in survivors of cardiac arrest (the Cascade Study). Am J Cardiol 72: 280-287

64. Dolack GL, for the CASCADE Investigators (1994) Clinical predictors of implantable cardioverter-defibrillator shocks (results of the CASCADE Trial). Am J Cardiol 73: 237-241

65. Newman D, Sauve MJ, Herre J et al (1992) Survival after implantation of the cardioverter defibrillator. Am J Cardiol 6: 899-903

66. Connolly SJ, Jent M, Roberts RS, Dorian P, Green MS, Klein GJ, Mitchell LB, Sheldon RS, Roy D (1993) Canadian Implantation Defibrillator Study (CIDS): study design and organization. Am J Cardiol 72: 103F-108F

67. AVID Investigators (1995) Antiarrhythmics versus implantable defibrillators (AVID): rationale, design and methods. Am J Cardiol 75:470-476

68. Zipes DP (1995) Are implantable cardioverter-defibrillators better than conventional antiarrhythmic drugs for survivors of cardiac arrest? Circulation 91: 2115-2117

New Antiarrhythmic Drugs for Ventricular Arrhythmias: Do They Work?

B. N. Singh

Department of Cardiology, Veterans Affairs Medical Center
of West Los Angeles, and the Department of Medicine, UCLA School of Medicine,
Los Angeles, USA

In the early 1960s, at the time Coronary Care Units (CCUs) were conceived and being set up as a way to reduce arrhythmia mortality by detecting, treating, and preventing ventricular arrhythmias, there were very few antiarrhythmic drugs available to the clinician – quinidine, procainamide, and lidocaine (1). Disopyramide was being developed and had not attained established usage. Digoxin was regarded as being an antiarrhythmic compound but its use in controlling ventricular tachyarrhythmias was never established. Thus, the field of antiarrhythmic drugs was dominated by drugs that acted fundamentally by delaying conduction via inhibition of sodium-channel activity. This was considered as having several major consequences. First, the delay in conduction and often complete block in certain tissues was thought to convert unidirectional to bidirectional block, thereby terminating and preventing reentrant tachycardia. Second, the block in conduction might be expected to markedly suppress premature ventricular contractions (PVCs) by preventing their propagation. It was consistent with the observation that the greater the propensity of a compound (e.g., class I agent) to block conduction, the higher its suppressant effect on PVCs. Third, it was realized that the refractory period of the ventricular myocardium may be prolonged by the blocking of sodium-channel activity by delaying its reactivation. Thus, the change in refractory period was time dependent when affected by drugs that selectively blocked sodium channels. It so happened that in the case of quinidine, the archetype of antiarrhythmic drugs, as well as in the case of procainamide and disopyramide, there was the additional property of lengthening repolarization, which in itself could prolong the refractory period and they constitute a discrete antifibrillatory mechanism. On the other hand, there has always been the theoretical possibility that excessive delay in conduction induced by sodium-channel blockers may create the substrate for reentrant ventricular tachycardia/ventricular fibrillation (VT/VF) as a proarrhythmic reaction (2, 3).

Later in the 1960s and during the decades that followed newer antiarrhythmic drugs with selective electropharmacological properties were synthesized (4-6).

The first were beta-blockers which neither slowed sodium-channel mediated conduction nor did they, as a class, prolong refractoriness in the ventricular myocardium to a significant degree. Yet, in numerous controlled clinical trials and in other less systematic obsevations, they have been shown to reduce sudden death (attributed to VT/VF), cardiac mortality and total mortality, in survivors of myocardial infarction (MI). They have been found to prolong survival in patients resuscitated from cardiac arrests (7) and in those with the long QT interval syndrome of the congenital type. All these beneficial effects are undoubtedly a class action (5). Clearly, these drugs work in reducing total mortality, possibly by preventing VF. Then followed the synthesis and characterization of class I agents which did not exhibit additional properties on repolarization nor on refractoriness – lidocaine congeners such as mexiletine and tocainide and aprindine or the so-called class Ic agents such as flecainide, encainide, and propafenone, among others. All such agents blocked sodium-channel activity to varying degrees and had somewhat different offset and onset kinetics of sodium-channel block. In general these are powerful suppressants of PVCs but given the context of serious cardiac disease, they all may increase mortality, presumably by inducing serious life-threatening ventricular arrhythmias (3, 6, 7). They may increase sudden . death and may produce incessant VT/VF which may be difficult to cardiovert or defibrillate. As a class these agents have not been shown to reduce mortality in any subset of patients with cardiac disease. Therefore, as far as mortality is concerned, it is clear that they do not work or work adversely.

A major recent focus has been on drugs that have appeared to work by prolonging cardiac repolarization (5, 6, 8). The prototypes have been sotalol and amiodarone; these are not new drugs, both having been synthesized about 1962, the first as a beta blocker and the second as a coronary vasodilator. The perceived effectiveness of these compounds to suppress ventricular tachyarrhythmias, their superiority in preventing recurrences of VT/VF in patients with symptomatic sustained VT/VF and in survivors of cardiac arrest (5, 6,

8) had led to the development of so-called pure class III agents. This has stemmed from the belief that the dominant action of these two compounds results from the lengthening of the action potential duration and refractoriness. They were developed in the belief that such newer compounds synthesized on the basis of selective targeting against myocardial membrane currents may be preferable antifibrillatory agents in terms of side effect profile while retaining much of the effectiveness of the complex prototypical molecules such as sotalol and amiodarone.

Against this background, a number of questions have arisen. Clearly, the most significant and certainly the most practical is the issue of whether the newer agents work, i.e., are they effective in relieving symptoms and/or prolonging survival? Both goals of therapy need to be addressed in stringently controlled clinical trials and not merely by the use of surrogate end points which have been used a great deal in the past to infer impact on mortality. In the case of asymptomatic ventricular arrhythmias, clearly the only goal of therapy is reduction in total mortality and the prolongation of survival. In considering old versus newer antiarrhythmic drugs with respect to the issue of whether they work, the separation boundary has become increasingly blurred as some of the beneficial actions of the older compounds on mortality have been found to be unrelated to arrhythmia suppression. Thus, one may logically suppress arrhythmias for relief of symptoms but such an approach may have little or no validity for the prolongation of survival. The salient aspects of these considerations form the basis of this paper, in which conclusions will be drawn on the strength of the newer data which bear on the often-asked question of whether antiarrhythmic drugs work in ventricular arrhythmias.

Sodium-Channel Blockers: Do They Work in Ventricular Arrhythmias?

There is now a substantive body of data which suggest that class I agents, as a class, do not prolong survival in patients with life-threatening ventricular arrhythmias and in patients with serious heart disease they are likely to increase mortality (3, 5-7). The "newer" agents (e.g., flecainide, encainide, propafeone), which tend to delay conduction and have relatively little effect on refractoriness, are powerful for suppressing spontaneously occurring ventricular arrhythmias documented on Holter recordings. The PVC suppressant effect appears to parallel increases in their ability to inhibit sodium-channel activity with a corresponding decrease in conduction velocity (9). The results of the Cardiac Arrhythmia Suppression Trials (CAST I & II) (10, 11) revealed an unexpected dichotomy between mortality and arrhythmia suppression, i.e., marked and predictable suppression of PVCs in the survivors of MI was accompanied by an increase in total and arrhythmia mortality. The data cast a serious doubt on PVC suppression as a valid or tenable surrogate end point for mortality. The dichotomy between the effect on mortality and arrhythmia suppression was entirely unexpected. In the event, the phenomenon has come to be of much relevance to the general field of arrhythmia control.

The results of the meta-analysis of randomized controlled studies have lent further support to the notion that class I agents have the potential to increase mortality in post-MI survivors (3, 9). The clinical data are also in accord with the experimental findings. For example, in an ischemic sudden death model (12), flecainide, quinidine, or lidocaine either had no protective effect or they facilitated the development of VF (12-15). In humans, these agents may stabilize the reentrant circuit, thereby facilitating the continued inducibility of VT by programmed electrical stimulation (16, 17). Thus, it appears that slowed conduction is conductive to the development of clinical VT (18). In humans, lidocaine and mexiletine (19, 20) may produce an excess of mortality in infarct survivors possibly by their proarrhythmic effects (3). Of note also are the findings of Rapaport and Remedios (21), who, in a post-MI patient follow-up study, found that mortality on antiarrhythmic agents (mostly procainamide and quinidine) was higher in the treated group than in patients not taking antiarrhythmic agents. Again, these data are in line with the meta-analytic data from patients with PVCs without recent MI in whom (22) quinidine produced a 2.5 – fold increase in mortality compared to placebo. Compared to beta-blockers or no treatment in survivors of cardiac arrest, class I agents have been found to be associated with a higher mortality rate (7). Higher mortality rate has also been found in patients given quinidine in atrial fibrillation when compared to placebo (23, 24).

Thus, overall, given the appropriate clinical setting, slowing of myocardial conduction by class I agents may lead to significant proarrhythmic effects which may have an adverse effect on mortality, especially in patients with diseased myocardial substrate. The data are compelling against the routine use of class I antiarrhythmic agents in patients at risk for sudden death. Their use in performing further randomized clinical trials to settle the issue more definitively is becoming increasingly controversial. It is improbable that such trials will be done in the future. Most clinicians are now finding it increasingly difficult to justify the continued use of class I agents in the suppression of ventricular arrhythmias in most, if not all, subsets of patients with significant structural heart disease.

It should also be emphasized that the largest number of patients presenting with VT/VF have significant structural heart disease. The question has therefore arisen as to whether class I agents can confer mortality benefit to this category of patients. There are no adequately controlled studies that suggest that they do. It is an intriguing therapeutic dilemma that class I agents, including the relatively newer agents such as flecainide, propafenone, and moricizine, have continued to remain approved indications for the treatment of VT/VF based on the data on efficacy demonstrated by serial drug testing using the criteria of noninducibility on drugs during programmed electrical stimulation (PES). It should be emphasized that the approval of these agents in VT/VF in the USA stemmed from observations of drug effects in responders versus nonresponders defined by PES and has not been validated against independent controls analogous to placebo. Thus, it is not clear whether these drugs are indeed superior to placebo and at least one of these compounds, propafenone, has been reported to produce a higher mortality than amiodarone, metroprol, or ICDs in patients resuscitated from cardiac arrest (25). Paradoxically, the newer class I agents such as flecainide and propafenone are no longer approved for the suppression of symptomatic PVCs in patients without structural heart disease where these agents in a similar setting but having supraventricular tachyarrhythmias have not been shown to increase total mortality (4-6). It may be concluded that the development of newer class I agents for the control of ventricular arrhythmias in patients with cardiac disease may be difficult to justify. While these agents clearly work in suppressing supraventricular tachyarrhythmias and maintain sinus rhythm in patients with atrial fibrillation and flutter, the use of these agents in patients with heart disease is likely to result in a net increase in mortality.

Suppression of VT/VF by Antiarrhythmic Drugs: Does It Result in Prolongation of Survival?

Suppression of manifest arrhythmias has been the cornerstone of the approaches to the reduction in arrhythmia mortality for many years. Such a notion has never been well validated. Now it is being challenged in light of increasing data to the contrary from controlled clinical trials. These trials have produced little evidence that suppression by antiarrhythmic drugs of manifest VT/VF or that induced by programmed electrical stimulation is predictive of a successful clinical outcome in terms of a favorable impact on mortality. Nor has a defined degree of suppression of ambient arrhythmias provided an index to predict a favorable impact on mortality due to ventricular arrhythmias. As indicated above, the results of the Cardiac Arrhythmic Suppression Trials (CAST I and II) revealed a striking dichotomy between suppression or elimination of premature ventricular contractions (PVCs) and mortality, i.e., increases in mortality despite marked suppression of PVCs (10, 11). If arrhythmia suppression and impact on mortality in the case of class I agents were dissociated in the case of one subset of patients at high risk of sudden death (e.g., postinfarct survivors), it is inherently improbable that such a relationship might be substantially different in another subset of patients if Holter-guided therapy were used as, for example in patients with VT/VF. The proarrhythmic reactions of class I drugs (discussed above) is likely to be greater in patients with manifest VT/VF than in the survivors of acute infarction. The issue is now further clouded by the outcome of the Electrophysiologic Versus Electrocardiographic Monitoring (ESVEM) trial (26, 27). There were several major findings. First, there was no significant difference between the two techniques in predicting the long-term outcome in terms of arrhythmia recurrence, sudden death, or total cardiovascular mortality. Second, comparisons of sotalol (the prototype class III agent with beta-blocking property) and six class I agents, collectively or individually, with respect to arrhythmia recurrence, sudden death, cardio-

vascular and total mortality, provided a significant difference in favor of sotalol. The arrhythmia recurrence rate of 21% on sotalol compared to 44% for class I agents ($p < 0.0007$) at 1 year is consistent with the notion that the effects of class I drugs on the suppression of inducible or spontaneous VT/VF are poorly predictive of the long-term outcome of drug treatment by the acute responses using so-called guided therapy. Furthermore, the fact that sotalol was not as effective as class I drugs (such as mexiletine) in suppressing nonsustained VT on Holter recordings but reduced mortality to a greater extent than did class I agents emphasizes again the dichotomy between arrhythmia suppression and total mortality. The fact that the techniques did not differ in predicting the outcome of drug therapy based on acute responses but the two classes of drugs did differ in this regard emphasizes drug-specific rather than technique-specific responses as the crucial determinants of the outcomes of pharmacologic therapy of VT/VF (2, 4-6). This is further supported by the results of the CASCADE Trial (28) in which survivors of cardiac arrest were randomized to Holter or PES-guided therapy involving class I agents versus amiodarone. Empirically given amiodarone was found to be superior to guided class I antiarrhythmic agents in terms of arrhythmia-free survival and cardiac and total mortality. Thus, sotalol was superior to class I agents in ESVEM and amiodarone superior to class I agents in CASCADE not because their effects could be predicted better with Holter monitoring or PES, but more likely that its electrophysiologic and pharmacodynamic effects "matched" better with the vulnerable substrate, in contrast to the possibility of a "mismatch" in the case of class I agents as clearly exemplified in CAST. However, the fact that both sotalol and amiodarone have been found to be superior to class I agents in terms of arrhythmia-free survival and possibly total mortality, the proof that they may be superior to placebo in terms of absolute mortality, is still lacking. Based on data from other subsets of patients, it is, however, likely that sotalol and amiodarone do in fact prolong survival by reducing arrhythmia mortality. It is becoming increasingly clear that to be able to demonstrate a favorable impact on arrhythmia mortality, controlled trials will need to focus on protocols in which the effects of drugs are compared to those of placebo in subsets of patients at high risk in whom no therapy has convincingly demonstrated a benefit by arrhythmia suppression; patients with manifest VT/VF protected by an ICD in both treatment limbs may need to be randomized to active drug and placebo. That arrhythmia suppression per se is unrelated to the issue of preventing symptoms, which clearly is an important therapeutic objective in many cases of ventricular arrhythmias, may have little or no role in the prolongation of survival by reducing total mortality in patients who already have manifest VT/VF or in those in whom there is a high probability of the arrhythmia developing. Recent data from heart failure studies, in particular the CHF STAT (29), has provided strong support for such an hypothesis. The data may indicate a general principle in antiarrhythmic therapy and be applicable to other subsets of patients in whom the presence of high density PVCs and nonsustained and sustained VT constitute important markers of increased mortality.

Amiodarone, Sotalol, Beta-Bockers: Do They Reduce Mortality in Patients at High Risk for Sudden Arrhythmic Death?

While the impact of amiodarone, sotalol, and beta-blockers in patients with manifest VT/VF and in survivors of cardiac arrest cannot be interpreted in terms of changes in absolute mortality because of the lack of placebo controls, there have been clinical trials in which the effects of these drugs in the so-called high-risk patients prone to arrhythmic deaths have been compared to those of patients on placebo. As indicated the best data are for beta-blockers in the survivors of MI (3, 9). The effects of sotalol, a beta-blocker with the additional property of lengthening repolarization, have been less decisive and may have stemmed from flaws in study design. Nevertheless, the drug did reduce reinfarction rate, as do most beta-blockers, and it did reduce total mortality by 18% (which did not reach statistical significance). The important issue here is that unlike class I agents, it did not increase mortality and mortality trends on the drug were in the direction of those seen with most beta-blockers. In the case of amiodarone, there have been a number of trials in the survivors of acute infarction, none reported that have been appropriately blinded. Most such trials (30) have indicated benefit in terms of total mortality as well as cardiac mortality. Two blinded studies (EMIAT and CAMIAT) (30) are ongoing. No such studies are ongoing or planned with dl-sotalol.

Perhaps the best model to test the hypothesis that antifibrillatory drugs have the potential to reduce arrhythmia mortality is the subset of cardiac patients with heart failure. It has long been recognized that patients with congestive cardiac failure and asymptomatic ventricular arrhythmias are at a particular risk for fatal cardiovascular events (31-33). This risk is further augmented by the presence of complex ventricular arrhythmias, and over 60% of patients with congestive heart failure have nonsustained ventricular tachycardia on Holter monitoring. The annual mortality is about 15% or higher, half the deaths being sudden and presumed to be arrhythmic in origin (31-33). No suppression trials testing the PVC hypothesis has been performed in heart failure. In light of the CAST trials, it is unlikely that conventional suppression trials are likely to be performed in patients with heart failure. However, controlled clinical trials in which drugs such as amiodarone, which are extremely potent in suppressing PVCs or nonsustained ventricular tachycardia (34), are of major interest.

The hypothesis that amiodarone will reduce total mortality in patients with moderate to severe congestive heart failure with asymptomatic ventricular arrhythmias (29) was therefore tested in a study that utilized a double-blind placebo-controlled protocol in which 674 patients with congestive heart failure with > 10 PVC's/h and left ventricular ejection fraction $\leq$ 40% were radomized to placebo (n = 338) and to amiodarone (n = 336). This study (CHF STAT) was performed under the sponsorship of the Veterans Affairs Co-operative Studies Division, Washington DC, USA. The median follow up was 45 (0 to 54) months. There was no significant difference (p = 0.60) in all-cause mortality between placebo and amiodarone. Among the placebo group, the actuarial 2-year survival was 70.8% (95% CI = 65.7 – 75.9); among the amiodarone patients the rate was 69.4% (95% CI = 64.2 – 74.6). There was also no significant difference between amiodarone and placebo on sudden death (p = 0.43), the corresponding 2-year survival figures being 81% for placebo and 85% for amiodarone. There was a trend in favor of amiodarone for reducing total mortality in patients with nonischemic cardiomyopathy (p = 0.07) but not in those with ischemic cardiomyopathy. Lower ejection fraction and the presence of ventricular tachycardia runs identified subjects with a higher mortality on placebo. Amiodarone was highly effective in suppressing premature ventricular contractions (with $\geq$ 80% suppression in 70% of patients) and in eliminating runs of ventricular tachycardia (67% free of VT runs at 2 weeks compared to 23% at baseline). The total mortality between the group in which the arrhythmias were suppressed versus those in which they were not was not significantly different. Amiodarone produced a sustained increase (over 40%) in left ventricular ejection fraction compared to baseline (p = 0.001) as well as to placebo (p = 0.0001); it reduced heart rate compared to baseline (p < 0.001) and to placebo (70 ± 12 bpm versus 79 ± 13 bpm; p < 0.0001).

In contrast, the study (35) from Argentina (Grupo de Estudio de la Sobrevida en la Insuficiencia Cardiaca en Argentina or GESICA) in which 516 patients with New York Heart Association Class III and IV heart failure were randomized to amiodarone (300 mg/day) and to standardized medical therapy revealed somewhat different findings. There was a 28% reduction in all-cause mortality, from 41.4% to 33.5% (95% CI = 4-45%; p = 0.024). Sudden death and death due to progressive heart failure appeared to be reduced to a similar extent (27% and 23%, respectively, p = 0.16) but did not reach statistical significance.

The reasons for the apparently marked difference between the mortality outcomes in CHF STAT and those in GESICA remain unclear. However, besides the blinded nature of CHF STAT, the most striking difference is the smaller proportion (39%) of the patients in GESICA who had coronary artery disease compared to that (70%) in the CHF STAT. Of note, in CHF STAT there was a favorable trend in total mortality in patients who had cardiac failure of nonischemic origin (p = 0.07). Whether this is the sole explanation for the differences in mortality between the two studies is uncertain. In this regard, the CHF STAT data on amiodarone, a powerful antiadrenergic agent with long-lasting effects (36), are similar to those of chronic beta-blockade with bisopropol in cardiac failure in 641 patients revealing no significant effect on total mortality (37). However, as in our trial with amiodarone, in the patients without previous MI (n = 338), there were 42 deaths out of 187 patients on placebo compared to 18 deaths on bisoprolol (22.5% versus 11.9% total mortality; p < 0.01).

CHF STAT was not an arrhythmia suppression

trial. Nevertheless, the powerful suppressant effect of amiodarone both on PVCs and on VT runs permitted an analysis of the relationship between suppression and mortality endpoints. Again, no difference in total mortality was found between the group in which ventricular arrhythmias were suppressed ["responders"] (i.e., 80% or greater suppression of PVCs and 100% suppression of VT runs) compared to those in which the arrhythmias were not suppressed ["nonresponders"]. The dichotomy between arrhythmia suppression and mortality (neutral in the case of amiodarone) casts further doubt on the validity of using Holter-guided therapy in predicting an effect on mortality in patients with reduced left ventricular ejection fraction and ventricular arrhythmias.

Antiarrhythmics of the Future: Simple Versus Complex Molecules

Considerable changes have occurred in the approaches to control VT and VF in the last 5 years. An important issue is the recognition that, as far as drug therapy is concerned, it is difficult to demonstrate that the time-honored antiarrhythmic agents have the potential to prolong survival by controlling VT/VF and, in fact, have the potential to increase mortality by their proarrhythmic reactions. This has led to a shift to agents with somewhat different properties characterized by the prolongation of repolarization and refractoriness of cardiac muscle in association with sympathetic inhibition (3-6). Some tentative conclusions can be drawn from the current state of knowledge. The data suggest that both sotalol and amiodarone are superior to class I agents and the continued use of class I agents in the control of VT/VF in patients with structural heart disease is questionable. If such a premise were to be accepted, the role of beta-blockers as monotherapy in patients with VT/VF remains to be determined (38) but the available data emphasize the significance of blunting sympathetic stimulation as an integral component of most, if not all, antiarrhythmics for controlling VT/VF. The data also suggest that while amiodarone and sotalol along with beta-blockers may now be considered as constituting the "best" medical therapy of VT/VF, they do fall considerably short of being the ideal agents. In the case of sotalol, the variable incidence of torsades de pointes and beta-blocker side effects continue to pose concerns; amiodarone has neither the beta-blocker side effects nor does it produce an appreciable incidence of torsades de pointes (39). The major deficiency of the drug is the complex array of side effects that develop during the course of therapy as a function of time especially in high doses.

To circumvent the perceived shortcomings of sotalol and amiodarone, there has been an intensive experimental and clinical research focus on simpler molecules which have the propensity to lengthen repolarization without any other major electrophysiologic effects. Such agents have been targeted against single or multiple repolarizing membrane currents (40). Most are specific blockers of the delayed rectifier potassium current, especially its rapid component (i_{kr}), E4031, dofetilide, sematilide, MK499, and the dextro-isomer of dl-sotalol (d-sotalol) being examples of the so-called "pure" class III agents. These agents selectively prolong repolarization and cardiac refractoriness without affecting myocardial excitability. They elevate the VF threshold and reduce the ventricular defibrillation threshold. They exert a weakly suppressant effect on premature ventricular contractions but are relatively potent in preventing the inducibility of VT and VF induced by programmed electrical stimulation. They are thought to exert their antifibrillatory activity by slowing VT, thereby preventing VF. In contrast to sodium-channel blockers, as a class, potassium-channel blockers do not exhibit negative inotropic actions but do produce a variable incidence of torsades de pointes.

Clearly, in evaluating their effectiveness as antifibrillatory agents, it is imperative to determine their net effect not only on sudden death but especially on total mortality, which cannot be inferred reliably from their influence on inducible VT/VF. At least in the case of one of the pure class III agents – d-sotalol – this has been determined in a double-blind, placebo-controlled study – Survival with Oral D-Sotalol (SWORD) involving high-risk patients after MI (41). This study was designed to enroll 6400 patients to test the hypothesis that d-sotalol would reduce total mortality in patients over 18 years of age with a left ventricular ejection fraction less than 40%; two subsets of patients were enrolled into the study. In the first were patients who had sustained MI within 42 days of the acute event and in the second subset were those who had incurred MI after 42 days at the time of entry into the study. The latter group were required to have had a documented history of cardiac failure (New York Heart Class II or III). Patients satisfying the entry criteria were randomized to placebo or to d-sotalol 100 mg bid which was increased to 200 mg bid if tolerated. The trial was stopped prematurely (because the boundary for harm was crossed) when 3119 patients had been enrolled (mean follow-up about 156 days). It was noteworthy that 42 (2.7%) died in the placebo group and 71 (4.6%) died in the group given d-sotalol (p = 0.005). There were no significant differences between the two groups, being about 30%; 29.2% of the patients enrolled into the study had recent MI and 70.8% had remote infarcts. It was also of note that the trend for mortality for both groups was similar for the remote as well as those with recent infarcts, with an increasing divergence of the survival curves as a function of time.

These data on the effects of d-sotalol are the first from the mortality trials in survivors of acute infarction involving pure class III compounds. It clearly shows a deleterious effect akin to those of the class I agents flecainide and encainide; the adverse effect on mortality was interpreted as being due to proarrhythmic reaction. A similar conclusion in the case of d-sotalol in SWORD is inescapable. It leads to the question of whether it might be a common property of most, if not all, pure class III agents, a possibility that remains to be confirmed or denied on the basis of data from similar studies in post-MI patients. In this regard, the outcome of an ongoing trial involving dofetilide being carried out in Denmark will be of major importance. For the present, it must be emphasized that the trial with dl-sotalol performed by Julian et al (42) was not adverse although there were some excess deaths on *dl*-sotalol compared to placebo during the early months of the study. At the end of the 12 months, sotalol had reduced total mortality by 18%, which did not, however, reach statistical significance. The fact that *dl*-sotalol, a potent beta-blocker (compared to *d*-sotalol), differs from the dextro-isomer in terms of the divergent effect on mortality emphasizes the importance of beta-blocking or antiadrenergic effect of antiarrhythmic drugs in mediating a salutary effect in survivors of acute MI. This has also been noted in the case of amiodarone which also is a potent sympathetic antagonist (30). Some tentative conclusions may be drawn from these observations. The outcome of the SWORD trial in which *d*-sotalol was used as a test agent against placebo, when considered in light of the beta-blocker data in the case of beta-blockers *dl*-sotalol and amiodarone suggest that attenuating sympathetic stimulation in survivors of acute infarction may be critical to arrhythmia mortality reduction. Furthermore, in this context, as indicated elsewhere (43), it would seem that complex molecules such as sotalol and amiodarone which encompass sympathetic antagonism as an integral component of their overall pharmacodynamic actions might be preferable to similar molecules developed to produce selective block of individual myocardial channels, receptors, or pumps. For the purposes of mortality reduction by preventing VF, it appears desirable that all newer antiarrhythmic molecules should be potent adrenergic antagonists. Such molecules are more likely to be effective in reducing mortality than those that appear to act principally by blocking a single ion channel or a component of a channel.

Conclusions

How ventricular arrhythmias should be treated is currently a rapidly changing scene that is and should be under continuous and close scrutiny. The goals and end points of therapy should be clearly defined. These are best done on the basis of data acquired from stringently controlled clinical trials. The results from such trials need to be incorporated into our thought processes and clinical decision making in the selection of regimens, pharmacologic and nonpharmacologic, for therapeutic use in the expectation of reducing mortality due to ventricular arrhythmias. While suppression of manifest arrhythmias is a desirable goal for reducting symptoms when they are related to the arrhythmias, efforts to suppress them for the purposes of prolonging survival remains an unproven hypothesis.

The requirements for demonstrating efficacy of newer agents are also becoming more stringent. The impact on mortality can only be demonstrated by adequately designed controlled trials. Newer trials need to take cognizance of the changing natural history of cardiovascular disease, especially the substrate for ventricular arrhythmias, the need for placebo-controlled trials, and the appropriate trial end points. In the case of asymptomatic arrhythmias the sole end point is clearly an improvement in mortality. The presence of arrhythmias in a particular setting in this instance

merely selected a subset of patients at high risk for arrhythmic deaths – patients with recent or remote myocardial infarction, heart failure, and cardiomyopathies, among others. In such subsets of patients the effects on total mortality have been determined with respect to beta-blockers, calcium-channel blockers, aspirin, angiotensin-converting enzyme (ACE) inhibitors, amiodarone, and certain antiarrhythmic drugs. Most such trials have utilized placebo controls. The availability of ICDs has provided an opportunity to use placebo controls even in patients with manifest VT/VF. It is clear that there are pharmacologic regimens which may not act directly on arrhythmias but which may have a substantial effect in either continuously modulating the arrhythmogenic influences on the substrate (e.g., beta-blockers) or which fundamentally alter the myocardium (ACE inhibitors or thrombolytics), thereby indirectly preventing the development of VF. An understanding of the mechanisms of the salutary effects of these classes of cardioactive compounds is critical since the use of such agents in patients at high risk for developing VF provides the largest scope for mortality reduction in patients with significant cardiac disease.

For controlling VT/VF a shift from class I agents to beta-blockers and to complex class III agents such as sotalol and amiodarone in recent years is occurring simultaneously as a shift from surrogate end points of arrhythmia suppression either on Holter or of arrhythmias induced by PES. An important realization from clinical trial end points has been that total mortality and indices of arrhythmia suppression have been divergent. This was dramatically illustrated by the findings in CAST with class I agents. This being the case, if one were to apply the data to VT/VF, it engenders considerable doubt whether antiarrhythmic drugs have been shown to prolong survival in patients with VT/VF in absolute terms. No longer does it appear reasonable to assume that in responders on the basis of PES studies mortality will be reduced. As far as guided drug therapy for VT/VF is concerned, it appears inherently unlikely that a drug might produce an increase in mortality in one subset of patients and a reduction in another, especially if the level of the left ventricular ejection fraction were comparable. For example, *d*-sotalol clearly increased mortality in high-risk post-MI survivors with low ejection fraction. Is it logical to believe that the drug might reduce mortality in patients with VT/VF if it is administered on the basis of PES-guided therapy? Such is the magnitude of the persisting dilemma of drug therapy in the case of VT/VF, a dilemma that has undoubtedly led to an increasing focus on the use of implantable devices in this setting. The advent of ICDs now permits controlled clinical trials which may indicate the true benefit (if any) of drug therapy in patients with symptomatic VT/VF. In these trials, ICDs may serve as the placebo arm of a randomized drug study. Controlled studies of these designs are not only desirable but are imperative for establishing the role of various treatment modalities in the control of VT/VF in patients with cardiac disease. The challenge is not only to synthesize ideal antifibrillatory agents but also to define precisely their net therapeutic effects on clinically relevant end points compared to no drug treatment (i.e., placebo) in patients with changing myocardial substrates. The availability of ICDs now permits such studies to be carried out without violating ethical principles of conducting controlled clinical trials.

Acknowledgment. This work was supported by the Medical Research Service of the Veterans Administration (Washington, DC) and the American Heart Association of the Greater Los Angeles Affiliate.

References

1. Singh BN (1992) Routine prophylactic lidocaine administration in acute myocardial infarction: an idea whose time is all but gone. Circulation 86: 1033-1035
2. Singh BN, Ahmed R (1994) Class III antiarrhythmic drugs. Curr Opin Cardiol 19: 12-19
3. Yusuf S, Teo KK (1991) Approaches to sudden death: need for fundamental re-evaluation. J Cardiovasc Electrophysiol 2: S233-S239
4. Ahmed R, Singh BN (1993) Antiarrhythmic drugs. Curr Opin Cardiol 8: 10-19
5. Singh BN (1993) Choice and chance in drug therapy of cardiac arrhythmias: technique versus drug – specific responses in evaluation of efficacy. Am J Cardiol 72: 114-124
6. Singh BN (1994) Whether antiarrhythmic drugs? In: Singh BN, Wellens HJJ, Hiraoka M (eds) Electropharmacological control of cardiac arrhythmias. To delay conduction or to prolong refractoriness? Futura, Mt Kisco, NY, pp 713-731
7. Hallstrom AP, Cobb LA, Yu BH, Weaver WD, Fahrenbruch CE (1991) An antiarrhythmic drug experience in 941 patients resuscitated from an initial cardiac arrest from 1970 and 1985. Am J Cardiol 68: 1025-1031
8. Singh BN (1988) Control of cardiac arrhythmias by lengthening repolarization. Futura, Mt Kisco, NY, pp 1-596
9. Teo KK, Yusuf S (1993) Overview of anti-arrhythmic drug trials: implications for anti-arrhythmic therapy. In: Singh BN, Dzau V, Woosley RA, Vanhoutte PM (eds), Cardiovascular pharmacology and therapeutics. Churchill-Livingstone, New York
10. The Cardiac Arrhythmia Suppression Trial (CAST) Investigators (1989) Preliminary report. Effect of encainide and flecainide on mortality in a randomized trial of arrhythmia suppression after myocardial infarction. N Engl J Med 321: 406-410
11. Cardiac Arrhythmia Suppression Trial II Investigators (1992) Ethmozine exerts an adverse effect on mortality in survivors of acute myocardial infarction. N Engl J Med 327: 227-233
12. Lynch JJ, Lucchesi BR (1987) How are animal models best used for the study of antiarrhythmic drugs? In: Hearse DJ, Mouring AS, Janse MJ (eds) Life-threatening arrhythmias during ischemia and infaction. Raven, New York, pp 169-196
13. Kou WH, Nelson SD, Lynch JJ, Montgomery DG, Di Carlo L, Lucchesi BR (1987) Effect of flecainide acetate on prevention on electrical induction of ventricular tachycardia and occurrence of ischemic ventricular fibrillation during the early post-myocardial infarction period. Evaluation in a conscious canine model of sudden death. J Am Coll Cardiol 9: 359-365
14. Patterson E, Lucchesi BR (1983) Quinidine gluconate in chronic myocardial ischemic injury. Differential effects in response to programmed stimulation and acute myocardial ischemia in the dog. Circulation 68: 111-118
15. Nattel S, Pedersen DH, Zipes DP (1981) Alterations in regional myocardial distribution and arrhythmogenic effects of aprindine produced by coronary artery occlusion in the dog. Cardiovasc Res 15: 80-86
16. Furuwaka T, Rozanski JJ, Monroe K, Gosselin AJ, Lister JR (1989) Efficacy of procainamide on ventricular tachycardia: relation to prolongation of refractoriness and slowing of conduction. Am Heart J 118: 702-708
17. Kus T, Dubue M, Lambert C, Shenasa M (1990) Efficacy of propafenone in preventing ventricular tachycardia, with insights from analysis of resetting response patterns. Am J Cardiol 15: 1229-1237
18. Stevenson WG, Weiss JN, Wiener I, Nademanee K (1989) Slow activation in the infarct scar relevance to the occurrence, detection, ablation of ventricular re-entry circuits results from myocardial infarction. Am Heart J 117: 452-467
19. MacMahan S, Collins R, Peto R, Koster RW, Yusuf S (1988) Effects of prophylactic lidocaine in suspected acute myocardial infarction. JAMA 20: 1910-1916
20. IMPACT Research Group (1984) International mexiletine and placebo anti-arrhythmic coronary trial. 1. Report in arrhythmias and other findings. J Am Coll Cardiol 4: 1148-1156
21. Rapaport E, Remedios P (1983) The high risk patient after recovery from myocardial infarction: recognition and management. J Am Coll Cardiol 1: 391-399
22. Morganroth J, Goin JE (1991) Quinidine – mortality in the short-to-medium term treatment of ventricular arrhythmias. Circulation 84: 1911-1983
23. Coplen SE, Antman EM, Berlin JA, Hewitt P, Chalmers TC (1990) Efficacy and safety of quinidine therapy for the maintenance of sinus rhythm after cardioversion. A meta-analysis of randomized control trials. Circulation 82: 1106-1116
24. Flaker GC, Blackshear JL, McBride R, Kronmal RA, Halperin JL, Hart RG (1992) Antiarrhythmic drug therapy and cardiac mortality in atrial fibrillation. J Am Coll Cardiol 20: 427-532
25. Siebels J, Cappato R, Ruppel R, Schneider R, Kuck KH and the CASH Investigators (1993) Preliminary results of the cardiac arrest study Hamburg (CASH). Am J Cardiol 72: 109F-113F
26. Mason JW and ESVEM Investigators (1993) A randomized comparison of electrophysiologic study to electrocardiographic monitoring for prediction of antiarrhythmic drug efficacy in patients with ventricular tachyarrhythmias. N Engl J Med 329: 445-451
27. Mason JW and ESVEM Investigators (1993) A comparison of sevent antiarrhythmic drugs in patients with ventricular tachyarrhythmias. N Engl J Med 329: 452-458
28. The CASCADE Investigators (1993) The Cascade Study – randomized anti-arrhythmic drug therapy in survivors of cardiac arrest in Seattle. Am J Cardiol 72: 280-287
29. Singh SN, Gross-Fisher S, Fletcher RD, Singh BN et al (1995) Amiodarone in patients with congestive heart failure and asymptomatic ventricular arrhythmias. N Engl J Med (in press)
30. Nademanee K, Singh BN, Stevenson WG, Weiss JN (1993) Amiodarone and post-MI patients. Circulation 88: 764-774
31. Holmes J, Kubo S, Cody R, Kligfield P (1985) Arrhythmias in ischemia and nonischemic dilated cardiomyopathy: prediction of mortality by ambulatory electrocardiography. Am J Cardiol 55: 146-151
32. Meinertz Te, Hoffman T, Kasper W et al (1984) Significance of ventricular arrhythmias in idiopathic cardiomyopathy. Am J Cardiol 53: 902-907
33. Van Olshausen K, Schafer A, Mehmel HC et al (1984) Ventricular arrhythmia in dilated cardiomyopathy. Br Heart J 51: 147-152
34. Salerno D, Gillingam KJ, Berry DA, Hodges M (1990) A comparison of antiarrhythmic drugs for the suppression of ventricular ectopic depolarization. A meta-analysis. Am Heart J 120: 340-349
35. Doval HC, Nul DR, Vancelli HO et al (1994) Randomized trial of low-dose amiodarone in severe congestive heart failure. Lancet 344: 493-498
36. Antimisiaris M, Sarma JSM, Schoenbaum MP et al (1995) Effects of amiodarone on the circardian rhythmicity and power spectral changes of heart rate and QT interval: significance for the control of sudden cardiac death. Amer Heart J 128: 884-891
37. CIBIS Investigators and Committees (1994) A randomized trial of beta-blockade in heart failure. The Cardiac Insufficiency Bisoprolol Study (CIBIS). Circulation 90: 1765-1773
38. Steinbeck G, Andersen D, Bach P et al (1992) A comparison of electrophysiologically anti-arrhythmic drug therapy with beta-blocker therapy in patients with symptomatic, sustained ventricular tachyarrhythmias. N Engl J Med 327: 987-992
39. Holnloser S, Klingenheben T, Singh BN (1994) Amiodarone-associated proarrhythmic effects: a review with special reference to torsades de pointes tachycardia. Ann Int Med 121: 529-535
40. The Sicilian Gambit (1994) A new approach to the classifica-

tions based on their actions on arrhythmogenic mechanisms. Circulation 84: 1915-1923

41. Julian DG, Jackson FS, Prescott RJ, Szekely P (1982) Control trial of sotalol for one year after myocardial infarction. Lancet 1: 1142-1146

42. Waldo AL, Camm AJ, De Ruyter H et al (1995) Preliminary results from the Survival with Oral D-Sotalol (SWORD) Trial. J Am Coll Cardiol 15A (abstr)

43. Singh BN, Ahmed R, Sen L (1993) Prolonging cardiac repolarization as an evolving antiarrhythmic principle. In: Escande D, Standen N (eds) K⁺ channels in cardiovascular medicine. Springer, Paris, pp 247-272

What Have We Learned from the SWORD Trial? Can Potassium Channel Blockers Reduce Sudden Cardiac Death?

P. J. Schwartz

Cattedra di Cardiologia, Università degli Studi di Pavia,
Policlinico San Matteo IRCCS, Pavia and
Istituto di Clinica Medica Generale e Terapia Medica
Università degli Studi, Milan, Italy

Introduction

On November 1, 1994, the SWORD (Survival With Oral D-sotalol) trial was terminated by the Steering Committee because of an excess mortality among the patients randomized to d-sotalol. Five years after the early termination of the Cardiac Arrhythmia Suppression Trial (CAST) for similar reasons, this event has caused further concern in the field of cardiac arrhythmias and electrophysiology and is raising questions about the availability of drugs that may reduce sudden cardiac death and also about the rationale and events that precede the initiation of large-scale clinical trials.

This article reviews the background of the SWORD trial and considers some of the reasons for its outcome. This analysis is limited by the impossibility of disclosing, at the moment of writing, very relevant information because the primary paper on SWORD has not yet been published.

Background

In the aftermath of CAST (1, 2), most drug companies abandoned the development of Na^+ channel blockers and concentrated their efforts on K^+ channel blockers. Let us examine what the reasoning was behind this move, because there is an important lesson to be learned by those interested in the pharmacologic prevention of sudden cardiac death and in the development and evaluation of antiarrhythmic drugs.

In addition to the well-established, but incomplete, protection offered by ß-adrenergic blocking agents the only antiarrhythmic drug that in the late 1980s still appeared to be promising was amiodarone. A few small-size studies (3, 4) had indeed reported a reduction in mortality with amiodarone, and two large-size studies, EMIAT (5) and CAMIAT (6), will report their final results on a total of 2700 postmyocardial infarction (MI) patients in 1996. Amiodarone is the prototype of class III antiarrhythmic drugs in the traditional Vaughan-Williams classification; this simplistic view has led many investigators and drug companies to incorrectly assume that all other class III antiarrhythmic agents share the same favorable characteristics of amiodarone but hopefully without its peculiar toxicity. As a consequence, the development of a large number of K^+ channel blockers was accelerated, and many of them (almokalant, ambasilide, azimilide, dofetilide, d-sotalol, risotilide, sematilide, E4031, MS-551, RP S8866, WAY-123-398) became either available for clinical investigation or are almost ready now. In the early 1990s, it was considered that for two of these compounds, d-sotalol and dofetilide, a sufficient amount of experimental and clinical data had been accumulated to justify their evaluation in a randomized clinical trial. Thus, Bristol-Myers-Squibb and Pfizer set in motion two major trials, SWORD and DIAMOND (Danish Investigation of Arrythmias and Mortality on Dofetilide).

As suggested above, the reasoning behind this decision was based, at least in part, on a series of oversimplifications that had already been challenged in the document produced in 1991 by a Task Force of the Working Group on Arrhythmias of the European Society of Cardiology called the "Sicilian Gambit" (7). The Sicilian Gambit, and its subsequent evolution (8, 9), pointed out that most antiarrhythmic drugs have a wide range of actions and that to consider them as belonging to a single class is a dangerous and misleading oversimplification. This was not the original intention of Vaughan-Williams, but this is the way his classification is being used, as indicated by the common reference to "class I antiarrhythmic drugs" or to "class III antiarrhythmic drugs." The Sicilian Gambit called attention to the fact that amiodarone does much more than to block the K^+ channels; as a matter of fact, it also blocks the Na^+ and the Ca^{2+} channels, albeit with a lower potency, and it has both α- and ß-adrenergic blocking effects in addition to an interesting coronary vasodilating effect. To assume that a drug that blocks solely the K^+ channel would produce the same effects as amiodarone is naive. On the other hand, there is scientific merit in attempting to assess the potential beneficial effect of a pure K^+ channel blocker. All too often concepts based on theory are proven wrong, and only a carefully conducted clinical trial can answer certain questions about drug efficacy and safety. The effect of prolonging ventricular refractoriness, which is the primary electrophysiologic effect of K⁺ channel blockers, is of major importance in preventing reentrant arrhythmias, and ischemic arrhythmias are usually reentrant in nature. Thus, a solid background for the assessment of K⁺ channel blockers was established. To carefully design a clinical trial which would assess the precise entity of the potential protective effect of K⁺ channel blockers was a necessary and important contribution to cardiology and to the understanding of the complex relation between manipulation of a single ionic channel and arrhythmogenicity in patients with ischemic heart disease. In this sense, the outcome of these trials was relatively unimportant because considerable progress in knowledge would be achieved by both a positive and a negative result.

This background is important because it explains two facts: (1) why leading drug companies have embarked on large clinical trials with K⁺ channel blockers and (2) why scientists who were, or who might have been, skeptical about the probability of success of these trials cooperated in their design and in carrying them out.

As of June 1995, DIAMOND is still ongoing, whereas SWORD was terminated in November 1994 because of excess mortality in the group receiving d-sotalol. In this brief article I will review data relevant to SWORD. I have to point out that, at the time of writing, the first presentation of the complete results of SWORD has not yet been published and therefore, like all the other members of the Steering Committee, I am bound to confidentiality and am not allowed to divulge the complete results. This is likely to be possible at the International Workshop on Cardiac Arrhythmias in October 1995.

SWORD Protocol

SWORD was designed as a multicenter study to assess the hypothesis that d-sotalol would reduce total mortality in two groups of patients who survived a myocardial infarction.

SWORD had planned to enroll 6400 patients at approximately 500 centers in 30 countries, including Europe, North and South America, South Africa, Australia, and New Zealand. These patients, all with left ventricular dysfunction (left ventricular ejection fraction less than 40%) and with a myocardial infarction, were included in two groups. Group 1 consisted of patients with an acute myocardial infarction 6-42 days prior to randomization with or without overt heart failure. Group 2 consisted of patients with a remote myocardial infarction occurring more than 42 days prior to randomization who also had a history of overt heart failure (New York Heart Association class II or III). The primary efficacy endpoint was total mortality; cardiac mortality was a secondary endpoint.

Among the exclusion criteria there was a QTc of more than 460 ms. The initial dosage was 100 mg twice daily for 1 week, to be increased to 200 mg twice daily if QTc had not exceeded 520 ms. The drug had to be discontinued whenever a QTc exceeding 560 ms was observed.

In estimating the sample size the following assumptions were made:
1. A trial duration of 3 years with a minimum patient follow-up of 18 months.
2. The acute and remote myocardial infarction patients will enter the study in a ratio of 2:1.
3. A cumulative average mortality of 17.7% in the placebo treated patients.
4. A 20% reduction in total mortality associated with d-sotalol.
5. A two-sided significance level of 0.05.
6. A power of 90%.

The sample estimate was based on one intent-to-treat analysis at the conclusion of the trial; however, the Data and Safety Monitoring Board was supposed to make periodic assessment with well-defined stopping rules, including differential boundaries for efficacy and harm, in order to allow termination of the trial before its completion if appropriate (10).

SWORD Outcome

As of November 1, 1994, a total of 3121 patients had been randomized in the SWORD trial with a mean follow-up of 146 days. The Data and Safety Monitoring Board recommended early termination of SWORD because the boundary for harm had been crossed (Z=2.8) and statistical significance had been reached (p=0.006). There was an increased mortality among the 1549 patients receiving d-sotalol (78 deaths, 5.0%) compared to the 1571 receiving placebo (48 deaths, 3.0%). This difference was present across all subgroups, even though it was markedly more present in some compared to others.

The unavoidable, and definite, conclusion of SWORD is that d-sotalol causes harm in patients with a prior myocardial infarction.

Is d-Sotalol Antifibrillatory?

A drug that aims at reducing mortality, and primarily sudden arrhythmic death, in patients with ischemic heart disease has to possess a marked antifibrillatory activity. Prior to initiation of a clinical trial, attention should be paid to experimental studies performed in preparations relevant to the clinical reality.

d-Sotalol had indeed been studied in two well accepted and established canine models of sudden cardiac death in conscious dogs with a healed myocardial infarction. Interestingly, the two studies provided opposite results.

Lucchesi and associates used a preparation based on the production of an occluding thrombus in the circumflex coronary artery of dogs 4-7 days after an anterior myocardial infarction (11,12). The study is performed while the dogs are at rest and, as the thrombus occlusion is irreversible, the only possible analysis is that based on group comparison. They reported a striking protective effect of d-sotalol. In two consecutive studies the incidence of ventricular fibrillation within the first 60 min after the appearance of electrocardiographic signs of acute myocardial ischemia was

20% (two out of ten) and 12.5% (one out of eight) among the dogs treated with *d*-sotalol, whereas it was 80% (eight out of ten) and 87% (seven out of eight) among the dogs treated with saline. These data were regarded as very encouraging for the initiation of a clinical trial with *d*-sotalol.

We studied *d*-sotalol in our own preparation for sudden death (13). This involves a brief ischemic episode, secondary to a 2-min occlusion of the circumflex coronary artery, in dogs with a 1 month old anterior myocardial infarction; this ischemic episode is produced toward the end of an exercise stress test. Thus, this model involves transient ischemia at the time of physiologic sympathetic activation. Whenever ventricular fibrillation occurs, the dogs are promptly defibrillated and can be tested again either in control conditions or after administration of several drugs. Another important feature of this preparation is the very high reproducibility of the outcome; this allows an internal control analysis.

Using this model, Vanoli et al (14) compared the protective effect of *d*-sotalol (*n*=10), of *d,l*-sotalol (*n*=9), and of propranolol (*n*=9) in the same dogs with a healed myocardial infarction. All these animals had developed ventricular fibrillation in the exercise and ischemia test performed in control conditions; based on our experience on several hundred postmyocardial infarction dogs, recurrence of fibrillation is expected in 92% of animals which repeat the test in control conditions. Propranolol and *d,l*-sotalol were effective in preventing ventricular fibrillation, as demonstrated by its recurrence in 44% and 33% of the animals, respectively. By contrast, ventricular fibrillation recurred in 90% of the dogs treated with *d*-sotalol (Fig. 1). Our conclusion was that *d*-sotalol does not reduce the risk for ventricular fibrillation during acute myocardial ischemia associated with sympathetic hyperactivity.

These results do not contradict the evidence that *d*-sotalol can effectively prevent the recurrence of life-threatening arrhythmias dependent on an anatomical substrate (11,12,15). However, they should alert us to the possibility that *d*-sotalol may not be able to reduce the risk for sudden death after myocardial infarction in those patients more likely to die because of the arrhythmogenic interaction between ischemic episodes and sympathetic activation. Most of these patients could probably be identified by the presence of markers of low vagal and high sympathetic activity, such as depressed baroreflex sensitivity (16-18) and reduced heart rate variability (19-21).

Why Does *d*-Sotalol Fail To Prevent Ventricular Fibrillation During Myocardial Ischemia and Symphathetic Activation?

The striking difference in results obtained with *d*-sotalol in the experiments conducted by Lynch et al (11,12) and by Vanoli et al (14) must be based on a sound pathophysiologic explanation. Searching for this explanation, we developed and tested the hypothesis that sympathetic excitation may interfere with the mechanism of action of K⁺ channel blockers. This concept has far-reaching theoretic and clinical implica-

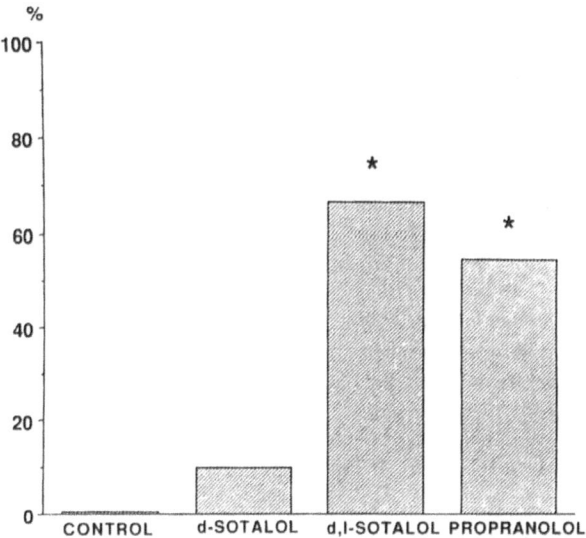

Fig. 1. Antiarrhythmic drug efficacy in preventing ventricular fibrillation during submaximal exercise and acute myocardial ischemia in ten dogs. All animals developed ventricular fibrillation during the control study. Survival (%) is defined as the absence of ventricular fibrillation during myocardial ischemia. Antiarrhythmic drug administration is described in the text. * $p < 0.05$

tions and certainly warrants adequate investigation.

Our hypothesis was based on the fact that the K⁺ current with the largest effect on ventricular repolarization, the delayed rectifier I_k, comprises two components: one rapidly activated (I_{kr}) and one slowly activated (I_{ks}) (22). I_{kr} is blocked by most of the traditional K⁺ channel blockers, such as *d*-sotalol, whereas I_{ks} is not blocked by *d*-sotalol and is activated by isoproterenol. Whenever sympathetic activity increases, I_{ks} becomes the predominant component of I_k (23). Thus, it might be postulated that in the presence of increased sympathetic activity, the sheer blockade of I_{kr} may have only a limited effect on action potential duration. We tested this hypothesis in two series of experiments performed in vivo and in vitro (24).

The in vivo experiments were conducted in anesthetized dogs in which the effect of left stellate ganglion stimulation on the monophasic action potential prolongation induced by *d*-sotalol was tested at constant heart rate. The in vitro experiments were conducted in isolated guinea pig ventricular myocytes: the effect of isoproterenol was tested on the action potential duration in the absence and in the presence of *d*-sotalol.

In control conditions, both in vivo and in vitro, adrenergic stimulation did not significantly change action potential duration. *d*-sotalol prolonged by 19% – 24% the action potential duration in the two experimental settings. Importantly, adrenergic activation reduced by 40% – 60% the prolongation of action potential duration produced by *d*-sotalol.

The inescapable conclusion of these experiments is that sympathetic activation counteracts the effect of K⁺ channel blockers on the duration of ventricular repolarization and may thus impair their primary antifibrillatory mechanism. The intriguing clinical implication was that K⁺ channel blockers might not be effective in protecting patients from malignant ischemic arrhythmias occurring in conditions of elevated sympathetic activity.

The relevance of these two studies to the outcome of the SWORD trial is obvious. It is reasonable to surmise that the results of SWORD may depend on the combination of a proarrhythmic effect (well known for all these compounds), more evident in the subgroup at lower risk, with a lack of protection in the subgroup at higher risk. Our experimental data, which have shown the inability of d-sotalol to prevent ischemia-induced ventricular fibrillation, contribute to explain the clinical result. They also demonstrate the validity of this specific animal preparation in providing information useful for the selection of the antiarrhythmic drugs most appropriate for being tested in a clinical trial.

References

1. The Cardiac Arrhythmia Suppression Trial (CAST) Investigators (1989) Preliminary report: effect of encainide and flecainide on mortality in a randomized trial of arrhythmia suppression after myocardial infarction. N Engl J Med 321:406-412
2. Task Force of the Working Group on Arrhythmias of the European Society of Cardiology (Akhtar M, Breithardt G, Camm AJ, Coumel P, Janse MJ, Lazzara R, Myerburg RJ, Schwartz PJ, Waldo AL, Wellens HJJ, Zipes DP) (1990) CAST and beyond. Implications of the Cardiac Arrhythmia Suppression Trial. Eur Heart J 11:194-199; Circulation 81: 1123-1127
3. Burkart F, Pfisterer M, Kiowski W, Follath F, Burckhardt D (1990) Effect of antiarrhythmic therapy on mortality in survivors of myocardial infarction with asymptomatic complex ventricular arrhythmias: Basel Antiarrhythmic Study of Infarct Survival (BASIS). J Am Coll Cardiol 16: 1711-1718
4. Ceremuzynski Y, Kleczar E, Krzeminska-Pakula M, Kuch J, Nartowicz E, Smielak-Korombel J, Dyduszynski A, Maciejewicz J, Zaleska T, Lazarczyk-Kedzia E, Motyka J, Paczkowska B, Sczaniecka O, Yusuf S (1992) Effect of amiodarone on mortality after myocardial infarction: a double-blind, placebo-controlled, pilot study. J Am Coll Cardiol 20:1056-1062
5. Schwartz PJ, Camm AJ, Frangin G, Janse MJ, Julian DG, Simon P, on behalf of the EMIAT Investigators (1994) Does amiodarone reduce sudden death and cardiac mortality after myocardial infarction? The European Myocardial Infarct Amiodarone Trial (EMIAT). Eur Heart J 15: 620-624
6. Cairns JA, Connolly SJ, Gent M, Roberts R (1991) Post-myocardial infarction mortality in patients with ventricular premature depolarizations. Canadian Amiodarone Myocardial Infarction Arrhythmia Trial Pilot Study. Circulation 84: 550-557
7. Task Force of the Working Group on Arrhythmias of the European Society of Cardiology (Bigger JT Jr, Breithardt G, Brown AM, Camm AJ, Carmeliet E, Fozzard HA, Hoffman BF, Janse MJ, Lazzara R, Mugelli A, Myerburg RJ, Roden DM, Rosen MR, Schwartz PJ, Strauss HC, Woosley RL, Zaza A) (1991) The Sicilian Gambit. A new approach to the classification of antiarrhythmic drugs based on their actions on arrhythmogenic mechanisms. Eur Heart J 12: 1112-1131 and Circulation 84: 1831-1851
8. Schwartz PJ, Zaza A (1992) The "Sicilian Gambit" revisited. Theory and practice. Eur Heart J 13 [Suppl F]: 23-29
9. Members of the Sicilian Gambit (Breithardt G, Camm AJ, Campbell RWF, Fozzard HA, Hoffman BF, Janse MJ, Lazzara R, Levy S, Myerburg RJ, Roden DM, Rosen MR, Schwartz PJ, Strauss HC, Waldo AL, Wit AL, Woosley RL, Zaza A, Zipes DP eds) (1994) Antiarrhythmic therapy: a pathophysiologic approach. Futura Armonk, p 337
10. Task Force of the Working Group on Arrhythmias of the European Society of Cardiology (Bigger JT Jr, Breithardt G, Camm AJ, DeMets DL, Furberg CD, Hallstrom A, Janse MJ, Julian DG, Lan KKG, Lazzara R, Marcus FI, Moss AJ, Schwartz PJ, Tijssen JGP, Waldo AL) (1994) The early termination of clinical trials: causes, consequences, and control. With special reference to trials in the field of arrhythmias and sudden death. Eur Heart J 15: 721-738 and Circulation 89: 2892-2907
11. Lynch JJ, Wilber DJ, Montgomery DG, Hsieh TM, Patterson E, Lucchesi BR (1984) Antiarrhythmic and antifibrillatory actions of the levo- and dextrorotatory isomers of sotalol. J Cardiovasc Pharmacol 6: 1132-1141
12. Lynch JJ, Coskey LA, Montgomery DG, Lucchesi BR (1985) Prevention of ventricular fibrillation by dextrorotatory sotalol in a conscious canine model of sudden coronary death. Am Heart J 109: 949-958
13. Schwartz PJ, Billman GE, Stone HL (1984) Autonomic mechanisms in ventricular fibrillation induced by myocardial ischemia during exercise in dogs with healed myocardial infarction. An experimental preparation for sudden cardiac death. Circulation 69: 790-800
14. Vanoli E, Hull SS Jr, Adamson PB, Foreman RD, Schwartz PJ (1995) K$^+$ channel blockade in the prevention of ventricular fibrillation due to acute ischemia and enhanced sympathetic activity. J Cardiovasc Pharmacol (in press)
15. Cobbe SM, Hoffman E, Ritzenhoff A, Brachmann J, Kubler W, Senges J (1983) Action of sotalol on potential reentrant pathways and ventricular tachyarrhythmias in conscious dogs in the late postmyocardial infarction phase. Circulation 68: 865-871
16. La Rovere MT, Specchia G, Mortara A, Schwartz PJ (1988) Baroreflex sensitivity, clinical correlates and cardiovascular mortality among patients with a first myocardial infarction. Circulation 78: 816-824
17. Farrell TG, Odemuyiwa O, Bashir Y, Cripps TR, Malik M, Ward DE, Camm AJ (1992) Prognostic value of baroreflex sensitivity testing after acute myocardial infarction. Br Heart J 67: 129-137
18. Schwartz PJ, La Rovere MT, Vanoli E (1992) Autonomic nervous system and sudden cardiac death. Circulation 85 [Suppl I]: I77-I91
19. Kleiger RE, Miller JP, Bigger JT Jr, Moss AJ, and the Multicenter Post-Infarction Research Group (1987) Decreased heart rate variability and its association with increased mortality after acute myocardial infarction. Am J Cardiol 59: 256-262
20. Farrell TJ, Bashir Y, Cripps T, Malik M, Poloniecki J, Bennett ED, Ward DE, Camm AJ (1991) Risk stratification for arrhythmic events in postinfarction patients based on heart rate variability, ambulatory electrocardiographic variables and the signal-average electrocardiogram. J Am Coll Cardiol 18: 687-697
21. Bigger JT Jr, Schwartz PJ (1994) Markers of vagal activity and the prediction of cardiac death after myocardial infarction. In: Levy MN, Schwartz PJ (eds) Vagal control of the heart: experimental basis and clinical implications. Futura, Armonk, pp 419-432
22. Sanguinetti MC, Jurkiewicz NK (1990) Two components of cardiac delayed rectifier K+ current. J Gen Physiol 96: 195-215
23. Sanguinetti MC, Jurkiewicz NK, Siegl PKS (1991) Isoproterenol antagonizes prolongation of refractory period by the class III antiarrhythmic agent E-4031 in guinea pig myocytes. Circ Res 68: 77-84
24. Vanoli E, Priori SG, Nakagawa H, Hirao K, Napolitano C, Diehl L, Lazzara R, Schwartz PJ (1995) Sympathetic activation, ventricular repolarization and I$_{kr}$ blockade: implications for the antifibrillatory efficacy of K$^+$ channel blockers. J Am Coll Cardiol 25:1609-1614

To Treat or Not To Treat Ventricular Arrhythmias in Dilated Cardiomyopathy?

D. Bracchetti, M. Mezzetti, G. Barbato, N. Franco, and G. Casella

Divisione di Cardiologia, Ospedale Maggiore, Bologna, Italy

Introduction

The management of patients (pts) with dilated cardiomyopathy (DC) and malignant ventricular arrhythmias (MVA), with particular attention to their treatment indication, should include a comprehensive clinical evaluation focusing on the potential role of triggering factors of rhythm disturbances. The clinical evaluation of the various interrelated adverse events that can precipitate MVA, as shown in Fig.1, is mandatory for the full understanding of the clinical problems of these pts. DC is characterized by a progressive dilatation of cardiac chambers, but principally of the left ventricle, together with poor and inadequate wall hypertrophy and severe reduction of myocardial contractility and overall ventricular function. Ischemic cardiomyopathy (ICM) and idiopathic cardiomyopathy (DCM) are the most common forms, but the etiology is often multifactorial. Death is caused

by progressive heart failure, with mortality rates ranging from 30% to 50% at 1 year from symptom onset, or sudden cardiac death (SCD) presumably resulting from arrhythmias, accounting for 28%-45% of fatal events (1, 2). SCD could be ascribed in most cases to ventricular tachycardia (VT) degenerating into ventricular fibrillation (VF; 3). Previous observations warrant addressing the issue of treatment of pts with DC and MVA.

Etiology and Pathogenesis

In DCM microscopic study reveals extensive areas of interstitial and perivascular fibrosis with small areas of necrosis and cellular infiltrate; in ICM discrete areas of scar tissue related to old myocardial infarction are prevalent. In addition, the dilatation of heart chambers causes an increase in wall stress and myocardial fiber

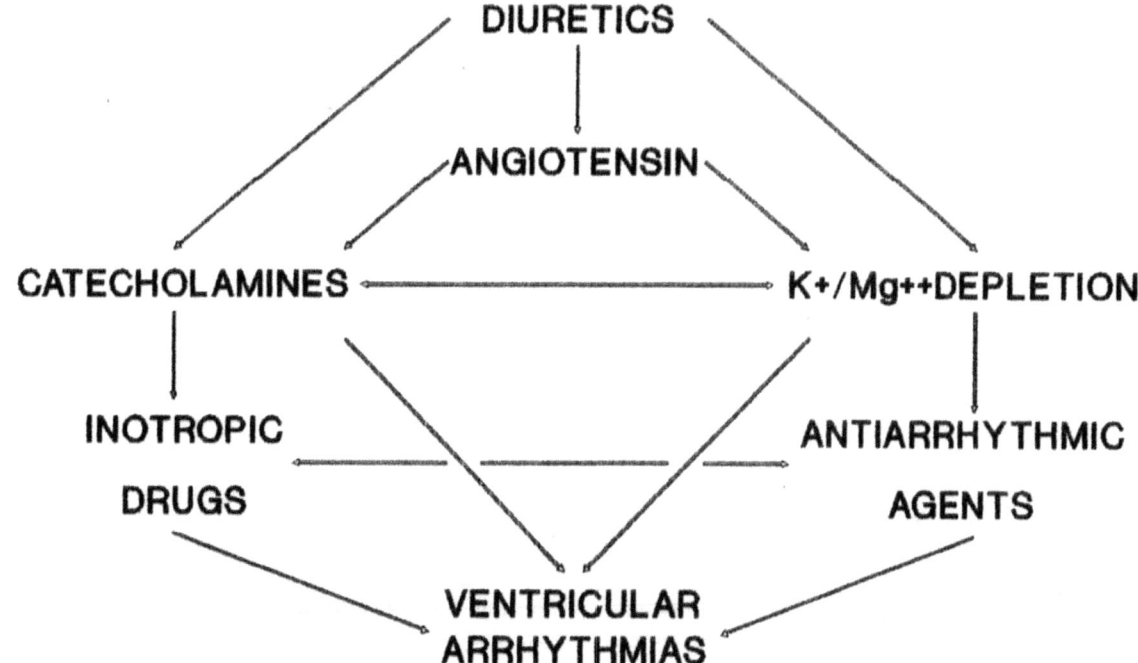

Fig. 1. Triggering factors of malignant ventricular arrhythmias

stretching. These histological and morphological changes could predispose to the development of rhythm disturbances such as bradyarrhythmias or tachyarrhythmias. Several mechanisms could be involved in the genesis of MVA in pts with DC:

– A reentrant circuit formed by the inhomogeneity of myocardial depolarization and conduction velocity within surrounding areas of active inflammation, fibrosis, or ischemia

– Enhanced automaticity secondary to myocardial stretching and increased transmural pressure

– Intracellular electrolyte fluxes consequent to diuretic therapy

Several triggering factors acting on this anatomical substrate can facilitate the emergence of MVA.

In pts with DC a direct arrhythmogenic effect could be ascribed to the enhanced sympathetic nervous tone and to circulating catecholamines, both inducing increase of myocardial oxygen consumption (potentially aggravating ischemia-related arrhythmias) and acute hypokalemia determined by a beta adrenergic mediated intracellular entry of potassium ions (4, 5). Moreover, activation of the renin-angiotensin-aldosterone system (6) in conditions of circulatory failure together with diuretic therapy raise the urinary excretion of magnesium and potassium ions. Drug therapy plays an important role as a triggering factor: digitalis and diuretics, for a long time considered the cornerstone in the management of heart failure, can both increase the prevalence of MVA (7). The proarrhythmic and negative inotropic effects of class 1A antiarrhythmic drugs are well established. The prognosis in pts with symptomatic DC is remarkably poor and appears related to the severity of the underlying myocardial disease; while there are many clinical and hemodynamic parameters that might predict a poor prognosis due to impending circulatory failure, it has been more difficult to predict which pts with DC might be at risk for arrhythmic SCD (8). Ventricular ectopic beats (VEB) and nonsustained ventricular tachycardia (NSVT) are detected at Holter monitoring (HM) in 70% and 20%-80% of pts with DC, respectively. The sensitivity of HM in detecting VEB and NSTV is high and appears to correlate to total cardiac deaths, but the specificity and predictive value with respect to arrhythmic SCD in DC pts appear to be low (9). It is difficult to make a uniform statement with regards to the prognostic significance of ventricular arrhythmias found on routine HM in predicting SCD. Antiarrhythmic therapy may be suitable for pts with aborted SCD or recurrent sustained VT but not in cases of asymptomatic MVA. Only in pts with VF or sustained VT, associated with a high incidence of VEB, the antiarrhythmic drug efficacy could be potentially predicted by a significant lowering of VEB at HM. The electrophysiologic mechanism of arrhythmia could be partially related to etiology. In ICM rather than DCM the presence of areas of scar tissue can facilitate the induction and maintainance of MVA on the basis of a reentrant circuit: nearly 70%-80% of pts with a history of clinical VT and VF had inducible MVA at baseline programmed electrical stimulation (PES) study (10). This group of pts has an improved prognosis if arrhythmia induced at baseline PES is subsequently suppressed by antiarrhythmic therapy (11). In pts with cardiomyopathy and a history of clinical

VT or VF, a standard PES protocol has a significantly lower yield, with sustained VT being inducible only in 50% of cases; in this group the inability to induce MVA by antiarrhythmic therapy at control PES is a marker of good prognosis (12). However, these pts represent only a small subset of all the pts with DCM (13). Prognostic significance of noninducibility of MVA at baseline PES in pts with symptomatic NSVT or clinical VT and VF is unknown and does not imply freedom from the risk of arrhythmia recurrence or SCD; in pts with asymptomatic MVA PES testing does not reliably stratify pts at risk for SCD (14). These pts could be treated either with antiarrhythmic drugs on an empirical basis or considered candidates for implantation of a cardioverter defibrillator (ICD). A complete PES evaluation is always strongly reccomended in pts with VF or sustained VT and DC, also for diagnostic purposes. Pts with DC and intraventricular conduction disturbances present with a relatively high incidence (6%-10%) of bundle branch reentry tachycardia (15). In this form of tachycardia the His-Purkinje system and a portion of the interventricular septum are involved in the reentry circuit; this tachycardia is usually very fast and the arrhythmia can degenerate into VF. In such cases, the diagnosis is by electrophysiologic study and catheter ablation treatment (16) of the right bundle branch is effective in 100% of cases.

Drug Therapy

In pts with DC the identification and treatment of all reversible factors playing a role in the genesis of arrhythmias is mandatory. Several questions have been raised in the last decade regarding the clinical efficacy and troublesome potential proarrhythmic effect of digoxin in particular. Encouraging data regarding digoxin therapy emerged from the recent RADIANCE and PROVED trials (17), carried out on in large patient populations; digoxin has an interesting balancing effect on the autonomic nervous system tone and a resulting reduction in renin secretion (18). Lown and Podrid (19) hypothesized a presumed direct antiarrhythmic effect of digoxin (well known for atrial fibrillation) in pts with heart failure that, however, has not been confirmed in recent controlled trials from which a trend toward higher mortality emerged. In our opinion the proarrhythmic effects of digoxin are more commonly observed in the presence of low potassium concentrations or could be ascribed to an increase in serum digoxin levels related to a reduction in the glomerular filtration rate in pts with transient impairment of ventricular function.

Antiarrhythmic Drugs

Caution should be exercised in the administration of antiarrhythmic drugs with their variable degree of negative inotropic effect to pts with heart failure and ventricular arrhythmias, since it may cause a hemodynamic impairment with further compromise of absorption, metabolism, and secretion rates. Furthermore, proarrhythmic effects are not only drug related (more often demonstrated for propafenone than for amiodarone) but also patient related, being more common in subjects with reduced ejection fraction (EF%) and complex ventricular

Table 1. Hemodynamic effects of antiarrythmic agents [modified from (30)]

Drug/group	Myocardial contractility	Peripheral vascular resistence	Cardiac output	Blood pressure
1A				
Quinidine	= ↓	= ↓	=	= ↓
Procainamide hydrochloride				
i.v.	= ↓	↓ ↓	= ↓	↓
o.s.	= ↓	= ↓	=	=
Disopyramide	↓ ↓	↑	↓ ↓	=
1B				
Lidocaine	=	=	=	=
Mexiletine	= ↓	=	=	=
1C				
Flecainide	↓ ↓	=	↓	= ↓
Propafenone	↓ ↓	= ↓	↓	= ↓
2				
ß-Blockers	↓ ↓	↑	↓	↓
3				
Amiodarone				
i.v.	↓	↓	↓	↓
o.s.	=	=	=	=
Sotalol hydrochloride	= ↓	= ↓	= ↓	= ↓
4				
Verapamil	↓ ↓	↓ ↓	= ↓	↓
Diltiazem hydrochloride	↓	↓ ↓	= ↓	= ↓

↑, decrease; ↓, increase; =, little or no definite effect; number of arrows represent relative intensity of effect.

arrhythmias. Considering the pharmacodynamic properties of antiarrhythmic drugs listed in Table 1, especially their negative inotropic action, cautious use is warranted in pts with heart failure and ventricular arrhythmias. From a practical point of view pharmacodynamic effects following acute intravenous administration are remarkably different from those related to long-standing oral treatment. In particular, the mild negative inotropic effect induced by intravenously administered amiodarone is not observed during chronic oral therapy, which is generally well tolerated in pts with heart failure, too.

The antiarrhythmic drugs of group 1 have more (disopyramide) or less (lidocaine and mexiletine) the same powerful negative inotropic effect. Group IC antiarrhythmic agents share a well-documented proarrhythmic and negative inotropic effect (more evident for flecainide). The significant reduction of myocardial contractility induced by antiarrhythmic agents should also limit their use in the treatment of pts with DC and sustained VT; in these cases overdrive pacing (OP) and DC shock are preferred.

Amiodarone. Teo and Yusuf, in a recent meta-analysis, compared the efficacy of antiarrhythmic drugs from analysis of data from 98 000 pts with ischemic cardiomyopathy enrolled in 138 trials (20): only amiodarone and ß-blockers proved to be effective drugs in reducing cardiac mortality. These data are of particular interest in pts with DC and heart failure with respect to the efficacy of orally administered amiodarone in reducing MVA and cardiac death with negligible negative inotropic effect. A later study by Neri et al. (21) found that amiodarone was effective in suppressing complex VEB on HM of pts with IDC. Herre et al. (22) in 1989 analyzed data fron 462 pts with heart disease of various etiology and ventricular arrhythmias and reported SCD reduction in pts treated

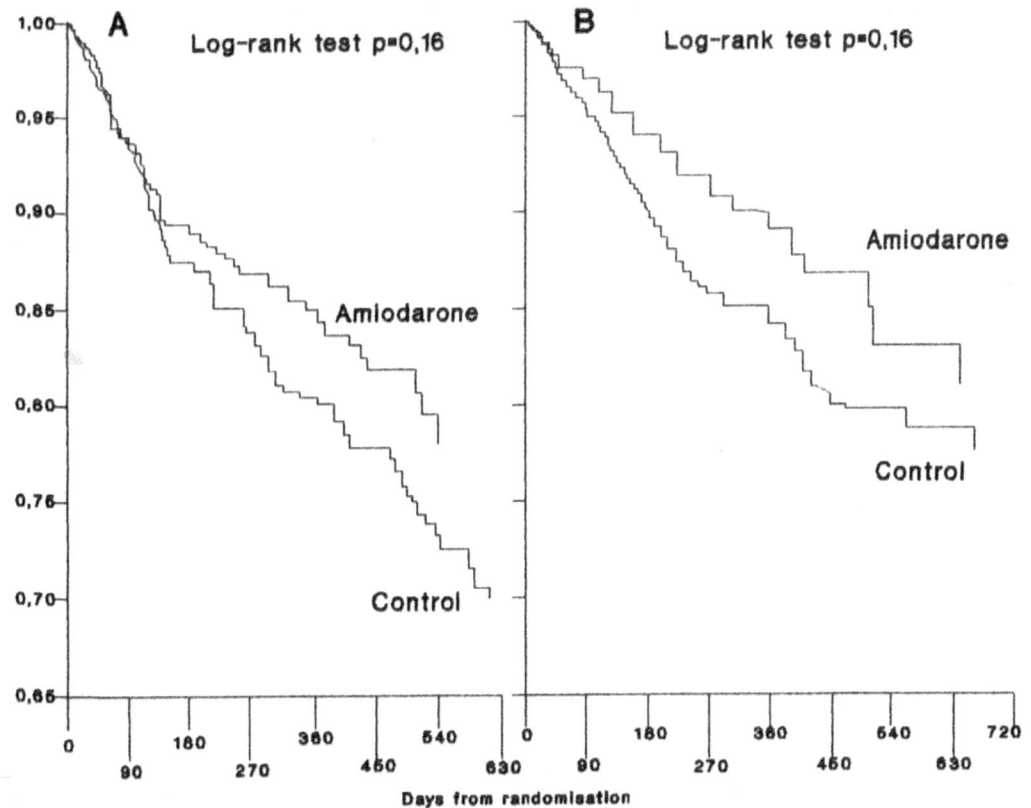

Fig. 2A, B. Survival rate curves over 24-month follow-up in the GESICA study, showing a trend toward reduction of death from progressive heart failure (A) and from sudden cardiac death (B). [From (25)]

with amiodarone. These positive results were confirmed by Ceremuzynski (23) and by the BASIS STUDY (24) with data obtained from pts with ischemic cardiomyopathy and previous myocardial infarction; in the latter amiodarone efficacy was demonstrated in pts with EF% greater than 40%, but not in the group with heart failure. Efficacy of 2-year low-dose amiodarone therapy in pts with heart failure, irrespective of the presence of ventricular arrhythmias, emerged from recent GESICA study data (25). Doval reported a reduction of SCD and of deaths related to progressive heart failure; only 12 pts withdrew from the study because the drug was poorly tolerated (Fig.2A, B). These results raise questions regarding the appropriate amiodarone administration as well as concerning the standard treatment regimen for pts with heart failure and ventricular arrhythmias. Data from the EMIAT study in postinfarction pts with EF% less than 30% (study ended in 1995) might possibly corroborate this orientation.

Angiotensin-Converting Enzyme Inhibitors. The angiotensin-converting enzyme (ACE) inhibitors captopril and enalapril have been shown to reduce mortality in pts with congestive heart failure (26). Several large scale trials in this decade evaluated the potential antiarrhythmic effect of ACE signaled in the previous report of Webster (27). In VHeFT II (28) enalapril significantly reduced the incidence of NSVT compared to pts treated with hydralazine and nitrosorbide; this study demonstrated a trend toward SCD reduction as supported by other trials. It could be concluded that there is an unquestionable reduction in the incidence of heart failure in the treated group and a trend toward the reduction of cardiac death, but there is not a clear demonstration of any antiarrhythmic action. Nevertheless, ACE inhibitors

do not induce the proarrhythmic effects observed for antiarrhythmic agents and inotropic drugs, reconfirming their safety in pts with congestive heart failure and ventricular arrhythmias.

ß-Blockers. ß-blockers can counteract the increase of sympathetic tone and of circulating catecholamine, representing a compensatory mechanism in patients with congestive heart failure; however, it is not often easy to titrate their dosage to the maximal clinical benefit without left ventricular function worsening. In an MDC study (29) performed in patients with DCM, metoprolol did not significantly reduce mortality when compared to placebo. In pts with ischemic cardiomiopathy and previous myocardial infarction, propranolol, metoprolol, and timolol were effective in reducing cardiac mortality even in the subset with low EF%. To date there is no argument for the routine use of ß-blockers in pts with DCM and MVA.

Personal Experience

We report our experience beginning in 1989 concerning the treatment of ventricular arrhythmia in patients with DC and heart failure. We evaluated the results obtained in the treatment of sustained VT and the prophylactic treatment of recurrences of VT and VF.

Our patient population consisted of pts with DC, mainly of ischemic etiology, with EF% < 35%, and left ventricular end-diastolic dimension > 65 mm.

Acute Treatment

Emergency treatment of acute sustained VT with restoration of sinus rhythm is mandatory because it

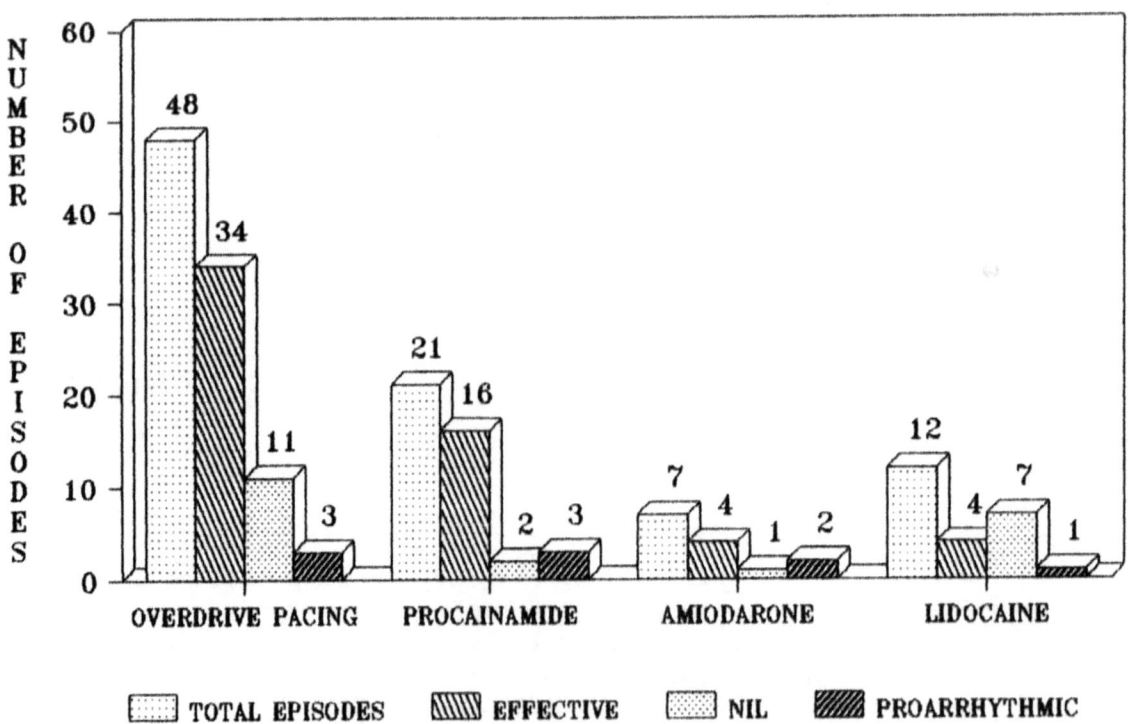

Fig. 3. Relative efficacy and safety of overdrive pacing and antiarrhythmic drug therapy in terminating acute sustained ventricular tachycardia with signs of hemodynamic decompensation

reduces the hemodynamic imbalance and prevents degeneration into VF. We evaluated the number of acute VT episodes, the incidence of heart failure during the arrhythmia, and the results in pts with DC and heart failure (group A: 35 pts) as compared with pts with normal ventricular function (group B: 19 pts). We observed 114 and 31 episodes of sustained monomorphic VT, respectively, in groups A and B with a mean number of episodes for pt of 3.25 and 1.6 ($p < 0.05$), respectively, in the two groups. Signs of hemodynamic deterioration were detected in 95/145 (65.5%) VT episodes with a significant prevalence in pts with EF% < 35% over pts with EF% > 35%, or 75/95 (78.9%) and 20/95 (21.1%), respectively. For the termination of sustained VT OP, antiarrhythmic drugs (procainamide in 21 episodes, lidocaine in 12, and amiodarone in seven) and DC shock were chosen in 48, 40, and seven episodes, respectively (Fig. 3). OP was more effective than antiarrhythmic drugs in restoring sinus rhythm, even if no statistical correlation was found: VT was terminated in 34/48 (70.8%) and 24/40 (60%) pts, respectively. Procainamide (effective in 16/21 episodes) and amiodarone (adequate in four of seven episodes) were significantly superior to lidocaine, which interrupted arrhythmia in four of 12 VT episodes. OP caused a lower incidence of proarrhythmic effects and hemodynamic deterioration than infusion of antiarrhythmic drugs (in three of 48 and six of 40 episodes, respectively), even if this was not statistically significant.

Chronic Treatment

Treatment with antiarrhythmic agents or implantation of an ICD should be considered as prophylaxis against arrhythmia recurrence and prevention of SCD in pts with DC and sustained VT or VF. The study population included 65 pts with structural heart disease and sustained VT or VF not related to acute myocardial infarction, electrolyte imbalance, or drug administration. After a complete clinical evaluation, pts underwent coronary arteriography with left ventriculography and PES study. ICM or DCM with severe left ventricular dysfunction (EF<35%) and a left ventricular end-diastolic dimension >65 was observed in 38 pts (58.4%). Pts were carefully followed clinically and admission to the cardiac care unit was immediately available in case of arrhythmia recurrence. The results of clinical evaluation and diagnostic testing show that 19 pts received empiric pharmacological therapy and 19 pts PES drug-guided therapy. ICD was implanted in nine pts; amiodarone and sotalol were prescribed in 19 (50%) and four (10.5%) pts, respectively; six pts were managed with combined antiarrhythmic agent therapy. During a mean 24± 20 months (Fig. 4) follow-up, two (5.2%) pts treated with antiarrhythmic agents died because of SCD while 12 pts (31.5%) died due to progressive heart failure (Fig. 4). Our data reveal that antiarrhythmic drug therapy (mainly amiodarone and sotalol) still plays an important role in the management of pts with left ventricular dysfunction at risk for arrhythmic SCD with an unclear indication for ICD implantation.

Therapeutic Indication and Conclusion

The management of pts with DC is complex and therapy should be principally aimed at preventing heart failure. The detection of MVA raises the following additional issues:

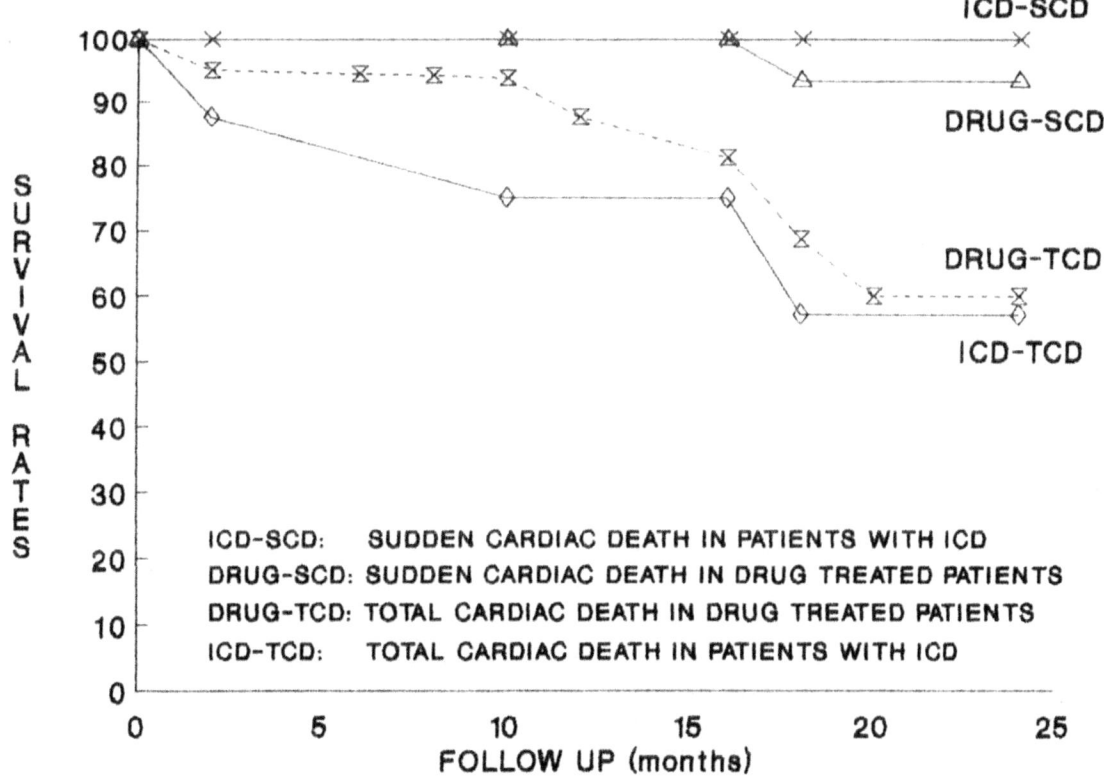

Fig. 4. Survival rate in patients with malignant ventricular arrhythmias and dilated cardiomyopathy with ejection fraction less than 35%

1. Careful evaluation of triggering factors
2. Contemporary use of drugs with indirect antiarrhythmic properties
3. Treatment of sustained VT or VF with restoration of sinus rhythm
4. Prophylaxis with antiarrhythmic agents (still a matter of debate)

Triggering Factors

As reported in the introduction, the control of triggering factors represents an important therapeutic step in the management of pts with DC, regardless of the presence and the type of ventricular arrhythmias detected by HM.

The proarrhythmic effect of hypokalemia is well accepted: in pts with heart failure, reduction of serum potassium level (specifically extracellular and intracellular potassium ratio) can be induced by diuretic therapy or by the enhancement of sympathetic tone. Thus hypokalemia potentially induced by diuretic therapy can trigger MVA in pts taking digoxin. Several drugs used to improve ventricular pump function can cause proarrhythmic effects. Reduction of glomerular filtration rate, consistent with transient impairment of ventricular function, can lead to an increase in digoxin serum levels.

Indirect Antiarrhythmic Effect

ACE inhibitors and probably ß-blockers play a role in the treatment of pts with DC and ventricular arrhythmias since they counteract the harmful effects of increased sympathetic tone and circulating catecholamines. While there are no doubts regarding the efficacy of ACE inhibitors in pts with DC and heart failure, there are no definite data supporting the administration of ß-blockers. The specific role of antiarrhythmic therapy is still to be considered.

Acute Treatment

Sustained VT in pts with DC should preferably be terminated with OP or DC shock, with some preference for OP since it avoids the negative inotropic effect of anesthetic drugs generally used for the countershock. The negative effect on myocardial contractility of antiarrhythmic agents greatly limits their use in the termination of sustained VT. In our experience, intravenous administration of amiodarone is effective and hemodynamically well tolerated. Lidocaine, traditionally considered the drug of choice for termination of sustained VT, rarely causes adverse hemodynamic effects, but is significantly less effective than procainamide or amiodarone in the restoration of sinus rhythm.

Chronic Treatment

According to the literature, the treatment of pts with DC and MVA should include ACE inhibitors (indirect antiarrhythmic effect). Among the antiarrhythmic agents only amiodarone appears to be effective in this patient population and data from GESICA supports

large-scale treatment with this drug. Nevertheless, if we consider inefficacy of antiarrhythmic drugs, the indications for ICD implantation should be evaluated for each individual pt; in fact, data from the literature show the high efficacy of this device in preventing SCD. In answer to the preliminary question, we can conclude that ventricular arrhythmias in pts symptomatic for hemodynamic impairment or at high risk for SCD should be treated with antiarrhythmic drugs (amiodarone) in addition to the standard heart failure therapy (ACE, etc.). In selected cases, ICD implantation must be considered.

References

1. Fuster V et al (1981) The natural history of idiopathic dilated cardiomyopathy. Am J Cardiol 47:525
2. Kannel WB, Plehn JF (1988) Cardiac failure and sudden death in the Framingham study. Am Heart J 115:869-875
3. Pratt CM et al (1983) Analysis of ambulatory electrocardiograms in 15 patients during spontaneous ventricular fibrillation with special reference to preceding arrhythmic events. J Am Coll Cardiol 2:789
4. Hollifield JW (1984) Potassium and magnesium abnormalities: diuretics and arrhythmias in hypertension. Am J Med 77:28
5. Brown MJ, Brown DC (1983) Hypokalemia from beta2-receptor stimulation by circulating epinephrine. N Engl J Med 309:1414
6. Cohn JN et al (1984) Plasma norepinephrine as guide to prognosis in patients with chronic congestive heart failure. N Engl J Med 311:819
7. Lazzara R et al (1988) Electrophysiological mechanisms for ventricular arrhythmias and sudden death in patients with chronic heart failure. Clin Cardiol 11:II-1
8. Packer M et al (1992) Lack of relation between ventricular arrhythmias and sudden death in patients with chronic heart failure. Circulation [Suppl 1] 85:50-56
9. Maskin CS et al (1984) High prevalence of nonsustained ventricular tachycardia in severe congestive heart failure. Am Heart J 107: 896-901
10. Morady F, Scheinman M (1983) Electrophysiologic testing in the management of survivors of out of hospital cardiac arrest. Am J Cardiol 51:85-90
11. Wilber JD, Garan H (1988) Out-of-hospital cardiac arrest: role of electrophysiologic testing in the prediction of long term outcome. N Engl J Med 318:19-24
12. Larsen L, Markham J (1994) Sudden death in idiopathic dilated cardiomyopathy: role of ventricular arrhythmias. PACE 16:1051-1059
13. Poll DS et al (1986) Usefulness of programmed stimulation in idiopathic dilated cardiomyopathy. Am J Cardiol: 58: 992-997
14. Zheutlin TA, Roth HC (1986) Programmed electrical stimulation to determine the need for antiarrhythmic therapy in patients with complex ventricular ectopic activity. Am Heart J 111:860-867
15. Tchou P, Blank Z (1989) Mechanism of inducible ventricular tachycardia in patients with idiopathic dilated cardiomyopathy. J Am Coll Cardiol 13:174A
16. Tchou P, Jazayeri M (1988) Transcatheter electrical ablation of the right bundle branch: a method of treating macro-reentrant ventricular tachycardia due to bundle branch reentry. Circulation 78:246
17. Packer M, Gheorghiade M (1993) Withdrawal of digoxin from patients with chronic heart failure treated with angiotensin-converting-enzyme inhibitors. N Engl J Med 829:1-7
18. Gheorghiade M, Ferguson B (1991) Digoxin: a neurohormonal modulator in heart failure? Circulation 84:2181-1816
19. Lown B, Podrid P (1977) Effect of digitalis drug on ventricular premature beats. N Engl J Med 296:301
20. Teo KK, Yusuf C (1993) Role of antiarrhythmic prophylaxis in acute myocardial infarction. JAMA 13:1589-1595
21. Neri R et al (1987) Ventricular arrhythmias in dilated cardiomyopathy: efficacy of amiodarone. Am Heart J 113:707

22. Herre J, Sauve M (1989) Long-term results of amiodarone therapy in patients with recurrent sustained ventricular tachycardia or ventricular fibrillation. J Am Coll Cardiol 13(2):442-449

23. Ceremuzynski Y, Kleczar E (1992) Effect of amiodarone on mortality after myocardial infarction. J Am Coll Cardiol 20:1056-1062

24. Burkart F, Pfisterer M (1990) Effect of antiarrhythmic therapy on mortality in survivors of myocardial with asymptomatic complex ventricular arrhythmias: Basel Antiarrhythmic Study of Infarct Survival (BASIS). J Am Coll Cardiol 16:1711-1718

25. Doval HC, Null DR (1994) Randomized trial of low dose amiodarone in severe congestive heart failure. Lancet 344:493-498

26. SOLVD Investigators (1992) Effect of enalapril on mortality and the development of heart failure in asymptomatic patients with reduced left ventricular ejection fraction. N Engl J Med 327:685-691

27. Webster MWI, Fitzpatrick MA (1985) Effects of enalapril on ventricular arrhythmias in congestive heart failure. Am J Cardiol 56:566-569

28. Cohn JN et al (1991) A comparison of enalapril with hydralazine-isosorbide dinitrate in the treatment of chronic congestive heart failure. N Engl J Med 325:303-308

29. Waagstein F, Bristow MR (1993) Beneficial effects of metoprolol in idiopathic dilated cardiomyopathy.Lancet 342:1441-1446

30. Block P (1983) Hemodynamic effects of antiarrhythmic agents. Am J Cardiol 52:14

Which Therapeutic Approach for Patients with Hypertrophic Cardiomyopathy and Ventricular Arrhythmias?

M. Di Biase, M.V. Pitzalis, G. Luzzi, C. Forleo, C.D. Dicandia, S. Favale, and P. Rizzon

Istituto di Cardiologia, Università degli Studi, Policlinico, Bari, Italy

Introduction

Sudden unexpected cardiac death is a common feature in the natural history of hypertrophic cardiomyopathy (HCM) and in some patients is the first clinical manifestation of the disease (1-4).

It has been reported that the incidence of sudden death in HCM is 2%-4% per year in adults and even higher, approximately 6% per year, in children and adolescents (5). These figures are exaggerated since they come from some selected referral centers; a more benign natural history is reported by nonspecialist institutions and in an identifiable subset of patients (6-9). Despite the controversial figures on the incidence of sudden death (mainly due to the broad clinical spectrum) there is no question that some patients are at increased risk.

Issues related to the nature and etiology of sudden death in HCM, and to the identification and treatment of patients at higher risk, have been the subject of numerous studies and debates. Although knowledge in these fields has increased over the past few years, many questions remain largely unresolved (10,11).

In this review, the objective of which is the definition of the best drug treatment for ventricular arrhythmias, attention will be focused on ventricular electrical instability, its role in the genesis of sudden cardiac death, and the usefulness of antiarrhythmic treatment.

Mechanisms Underlying Sudden Cardiac Death in HCM

Hemodynamic Mechanisms

An increased ventricular rate secondary to sinus tachycardia or atrial arrhythmias (fibrillation, flutter, or tachycardia) may be associated with hypotension, ischemia, symptoms of angina, and impaired consciousness; this may be due to the coexistence of enhanced atrioventricular (AV) nodal conduction (12,13), accessory bypass tracts (14), or increased sympathetic tone. Reduced diastolic filling, the reduced size of left ven-

tricular cavity, and abnormal vascular response reported in these patients (15), lead to cardiac arrest.

Electrical Mechanisms

1. *Transformation of a supraventricular arrhythmia in ventricular fibrillation.* In the simultaneous presence of an atrial arrhythmia and an accessory pathway, impulses could reach the ventricle during incomplete recovery, create areas of slow conduction, and block and induce ventricular tachycardia or fibrillation (12,16).
2. *Induction of Ventricular Tachycardia or Fibrillation by Timed Ventricular Premature Beats.* The occurrence of premature ventricular beats and susceptibility to ventricular fibrillation could be enhanced by transient myocardial ischemia and increased sympathetic tone.

Bradyarrhythmias

Bradyarrhythmias are mainly represented by a complete AV block or a sinus arrest.

Other mechanisms

The dynamic obstruction of the left ventricular outflow tract during effort and severe hypotension, due to ventricular baroreflex or induced by exercise and mediated by an abnormal vascular response, have also been suggested as underlying mechanisms of sudden cardiac death.

Prevalence of Ventricular Arrhythmias

Ventricular arrhythmias have been observed by 24-h Holter monitoring in about two thirds of patients, and nonsustained ventricular tachycardia (VT) has been reported in between 19% and 27% of adult patients (11, 17). Short runs of nonsustained VT are recorded in about half of the patients after 5 days of in hospital ambulatory telemetry electrocardiographic monitoring (18).

Nonsustained VT is frequently asymptomatic. Its rate is slow (about 140 beats/min), and it frequently follows a period of relative bradycardia, is not associated with ST changes or QT alterations, and there is considerable variation in QRS morphology.

To date, the mechanisms underlying ventricular arrhythmias in patients with HCM are not completely understood; moreover, the sequence by which these generally nonsustained arrhythmias lead to sudden death has not been defined.

The cellular electrophysiological modifications induced by hypertrophy, such as the increase in the duration of action potential, or the occurrence of delayed afterdepolarizations and triggered activity, may be responsible for ventricular arrhythmias as a result of the conduction alterations sometimes observed during the development of hypertrophy, particularly those dependent on sympathetic nervous system activity (19,20).

Disarray may cause dispersion of ventricular activation due to changes in fiber caliber, tortuosity and fibrosis, and so create the substrate for reentrant tachycardias (21). Since the incidence of arrhythmias increases with age, it has been suggested that their presence is not simply secondary to myocyte disarray but also due to myocyte replacement fibrosis as well as interstitial fibrosis (22).

Prognostic Significance of Ventricular Arrhythmias

In 1981 two independent studies (11,17) reported a strong association between nonsustained VT and sudden cardiac death in patients with HCM. In particular, adult patients had a sevenfold increased risk of sudden death within 3 years with high negative (97%) and low predictive accuracy (22%). These data from tertiary referred centers, probably enrolling most of the worst extremes of the disease spectrum, suggested that patients with nonsustained VT at Holter monitoring should be treated with antiarrhythmic therapy.

More recently, doubts have been raised regarding the possibility that these data can be applied to a population that more closely reflects the characteristics of the overall group of HCM patients (6-9).

Spirito et al. in 1994 (9) reported on 151 asymptomatic or mildly symptomatic patients with HCM. Forty-two had nonsustained VT at Holter monitoring and their sudden death rate was 1.4% per year; the figure was 0.6% in patients without nonsustained VT. On the basis of these data, the authors suggested that the sole presence of nonsustained VT should not in itself be considered an indication for antiarrhythmic treatment.

Kofflard et al. (8) reported an annual mortality rate of 1% in a large clinical population.

Although it can be presumed that nonsustained VT is a marker of arrhythmic potential, this finding requires more detailed characterization to identify the high risk cohort of patients who should receive antiarrhythmic therapy or, failing that, other therapies, such as the implant of cardioverter defibrillator (ICD) or myectomy.

Methods Allowing Identification of High-Risk Patients

Electrophysiologic Study

Fananapazir et al. performed electrophysiologic studies in a series of patients with HCM (23). Using a protocol which utilizes up to three extra stimuli, stimulation in the right and left ventricle and three differently paced ventricular cycle lengths, these authors produced nonsustained VT in 14% and sustained VT in 43% of patients; monomorphic VT was induced in 10%, and polymorphic VT or ventricular fibrillation in 33%. Because of the aggressive protocol (which lowers specificity), the induction of polymorphic VT, which frequently degenerated into ventricular fibrillation, and the fact that only a minority of the inducible patients will die suddenly in subsequent years, it can be suggested that the positive predictive accuracy of this method is low. Notwithstanding the highly significant association between the inducibility of sustained VT and a history of cardiac arrest or syncope (24), this method is not suitable for extensive and routine use and is not indicated for a large general HCM population.

A new method, which assesses the inhomogeneity of intramyocardial conduction, has more recently shown that the early onset of electrogram fractionation is associated with sudden death (25) but the data from this study need confirmation in a large series of patients.

Since the currently used electrophysiologic methods do not allow definitive conclusions to be drawn, the electrophysiologic approach should be limited to those HCM patients with nonsustained VT at Holter monitoring and should give more information regarding the substrate and intramyocardial conduction disturbances than the poorly specific inducibility of ventricular arrhythmias.

Electrophysiologic study alone should also be used to evaluate the presence of sinus node dysfunction or AV conduction abnormalities (in the AV node, His bundle, and His-Purkinje system), enhanced AV node conduction and accessory bypass tracts.

Signal-Averaged Electrocardiogram

Cripp et al. (26) utilized signal-averaged electrocardiography to define the prognosis of patients with HCM. In this study there was a significant association between the prevalence of nonsustained VT on 48-h Holter monitoring and abnormal signal-averaged ECG. Of four patients with a history of cardiac arrest, three had an abnormal signal-averaged ECG. In the same study there was no association between an abnormal signal-averaged ECG and a family history of premature sudden cardiac death or history of syncope or symptomatic status.

Since this lack of correlation is troublesome, it can be concluded that the abnormal signal-averaged ECG may be a useful adjunct to the noninvasive assessment of patients with HCM and nonsustained VT at Holter monitoring but it does not help to select a cohort of patients at higher risk of sudden cardiac death.

Electrophysiologic Testing and Other Variables

In a recent study of Fananazapir et al. (27), it was demonstrated that there was a highly significant correlation between induction of sustained ventricular arrhythmias and symptoms of impaired consciousness (cardiac arrest, syncope or presyncope). An adverse cardiac event was observed in 18% of these individuals, whereas the figure was 3% when ventricular arrhythmias were not induced.

In the same study, the value of 31 clinical, hemodynamic, electrophysiologic, and electrocardiographic variables was tested: only the induction of sustained ventricular arrhythmias at baseline and a history of cardiac arrest or syncope were identified as significant predictors of subsequent cardiac events by logistic regression analysis. This study supports the evidence that risk stratification in patients with HCM should be done by means of the close evaluation of electrophysiologic and clinical parameters.

Patients Surviving Cardiac Arrest

In the study by Cecchi et al. (28), which involved 33 patients with HCM who survived cardiac arrest during a follow-up period of between 17 months and 22 years (mean 7 years), 22 were alive and 16 had remained asymptomatic or mildly symptomatic.

No data were collected regarding the presence of ventricular arrhythmias in the surviving patients or in those who died.

In Fananapazir and Epstein's study (24) of 30 survivors of cardiac arrest, the incidence of nonsustained VT at Holter monitoring was low (39%). There was no statistically significant difference in age between the two groups, while the inducibility of sustained ventricular arrhythmias was 77% in patients with and 65% in patients without sustained ventricular arrhythmias. From these data it can be concluded that there is no evidence that the incidence of nonsustained VT is higher in patients who have experienced a cardiac arrest.

Antiarrhythmic Drugs for Patients with HCM

As various electrophysiologic mechanisms may be involved in the genesis of ventricular arrhythmias, and the risk of sudden death being different in symptomatic and asymptomatic patients, the therapeutic approach towards ventricular arrhythmias needs to be personalized. Drug therapy, surgical therapy, electrical device therapy and even ablative therapy may be the best option in an individual patient.

ß-Adrenergic Blockers. ß-Adrenergic blockers (propanolol in particular) have been the mainstay of treatment for over 25 year. However, no adequate, controlled studies have shown that ß-adrenergic blocker therapy has a beneficial effect on survival. Most studies have shown that, when treated with ß-adrenergic blockers, there is a mortality rate of 15%-20% in patients with New York Heart Association (NYHA) class III and IV disease; those with NYHA class I and II disease have a mortality rate of 5%-10% (29). Considering the current literature, McKenna et al. (30) concluded that ß-adrenergic blocker therapy may improve symptoms but does not prevent sudden cardiac death.

Calcium Channel Antagonists. Calcium channel antagonists have been advocated to improve symptoms, in-crease exercise tolerance, reverse myocardial hypertrophy and improve diastolic relaxation and filling.

The in vitro effects of verapamil on muscle thickness and arrhythmias provide an attractive theoretical basis for its clinical use in patients with HCM. However, these desirable antiarrhythmic effects were not seen clinically (30). Serious ventricular arrhythmias are positively correlated with impaired septal motion, but not with ventricular wall thickness (31). Pelliccia et al. (32) have recently reported the favorable effect of verapamil in reducing the incidence of sudden cardiac death in HCM. Of the 101 patients included in this study, three who were taking oral verapamil died suddenly over a 5-year follow-up period, as against eight patients treated with oral propanolol. These results were not statistically significant.

Class I Antiarrhythmic Drugs. Class I agents, disopyramide and propafenone in particular, have been used with success to control heart rate in atrial fibrillation and obtain "chemical cardioversion" back to sinus rhythm in HCM patients. Moreover, a number of investigators have shown that intravenous disopyramide causes a significant drop in the left ventricular outflow tract gradient and an increase in cardiac output (33). However, no studies have yet shown either a clear benefit on survival or a reduction in ventricular arrhythmias.

Amiodarone. Amiodarone is the most widely used drug in patients with HCM. It has been used for its antiarrhythmic and hemodynamic effects, and has also been shown to be able to reduce the symptoms caused by left ventricular outflow tract obstruction, to increase exercise tolerance, and improve left ventricular compliance and diastolic filling (34).

Dritsas et al. (35) have reported that amiodarone prolongs corrected QT(QTc) while reducing QTc dispersion in patients with HCM.

In 1985, McKenna et al. (36) demonstrated that low doses of amiodarone could prevent sudden death in patients with nonsustained VT at Holter monitoring. Treatment with amiodarone in 21 asymptomatic or mild to moderately symptomatic patients with HCM suppressed VT during repeat 24-h Holter monitoring periods and prevented sudden death during a 3-year follow-up. The mortality in this group of patients was similar to that in patients without nonsustained VT. In the group of patients with sustained VT treated with conventional therapy, mortality was about 20%.

These findings suggested that all patients with HCM and nonsustained VT detected at Holter monitoring should be treated indefinitely and empirically with oral amiodarone to prevent sudden cardiac death. This approach implies that there is no need for electrophysiologic study to evaluate whether, during treatment, individual patients have an arrhythmogenic left ventricular substrate capable of sustaining a more malignant ventricular arrhythmia, or whether there is a conduction abnormality that may be exacerbated by amiodarone.

This empirical approach to the treatment of subjects with HCM and nonsustained VT has not been shared by other investigators.

In a retrospective study of 50 patients with HCM, who had received 2-month empiric treatment with high doses of amiodarone (400 mg/day), Fananapazir et al. (37) observed a statistically significant reduction in the number of patients with nonsustained VT (4% versus 42%); however, during the 6-month follow-up, the mortality in patients with nonsustained VT was much higher (38%) than that in patients without nonsustained VT (3%).

This study demonstrated that high doses of amiodarone do not prevent sudden death in patients with symptoms refractory to ß-blockers and nonsustained VT. These conflicting results could be explained by an effect of amiodarone on refractoriness and conduction which leads to abnormal AV nodal conduction and an increased inducibility of ventricular arrhythmias during electrophysiologic study.

Despite the good prognosis of mildly asymptomatic patients with nonsustained VT, the lack of prospective studies demonstrating the favorable or adverse effects of this drug in selected cohorts of patients with nonsustained VT, as well as its side effects on young people or adolescents, suggest the conclusion that the efficacy of amiodarone in preventing sudden cardiac death in HCM has not been established. Treatment with amiodarone can be recommended only for young patients with nonsustained VT, with a familiar a history of sudden death and with syncope who are at highest risk.

Although sustained ventricular tachycardias are rare in HCM, and frequently associated with ventricular aneurysm, amiodarone could be used for the treatment of these arrhythmias (38). Electrophysiologic testing is needed in order to evaluate efficacy of the drug.

Amiodarone could be used in patients with an implanted defibrillator to reduce the daily number of nonsustained VT, slow their rate, and reduce the device shocks. Amiodarone could also be used in patients submitted to surgical treatment and recurrent episodes of nonsustained VT.

Sotalol. Sotalol is a unique antiarrhythmic drug that has a ß-blocking effect and prolongs action potentials. Its usefulness in treating patients with HCM and ventricular arrhythmias is unclear.

Tendera et al. (39) evaluated the effect of sotalol on exercise tolerance and the incidence of arrhythmias in 30 patients with HCM; in the short-term, the drug was able to improve exercise tolerance significantly and reduce the incidence of both supraventricular and ventricular tachyarrhythmias.

Long-term controlled investigations should be performed in order to obtain further insights into its safety and efficacy.

Conclusion

In order to briefly answer the question as to which therapeutic approach should be used in patients with HCM and ventricular arrhythmias, analysis of the data allows the following conclusions to be drawn:

1. Adult patients with nonsustained VT and no or minor/mild symptoms have a good prognosis (1.4% annual mortality) and probably do not need chronic treatment because:

– Amiodarone has side effects and there are conflicting results concerning its ability to prevent sudden death. The available data come from tertiary referring centers who used different dosages of the drug.

– There is still no sufficient information on the effects of other types of drugs.

2. Adult patients with severe symptoms and nonsustained VT should receive low doses of amiodarone since the incidence of sudden death in this group of patients is high (2.4% per year) and the results of one study showed a reduction in the sudden death rate with this type of treatment.

3. Adult patients with previous cardiac arrest should receive low doses of amiodarone. In the case of the persistent inducibility of sustained ventricular arrhythmias during treatment, they should undergo defibrillator implantation.

4. Young patients and adolescents should receive low doses of amiodarone if there is a familial history of sudden death and syncope.

5. Sotalol and amiodarone could be administered to patients with an implanted defibrillator or submitted to surgical treatment in order to reduce the recurrences of ventricular arrhythmias.

6. Patients with accessory bypass tracts and atrial arrhythmias should be treated with amiodarone, sotalol, or class I antiarrhythmic agents in order to prevent the transformation of a supraventricular arrhythmia into a ventricular fibrillation.

In the future patients with HCM should be more appropriately stratified in order to assess the role of noninvasive and invasive investigations in identifying patients at higher risk of sudden cardiac death, the need for treatment, and the most appropriate one (40).

References

1. Frank S, Braunwald E (1968) Idiopathic hypertrophic subaortic stenosis: clinical analysis of 126 patients with an emphasis on the natural history. Circulation 37:759 788
2. McKenna W, Deanfield J, Farouqui A, England D, Oakley CM, Goodwin JF (1981) Prognosis in hypertrophic cardiomyopathy: role of age and clinical, electrocardiographic and hemodynamic features. Am J Cardiol 47:532-538
3. Maron BJ, Bonow RO, Cannon RO III, Leon MB, Epstein SE (1987) Hypertrophic cardiomyopathy: interrelations of clinical manifestations, pathophysiology and therapy. N Engl J Med 316:780-789,844-852
4. Maron BJ, Roberts WC, Epstein SE (1982) Sudden death in hypertrophic cardiomyopathy: a profile of 78 patients. Circulation 67:1388-1394
5. McKenna WJ, Goodwin JF (1981) The natural history of hypertrophic cardiomyopathy. In: Harvey P (ed) Current problems in cardiology, vol 6. Year Book Medical, Chicago, pp 5-26
6. Shapiro LM, Zezulka N (1983) Hypertrophic cardiomyopathy: a common disease with a good prognosis: five year experience of a district general hospital. Br Heart J 50:530-533
7. Spirito P, Chiarella F, Carratino L, Zoni-Berisso M, Bellotti P, Vecchio C (1989) Clinical course and prognosis of hypertrophic cardiomyopathy in an outpatient population. N Engl J Med 320:749-755
8. Kofflard MJ, Waldstein DJ, Vos J, Folkert J, Cate T(1993) Prognosis in hypertrophic cardiomyopathy observed in a large clinic population. Am J Cardiol. 72:939-943

9. Spirito P, Rapezzi C, Autore C, Bruzzi P, Bellone P, Ortolani P, Fragola PV, Chiarella F, Zoni-Berisso M, Branzi A, Cannata D, Magnani B, Vecchio C (1994) Prognosis of asymptomatic patients with hypertrophic cadiomyopathy and nonsustained ventricular tachycardia. Circulation 90:2743-2747

10. Maron BJ, Roberts WC, Edwards JE, McAllister HA Jr, Foley DD, Epstein SE (1978) Sudden death in patients with hypertrophic cardiomyopathy: characterization of 26 patients without functional limitation. Am J Cardiol 41:803-810

11. McKenna WJ, England D, Doi YL, Deanfield JE, Oakley CM, Goodwin JF (1981) Arrhythmia in hypertrophic cardiomyopathy I: influence on prognosis. Br Heart J 46:168-172

12. Favale S, Minafra F, Rizzo U, Di Biase M, Rizzon P (1987) Ventricular fibrillation induced by transesophageal atrial pacing in hypertrophic cardiomyopathy. Eur Heart J 8:912-916

13. Stafford WJ, Trohman RG, Bilsker M, Zaman L, Castellanos A, Myerburg RJ (1986) Cardiac arrest in an adolescent with atrial fibrillation and hypertrophic cardiomyopathy. J Am Coll Cardiol 7:701-704

14. Krikler DM, Davies MJ, Rowland E, Goodwin JF, Evans RC, Shaw DB (1980) Sudden death in hypertrophic cardiomyopathy: associated accessory atrioventricular pathways. Br Heart J 43:245-251

15. Frenneaux MP, Counihan PJ, Webb D, McKenna WJ (1989) Evidence for an abnormal vasodilator response in hypertrophic cardiomyopathy. J Am Coll Cardiol 13:117A

16. Madariaga I, Carmona JR, Mateas FR, Lezaun R, De Los Arcos E (1994) Supraventricular arrhythmia as the cause of sudden death in hypertrophic cardiomyopathy. Eur Heart J 15:134-137

17. Maron BJ, Savage DD, Wolfson JK, Epstein SE (1981) Prognostic significance of 24-hour ambulatory electrocardiographic monitoring in patients with hypertrophic cardiomyopathy: a prospective study. Am J Cardiol 48:252-257

18. Fananapazir L, Epstein SE, Epstein ND (1991) Investigation and clinical significance of arrhythmias in patients with hypertrophic cardiomyopathy. J Cardiovasc Electrophysiol 2:525-530

19. Aronson R (1991) Mechanisms of arrhythmias in ventricular hypertrophy. J Cardiovasc Electrophysiol 2:249-261

20. Charpentier F, Baudet S, Le Marec H (1991) Triggered activity as a possible mechanism for arrhythmias in ventricular hypertrophy. Pace 14:1735-1741

21. Samuarez RC, Panagos A, De Belder M, Simpson I, Camm AJ, McKenna WJ (1992) Abnormal intraventricular conduction in patients with hypertrophic cardiomyopathy and out of hospital ventricular fibrillation. J Am Coll Cardiol 19:367A (Abstr)

22. McKenna WJ, Sadoul N, Slade AKB, Samuarez RC (1994) The prognostic significance of nonsustained ventricular tachycardia in hypertrophic cardiomyopathy. Circulation 1994 90:3115-3117

23. Fananapazir L, Tracy CM, Leon MB, Winkler JB, Cannon III RO, Bonow RO, Maron BJ, Epstein SE (1989) Electrophysiologic abnormalities in hypertrophic cardiomyopathy: a consecutive analysis in 155 patients. Circulation 80:1259-1268

24. Fananapazir L, Epstein S (1991) Value of electrophysiologic studies in hypertrophic cardiomyopathy treated with amiodarone. Am J Cardiol 67:175-182

25. Samuarez RC, Camm AJ, Panagos A, Gill JS, Stewart JT, De Belder MA, Simpson IA, McKenna WJ (1992) Ventricular fibrillation in hypertrophic cardiomyopathy is associated with increased fractionation of paced right ventricular electrograms. Circulation 86:467-474

26. Cripp TR, Peter J, Counihan MB, Frenneaux MP, Ward DE, Camm J, Mckenna WJ (1990) Signal-averaged electrocardiography in hypertrophic cardiomyopathy. J Am Coll Cardiol 15:956-961

27. Fananapazir L, Chang AC, Epstein SE, MCAreavey D (1992) Prognostic determinants in hypertrophic cardiomyopathy: prospective evaluation of a therapeutic strategy based on clinical, Holter, hemodynamic and electrophysiological findings. Circulation 86:730-740

28. Cecchi F, Maron BJ, Epstein SE (1989) Long-term outcome of patients with hypertrophic cardiomyopathy successfully resuscitated after cardiac arrest. J Am Coll Cardiol 13:1283-1288

29. McKenna WJ (1988) The natural history of hypertrophic cardiomyopathy. In: Cardiomyopathies: clinical presentation, differential diagnosis and management. Cardiovasc Clin. 4:135-149

30. McKenna WJ, Harris L, Perez G, Kriker DM, Oakley C, Goodwin JK (1981) Arrhythmia in hypertrophic cardiomyopathy II: comparison of amiodarone and verapamil in treatment. Br Heart J 46:173-178

31. Doi YL, McKenna WJ, Chetty S, Oakley CM, Goodwin JF (1980) Prediction of mortality and serious ventricular arrhythmia in hypertrophic cardiomyopathy: an echocardiographic study. Br Heart J 44:150-157

32. Pelliccia F, Cianfocca C, Romeo F (1990) Hypertrophic cardiomyopathy: long term effects of propanolol versus verapamil in preventing sudden death in "low risk" patients. Cardiovasc Drugs Ther 4:1515-1518

33. Sherrid M, Delia E, Dwyer E (1988) Oral disopyramide therapy for obstructive hypertrophic cardiomyopathy. Am J Cardiol 62:1085-1088

34. Blanchard DG, Ross J (1991) Hypertrophic cardiomyopathy: prognosis with medical or surgical therapy. Clin Cardiol 14:11-19

35. Dritsas A, Gilligan D, Nihoyannopoulos P, Oakley CM (1992) Amiodarone reduces QT dispersion in patients with hypertrophic cardiomyopathy. Int J Cardiol 36:345-349

36. McKenna WJ, Oakley CM, Krikler DM, Goodwin JF (1985) Improved survival with amiodarone in patients with hypertrophic cardiomyopathy and ventricular tachycardia. Br Heart J 53:412-416

37. Fananapazir L, Leon MB, Bonow RO, Tracy CM, Cannon III RO, Epstein SE (1991) Sudden death during empiric amiodarone therapy in symptomatic hypertrophic cardiomyopathy. Am J Cardiol 67:169-174

38. Alfonso F, Frenneaux M, McKenna WJ (1989) Clinical sustained monomorphic ventricular tachycardia in hypertrophic cardiomyopathy: association with left ventricular apical aneurysm. Br Heart J 61:178-181

39. Tendera M, Wycisk A, Schneeweiss A, Polonski L, Wodniecki J (1993) Effect of sotalol on arrhythmias and exercise tolerance in patients with hypertrophic cardiomyopathy. Cardiology 82:335-342

40. DeRose J, Banas JS, Winters SL (1994) Current perspectives on sudden cardiac death in hypertrophic cardiomyopathy. Progr Cardiovasc Dis 36:475-484

Radiofrequency Catheter Ablation of Ventricular Tachycardia in Patients with Structural Heart Disease: Pathophysiologic Considerations to Simplify the Selection of the Target Sites

J. Farré, J.M. Rubio, A. Negrete, M. Nogueira, and J. Romero

Electrophysiology Laboratory Arrhythmia and Coronary Care Units,
Servicio de Cardiología, Fundación Jiménez Díaz,
Madrid, Spain

Introduction

Atrionodal reentrant tachycardias and tachyarrhythmias related to accessory atrioventricular pathways can be successfully treated with radiofrequency catheter ablation (RFCA) techniques with a low incidence of complications (1-4). In patients with ventricular tachycardia (VT), RFCA faces clinical, electrophysiologic, anatomic, and methodologic difficulties not found in the above two situations (Table 1). To be amenable to RFCA, the clinically occurring VT has to be reproducibly inducible in the electrophysiology laboratory, well tolerated, and sustained enough to be mappable.

Table 1. Difficulties in RFCA in patients with VT

1. Clinical	VT has to be hemodynamically well tolerated
2. Electrophysiologic	VT has to be Due to a mechanism enabling its reproducible induction in the laboratory (with electrical stimulation techniques or isoprenaline) Prolonged enough to permit catheter mapping
3. Anatomical	Site of origin or an essential component of the VT pathway must be Subendocardial Relatively narrow isthmus of tissue The number of VT with different sites of origin or reentry pathway mechanisms should be relatively low
4. Methodologic	Identification of markers for RFCA that are both sensitive and predictive for success Suggested guides for VT RFCA Earliest endocardial activation Pace mapping Isolated mid-diastolic potentials Concealed entrainment Analysis of resetting and postpacing pause during VT Analysis of the stimulus-QRS during concealed entrainment as compared with the interval mid-diastolic potential QRS onset of VT

RFCA, radiofrequency catheter ablation; VT, ventricular tachycardia.

In addition, due to the limited depth of the lesion produced with current RFCA techniques, the site of origin of the VT, if the latter is due to a focal mechanism, or an essential link of its reentry pathway have to be relatively subendocardial. Finally, the patient ideally should not have too many morphologically distinct VT, particularly if they come from very distant ventricular sites or if catheter manipulation during mapping of one morphology frequently leads to a different VT and, on approaching the latter, the former VT or a different one is elicited. To these difficulties we must add methodologic problems to identify with certainty the site of successful application of RF current. RFCA of VT has been based so far on the results of several mapping and pacing techniques such as (a) endocardial catheter electrode mapping to determine the site of earliest activation (5,6), (b) reproduction with endocardial pacing techniques of the VT morphology (pace mapping; 7-9), (c) demonstration of the phenomenon of concealed entrainment or as termed by Stevenson et al. "entrainment with concealed fusion" (10-17), and (d) identification of mid-diastolic potentials whose participation in the VT pathway is validated analyzing the phenomenon of resetting, concealed entrainment, and the duration of the postpacing interval (14-18).

The major problems in relation to RFCA of VT are (a) that our understanding of the underlying pathophysiologic mechanisms of the arrhythmia is incomplete, (b) that the methodology customarily used to identify the site of successful ablation is time consuming and demands prolonged catheter stability (10-18), (c) that we lack visual markers similar to those used to ablate the so-called slow atrionodal pathway or accessory atrioventricular pathways (1-3, 19-23), and (d) last but not least, that some forms of VT may have intramural and/or epicardial origins or pathways not reachable with current RFCA technology (24-32). Stevenson et al. have recently studied the value of several criteria to predict VT interruption during RF current application (16). As shown in Table 2, the most commonly used criteria to localize the site of successful application in postmyocardial infarction VT had a very poor predictive value. This indicates the need of

Table 2. Predictors of VT termination by RF current application (16)

Criteria	PPV
ECF	17%
PPI-VT cycle < 30 ms	20%
Isolated cycle DP or CEA	32%
ECF and PPI-VT cycle < 30 ms	25%
ECF and DP/CEA	45%

VT, ventricular tachycardia; RF, radiofrequency; ECF, entrainment with concealed fusion; PPI, postpacing interval; DP, diastolic potential; CEA, continuous electric activity.

improving our current methodology in order to be able to simplify RFCA in patients with VT and structural heart disease. Apart from these improvements in the methodology of the electrophysiologic selection of the ablation targets, it is possible that new technologic developments in the field of RF current application or catheter design will further enhance the role of catheter ablation techniques in the treatment of mappable VT.

Pathophysiological Considerations in Patients with a Healed Myocardial Infarction

VT in patients with underlying organic heart disease, particularly a postmyocardial infarction scar, is thought to be due to reentry. Although initial views on postmyocardial infarction VT suggested that they were based on a reentry mechanism mainly involving subendocardial regions in the border of the scar tissue (5, 7, 24-26), subsequent studies have questioned the universal value of this assumption (27-34). Svenson et al. demonstrated that 15% of the 85 VTs terminated by laser photocoagulation required an epicardial application of the energy (27). These investigators found that predictors for an epicardial substrate were the absence of a ventricular aneurysm and infarctions in the posteroinferior regions. Littmann et al. have shown that some VT in postmyocardial infarction patients can be due to subepicardial reentrant circuits incorporating surviving myocardial fibers in the epicardial border zone (28). Kaltenbrunner et al., using intraoperative epicardial and endocardial mapping techniques, suggested that VT in patients with myocardial infarction could be due to substrates involving subepicardial and deep septal layers in up to 32% of the 47 VTs induced in 28 patients (29). This type of VT would not be amenable to current RFCA techniques.

De Bakker et al. have made important observations in VT related to a chronic myocardial infarction (30-32). In their initial report on 72 patients with postmyocardial infarction VT in whom they recorded intraoperatively the endocardial electrical activity from 64 electrodes covering the surface of a balloon, they found an endocardial site of origin in 136 of the 139 mapped VTs (98%) from which the activation wavefront spread centrifugally (30). This focal pattern of endocardial activation contrasts with that observed in very few instances (three VTs in this report) in which endocardial activation seems to circulate around the anatomical obstacle of the scar tissue. We agree with their interpretation that this site of origin represented the endocardial breakthrough since (a) in 12 cases a second site of origin was found and (b) on reviewing their recordings (not mentioned by the authors) (Fig. 4 in reference 30) the near DC unipolar electrogram at the site of origin shows a QS morphology whose onset starts some 60-70 ms before the fastest intrinsic deflection, taken as activation time 0; therefore, the earliest breakthrough in this example and in some other instances should be at another unexplored site, either endocardially, intramurally, or epicardially. They also found a silent gap between the latest endocardial activity and the activation of the site of origin of the next beat, thus indicating that an unexplored route (intramural or endocardial but undetected) existed to fill this electric silence (30). Indeed, in 24 of the 136 maps with one or two endocardial sites of origin, the onset of the main deflection at the endocardial breakthrough point was preceded by the recording in one or more balloon leads of small deflections that the authors termed "presystolic activity"; in three VTs these deflections were detected at several sites and an endocardial route of propagation could be tentatively reconstructed; sometimes Purkinje spikes were recorded at the same sites during sinus rhythm and it was suggested that Purkinje fibers might have participated in the maintenance of VT in these instances. In addition, they also performed extensive mapping in two isolated, Langerdorff-perfused hearts, from patients with VT who underwent cardiac transplant. An intrascar route consisting of surviving myocardial fibers and electrically connecting areas of remaining myocardium was also demonstrated in these two isolated Langerdorff-perfused hearts in which the activation wavefront, represented by small sharp deflections, seemed to spread through a tract of surviving myocardial fibers over the infarcted zone; histologic studies in these hearts showed a continuous zone of viable myocardial fibers within the infarcted area connecting remaining tissue (30).

De Bakker et al. subsequently reported on their observations in 15 hearts from patients with chronic myocardial infarctions who underwent cardiac transplantation and were studied in a Langerdorff-perfused set up (31). Fifteen monomorphic sustained VTs were induced in nine hearts and endocardial and epicardial recordings were obtained in 10 VTs. In three VTs the earliest epicardial and endocardial activation was almost simultaneous whereas in the remaining seven VTs the epicardial breakthrough was recorded ≥20 ms after the earliest endocardial activation. This earliest site was located within 2 cm of the border of the infarct. The earliest and latest endocardial sites were connected through the scar tissue by bands of surviving myocardial fibers that at certain points in their course could be more than 5-7 mm deep in relation to the endocardial surface (see Fig. 4 in reference 31). These connecting tracts may run subendocardially, intramurally, and even subepicardially. In one heart the connecting tract seemed to be used orthodromically and antidromically in two morphologically distinct VTs. More than one tract of surviving tissue may transverse an infarct zone and connect the remaining healthy myocardium at either side of the scar. In hearts where the silent gap between the earliest and latest endocardial activations lasted for more than 150 ms the orientation of the fibers of the connecting intrascar surviving bundles was perpendicular to the line between the two gap points, in contrast with a parallel fiber orientation found in hearts where the silent gap was in the range of 30 ms (31). In hearts in which the silent gap lasted between 60 and 150 ms the orientation of the surviving fibers varied along the area of delay (31).

In a third study, De Bakker et al. reported on their intraoperative endocardial mapping observations in 20 patients with postmyocardial infarction VT in whom diastolic potentials were recorded at three or more sites during at least one episode of sustained tachycardia (32). A total of 46 different sustained uniform VT were mapped and in all of them the endocardial activation spread centrifugally from a rather circumscribed area (< 6 cm²; so called focal pattern). In 27 morphologically distinct VTs, diastolic potentials were recorded in three to 12 different endocardial sites (Table 3). The rest of their findings during endocardial mapping are also summarized in Table 3. The diastolic potentials started from sites of late activation of one VT beat and moved towards the area of earliest endocardial activation of the next cycle, further supporting the concept of a macroreentry using isolated tracts of surviving tissue within the area of infarction and the remaining healthy myocardium (32). In several cases in this study the area with diastolic potentials during VT was very extensive, suggesting that the intrascar limb of the reentrant pathway can be wide or composed of several tracts or, at least in our opinion, that part of these diastolic potentials reflect deadend pathways also activated orthodromically but not contributing to the completion of the circus movement. Our latter argument might be supported by the analysis of data shown by De Bakker et al. (Fig. 3 in reference 32) which suggests that, close to the site of entry of the activation wavefront into the compromised tissue, the area with diastolic potentials is wider than that at the border of the exit site (32).

The group of Cain in Saint Louis provided further evidence of the complexity of VT in patients with an old myocardial infarction, suggesting that they can be due to

intramural reentry as well as to a focal mechanism that, on occasions, is subendocardially located (33). Their conclusions regarding the potential focal mechanism were based on the lack of continuous electric activity between the end of one VT beat and the onset of the subsequent one during intramural three-dimensional high-density intraoperative mapping studies (39 needles with four pairs of electrodes each). This very impressive mapping density is possibly not sufficient to exclude either microscopic bands (especially if they are subendocardial and tortuous since true endocardial mapping was not performed in this study) connecting the terminal portions of the QRS complex of the VT with the next beat or a reentry mechanism among structures contained within 1 cm². These so-called focal VTs were also induced by programmed electrical stimulation; since chronic recurrent sustained VT rarely responds to verapamil (35), it is very unlikely that the focal tachycardias described by Pogwizd et al. (33) are due to triggered activity rather than to a form of reentry. Better documented, in our opinion, is the existence in the patients reported by Pogwizd et al. of intramural circuits that can incorporate as a limb of the reentry pathway a subendocardial bond of surviving myocardium localized over the scar tissue while others lack this endocardial element (33). In some of their patients with multiple morphologically distinct VT, both a macro-reentrant and a focal mechanism were identified (33). Pathologic examinations of the resected areas suggested that the structural factors leading to intramural reentry were: (a) a transverse fiber orientation relative to the spread of activation resulting in slow conduction, (b) the presence of interstitial fibrosis also resulting in slowing of conduction velocity most likely due to myocyte uncoupling, (c) the interface of peri-infarct region and adjacent, hypertrophic, noninfarcted myocardium that was the plane of functional block and the site of exit of the VT, and (d) the scar tissue that was the site of fixed conduction block. In some cases the macro-reentrant intramural pathway could have a length of 14 cm. Also of interest are their pathologic findings in the two patients in whom the site of origin of the apparently focal VT was included in the resected tissue. In both instances the VT focus consisted of an extensively thickened and fibrotic subendocardial tissue with strands of residual surviving subendocardial muscular bundles and Purkinje fibers (33).

Theoretical Considerations To Improve RFCA of VT

The above studies suggest that in patients with an old myocardial infarction the development of VT is based on complex pathophysiologic mechanisms. Initial catheter mapping studies identified as the site of origin of VT the area where the earliest diastolic (presystolic) activity was recorded (5-7, 26, 36, 37). This concept has to be abandoned; if the mechanism of VT is macroreentry, the site of earliest presystolic activity (a) may or may not belong to the reentry pathway, or (b) if it is part of the area of slow conduction, its relation to the VT is the same as that of other elements of this tract that are activated subsequently in the tachycardia cycle.

The traditional approach to perform catheter ablation of VT in patients with underlying structural heart

Table 3. Findings during intraoperative endocardial mapping in postmyocardial infarction VT with a focal pattern of endocardial activation (32)

	Min	Max	Mean
VT sites with DP	3	12	4.7
Timing (ms) of earliest DP relative to endocardial ES	36	188	91
Distance (cm) between the earliest DP and endocardial ES	0	8.5	4.2
Time interval (ms) between latest endocardial activation and earliest DP	10	175	52
Distance (cm) between sites of latest activation and ES	0	4.8	2.1

VT, ventricular tachycardia; DP, diastolic potentials; ES, exit site.

disease was to identify the so-called area of slow conduction (6, 11, 12-18). Application of RF current at sites with diastolic potentials has been shown to have a low predictive value for success (Table 2; 16). Many of these diastolic potentials can be related to deadend pathways or bystanders not contributing to the mechanism of VT. In this section we offer some preliminary views on our approach to VT ablation in patients with organic heart disease (42-44).

Significance of the Earliest Diastolic Potential

From the discussion of the aforementioned intraoperative mapping studies it is evident that it is incorrect to consider as site of origin the endocardial zone at which the earliest diastolic potential is recorded. The earliest diastolic potential in patients with VT and structural heart disease, if it belongs to the tachycardia pathway, represents the activation of one of the most proximal

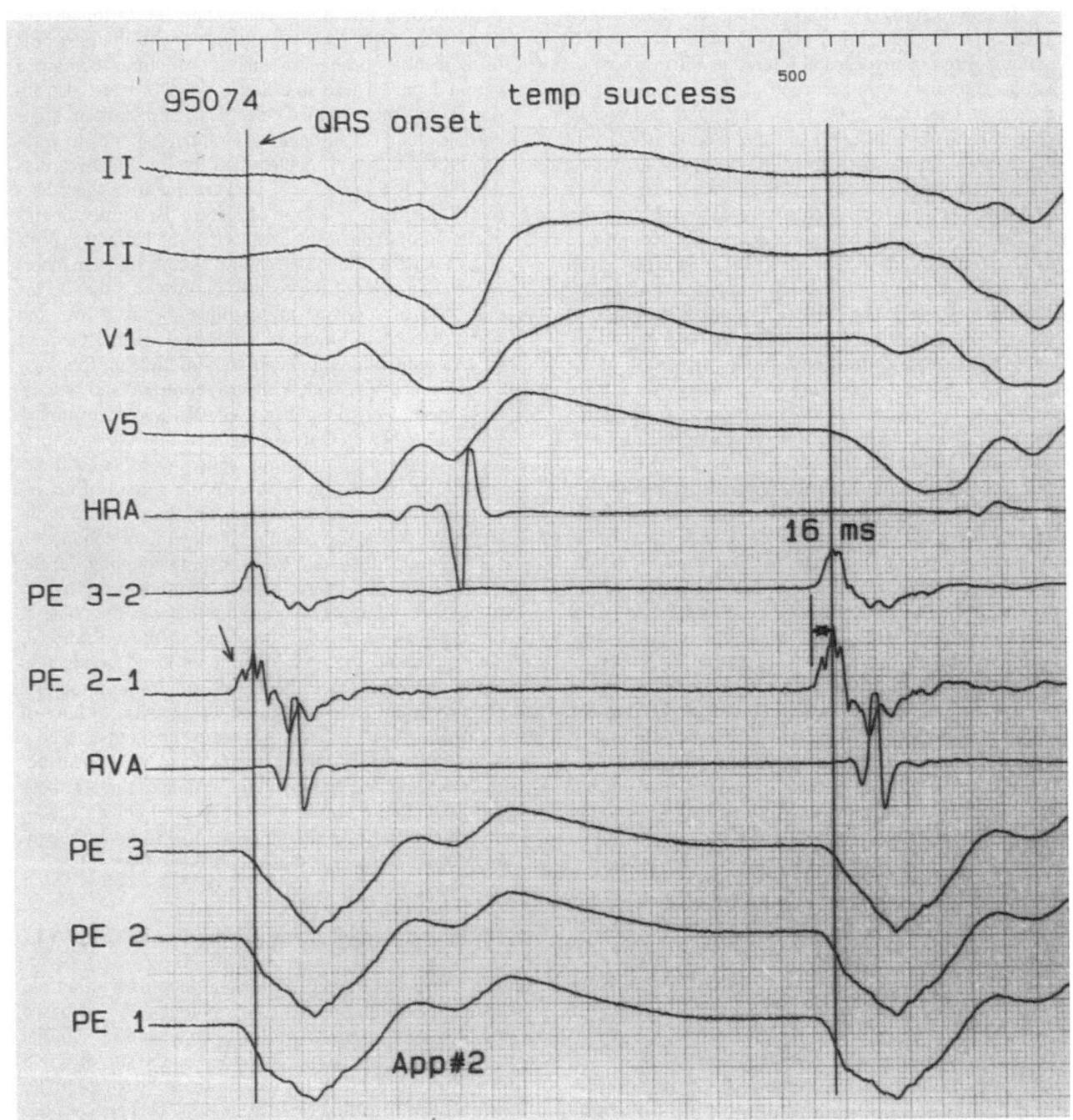

Fig. 1. Example of exit site in a patient with an incessant ventricular tachycardia (VT) in relation to a chronic anterior wall myocardial infarction with an anteroapical aneurysm. The *vertical line* was traced to signal the onset of the QRS complex in the surface 12-lead ECG during tachycardia. Note that the near DC unipolar recordings from the three distal probing electrodes (PE3, PE2, and PE1, respectively) show a QS-like negative deflection whose onset preceded that of the QRS complex in V5 by 16 ms. The distal bipolar filtered (30-500 Hz) electrogram from the probing electrode (PE 2-1) also shows presystolic activity. Application of radiofrequency (RF) current at this site resulted in interruption of VT that was noninducible for a few minutes. The location of the ablation catheter is shown in Fig. 2 (*upper two panels*). Note that the downslope of the QS unipolar waveform in lead PE1 was relatively slow, thus indicating that the real exit site was at a certain distance (most likely intramurally in the septum). Successive applications at this site always resulted in termination of VT that could be reinduced after a few minutes. Extensive mapping near this site did not disclose the presence of single or multiple sharp deflections preceding the QS in the unipolar recording

elements of the slow conducting limb of the circuit. Although this has not been studied systematically, some of the examples provided by De Bakker et al. (32) as well as theoretical considerations suggest that the earliest diastolic potentials have higher statistical chances of representing bystanders than presystolic sharp deflections close to the exist site (see below). That this assumption is probably true is further suggested by the fact that application of DC current shock at these earliest sites was frequently ineffective (36-39). In the study by Stevenson et al. (16) sites resulting in VT termination by RF current showed electrograms that were located close to the onset of the tachycardia QRS complex most of the time (either within the one third of the cycle preceding the QRS onset, at the onset, or immediately after the beginning of the QRS).

Exit Site

We define the exit site as the point at which the earliest unipolar QS-like endocardial electrogram is recorded during catheter electrode mapping (Figs. 1-4). When its initial downslope is fast, the earliest site is probably subendocardial; if the negative initial downslope is slow and we are in good contact with the endocardial surface, all the electric forces go away from the probing electrode, thus suggesting that we are over the scar tissue and that the earliest activation of the remaining normal myocardium (the real exit site) is at a certain distance, either endocardially, intramurally, or epicardially (Figs. 1, 3, panel B). If after extensive catheter electrode mapping no unipolar QS-like electrogram with initial fast intrinsic deflections are found, the real exit point is most likely intramural or epicardial.

Theoretically speaking, this exit site should be coincidental with the onset of the QRS complex of the VT in the surface ECG. The QRS onset of VT is an essential reference for catheter electrode mapping to perform RFCA. The onset of the QRS during VT is not simultaneous in all 12 ECG leads so that the first task should be to look for the lead or leads showing the earliest QRS onset (Figs. 1, 3); these leads, rather than a standard group of ECG leads, should be used as a reference (V3, V4, and V5 in the example of Fig. 3). Stevenson et al. demonstrated that during pacing at left ventricular sites with normal electrograms, the earliest QRS could be detected as late as 40 ms after the

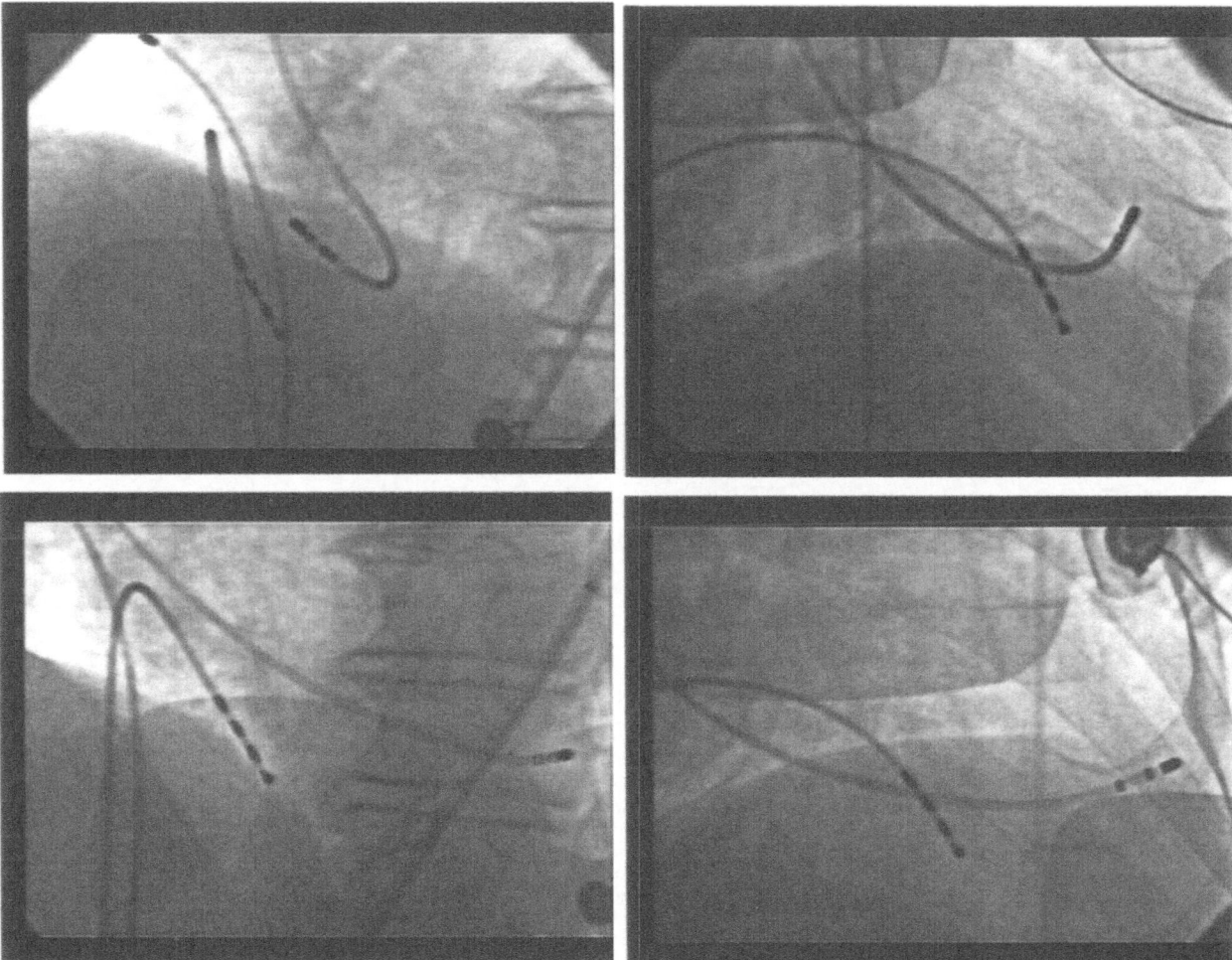

Fig. 2. Same patient as in Fig. 1. Digital cine-fluorograms obtained in left anterior oblique (*left panels*) and right anterior oblique projections (*right panels*). The *upper two panels* illustrate the position of the ablation catheter at the site shown in Fig. 1. The catheter was placed at the midanteroseptal border of the aneurysm. As mentioned before, several applications of radiofrequency (RF) current at this site interrupted the ventricular tachycardia (VT) and made it noninducible for a variable number of minutes (depending on the duration of the RF pulse). In the *lower two panels* we present the position of the ablation catheter at the site of permanent success (see also Figs. 3, 4). As it can be observed, particularly comparing both left anterior oblique projections (*left panels*) the permanently successful site was several centimeters away from the exit site, at the posterolateral border of the aneurysm

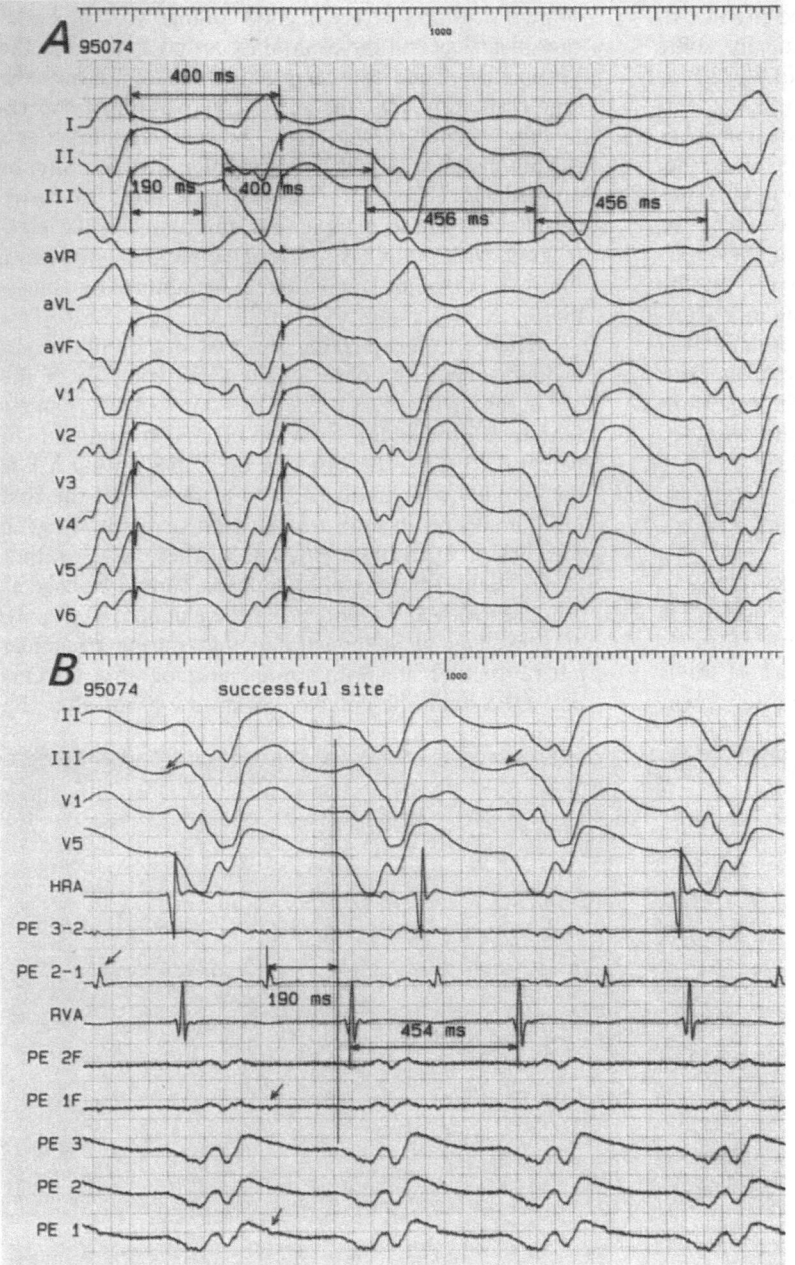

Fig. 3 A, B. Same patient as in Figs. 1, 2. **A** concealed entrainment or entrainment with concealed fusion at the site of successful ablation. Note that the QRS complexes during concealed entrainment are identical to those of the ventricular tachycardia (VT) in all 12 surface ECG leads. **B** Catheter electrode mapping at this site. Also note that a bipolar deflection was recorded from the distal pair of electrodes of the probing catheter (PE 2-1, see *arrow*). We present in **B** not only the unfiltered (near DC, 0.1-500 Hz) unipolar recordings from PE3, PE2, and PE1 but also the filtered (30-500 Hz) unipolar recordings from electrodes 1 and 2 (PE 1F and PE 2F, respectively). The following observations are worth noting: (1) although the near-DC unipolar recordings also show a QS-like negative configuration, (a) the onset of this QS waveform does not precede the onset of the QRS complex in the surface ECG, (b) the initial negativity of these QS unipolar waves is even slower than the one recorded at the site shown in Fig. 1, thus suggesting that we are even further from the exit point of this VT; (2) the sharpest spike recorded in lead PE 2-1 is mainly obtained from the distal ablating electrode (1) as pointed by the *arrows* in leads PE 1F and PE 1 (3) the distance from this sharp spike to the onset of the QRS complex in the surface ECG was 190 ms (**B**), the same as the distance from the stimulus artifact to the onset of the QRS complex during concealed entrainment (**A**)

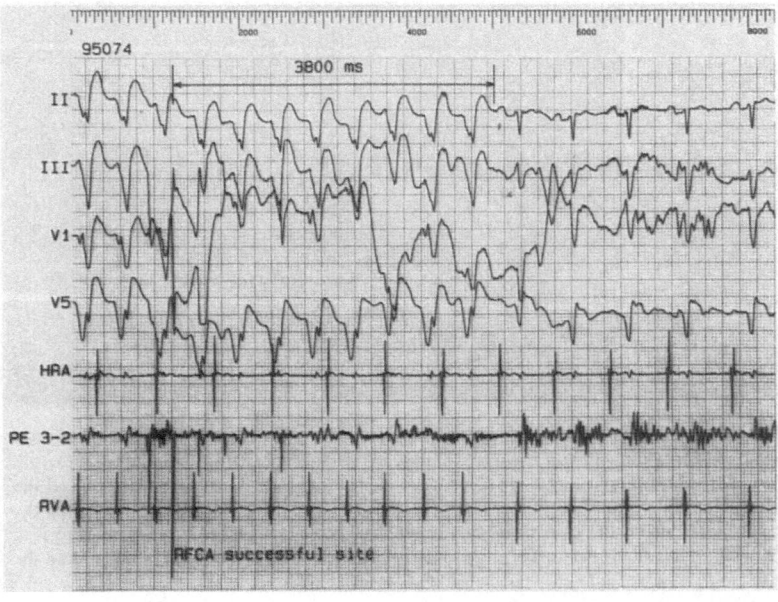

Fig. 4. Same patient as in Figs. 1-3. Application of radiofrequency (RF) current at the site shown in Fig. 3 resulted in the interruption of ventricular tachycardia (VT) in less that 4 s. VT that clinically was incessant and after the initial ablation attempts over the septal exit site very easily inducible with straight ventricular pacing became noninducible with programmed ventricular stimulation from the right and left ventricles using up to four consecutive extrastimuli and has not recurred during a period of more than 4 months of follow-up with repeated Holter and exercise tests

stimulus artifact (40). This indicates that the real exit site (according to our definition) should precede the onset of the QRS complex in the ECG (Fig. 1).

Targets for RFCA: Subendocardial Surviving Isthmus Essential for the Maintenance of VT

The exit site has to be connected to a narrow isthmus of tissue within the compromised myocardium; this isthmus can be endocardial, intramural, or epicardial. For the aforementioned reasons, the closer to the exit site the lower the chances that this isthmus will represent a bystander. The second step, therefore, is to look for fast, sharp deflections close to the area where the unipolar electrograms show QS-like, pre-QRS electrograms (Fig. 5). Absence of fast deflections immediately preceding or coincidental with these QS-like unipolar electrograms can indicate an inappropriate mapping technique or that the distal connecting limb is not subendocardial (41) (Fig. 1). When these sharp potentials are found (usually some 40-90 ms preceding the onset of the QRS in the surface ECG) and the VT morphology is reproduced in the 12 surface ECG leads (particularly if concealed entrainment is demonstrated) (Figs. 5, 6) application of RF current usually results in the immediate termination of VT (Fig. 7). Some of these potentials are so sharp that they resemble Purkinje fiber depolarizations. It is well known that Purkinje fibers survive

the myocardial infarction; should some of these surviving Purkinje fibers participate as connecting bonds between the slow intrascar pathway and the healthy remaining myocardium, they will be the ideal targets for RFCA since nothing is more subendocardial and of a diameter susceptible to the lesions produced by RF energy than a Purkinje bundle. Only occasionally have we been able to register at the site of successful VT ablation sharp potentials also preceding the QRS onset during sinus rhythm, thus suggesting that they indeed represent activation of Purkinje fibers.

As shown by Pogwizd et al. some macro-reentrant circuits responsible for VT can have only a subendocardial reflection and the rest of the reentry pathway an intramural course (33). This type of VT enables RFCA to be performed at points that are very distant from the so-called exit site. At the exit site no fast spikes are identified preceding the QRS onset, and, under these circumstances, isolated mid-diastolic sharp potentials representing surviving tissue that might be a link in the tachycardia pathway should be searched for (Fig. 3). The chances of damaging the normal myocardium by applying RF current at these sites are scanty since the underlying tissue (apart from the one generating the sharp deflections) is a noncontractile scar. RF current could be applied or pacing can be performed to demonstrate concealed entrainment (entrainment with concealed fusion), a distance between

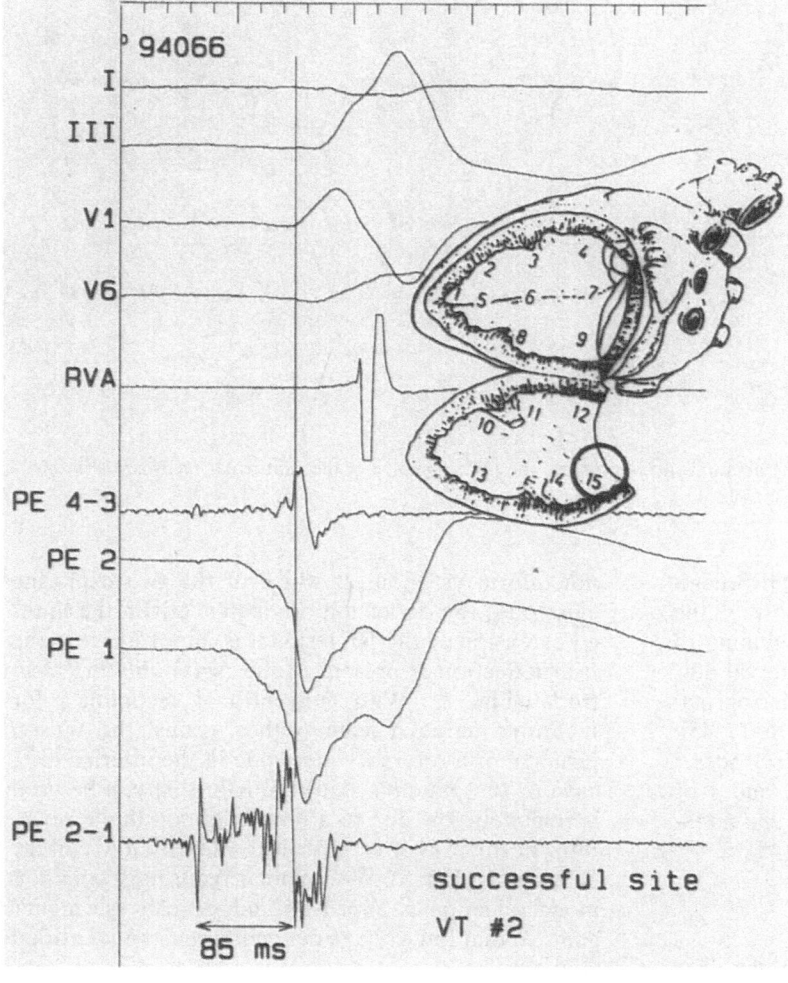

Fig. 5. Sharp bipolar deflections recorded preceding the onset of the QRS complex during ventricular tachycardia (VT; this patient, who had an anterolateral postinfarction aneurysm, had two additional VTs ablated in the same session). Note that the unipolar electrograms of the distal two electrodes of the probing catheter (PE 2 and PE 1, respectively) present a QS-like configuration although the initial negativity that precedes the onset of the QRS in the surface ECG shows a rather slow downslope, thus suggesting that the exit site was most likely intramural. Preceding this negativity multiple sharp spikes were recorded

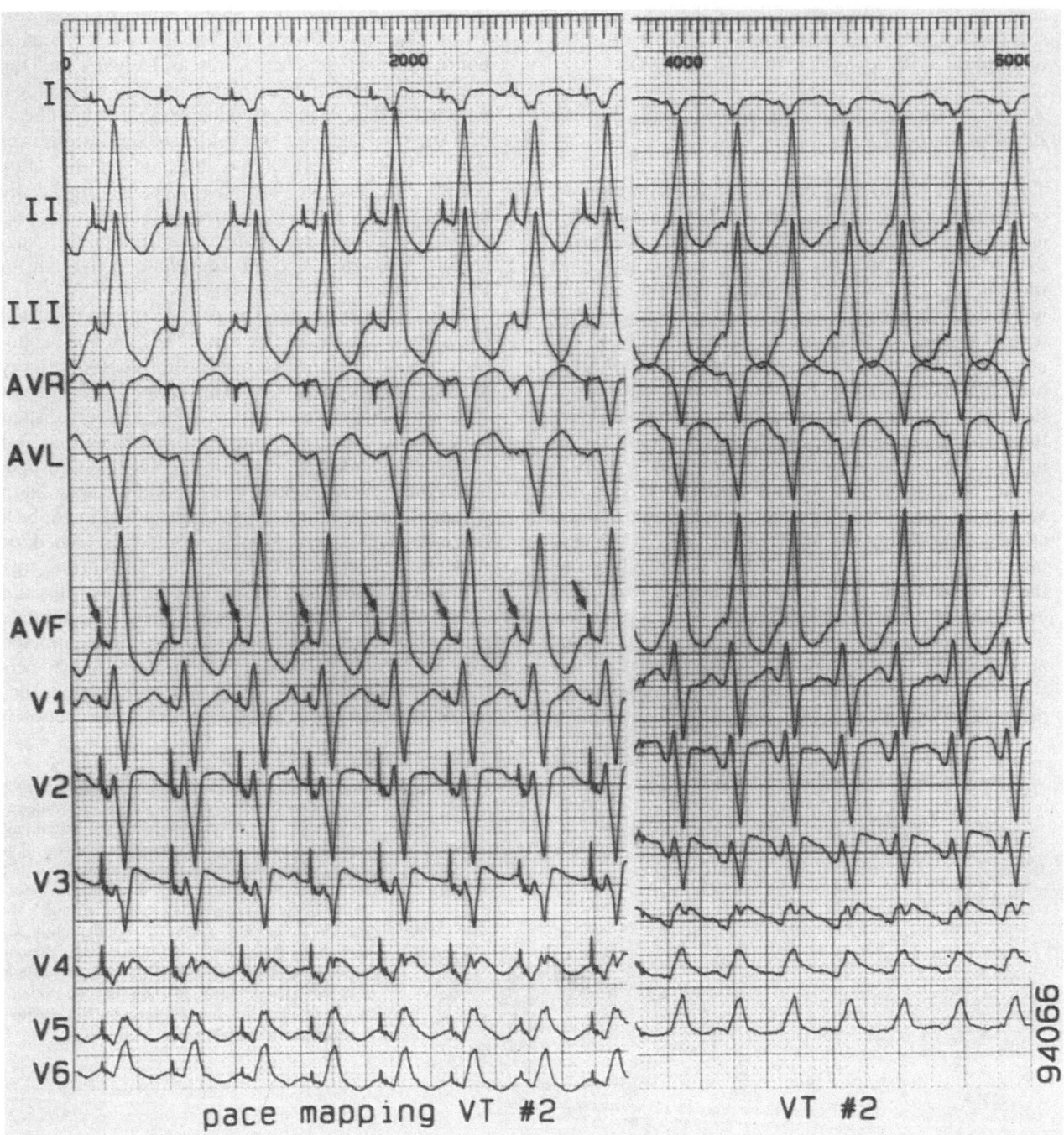

Fig. 6. Same patient as in Fig. 5. Pace mapping at the ablation site reproduced the QRS complex of the ventricular tachycardia in the 12 ECG leads

the stimulus artifact, and the onset of the QRS complex similar (<20 ms) to the time interval between the discrete mid-diastolic potential and the beginning of the next QRS of the VT, or a postpacing interval during entrainment with concealed fusion that is approximately equal to the VT cycle length (Fig. 3; 16, 17, 45). Pacing should not be performed between electrodes 1 and 2 but preferably between electrodes 1 and 4 or even better between the distal electrode (1) and an indifferent electrode in the inferior vena cava (45).

Additional Value of Unipolar Recordings

The recording of these fast bipolar deflections does not inform us about at which of the two exploring electrodes the deflection originates. Given the limited extension of the RF lesion it is important that the fast deflection is present in the distal ablating electrode (Fig. 3). With conventional techniques for recording unipolar leads (either against the Wilson terminal or a reference electrode in the inferior vena cava or the patient's skin) the gain that can be used is relatively low due to a poor common mode rejection. In this way it is difficult to identify low voltage deflections (Fig. 5). With bipolar recordings common mode rejection is improved and we can use higher gains so that low voltage deflections can be identified (Fig. 5).

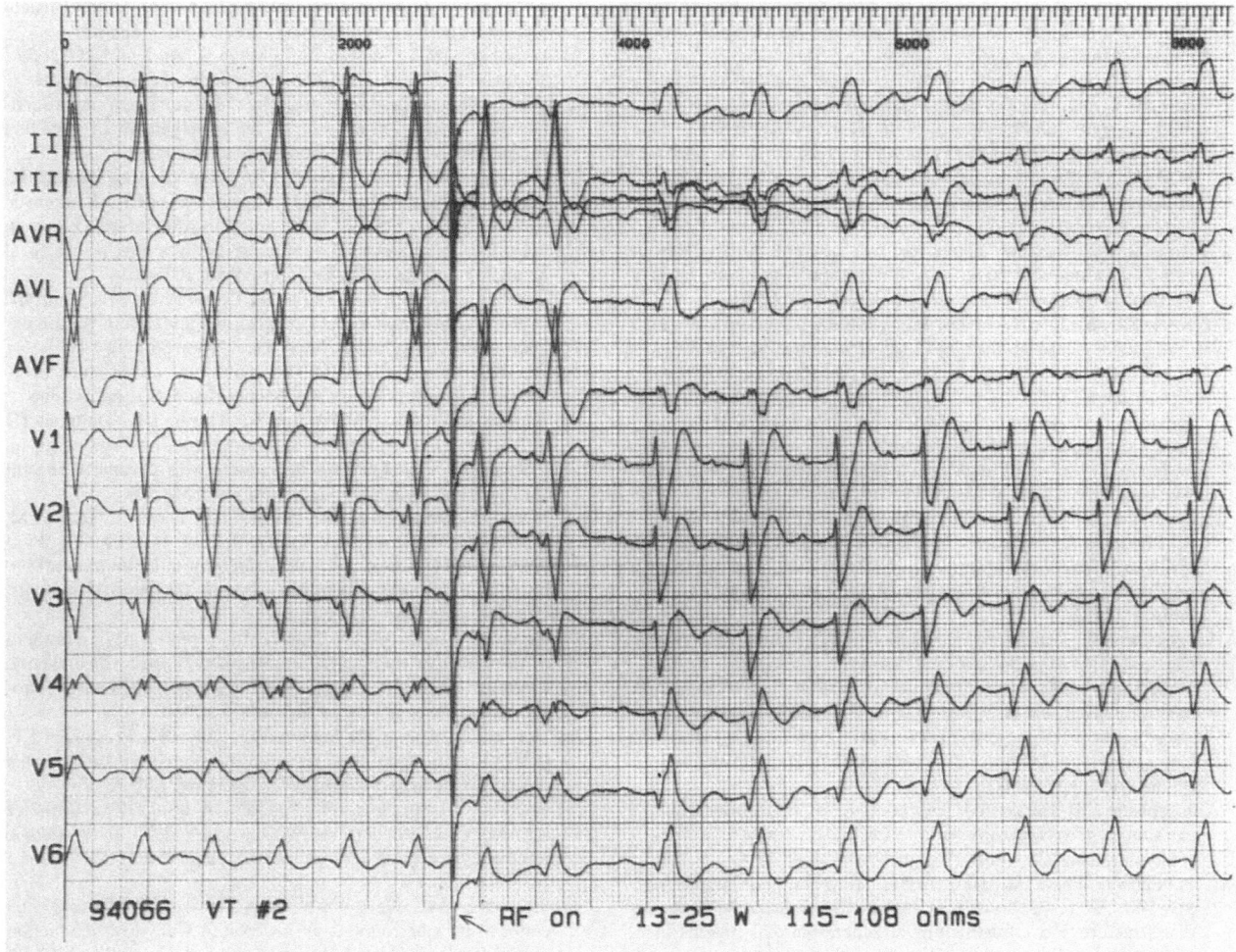

Fig. 7. Same patient as in Figs. 5, 6. Application of radiofrequency *current* during ventricular tachycardia (*VT*) at the site shown in Fig. 5 resulted in the immediate interruption of the VT that could not be reinduced subsequently

References

1. Jackman WM, Wang X, Friday J, Roman CA, Moulton KP, Beckman KJ, McClelland JH, Twidale N, Hazlitt HA, Prior MI, Margolis PD, Calame JD, Overholt ED, Lazzara R (1991) Catheter ablation of accessory atrioventricular pathways (Wolff-Parkinson-White syndrome) by radiofrequency current. N Engl J Med 324:-1605-1611
2. Kuck KH, Schlüter M, Geiger M, Siebels J, Duckeck W (1991) Radiofrequency current catheter ablation of accessory atrioventricular pathways. Lancet 337:1557-1561
3. Jackman WM, Beckman KJ, McClelland JH, Wnag X, Friday KJ, Roman CA, Moulton KP, Twidale N, Hazlitt HA, Prior MI, Oren J, Overholt ED, Lazzara R (1992) Treatment of supraventricular tachycardia due to atrioventricular nodal reentry by radiofrequency catheter ablation of slow-pathway conduction. N Engl J Med 327:313-318
4. Hindricks G on Behalf of the MERFS Investigators (1993). The Multicentre European Radiofrequency Survey (MERFS): complications of radiofrequency catheter ablation of arrhythmias. Eur Heart J 14: 1644-1653
5. Josephson ME, Horowitz LN, Scott R et al (1982) Role of catheter mapping in the preoperative evaluation of ventricular tachycardia. Am J Cardiol 49: 207-220
6. Kuck KH, Schlüter M, Geiger M, Siebels J (1991) Successful catheter ablation of human ventricular tachycardia with radiofrequency current guided by endocardial mapping of the area of slow conduction. PACE 14: 1060-1071
7. Josephson ME, Waxman HL, Cain ME et al (1982) Ventricular activation during endocardial pacing. II: role of pace-mapping to localize origin of ventricular tachycardia. Am J Cardiol 50: 11-20

8. Klein LS, Shih HT, Hackett K et al (1992) Radiofrequency catheter ablation of ventricular tachycardia in patients without structural heart disease. Circulation 85: 1666-1674
9. Morady F, Kadish AH, DiCarlo L et al (1990) Long-term results of catheter ablation of idiopathic right ventricular tachycardia. Circulation 82: 2093-2099
10. Okumura K, Henthorn RW, Epstein AE et al (1985) Further observations on transient entrainment: importance of pacing site and properties of the components of the reentry circuit. Circulation 72: 1293-1307
11. Frank R, Tonet JL, Kounde S et al (1987) Localization of the area of slow conduction during ventricular tachycardia. In: Brugada P, Wellens HJJ (eds) Cardiac arrhythmias: where to go from here? Futura, Mount Kisco, NY, pp 191-208
12. Okumura K, Oldshansky B, Henthorn RW et al (1987) Demonstration of the presence of slow conduction during sustained ventricular tachycardia in man: use of transient entrainment of the tachycardia. Circulation 75: 369-378
13. Morady F, Frank R, Kou WH et al (1988) Identification and catheter ablation of a zone of slow conduction in the reentrant circuit of ventricular tachycardia in humans. J Am Coll Cardiol 11: 775-782
14. Morady F, Kadish A, Rosenkeck S, Calkins H, Kou WH, De Buitleir M, Sousa J (1991) Concealed entrainment as a guide for catheter ablation of ventricular tachycardia in patients with prior myocardial infarction. J Am Coll Cardiol 17: 678-689
15. Morady F, Harvey M, Kalbfleisch SJ, El-Atassi R, Calkins H, Lamberg JJ (1993) Radiofrequency ablation of ventricular tachycardia in patients with coronary artery disease. Circulation 87: 363-372
16. Stevenson WG, Khan H, Sager P, Saxon LA, Middlekauff HR, Natterson PD, Wiener I (1993) Identification of reentry circuit

sites during catheter mapping and radiofrequency ablation of ventricular tachycardia late after myocardial infarction. Circulation 88: 1647-1670

17. Khan HH, Stevenson WG (1994) Activation times in and adjacent to reentry circuits during entrainment: implications for mapping ventricular tachycardia. Am Heart J 127: 833-842

18. Fitzgerald DM, Friday KJ, Wah JAYL, Lazzara R, Jackman WM (1988) Electrogram patterns predicting successful catheter ablation of ventricular tachycardia. Circulation 77: 806-814

19. Jackman WM, Friday KJ, Yeung Lai-Wah JA, Fitzgerald DM, Bowman AJ, Stelzer P, Harrison L, Lazzara R (1988) New catheter technique for recording left free wall accessory atrioventricular pathway activation. Circulation 78: 598-610

20. Kuck KH, Schlüter M (1991) Single catheter approach to radiofrequency current ablation of left sided accessory pathways in patients with the Wolff Parkinson White syndrome. Circulation 84: 2366-2375

21. Jackman WM, Beckman KJ, McClelland JH et al (1992) Treatment of supraventricular tachycardia due to atrioventricular nodal reentry by radiofrequency catheter ablation of slow-pathway conduction. N Engl J Med 327: 313-316

22. Haissaguerre M, Gaita F, Fisher B, Commenges D, Monserrat P, d'Ivernois C, Lemetayer P, Earin JF (1992) Elimination of atrioventricular nodal reentrant tachycardia using discrete slow potentials to guide application of radiofrequency energy. Circulation 85: 2162-2175

23. Jackman WM, Nakagawa H, Heidbüchel H, Beckman KJ, McClelland JH, Lazzara R (1995) Three forms of atrioventricular nodal (junctional) reentrant tachycardia: differential diagnosis, electrophysiological characteristics, and implications for anatomy of the reentrant circuit. In: Zipes DP, Jalife J (eds) Cardiac electrophysiology: from cell to bedside, 2nd edn. Saunders, Philadelphia, pp 620-637

24. Josephson ME, Harken AH, Horowitz LN (1979) Endocardial excision: a new surgical technique for the treatment of recurrent ventricular tachycardia. Circulation 41: 1035-1044

25. Fenoglio JJ, Pham TD, Harken AH, Horowitz LN, Josephson ME, Wit AL (1983) Recurrent sustained ventricular tachycardia: structure and ultrastructure of subendocardial regions in which tachycardia originates. Circulation 68: 518-533

26. Miller JM, Harken AH, Hargrove WC, Josephson ME (1985) Pattern of endocardial activation during sustained ventricular tachycardia. J Am Coll Cardiol 6: 1280-1287

27. Svenson RH, Littmann L, Gallagher JJ, Selle JG, Zimmern SH, Fedor JM, Colavita PG (1990) Termination of ventricular tachycardia with epicardial laser photocoagulation: a clinical comparison with patients undergoing successful endocardial photocoagulation alone. J Am Coll Cardiol 15: 163-170

28. Littmann L, Svenson RH, Gallagher JJ, Selle JG, Zimmern SH, Fedor JM, Colavita PG (1991) Functional role of the epicardium in postinfarction ventricular tachycardia. Observations derived from computerized epicardial activation mapping, entrainment, and epicardial laser photoablation. Circulation 83: 1577-1591

29. Kaltenbrunner W, Cardinal R, Dubuc M, Shenasa M, Nadeau R, Tremblay G, Vermeulen M, Savard P, Pagé PL (1991) Epicardial and endocardial mapping of ventricular tachycardia in patients with myocardial infarction. Is the origin of tachycardia always subendocardially localized? Circulation 84: 1058-1071

30. DeBakker JMT, Van Cappelle FJL, Janse MJ, Wilde AAM, Coronel R, Becker AE, Dingemans KP, Van Hemel NM, Hauer RNW (1988) Reentry as cause of ventricular tachycardia

in patients with chronic ischemic heart disease. Electrophysiologic and anatomic correlations. Circulation 77: 589-606

31. DeBakker JMT, Coronel R, Tasseron S, Wilde AAM, Opthof T, Janse MJ, Van Cappelle FJL, Becker AE, Jambroes G (1990) Ventricular tachycardia in the infarcted, Langerdorff-perfused, human heart: role of the arrangement of surviving cardiac fibers. J Am Coll Cardiol 15: 1594-1607

32. DeBakker JMT, Van Cappelle FJL, Janse MJ, Van Hemel NM, Hauer RNW, Defauw JJAM, Vermeulen FEE, Bakker de Wekker PFA (1991) Macroreentry in the infarcted human heart: the mechanism of ventricular tachycardias with a focal activation pattern. J Am Coll Cardiol 18: 1005-1014

33. Pogwizd SM, Hoyt RH, Saffitz JE, Corr PB, Cox JL, Cain ME (1992) Reentrant and focal mechanisms underlying ventricular tachycardia in the human heart. Circulation 86:1872-1887

34. Wit AL, Janse MJ (1993) The ventricular arrhythmias of ischemia and infarction. Futura, Mount Kisco, NY, pp 267-356

35. Wellens HJJ, Bär FWHM, Lie KI, Duren DR, Dohmen HJ (1977) Effect of procainamide, propranolol and verapamil on mechanism of tachycardia in patients with chronic recurrent ventricular tachycardia. Am J Cardiol 40: 579-585

36. Morady F, Scheinman MM, DiCarlo LA, Davis JC, Herve JM, Griffin JC, Winstomn SA, De Buitleir M, Hautler CB, Wahr JA, Kou WH, Nelson SD (1987) Catheter ablation of ventricular tachycardia with intracardiac shocks: results in 33 patients. Circulation 75: 1037-1049

37. Garan H, Kuchar D, Freeman C et al (1988) Early assessment of the effect of map-guided transcatheter intracardiac electric shock on sustained ventricular tachycardia secondary to coronary artery disease. Am J Cardiol 61: 1018-1023

38. Hauer RW, Robles De Medina EO, Kuijer PJ, Westerhof PW (1989) Electrode catheter ablation for ventricular tachycardia: efficacy of a single cathodal shock. Br Heart J 61: 38-45

39. Borgreffe M, Breithardt G, Podczeck A et al (1990) Catheter ablation of ventricular tachycardia using defibrillator pulses: electrophysiological findings and long-term results. Eur Heart J 10: 591-601

40. Stevenson WG, Weiss JN, Wiener I et al (1989) Fractionated endocardial electrograms are associated with slow conduction in humans: evidence from pace mapping. J Am Coll Cardiol 13: 369-376

41. Farré J, Grande A, Martinell J, Fraile J, Ramírez JA, Rábago G (1987) Atrial unipolar waveform analysis during retrograde conduction over left-sided accessory atrioventri-cular pathways. In: Brugada P, Wellens HJJ (eds) Cardiac arrhythmias: where to go from here? Futura, Mount Kisko, NY, pp 243-269

42. Farré J, Asso A, Monteiro F, Castro J, Pérez-Casas ML, Pérez PP, Buj R, Aguado E (1994) Ventricular tachycardia potential: a new visual catheter electrode mapping marker for radiofrequency catheter ablation. Eur Heart J 15 [Suppl]: 244 (abstr)

43. Asso A, Farré J, Monteiro F, Castro J, Negrete A, Romero J (1994) Radiofrequency catheter ablation of ventricular tachycardia in arrhythmogenic right ventricular dysplasia. Eur Heart J 15: 542 (abstr)

44. Asso A, Farré J, Zayas R, Negrete A, Cabrera JA, Romero J (1995) Radiofrequency catheter ablation of ventricular tachycardia in patients with arrhythmogenic right ventricular dysplasia. J Am Coll Cardiol 25 [Suppl]: 315A (abstr)

45. Stevenson WG (1995) Catheter mapping of ventricular tachycardia. In: Zipes DP, Jalife J (eds) Cardiac electrophysiology: from cell to bedside, 2nd edn. Saunders Philadelphia, pp 1093-1112

IMPLANTABLE DEFIBRILLATORS

Is Total Mortality Really Reduced by the Implantable Cardioverter Defibrillator?

S. Nisam

Medical Science CPI/Guidant Europe, Zaventem, Belgium

Introduction: Why the Controversy?

The fact that the implantable cardioverter defibrillator (ICD) has reduced arrhythmic sudden death to about 1% per year is no longer contested. Irrefutable dramatic evidence of this phenomenon comes from the stored electrograms, which have visually captured the interruptions of countless episodes of malignant sustained arrhythmias in thousands of patients. But these patients have sick hearts, and the question asked by some – and which we will address here – is whether this reduction in sudden death translates to an overall, meaningful benefit in overall survival.

Implicit in questioning whether the ICD improves overall survival is the contention that the patient's *mode of death* is merely being converted from sudden to nonsudden death (1,2). This argument implies that the timing of the patient's actual demise, following the occurrence of life-saving ICD therapy, is essentially simultaneous – or at the best a few days or weeks later. It is certainly true that patients with heart failure or cardiomyopathy often present with inconvertible arrhythmias as an end stage (Fig. 1). The major fallacy in the "converts mode of death" theory is that it precludes the possibility of life-threatening ventricular tachycardia (VT) / ventricular fibrillation (VF) *months and years prior* to the terminal event, as illustrated in this example. This question is closely tied to *patient selection* for ICD therapy. Levine et al. demonstrated that NYHA Class IV patients survived barely a month following appropriate ICD shocks; whereas the "prolongation" in life for the class I patients averaged 32.8 months (3). Another problem with the "conversion" premise is that it overlooks the fact that most ICD recipients have their VT efficaciously interrupted by antitachycardia pacing (ATP) *before* these stable VTs degenerate to the ultimate lethal arrhythmias.

Evidence That the ICD Improves Survival

The evidence that the ICD improves survival, as we will show, is ample from multiple investigations and covering various patients populations; it has remained consistent from the earliest reports over a decade ago through more recent studies. In the early days of ICD therapy, Fogoros et al. examined the total survival of fifty patients with VT or VF who were *syncopal* during their arrhythmias and found nonresponsive to electrophysiologically (EP) guided antiarrhythmic drugs (4). Twenty-nine were treated with amiodarone and an ICD; but due to manufacturing problems during approximately 1 year, 21 patients were discharged on amiodarone alone. The two cohorts were similar in terms of all the critical risk factors (age, left ventricular ejection fraction - LVEF, etc.). Actuarial analysis at 2 years revealed 37% total mortality in the patients on

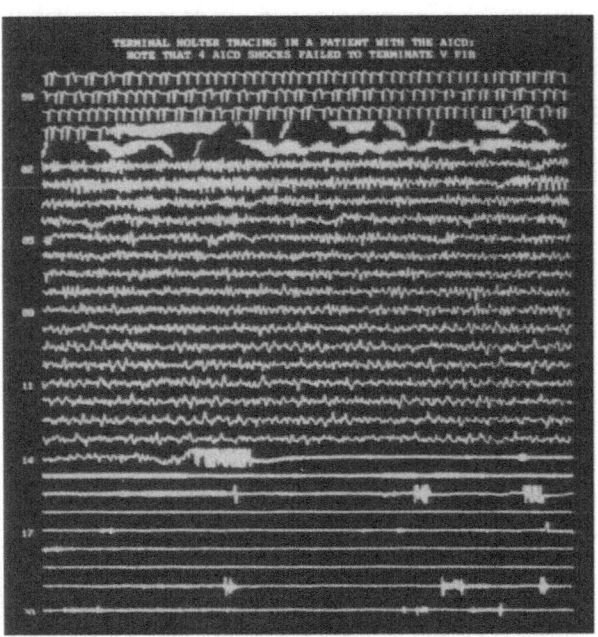

Fig. 1. Holter recording of terminal arrhythmia for a patient implanted 2 years earlier with an automatic implantable cardioverter defibrillator. The *top of the tracing* shows that ventricular flutter/fibrillation subsisted despite four shocks from the device. During the preceding 2 years, the patient had received eight appropriate shocks, terminating similar rhythms. (Courtesy of Dr. R. Luceri, Ft. Lauderdale, FL, USA)

AICD Survival Benefit

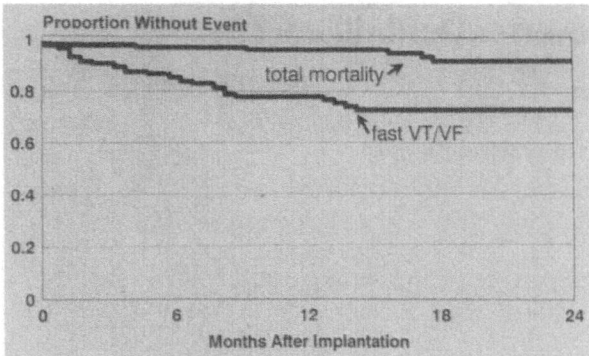

Fig. 2. Actuarial curves for freedom from overall mortality (*top tracing*) and from fast (presumably life-threatening) ventricular tachyarrhythmias (*lower tracing*) for 183 patients implanted with ICDs. *Fast VT/VF*, ventricular tachycardia/fibrillation at rates exceeding 240 bpm, and confirmed by device electrograms and/or R-R interval counters to be of ventricular origin and sustained. (Courtesy of D. M. Block, Münster, Germany)

amiodarone alone compared to 5% in the apparently matched ICD cohort. Importantly, the actuarial rate of appropriate shocks in the ICD group was nearly coincident with the actual rate of deaths in the amiodarone group! In the mid-1980s Newman et al. initiated a "matched case control" study in which the survival of 60 patients receiving ICDs was compared to 120 equally matched patients who received amiodarone (5). The 3-year actuarial analysis revealed 31% lower mortality ($p \leq .01$) in the ICD cohort. Böcker and coworkers (6) carried out one of the most scientifically rigorous studies: they restricted their analysis to consecutive patients receiving exclusively third-generation ICDs having stored electrograms and/or R-R interval counters, and they defined their endpoint for probable death as sustained VT/VF at rates > 240 BPM. In an update of that report (M. Block, personal communication), now through 2 years and covering 183 patients, their actuarial analysis found 8% total mortality at 24 months, versus 27% projected on the basis of these rapid sustained episodes of VT/VF (Fig. 2). In response to the converts mode of death argument, these investigators explicitly pointed out that their patients were not dying within a short time following the conversion by the ICD of these life-threatening rhythms. Schlepper et al., using an almost identical study design (VT > 230 BPM + electrogram verification), reached similar conclusions in their series of 167 patients, followed up over 5 years (7).

In yet another major study, CASCADE (Cardiac Arrest in Seattle: Conventional versus Amiodarone Drug Evaluation), analysis of the early results versus those published later is very revealing (8,9). In the initial report, the patient generally did not get implantable defibrillators, and the authors reported 17% cardiac arrest at 1 year and 35% at 3 years. Due to this unacceptably high mortality, the investigators *changed the study design* so that most subsequent patients received ICDs. They conluded, "Future studies should concentrate on the success of amiodarone treatment compared with placebo in patients who have an implanted cardioverter/defibrillator in whom it would be ethical to withhold drug treatment" (9).

Powell et al. retrospectively analyzed the long-term outcome of 331 cardiac arrest survivors treated at two U.S. institutions, one on the east coast and the other on the west coast (10). One hundred eighty-one received EP-guided drug therapy, the remaining 150 received ICDs – usually as a result of no effective drug being found. Not unexpectedly, the drug cohort seemed to represent a significantly lower risk profile, with a mean EF of .45 versus .35 for the ICD group (p <.0001); pulmonary wedge pressure was 12.7 mmH in the ICD patients versus 9.4 in the antiarrhythmic drug group ($p < .0002$), and 22% of patients were revascularized in the ICD group versus 37% in the patients on drug therapy ($p < .0001$). Nevertheless, the overall survival was 74% in the ICD patients versus 63% in the drug cohort. The authors declared, *"Despite this bias and the anticipated increase in non sudden cardiac deaths due to pump dysfunction in defibrillator recipients, a reduction in total mortality was observed in the defibrillator group"*. This same study is very enlightening for the question of patient selection: in patients with EF > 40%, drugs did just as well as the ICD through 3 years (actuarial), and it was only at 5 years that the ICD showed significantly better survival, 96% versus 82%. (The authors speculated that this higher mortality in the drug cohort was due to late drug failure or change of substrate.) On the other hand, in the poor EF group (EF < 40%), the better survival for the ICD group was manifest early and throughout the follow-up: 94% versus 86% at 1 year, 64% versus 43% at 5 years.

Hypothesis: The ICD Does *Not* Prolong Life

Let us examine this *contrary* hypothesis, on the basis of available data.

Evidence from Electrograms

Looking at electrograms of a sustained, extremely rapid VT in a patient with compromised left ventricular function (LVF), this would mean that this patient would have survived that (and possibly many similar) episodes *without the ICD*, or that the ICD truly *momentarily* saved the patient from sudden cardiac death, but he would go on to die with no meaningful extension of his life.

Clinical experience does not support either of these conclusions.

Comparing Survival of Patients With and Without Shocks

Multiple series [Myerburg (11), Mehta (12), Levine (13), and others] show 50%+ of their patients receiving appropriate shocks, and that these shocked patients have the same survival as the remaining nonshocked patients. There were no significant differences in the risk profiles (LVEF, etc.) between those who received shocks compared to those who did not. Those who died in the latter group succumbed of "natural" causes, i.e., the ICD played no role. So did the shocked patients, but in their case *later*, due to the ICD preventing *premature* arrhythmic deaths. Are we to believe that the shocks responding to and quickly terminating (often multiple) episodes of VT/VF contributed *nothing* to allowing these patients to live out their life until congestive heart failure (CHF) took over? Is it not much more plausible to accept that the shocks ended these electrical cardiac accidents, for many patients on numerous occasions, and prolonged their lives from date of shock to death?

Patients with Extremely Rapid, Sustained VTs/VFs

Looking at Böcker's study (6; documented sustained VT > 240 BPM = death), would these patients have achieved 92% survival through 2 years in the absence of these shocks? This is highly unlikely. Furthermore, their survival aftershock was not hours or days, but rather months or years; nearly all were still alive at 24 months! These results are further supported by Schlepper et al.'s similar study, which showed 85% of their patients still alive at 5 years (7).

Retrospective Studies

Powell et al. (10) reported for patients with EF ≥ 40% that the survival of ICD-treated patients was 96% at 5 years, compared to 82% for drug-treated patients. For the EF < 40%, survival for ICD compared to drug-treated patients was 94% versus 86% at 1 year and 64% versus 43% at 5 years. Why this difference? If the ICD was not the reason, was the higher mortality due to the drugs? (But these were precisely the drugs which had rendered these patients' previously inducible VTs non-inducible!)

Prospective Randomized Study

A very recently published study by Wever et al. dramatically reinforces all the above findings (13). Sixty patients resuscitated from cardiac arrest were randomized to ICD versus "conventional" therapy. The results showed ICD patients with 13% overall mortality at 2 year follow-up, compared to 35% for the drug cohort. The authors emphasized that, while amiodarone was only used in two patients, it is highly improbable – based on their own and others' experience with that drug – that this factor would have significantly changed the final outcome.

Discussion

There are many other studies with similar results. Importantly, there are no studies showing the contrary though some (usually from early series with high rates of perioperative mortality) show less *relative* benefit for the patient receiving an ICD (1,14). Skeptics point to the lack of a controlled randomized study as lack of substantial evidence that the ICD prolongs survival (2,15). (The same could be said, by the way, about cardiac pacemakers, penicillin, radiofrequency ablation for Wolff-Parkinson-White syndrome, and a multitude of well-established medical therapies...) The problems with a randomized study of the ICD in patients with previous cardiac arrest or syncopal VT have been well elucidated in recent editorials by Fogoros (16) and Sweeney and Ruskin (17). The latter article pointed out that a study designed to prove that ICDs improve survival (e.g., versus amiodarone) would – in patients with well-preserved LVF – likely require 1000 or so patients and up to 5 years of follow-up! At the other extreme, the *indiscriminate* (for that is exactly what a randomized trial requires) implantation of ICDs in patients with very poor LVF would give the ICD very little chance to show benefit, since such patients' competing risk of dying from heart failure predominates. ICD implantation would be contraindicated in such patients at most institutions.

There is ample opportunity for *both* these types of *selection bias* to enter any such trial (including, of course *AVID* (antiarrythmic drugs versus implantable defibrillator) (18). Imagine that one third of the 1200 patients to be enrolled in AVID belong to the low-risk category, a second third to the category characterized by high risk of CHF death, and the remaining third representative of a typical ICD cohort. Table 1 projects our *estimates* of 2-year actuarial mortality rates for these three groups. (The nonsudden death rate, especially for group B, is projected as *higher* for ICD patients, a phenomenon observed in many series, and one which reflects the fact that, as these patients are "saved" from sudden death, their risk for CHF death augments over time.) For all 1200 patients, the ICD's superiority is "only" 17.6%, well under the objective set by AVID to demonstrate statistical significance. Furthermore, if some patients "cross over" to ICD therapy following VT recurrences on amiodarone or sotalol, their subsequent

Table 1. Hypothetical mortality rates[a] (%, for actuarial 2 years)
(Potential scenario for enrollment in the AVID study)

Causes of death	A (n = 400)		B (n = 400)		C (n = 400)		All (n = 1200)	
	Drugs	ICD	Drugs	ICD	Drugs	ICD	Drugs	ICD
SCD	5	1	13	4	12	2	10	2.3
Cardiac + other non-SCD	9	10	27	33	19	20	18.3	21.0
Total mortality	14	11	40	37	31	22	28.3	23.3
ICD better by (%)	21.4		7.5		29		17.6	

A, low-risk; e.g., noninducible (baseline) and good left ventricular function;
B, enrolled patients with high comorbidity, e.g., high risk of déath from heart failure;
C, typical, current ICD population;
ICD, implantable cardioverter defibrillator; SCD, sudden cardiac death
[a] Influence of *crossovers not* reflected in these projections.

protection (by the ICD) will continue to be attributed to the drugs, on the "intention-to-treat" analysis. This would in effect lower the sudden cardiac death rate, hence the overall mortality rate, of the drug cohort, thus further diminishing the ICD advantage. Group C, which we have designated as typical ICD patients today, shows a good improvement, 29%, but the sample size would probably be insufficient to make this statistically significant.

Concern about patient selection bias is precisely the reason why the investigators have instituted a "registry". Unfortunately, there are multiple ways for eligible patients to bypass the registry; furthermore, once the study results come out, even if the registry should show that the patients entered are not necessarily representative of most current ICD candidates, it will be very difficult to change people's initial perceptions, particularly administration and third-party payers, who will be less interested in the *fine print*.

Conclusions

As the near elimination of *sudden death* by the ICD is undisputed, the question "does ICD prolong life?" really implies that ICD therapy simply converts patients' *mode* of death from sudden to nonsudden (e.g., CHF), with little or no extension of life. This conversion theory is refuted by multiple reports, showing that death *imminently* following successful ICD therapy is rare and by the fact that patients who do receive shocks live just as long as those free of VT/VF, implying (*strongly*) that the ICD simply eradicated these *premature* causes of death, allowing the patient to live out his or her life.

Furthermore, this theory overlooks the role of ATP therapy in *preventing* the degeneration of stable VT into polymorphic VT or VF. The *AVID* study runs a considerable possibility of patient selection bias, by enrolling low-risk patients often well protected by drugs and, at the other extreme, those with significant competing CHF risk. This bias, combined with patients crossing over from drugs to ICDs, makes it unlikely for ICD therapy to show benefit. Unfortunately, the study is not sufficiently powered to demonstrate which, if any, specific subgroups do benefit from the ICD. In summary, there is overwhelming clinical evidence, from multiple sources, demonstrating that the ICD prolongs life in appropriately selected patients. It does so by preventing sudden death and often by terminating arrhythmias which would lead to cardiac arrest. The *degree* of the ICD's contribution to survival depends largely on patient selection. Questions concerning *quality of life, cost-effectiveness,* role of concomitant drug or ablative therapy, the ICD's role in *prophylaxis,* and many others are legitimate questions which warrant ongoing and future research efforts.

Acknowledgment. The author wishes to acknowledge the expert counsel of *Dr. Rich Fogoros*, Pittsburgh, PA, for portions of this article.

References

1. Kim, S, Fisher J, Furman S et al (1991) Benefits of implantable defibrillators are overestimated by sudden death rates and better represented by the total arrhythmic death rate. J Am Coll Cardiol 17: 1587-1592
2. Kim S (1993) Implantable defibrillator therapy: does it really prolong life? How can we prove it? Am J Cardiol 71: 1213-1218
3. Levine J, Mellits E, Baumgardner R, Veltri E et al (1991) Predictors of first discharge and subsequent survival in patients with automatic implantable cardioverter defibrillators. Circulation 84 : 558-566
4. Fogoros R, Fiedler S, Elson J (1987) The automatic implantable cardioverter defibrillator in drug-refractory ventricular arrhythmias. Ann Intern Med 107 : 635-641
5. Newman D, Sauve J, Herre J et al (1992) Survival after implantation of the cardioverter defibrillator. Am J Cardiol 69: 889-903
6. Böcker D, Block M, Isbruch F, Wietholt D et al (1993) Do patients with an implantable defibrillator live longer? J Am Coll Cardiol 21:1638-1644
7. Schlepper M, Neuzner J, Pitschner H (1995) Implantable cardioverter defibrillator: effect on survival. PACE 18: 569-578
8. Greene H, CASCADE Investigators (1991) Cardiac arrest in Seattle: conventional versus amiodarone drug evaluation: the Cascade Study. Am J Cardiol 67: 578-584
9. CASCADE Investigators (1993) Randomized antiarrhythmic drug therapy in survivors of cardiac arrest (the CASCADE Study). Am J Cardiol 72: 280-287
10. Powell A, Finkelstein D, Garan H et al (1993) Influence of implantable cardioverter-defibrillators on the long-term prognosis of survivors of out-of-hospital cardiac arrest. Circulation 88: 1083-1092
11. Myerburg R, Luceri R, Thurer R et al (1989) Time to first shock and clinical outcome in patients receiving an automatic implantable cardioverter defibrillator. J Am Coll Cardiol 14 : 508-514
12. Mehta D, Saksena S, Krol R (1992) Survival of implantable cardioverter-defibrillator recipients: role of left ventricular function and its relationship to device use. Am Heart J 124: 1608-1614
13. Wever E, Hauer R, Van Capelle F et al (1995) Randomized study of implantable defibrillator as first-choice therapy versus conventional strategy in postinfarct sudden death survivors. Circulation 91:2195-2203
14. Gartman D, Bardy G, Allen M et al (1990) Short-term morbidity and mortality of implantation of automatic implantable cardioverter-defibrillator. J Thorac Cardiovasc Surg. 100 : 353-359
15. Connolly S, Yusuf S (1992) Evaluation of the implantable cardioverter defibrillator in survivors of cardiac arrest: the need for randomized trials. Am J Cardiol 69: 959-962
16. Fogoros R (1994) An AVID Dissent (Editorial). PACE 17:1707-1710
17. Sweeney M, Ruskin J (1994) Mortality benefits and the implantable cardioverter defibrillator. Circulation 89: 1851-1858
18. Greene H (1994) Antiarrhythmic drugs versus implantable defibrillators: the need for a randomized controlled study. Am Heart J 127: 1171-1178

What Are the Acute and Long-Term Results of Transvenous Implantable Cardioverter Defibrillators?

G. Gasparini, A. Raviele, and S. Themistoclakis

for the Italian Endotak Investigator Group*

Divisione di Cardiologia, Ospedale Umberto I, Mestre-Venice, Italy

The clinical experience with implantable cardioverter defibrillators (ICD) has been limited for many years almost exclusively to devices requiring thoracotomy for placement of one or more epicardial electrodes. This has generated a significant perioperative mortality and morbidity (1,2) and has reduced the widespread clinical application of such a therapy. In the last few years, different transvenous systems have been developed and introduced into clinical practice (3-12). One of these systems (Endotak, CPI, St Paul, MN, USA) has been extensively evaluated in Italy since 1990 by means of a multicenter trial (37 centers). In this paper the results of this trial are reported.

Methods

Between October 1990 and July 1994 a total of 307 patients were enrolled by the 37 participating centers in the Italian Endotak multicenter trial. The indications for ICD implantation were: (a) documented cardiac arrest due to ventricular tachyarrhythmia unrelated to transient or reversible clinical events; (b) sustained ventricular tachycardia either spontaneously recurring or still inducible despite drug therapy.

The CPI Endotak lead system, which has been described in previous reports (3-7, 10, 12), consists of an endocardial electrode catheter (Endotak C), a subcutaneous/submuscolar patch electrode (Endotak SQ), or a subcutaneous lead array (SQ array) and a connector (Endotak Y). The pulse generators used in this trial were the CPI Ventak models (P, P2, PRX, PRX2). The implantation procedure has been extensively described in previous papers (3-5, 13).

The defibrillation threshold (DFT; defined as the lowest converting energy) was established provided that the clinical condition of the patient was sufficiently stable to allow it. Otherwise, only the capability of the implanting system to defibrillate with a safety margin (at least 10 J less than the maximum power of the

ICD) was assessed. Initial defibrillation attempts were with 20 J. If ventricular fibrillation was successfully interrupted with this energy, termination was then attempted at progressively lower energies with 5-J reductions until the first failure occurred. Successful conversion at 5 J was generally accepted without further attempts. If the first shock at 20 J failed, the endocardial electrode was repositioned and/or the SQ patch or SQ array was inserted to test different lead configurations and to lower the DFT. A lead configuration was considered to be appropriate for permanent implantation if at least one successful conversion occurred at 20 J with a 30-J pulse generator (Ventak P) or if at least one successful conversion occurred at 25 J with a 35-J pulse generator (Ventak P2, PRX, PRX2). In the case of DFT with an inadequate safety margin (less than 10 J) the decision to definitively implant the system with an endocardial approach was left to the implanting physician.

In most patients prior to hospital discharge and/or 8-12 weeks after implantation, the ability of the implanted system to correctly sense and to convert ventricular fibrillation was tested in the electrophysiology laboratory. Subsequently, follow-up outpatient visits were scheduled every 2 – 3 months.

Definition of Terms

The terms involved were defined as followed: *perioperative mortality*, death from any cause within 30 days after ICD implantation; *sudden cardiac death mortality*, instantaneous (within 5 min from the onset of symptoms) or unwitnessed death, usually during sleep; *non-sudden cardiac death mortality*, witnessed death determined to be cardiac in nature and occurring not instantaneously; *cardiac death mortality*, sudden and non sudden cardiac deaths; *total mortality*, deaths from all causes; *appropriate ICD shocks*, shocks associated with documented ventricular tachyarrhythmia or those that were preceded by symptoms of severe dizziness, presyncope or syncope; *inappropriate shocks*, shocks associated with documented supraventricular tachyarrhythmias or sinus tachycardia or those that were not preceded by specific symptoms.

* *The list of investigators is reported in the Appendix of the original work published in PACE (1995) 18:599-608.*

Statistics

The data are presented as mean values ± SD unless otherwise specified. Life table analysis and actuarial analysis were performed using the Kaplan-Meier method. Differences in continuous variables were computed by means of the Wilcoxon test, and groups were compared by means of the chi-square test. Multivariate analysis was performed using logistic regression analysis with the method of backward regression.

Differences were considered statistically significant at $p < 0.05$.

Results

The clinical characteristics of the patient population are summarized in Table 1. Chronic ischemic heart disease was present in 205 patients (66.5%). The mean left ventricular ejection fraction was 33.3 ± 12.7% (range, 10% – 81%). The presenting arrhythmia was ventricular tachycardia in 172 cases (56%), ventricular fibrillation in 130 (42.5%), and unknown in five (1.5%). Each patient underwent a mean of 2.0±1.2 (range, 0 – 6) unsuccessful drug trials before ICD implantation. At least one pharmacologic agent was tested in 251 of 278 (90%) patients in whom data on drug therapy were available. Amiodarone was tested in the majority of these cases (237 of 278, 85%).

A total of 112 patients (36.5%) received a pulse generator capable of delivering monophasic shocks (models Ventak P and PRX) and 195 (63.5%) a pulse generator capable of delivering biphasic shocks (models Ventak P2 and PRX2). In 216 patients (73%) the implanted device did not have antitachycardia pacing capability (models Ventak P and P2) and in 91 (27%) it did (models Ventak PRX and PRX2).

Transvenous lead system implantation was done in 306 of the 307 patients (99.7%). The mean DFT for all 307 patients was 16.9 ± 5.7 J. The DFT (stepwise reduction until failure) was determined in 133 patients (43%). The mean value of DFT was significantly lower in patients that received biphasic shocks than in patients that received monophasic shocks (15.3 ± 5.2 J versus 19.6 ± 5.4 J; $p < 0.0001$). The remaining 173 patients (57%) were implanted with the Endotak system without assessing the DFT. All of them had ventricular fibrillation induced and successfully interrupted at least once at 20-25 J. The DFT showed a safety margin of at least 10 J vis-à-vis the maximum power of the ICD in 287 of the 307 patients (93.5%). The percentage of subjects that had a safety margin of ten or more was significantly higher among patients tested with biphasic than with monophasic shocks (192 of 195, 98% versus 95 of 112, 85%; $p < 0.0001$). Nineteen patients (6.2%) had an inadequate safety margin (i.e., less than 10 J). All of these 19 patients were definitively implanted with the Endotak system. In one patient (0.3%) the DFT exceeded the maximum power of the ICD; in this patient a mixed approach was utilized, consisting in the implantation of an epicardial patch in conjunction with the endocardial catheter.

Apart from a monophasic morphology of waveform shock, other variables were associated with a low safety margin, as reported in Table 2.

Among the 306 patients that finally received the Endotak system, lead configuration 3 was implanted in 164 (53%), lead configuration 2 in 134 (44%), and lead configuration 1 in four (1.3%). In four patients (1.3%) the type of configuration used was not reported. The percentage of subjects in whom an endocardial lead without the need for an SQ patch or SQ array (configuration 3) was 81% (158 of 195) in patients whose pulse generator was capable of delivering biphasic shocks.

The implanted defibrillation system was retested before hospital discharge and after 2-3 months of follow-up in 141 (46%) and 51 (17%) patients, respectively. In all patients the induced ventricular fibrillation was correctly sensed and terminated by the ICD.

No perioperative deaths occurred. Thirty patients (9.9%) developed early complications within a 30-day

Table 1. Clinical characteristics of patients ($n = 307$)

Characteristics	Patients	
	(n)	(%)
Men	267	87.0
Women	40	13.0
Organic heart disease	305	99.3
Coronary artery disease	205	66.5
Dilated cardiomyopathy	64	21.0
Hypertrophic cardiomyopathy	5	1.6
Arrhythmogenic RVD	14	4.6
Other heart disease	17	5.6
Presenting arrhythmia		
Sustained ventricular tachycardia	172	56.0
Syncopal	120	39.0
Not syncopal	52	17.0
Ventricular fibrillation	130	42.5
Not reported	5	1.5
Inducibility at baseline EPS	245/279	88.0
Refractory to drugs	251/278	90.0
Amiodarone therapy	237/278	85.0

The mean age was 57.5 years, the mean left ventricular ejection fraction (LVEF) was 33.3%, and the mean number of drug trials was two.
EPS, electrophysiologic study; RVD: right ventricular dysplasia.

Table 2. Factors associated with a high defibrillation threshold (DFT) at implantation

	Patients with DFT ≤ 20-25 J ($n = 287$)	Patients with DFT > 20-25 J ($n = 20$)
Monophasic shock (%)*	33	85
NYHA class higher than 2 (%)**	22	47
Mean LVEF (%)***	34 ± 13	29 ± 14
Mean number of drugs tested***	2.2 ± 1.2	1.4 ± 1.0
VF as presenting Arrhythmia (%)**	40	63

DFT, defibrillation threshold; LVEF, left ventricular ejection fraction; NYHA, New York Heart Association; VF, ventricular fibrillation.
* $p < 0.0001$ (univariate and multivariate)
** $p < 0.05$ (univariate); $p < 0.01$ (multivariate)
*** $p < 0.05$ (univariate); p, not significant (multivariate)

interval after ICD implantation (Table 3). Eight of these patients (2.7%) required surgical intervention.

Complete follow-up data are available for 271 patients. A total of 146 of these patients (54%) were discharged from the hospital on antiarrhythmic drug therapy.

The mean duration of follow-up was 14.5 ± 10.2 months (range, 1 – 38 months). During this period (Table 4), 30 patients (11%) died, six (2.2%) from sudden cardiac death, 21 (7.7%) from non-sudden cardiac death, and three (1.1%) from a noncardiac death. As shown in Table 5, the cumulative probability of survival at 12 and 36 months of follow-up was 98% and 96% for sudden death, 91.2% and 82% for cardiac death, and 90% and 80% for total death, respectively. Patients who died from a cardiac cause were significantly older than the remaining patients (mean age, 64.2 ± 9.0 years versus 56.8 ± 13.4 years, respectively; $p < 0.0001$). Moreover, they had a lower left ventricular ejection fraction (29.8 ± 12% versus 34.1 ± 13%; $p < 0.05$) and higher NYHA functional class ($p < 0.01$).

During the follow-up period, 157 patients (58%) received at least one spontaneous shock (range, one to 290 shocks; mean, 13.3 shocks per patient). The shocks were considered appropriate in 74% of the episodes and inappropriate in 26%. A total of 94 patients (60%) received only appropriate shocks, 17 (11%) only inappropriate shocks and 46 (29%) both appropriate and inappropriate shocks. The mean time to the first appropriate shock was 4.4 ± 5.1 months (range, 0 – 30 months). By life-table analysis (Table 5), the cumulative incidence of first appropriate shock occurrence was 57% and 72% at 12 and 36 months of follow-up and that of first inappropriate shock occurrence, 31% and 38% at the same time intervals, respectively. A left ventricular ejection fraction greater than 30% and a higher NYHA functional class were both predictive of an high recurrence rate of appropriate shocks ($p < 0.05$ and $p < 0.001$, respective-

ly). Patients with inappropriate shocks were taking antiarrhythmic drugs more frequently than the remaining patients (70% versus 49%, $p < 0.05$).

Late complications occurred in 14 patients (5.1%) (Table 6). Twelve of these patients (4.4%) required surgical intervention. Interestingly, the lead insulation break, always responsible for oversensing problems and inappropriate shocks, occurred at the level of the abdominal pocket, where the yoke joins with the connectors, in five patients (2.0%) and at the level of subclavicular area where the clavicle crosses the first rib in one patient (0.3%). The mean time between ICD implant and lead insulation break was 17.8 ± 6.0 months (range, 11 – 30 months).

The 19 patients that were definitively implanted with the Endotak system, despite the DFT showing an inadequate safety margin at implantation, had a significantly higher incidence of cardiac death during the follow-up compared to the remaining patients (25% versus 8.7%, $p < 0.05$). In contrast, sudden death mortality and appropriate and inappropriate shock occurrence rates were similar in the two groups of patients.

Conclusion

In summary the main findings of the present study are the following:

1. The Endotak lead system is permanently implantable with an adequate safety margin in 93.5% of cases; implantation is possible with an endocardial lead alone without the need for an additional SQ patch or SQ array in 53% of cases. These values increase to 98% and 81%, respectively, when a device capable of delivering a biphasic shock is used.

Table 3. Early complications after implantable cardioverter defibrillator (ICD) implant (within 30-day interval)

	Patients	
	(n)	(%)
Cerebrovascular accident	2	0.7
Pulmonary embolism	1	0.3
Pneumothorax	3	1.0
Paralytic ileum	2	0.7
Pocket infection[a]	4	1.3
Pocket hematoma[b]	9	2.9
Lead dislodgment[c]	9	2.9

[a]Requiring ICD explantation in two patients (0.7%).
[b]Requiring surgical revision in one patient (0.3%).
[c]Requiring lead repositioning in five patients (1.7%).

Table 4. Patient mortality (271 patients with complete follow-up data)

	Patients	
	(n)	(%)
Perioperative mortality	0	0
Sudden death	6	2.2
Cardiac death	21	7.7
Noncardiac death	3	1.1
Total death	30	11

Table 5. Kaplan-Meier actuarial event-free rates (%)

	6 month	12 month	24 month	36 month
Sudden death	98	98	96	96
Cardiac death	95.6	91.2	82	82
Total death	94.6	90	80	80
Appropriate shock	47	43	34	28
Inappropriate shock	73	69	62	62
Any shock	43	37	28	23

Table 6. Late complications[a]

	Patients	
	(n)	(%)
Superior vena cava thrombosis	2	0.7
Pocket infection[b]	2	0.7
Lead dislodgment[c]	2	0.7
Sensing pin disconnection[d]	2	0.7
Lead insulation break[e]	6	2.3

[a] One month or more after implantable cardioverter defibrillator (ICD) implantation.
[b] Requiring ICD explantation in both.
[c] Requiring lead repositioning in both.
[d] Requiring ICD replacement in both.
[e] Requiring Endotak lead repair in one patient (0.3%), insertion of a second endocardial lead for sensing in four patients (1.4%), and Endotak lead removal and epicardial leads and patches placement in one patient (0.3%).

2. The implantation is not associated with perioperative mortality, and the incidence of early complications is small (about 10%).

3. The clinical outcome of the implanted patients is satisfactory. The 1- and 3-year actuarial incidences of sudden death are 2% and 4%, respectively, and that of total death 10% and 20%, respectively.

4. The long-term efficacy and reliability of the system is good, with a high cumulative recurrence rate of appropriate shocks (57% and 72% at 1 and 3 years, respectively) and a relatively low incidence of ICD related problems.

In conclusion, the results of this study show that the CPI Endotak lead system may be implanted with a good safety margin and utilizing only the endocardial lead in almost all patients, provided that a device capable of delivering a biphasic shock is used. Implantation is safe, easy, and not complicated by major problems. The long-term performance, efficacy, and reliability of the system is good, with a relatively low incidence of sudden death, cardiac death, and total mortality. Late complications are rare, and the integrity of the system seems to remain unchanged during a relatively long period of time in the vast majority of patients.

References

1. Mosteller RD, Lehman MH, Thomas AC, Jackson K and Participating Investigators (1991) Operative mortality with implantation of the automatic cardioverter-defibrillator. Am J Cardiol 68: 1340-1345
2. Grimm W, Flores BF, Marchlinski FE (1993) Complications of implantable cardioverter defibrillator therapy: follow-up of 241 patients. PACE 16: 218-222
3. Saksena S, Parsonnet V (1988) Implantation of a cardioverter-defibrillator without thoracotomy using a triple electrode system. JAMA 259: 69-72
4. Tullo NG, Saksena S, Krol KB, Mauro AM, Kunecz D (1990) Management of complications associated with a first-generation endocardial defibrillation lead system for implantable cardioverter-defibrillators. Am J Cardiol 66: 411-415
5. McCowan R, Maloney J, Wilkoff B et al (1991) Automatic implantable cardioverter-defibrillator implantation without thoracotomy using an endocardial and submuscolar patch system. J Am Coll Cardiol 17: 415-421
6. Hauser RG, Kurschinski DT, McVeigh K, Thomas A, Mower MM (1993) Clinical results with nonthoracotomy ICD system. PACE 16: 141-152
7. Neuzner J for the European Ventak P2 Investigator Group (1994) Clinical experience with a new cardioverter defibrillator capable of biphasic waveform pulse and enhanced data storage: results of a prospective multicenter study. PACE 17: 1243-1255
8. Bardy GH, Hofer B, Johnson G (1993) Implantable transvenous cardioverter-defibrillators. Circulation 87: 1152-1168
9. Saksena S for the PCD Investigator Group (1994) Clinical outcome of patients with malignant ventricular tachyarrhythmias and a multiprogrammable implantable cardioverter-defibrillator with and without thoracotomy: an international multicenter study. J Am Coll Cardiol 23: 1521-1530
10. Bardy GH, Johnson G, Poole JE et al (1993) A simplified, single lead unipolar transvenous cardioversion-defibrillation system. Circulation 88: 543-547
11. Sra JS, Natale A, Axtell K et al (1994) Experience with two different nonthoracotomy system for implantable defibrillator in 170 patients. PACE 17: 1741-1750
12. Brachmann J, Sterns LD, Hilbel T et al (1994) Acute efficacy and chronic follow-up with non-thoracotomy third generation implantable defibrillators. PACE 17: 499-505
13. Jordaens L, Vertongen P, Van Belleghem Y (1993) A subcutaneous lead array for implantable cardioverter defibrillators. PACE 16: 1429-1433

How To Prevent or Avoid Inappropriate Implantable Cardioverter Defibrillator Shocks?

A. Auricchio and H. Klein

Klinik für Kardiologie, Angiologie und Pulmologie, Medizinische Fakultät,
Otto-Von-Guericke-Universität, Magdeburg, Germany

Multiple reports from different institutions around the world have definitively demonstrated the efficacy of implantable cardioverter defibrillator (ICD) in the treatment of malignant ventricular tachyarrhythmias and in the prevention of sudden cardiac death. Despite efforts to reduce defibrillator size and defibrillation threshold while continuing to provide more sophisticated tiered therapy, inappropriate ICD discharges remain a relatively frequent clinical problem; in fact, it has been reported that about one-third of all shocks are delivered for reasons other than ventricular tachyarrhythmias. Frequent ICD shocks can cause pain and may impair ventricular function and quality-of-life of patients with an ICD. Repetitive activations may also determine early battery depeletion or finally be proarrhythmic (1) and even fatal (2).

Diagnosis of inappropriate ICD disharge is based on (a) the documentation of a delivered shock and on (b) the demonstration of the cardiac rhythm, which by definition should not be a sustained episode of ventricular tachycardia (VT) or fibrillation (VF) before or during the ICD discharge. Until recently, the diagnosis of inappropriate shocks has mainly been made on the basis of clinical symptoms; however, several reports have demonstrated that symptoms are not reliable either for identifying the type of arrhythmia or for qualifying the appropriateness of ICD discharge (3, 4). Thus, there have been cases of ICD patients imagining or dreaming of shocks that never took place (5). A difficult clinical question is the significance of an ICD discharge in an asymptomatic patient – which by no means is proof that the shock was inappropriate, since it is well known that up to 30% of "inappropriately" delivered shocks are subsequently validated as appropriate by means of stored intracardiac electrograms (IEGM) (6, 7). The clinical history – whether the patient received single discharges or repetitive shocks over a few hours – can often lead to a correct diagnosis. The occurrence of single shocks is typical of ICD discharges for VT, whereas repetitive shocks often indicate inappropriate shocks. However, exceptions to this rule exist; incessant VT$_s$ or recurrent VT$_s$ due to electrolyte imbalance, ischemia, proarrhythmic effects

of an antiarrhythmic drug, or worsening of congestive heart failure could continuously trigger the device, appearing as repetitive firing, thus simulating an episode of supraventricular arrhythmias.

It is largely accepted that symptoms such as palpitation, dizziness, or even presyncope are less specific and less sensitive for ventricular tachyarrhythmias, occurring with similar frequency during supraventricular as well as ventricular arrhythmias (6, 7). Unlike these "classical" symptoms of arrhythmias (i.e., palpitation, dizziness, etc.), we recently reported that the sudden onset of a warm feeling arising from the epigastrum and/or a generalized "hot flush" is more frequently associated with ventricular tachyarrhythmias (6). Because of the lack of correlation between symptoms and sustained VT or VF, the implication is that for the diagnosis of inappropriate shocks an electrocardiogram (ECG) documentation at the time of ICD discharges is absolutely necessary.

Until the recent introduction of stored IEGM, inappropriate ICD therapy was occasionally documented by fortuitous ECG recordings at the time of ICD discharge. The telemetry for most current ICD$_s$ provides detailed therapy information as well as IEGM preceding and leading up to the shock (Fig. 1). Once it is clear that shocks have occurred, it is necessary to determine their etiology. The use of IEGM has considerably

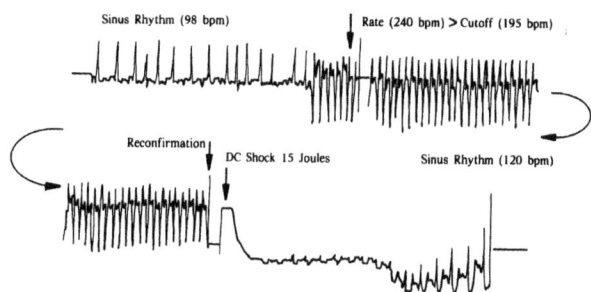

Fig. 1. Intracardiac stored electrogram recorded in a patient affected by a dilatative cardiomyopathy, resuscitated from a cardiac arrest and implanted with a two-zone device (Ventak P2, CPI). The device was triggered by a spontaneous episode of sustained ventricular monomorphic tachycardia (240 bpm) which was terminated by a single shock at 15 J

enhanced the diagnostic process and helped in troubleshooting.

Two different modalities of IEGM recordings have been implemented in the most recent generation of devices: the "far-field" IEGM recorded from endocardial shock lead (Fig. 1) and the short rate-sensing bipolar IEGM (Fig. 2). The far-field IEGM$_s$ provide clearer recordings of the atrial and ventricular relationship than the short rate-sensing bipolar IEGM$_s$ and are more sensitive and specific, thus more helpful, for determining the appropriateness of ICD therapy (8). Additional differences and advantages of each system have been extensively discussed elsewhere and are beyond the scope of this chapter (9).

Possible causes of inappropriate ICD discharge are listed in Table 1; they can be categorized by (a) problems of the discrimination algorithm, (b) problems of detection algorithm, or (c) hardware problems. Among the three, discrimination algorithm has been most frequently reported as the cause of inappropriate ICD discharge.

Discrimination Algorithm

Inappropriate detection of atrial fibrillation and sinus tachycardia is still a significant problem even in the third-generation devices with antitachycardia pacing (ATP). With slower VT, the probability of rate overlap between the target rate of VT and supraventricular arrhythmias is quite common. Cardioversion may induce atrial fibrillation, which may in turn be detected as VT and then treated by pacing or direct current (DC) shock, with the risk of reinitiating VT or even VF. Such repetitive cycles have been reported and may have a fatal outcome. Among the causes of inappropriate shocks, sinus tachycardia occurs in about 9% of patients (10); it occurs most commonly in patients with slow VT due to overlap between the lowest programmed zone of therapy and the maximum sinus heart rate. Since ATP schemes are frequently used in the lowest zone, sinus tachycardia could trigger ATP leading to VT or VF. Inappropriate shocks for sinus tachycardia have also been described with the one-zone device, especially in young patients who are capable of a high sinus rate during physical activity. Another discrimination criterion is therefore necessary, i.e., the sudden onset criterion. This is an optional detection feature available in most of the most recent generation of ICD. The "sudden onset" criterion attempts to discriminate sinus tachycardia, which accelerates slowly, from VT, which in contrast begins abruptly (11, 12).

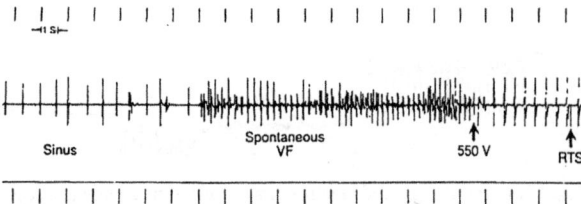

Fig. 2. Spontaneous episode of ventricular fibrillation (*VF*) in a patient implanted with a Cadence V100 (Ventritex). The device correctly identified the arrhythmia, which was promptly terminated by single DC shock. *RTS*, return to sinus.

Table 1. Possible etiology of inappropriate implantable cardioverter defibrillator (ICD) therapy

Discrimination algorithm
  Sinus tachycardia
  Sustained or paroxysmal atrial flutter or fibrillation, with rapid
    ventricular conduction
  Nonsustained ventricular tachycardia

Detection algorithm
  T wave or P wave oversensing
  Pacemaker "spike" or evoked potentials

Hardware problems
  Lead fracture, insulation break, loose set screws, dislodgment
  Detection algorithms
  Outside source (EMI, MRI, electrocautery)

EMI, electromagnetic interference; MRI, magnetic resonance imaging.

When the sudden onset criterion is "on," VT detection will not occur unless the onset algorithm is satisfied; some ICD use a percentage of rate change calculated either as an average of the four most recent events (PCD Jewel, Medtronic) or as the difference between adjacent intervals for the five intervals on each side of the lowest rate boundary (Ventak Prx, CPI); others require a sudden onset delta in milliseconds (Cadence, Ventritex). Regardless of the ICD programming, the use of sudden onset as a criterion appears to be able to reduce significantly the incidence of ICD activation (13, 14). In fact, Swerdlow et al. (12), analyzing the value of sudden onset in rejecting sinus acceleration, found a most appropriate mean value of 84% for the PCD onset ratio algorithm. By programming an onset ratio of 87%, they prevented inappropriate detection of sinus acceleration during follow-up and provided a substantial safety margin above the values that permitted detection of all episodes of VF. Similarly, Pitschner et al. (13), using the Ventak Prx2 algorithm programmed at a value of 10%, avoided device intervention in sinus tachycardia without affecting the sensitivity of VT detection.

More frequently inappropriate shocks are due to recurrent paroxysmal episodes of sustained supraventricular tachyarrhythmias, i.e., atrial flutter or fibrillation with rapid conduction to the ventricles exceeding the programmed cutoff rates. In fact, using stored IEGM to verify the cause of inappropriate shocks, Neuzner et al. (3) recently reported that atrial fibrillation accounts for 86% of all inappropriate ICD discharged. Data supporting the diagnosis of inappropriate discharge comes first and foremost from knowledge or investigation of the patients' susceptibility to such rhythm and whether their atrial fibrillation could result in ventricular rates that could trigger the ICD. Since all ICD detection algorithms are based on "rate," correct counting of the number or the R-R intervals is most important. Thus any arrhythmia that has a heart rate higher than the programmed cutoff rate, regardless of its origin, will trigger the ICD to an alert position; then, when the programmed duration delay is satisfied, the ICD will start capacitor charging and finally, after fulfilling the reconfirmation algorithm, will deliver the therapy. Since heart rate at the beginning of an episode of paroxysmal atrial fibrillation or flutter is generally high (150-170 bpm), this leads to early activation of the device.

From a clinical point of view, it is possible to reduce the number of inappropriate shocks by using antiarrhythmic drugs, selecting additional criteria, such as stability rate, or even by interruption or modulation of the atrioventricular conduction. Although both antiarrhythmic drugs and selection of the rate stability criterion are valid options, each can potentially have a negative impact on ICD efficacy. In fact, the use of antiarrhythmic drugs can slow down the VT rate, thus potentially affecting ATP, or can modify the pacing/defibrillation threshold. We also have to bear in mind that antiarrhythmic drugs may become proarrhythmic. Selection of rate stability could potentially lead to VT being missed (15, 16).

Digitalis is one of the most commonly used drugs for controlling heart rate during atrial fibrillation at rest, but it often fails to adequately control the ventricular response during exercise. Beta blockers and calcium antagonists may be very useful antiarrhythmic drugs for reducing heart rate both at rest and during exercise as well as for preventing the recurrence of atrial tachyarrhythmias. Since a large proportion of patients with an ICD have poor ventricular function and are in NYHA (New York Heart Association) class II-III (17), and therefore in need of inotropic and lusitropic support, our preference is the use of these drugs as the first option with subsequent addition of amiodarone.

Radiofrequency ablation of the atrioventricular node in order to create complete atrio-ventricular block has been proposed as an alternative therapy to antiarrhythmic drug use, but has rarely been performed in patients with an ICD. This is probably related to the lack of either dual-chamber pacing and/or activity-controlled pacing even in the modern ICD generation. Recently, modulation of the atrioventricular node has been proposed as a more effective therapy instead of complete interruption of the atrioventricular conduction during atrial fibrillation (18). Although modulation of the atrioventricular node could be a useful technique, no data are available, at the present time, in patients with cardioverter-defibrillators.

Stability is an optional detection feature available in many commercially available ICD. The main objective of this algorithm is to reject atrial fibrillation that conducts rapidly to the ventricle with a rather wide R-R variability. Other rhythms, such as polymorphic nonsustained VT and complex ventricular ectopy, which usually do not respond well to APT therapy may also be rejected. Studies on VT rate variability revealed a mean cycle length difference of about 7% (19) at its onset, decreasing over time (20); in addition, slower VT had more variability in the R-R cycle length, and 45% of all VT stabilized within the first 15 beats (21). Although algorithms for stability criterion of different devices have similar endpoints, we should be aware of some possibly significant differences in the algorithms present in various devices. The difference in device algorithms may translate into fairly important clinical differences and thus comparison among published studies may be difficult (12, 22). Since the rate stability algorithm influences device sensitivity, selection of an appropriate parameter is crucial; at the present time, it is selected empirically and therefore

represents an enormous source of error. Some recent ICD (Ventak Prx2 and Prx3, CPI) automatically generate sudden onset and stability rate valued (even if they are not selected) when the device is activated by a spontaneously occurring arrhythmia. The use of these values in combination with IEGM facilitates considerably the selection of the most appropriate values (13).

An unresolved problem for supraventricular arrhythmia discrimination is the occurrence of atrial flutter with rapid stable conduction to the ventricle. This type of supraventricular arrhythmia is very difficult to distinguish from VT using current algorithms because it fulfills similar criteria for sudden onset and rate stability as VT. Therefore, at the present time, no reliable method exists other than pharmacologic control of ventricular rate or of the flutter circuit ablation or modulation of the atrioventricular node.

Another, fortunately rare, source of inappropriate ICD discharge is nonsustained VT, i.e., a VT that terminates spontaneously prior to ICD discharge. Due to the possibility of retrieving stored IEGM, it has been identified as a seldom, but existing cause of inappropriate discharge. According to a recently published series (23), these events could account for 10% of all ICD shocks detected by first- and second-generation device. The main reason for inappropriate shocks is the lack of programmability of a detection delay as well as a reconfirmation algorithm during and after the capacitor charging. Although significantly diminished by the introduction of programmable detection delays and of device commitment, inappropriate discharges still occur. Severe symptoms and possibly a rise in the ventricular cardioversion defibrillation threshold can occur by significantly prolonging the detection delay; careful evaluation of the hemodynamics during induced ventricular tachyarrhythmias is needed before altering the detection delay. In particular, a noncommitted therapy has a great advantage over the prolongation of detection delay. The reconfirmation algorithm requires confirmation of the detected arrhythmia prior to shock delivery and will abort the therapy if the rate criterion is no longer fulfilled. Almost all devices are now able to reconfirm the actual arrhythmia prior to discharge (Fig. 3). The detection delay and the device commitment feature, however, should not be considered as alternatives, but as complementary features.

Detection Algorithm

One particular problem for inappropriate ICD shocks are pacemaker–defibrillator interactions. The first generation of ICD had no antibradycardia pacing features, which not rarely become necessary. Since the conventional pacemaker has a fixed sensing gain, VT or VF could not be recognized appropriately; therefore, the pacemaker paced during the ongoing ventricular tachyarrhythmias and thus prevented the pacing spike being taken as an R wave. In contrast, oversensing of atrial and ventricular pacemaker spikes by ICD could alert the device and again generate inappropriate discharges. The pacemaker–defibrillator interaction has mostly been overcome by the third-generation ICD

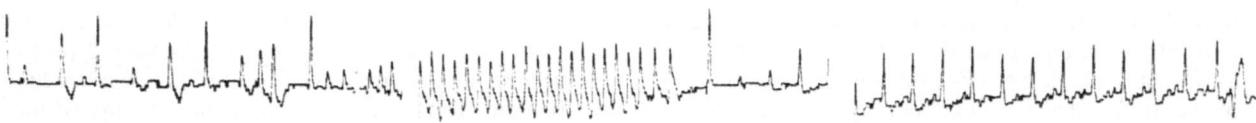

↓10 mm/s

Fig. 3. Spontaneous episode of rapid ventricular tachycardia (203 bpm) which was detected by the device. The reconfirmation algorithm of the implantable cardioverter-defibrillator (Ventak Prx2) was activated and continuously monitored the rate of the ongoing tachycardia. Since the tachycardia spontaneously terminated during the charging phase, the reconfirmation algorithm stopped it, and after the restoration of sinus rhythm (82 bpm), the shock was internally diverted

systems, which have the capability for bradycardia pacing as well as ATP and cardioversion/defibrillation (24, 25). However, pacemaker-defibrillator interactions still occur in third-generation devices (26), most specifically in the Ventritex Cadence tiered therapy defibrillator system (Ventritex, Inc). Analysis of real time and stored IEGM not rarely revealed intermittent high-frequency, large-amplitude noise as well as oversensing of maximally gained R and T waves as a result of a feature of the Cadence device itself (26). The Cadence models use an automatic gain circuit to sense incoming signals. During pacing for bradycardia, the sensitivity is maximally increased to prevent undersensing of an arrhythmia with small-amplitude signals (Fig. 4). Signals of a different nature, such as muscular noise and P or T waves can be sensed as VT or VF, thus activating the device (Fig. 4) and eventually leading to inappropriate DC shock. Reprogramming of the device by prolonging the postpacing refractory period, implantation of a separate permanent pacemaker, or using a different device are possible solutions to avoid further inappropriate ICD activations.

Hardware Failure

Hardware failure can lead to inappropriate ICD discharges, inadequate discharges, or missing of the arrhythmia. Several different failure modalities have been described, including lead fracture or dislodgment (27, 28), connector insulation or fracture, sensing of electrical or magnet interference (29), or, on rare occasions, device malfunction (30, 31).

Most commonly, a lead fracture or dislodgment is responsible for repetitive inappropriate ICD discharges. Chest X-rays are most important to access the integrity of a lead system; stored and real-time IEGM also provide important information and the correct "failure" diagnosis. Finally, telemetric analysis of shock and/or pacing impedance and sensing provide detailed clues for a definitive diagnosis; infinite lead impedance – quite often intermittently – is indicative of a lead fracture, whereas insulation breaks will be associated with an abnormally low impedance. It is extremely important in cases of frequent inappropriate discharges as well as after a missed arrhythmia episode to analyze sensing and impedance of the pacing and shock lead. In the case of an isolated pacing problem, the implantation of a separate conventional pacing lead might become necessary instead of implanting ex novo defibrillation and pacing leads.

One example of combined sensing and pacing failure is presented in Fig. 5. The patient was implanted with a Ventak P2 and Endotak lead (CPI). One year

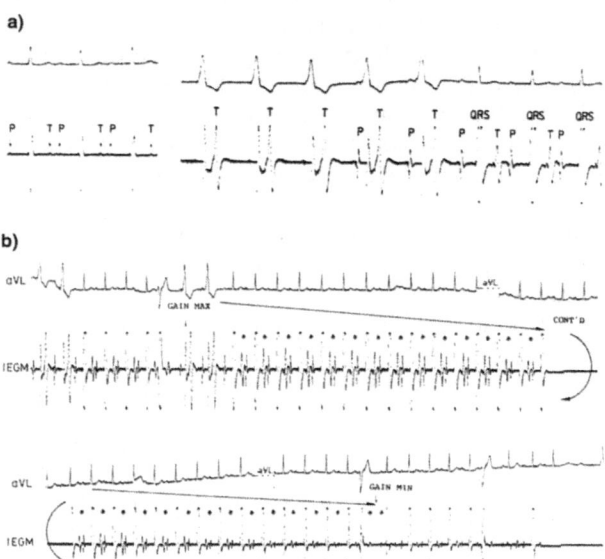

Fig. 4a,b. Stored intracardiac electrograms recorded in a patient implanted with a Cadence V100 V (Ventritex) receiving several documented inappropriate shocks. In sinus rhythm a large-amplitude R signal is evident, followed by two low-amplitude signals, corresponding to the T and P wave. During pacing (90 bpm), the automatic gain control of the Cadence maximally increases its sensitivity in order to prevent undersensing of any ventricular tachycardia (VT) or ventricular fibrillation (VF). By doing so, the small-amplitude signals (noted in sinus rhythm) were amplified with the result of a double count (QRS complex and T wave) which was still below the programmed cutoff rate (**a**). However, when the pacing rate was programmed to a value (55 bpm) similar to that of the sinus rhythm (56-58 bpm), soon after a ventricular pacing beat the device maximally increased the gain leading the triple count (QRS complex, P and T wave) which reached the cutoff rate of the device and activated it. Due to the slow decrease of the implantable cardioverter defibrillator (ICD) automatic gain control and the recurrence of pacing spike, the device reconfirmed the presence of the ventricular arrhythmia (but in reality the ICD continued to have a triple count) and could theoretically deliver a shock

after the first ICD implantation, the patient reported frequent device activations preceded by a dizzy spell or presyncope. Some of those device activations, which have been documented, were judged to be appropriate because of VT and VF. The analysis of counters, however, also demonstrated frequent, non-reconfirmed VT episodes. The clinical history prevented suspicion of inappropriate ICD interventions. The analysis of the shock impedance, however, demonstrated a sudden reduction of shock impedance while the pacing impedance was unchanged. The analysis of stored IEGM revealed sensing noise and pacing inhibition, due to a lead breakage of the distal shock coil. Because CPI devices use integrated bipolar endocardial sensing, the isolated rupture of the connection to the distal coil caused modification of pacing and shock impedance. Replacement of the shock lead and pacing lead com-

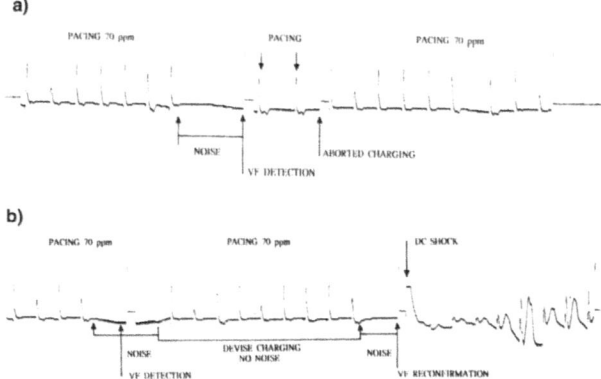

a)

b)

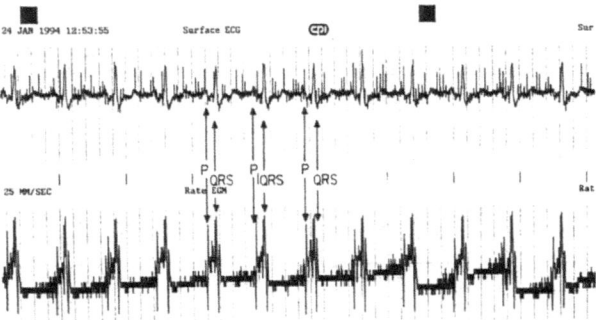

Fig. 6. Intracardiac electrogram (*EGM, bottom*) and surface electrocardiogram (*ECG, top*) in a patient experiencing recurrent implantable cardioverter defibrillator (ICD) discharges. Double sensing, P and QRS, due to macroscopic lead dislodgement was evident.

Fig. 5a,b. Stored intracardiac electrograms (IEGM) documenting lead defect. The patient with a chronic atrial fibrillation and low ventricular response (40 bpm) was pacemaker dependent (VVI at 70 bpm). Because of the insulation defect of the electrical connection to the distal coil of the Endotak, noise was detected by the device; this noise was recognized as ventricular fibrillation (*VF*), which inhibited pacing and triggered the device (**a, b**). Because the insulation breaks were intermittent and most likely related to body movements, the disappearance of the noise led to pacing resumption, while the reconfirmation algorithm detected the restoration of a regular rhythm and terminated the capacitor charging (**a**). In contrast, in **b**, the pacing was once again inhibited because of the reappearance of electrical noise while the reconfirmation algorithm redetected the persistence of ventricular fibrillation (noise) with the result of implantable cardioverter defibrillator (ICD) discharge. *DC*, direct current

pletely abolished inadequate ICD function. Lead dislodgment is a fairly common source of hardware failure; it can cause double counting of P or T waves (Fig. 6). On rare occasions, the lead dislodgment within the atrium can lead to mechanical induction of atrial fibrillation or flutter. Lead repositioning is most often an effective and sufficient maneuver to overcome this problem.

Detection Algorithm Failure

The detection algorithms themselves and their application through programming steps can lead to inappropriate shocks or inadequate interference of ATP. The occurrence of these shortcomings can usually be established from the device itself. Diagnosis of this failure remains important, since frequent aborted shocks can reduce the battery life considerably. This particular type of failure occurs mainly in an attempt to achieve 100% sensitivity for the detection of potentially dangerous arrhythmias, thus possibly inadvertently oversensitizing the device's detection parameters. Reprogramming the device is most often sufficient to eliminate this device failure.

Conclusion

We believe that inappropriate shocks continue to be a major problem in patients implanted with a cardioverter defibrillator for various types of ventricular tachyarrhythmias. Extensive programmability, misuse of ATP, and poor understanding of the underlying arrhythmia mechanism increases the likelihood of inappropriate discharges. Systematic troubleshooting involves categorizing the observed (or suspected) prob-

lems, and leads to appropriate measures being taken to avoid further failures. Paroxysmal supraventricular arrhythmias represent the most common source of inappropriate discharges, and a variety of helpful measures are available. Improvement of discriminating algorithms, the introduction of separate atrial and ventricular sensing leads, or better morphologic analysis of far-field IEGM might provide an acceptable solution in the near future. Furthermore, alternative options such as modulation of the atrioventricular node either pharmacologically or electrically are often useful methods. Finally, intensive cooperation between ICD engineers and manufacturers and implanting physicians will maximize the benefits from the use of all the available programmable modalities, which are often difficult to understand or to apply.

References

1. Cohen TJ, Chien WW, Lurie KG et al (1991) Implantable cardioverter defibrillator proarrhythmia: case report and review of the literature. Pace Pacing Clin Electrophysiol 14: 1326
2. Birgesdotted-Green U, Rosenqvist M, Lindemann FW et al (1991) Holter documented sudden death in a patient with an implanted defibrillation. Pace Pacing Clin Electrophysiol 15: 1008
3. Neuzner J (1994) Clinical experience with a new cardioverter defibrillator capable of biphasic waveform pulse and enhanced data storage: results of a prospective multicenter study. European Ventak P2 Investigator Group. Pace Pacing Clin Electrophysiol 17: 1243
4. Marchilinski FE, Gottlieb CD, Sarter B et al (1993) ICD data storage: value in arrhythmia management. Pace Pacing Clin Electrophysiol 16: 527
5. Kowey P, Marinchak R, Rial S (1992) Things that go back in the night. N Engl J Med 327: 1884
6. Auricchio A, Scafuri A, Auricchio U et al (1994) Sintomi ed eventi aritmici in pazienti portatori di defibrillatore automatico impiantabile. G Ital Cardiol 24: 1567
7. Hook BG, Marchilinski FE (1991) Value of ventricular electrogram recordings in the diagnosis of arrhythmias precipitating electrical device shock therapy. J Am Coll Cardiol 17: 985
8. Block M, Isbruch F, Clerc G (1992) ECG's of defibrillation electrodes yield more information than ECG's of sensing electrodes. Eur J Cardiac Pacing Electrophysiol 2: A122 (abstr)
9. Olson WH (1994) Tachyarrhythmia sensing and detection. In: Singer I (ed) Implantable cardioverter defibrillator. Futura, New York, pp 71-108
10. Grimm W, Flores BF, Marchilinski FE (1992) Electrocardiographically documented unnecessary, spontaneous shocks in 241 patients with implantable cardioverter defibrillators. Pace 15: 1667
11. Olson WH, Bardy GH, Mehra R et al (1987) Comparison of

different onset and stability algorhithm for detection of spontaneous ventricular arrhythmias. Pace 10: 439

12. Swerdlow CD, Chen PS, Kass RM et al (1994) Discrimination of ventricular tachycardia from sinus tachycardia and atrial fibrillation in a tiered-therapy cardioverter-defibrillator. J Am Coll Cardiol 23: 1342
13. Pitschner H, Neuzner J, König S et al (1994) "Sudden onset" and "rate stability" in cardioverter-defibrillator therapy: optimized programming for enhanced specificity, in tachyarrhythmia detection. Eur J Cardiac Pacing Electrophysiol 4: 126 (abstr)
14. Himmrich E, Liebrich A, Treese N et al (1994) Onset pattern of ventricular tachycardia in patients with implantable cardioverter defibrillator using stored electrograms. Eur J Cardiac Pacing Electrophysiol 4: 126 (abstr)
15. Bardy GH, Hoffer B, Johnson G et al (1993) Implantable transvenous cardioverter-defibrillators. Circulation 87: 1152
16. Fromer M, Schlappfer J, Fisher A et al (1991) Experience with a new implantable pacer-cardioverter-defibrillator for the therapy of recurrent sustained ventricular tachyarrhythmia: a step toward a universal ventricular tachyarrhythmia control device. Pace 14: 1288
17. Nisam S, Mower MM, Thomas A et al (1993) Patient survival comparison in three generations of automatic implantable cardioverter defibrillators: review of 12 years, 25.000 patients. Pace 16: 174
18. Williamson BD, Man KC, Daoud E et al (1994) Radiofrequency catheter modification of atrioventricular conduction to control the ventricular rate during atrial fibrillation. N Engl J Med 331: 910
19. Geibel A, Zehender M, Brugada P et al (1988) Changes in cycle length at the onset of sustained tachycardias – importance for antitachycardic pacing. Am Heart J 115: 588
20. Volosin KJ, Beauregard LM, Fabiszewski R et al (1991) Spontaneous changes in ventricular tachycardia cycle length. J Am Coll Cardiol 17: 409
21. Olson WH, Bardy GH (1986) Cycle length and morphology patterns at the onset of spontaneous ventricular arrhythmias. Pace 9: 284
22. Higgins SL, Lee RS, Farmer CE et al (1993) Stability: ICD detection criteria useful in discriminating atrial fibrillation from ventricular tachycardia. Pace 17:210 (abstr)
23. Hurwitz JL, Hook BG, Flores BT et al (1993) Importance of abortive shock capability with electrogram storage in cardioverter-defibrillator device. J Am Coll Cardiol 21: 895
24. Epstein AE, Kay GN, Plumb VJ et al (1989) Combined automatic implantable cardioverter-defibrillator and pacemaker systems: implantation techniques and follow-up. J Am Coll Cardiol 13: 12
25. Marchilinski FE, Flores BT, Buxton AE et al (1986) The automatic implantable cardioverter-defibrillator: efficacy, complications and device failures. Ann Intern Med 104: 481
26. Kelly PA, Mann DE, Damle RS et al (1994) Oversensing during ventricular pacing in patients with a third-generation implantable cardioverter-defibrillator. J Am Coll Cardiol 23: 1531
27. Metha D, Lipsius M, Suri RS et al (1992) Twiddler's syndrome with the implantable cardioverter defibrillator. Am Heart J 4: 1079
28. Chapman PD, Troup P (1992) The automatic implantable cardioverter/defibrillator: evaluating suspected inappropriate shocks. J Am Coll Cardiol 7: 1075
29. Kim SG, Furman S, Matos JA et al (1987) Automatic implantable cardioverter-defibrillator: inadvertant discharges during permanent pacemaker magnet tests. Pace 10: 579
30. Maloney J, Masterson M, Khours D et al (1991) Clinical performance of the implantable cardioverter defibrillator: electrocardiographic documentation of 101 spontaneous discharges. Pace 14: 280
31. Sulke N, Holt P, Bostock et al (1988) Inappropriate discharge by the implantable cardioverter/defibrillator during postoperative testing: implication for intraoperative assessment. Ann Intern Med 109: 529

What Have We Learned from Stored Implantable Cardioverter Defibrillator Electrocardiograms about the Mechanism of Sudden Death?

B.D. Gonska, A. Schaumann, and S. Purrer

Department of Cardiology, University Hospital Göttingen,
Göttingen, Germany

Introduction

The prevention of sudden cardiac death is an unsolved problem in modern cardiology. It is estimated that about 200 000-400 000 people in the United States and about 90 000 in Germany die as a result of sudden cardiac death per year (1,2). First insights into the electrical events causing sudden death were reported by MacWilliams in 1889 (3) and Lewis in 1915 (4), who found an association between ventricular fibrillation (VF) and sudden cardiac death. Large-scale epidemiologic studies revealed that ventricular tachyarrhythmias contribute in about 80% and bradyarrhythmias in about 20% of cases to this serious clinical event (5,6).

The initial rhythm that can be identified in a patient with cardiovascular collapse depends on the time between loss of consciousness and the first electrocardiogram (ECG) recording. When the time elapsed is not known, the inital rhythm recorded is VF in 40%, asystole in another 40%, electromechanical dissociation in 20%, while ventricular tachycardia (VT) is only documented in 1% of the patients (7).When the time from collapse to rhythm identification is less than 4 min, VF can be documented in 95% and asystole for 5% of the patients; if the rhythm is only documented 12-15 min thereafter, VF can be found in about 70% and asystole in the remaining 30% (8). Thus it can be assumed that electromechanical dissociation and asystole are the result of a prolonged episode of VF and concomitant hypoxia. Survival rates of patients with sudden cardiac death indirectly support this assumption. In patients in whom the initial rhythm identified was VF, the long-term survival rate was 25%, while it was only 6% in patients in whom electromechanical dissociation was present and 1% in those with asystole at the time of recording (9).

Monomorphic VT has rarely been observed at the time of sudden cardiac death (7,10). This suggests that this arrhythmia does not in general precede VF. On the other hand, ambulatory ECG monitoring stressed the significance of VT as the initial rhythm of subsequent sudden cardiac death (11-17). However, these observations are limited due to the fact that, in most of the studies, polymorphic VT and ventricular flutter were only classified as VT and, furthermore, because most of these recordings were obtained while assessing antiarrhythmic drug therapy, which may cause proarrhythmia, such as torsade de pointes. All these patients had already exhibited symptoms such as palpitations, syncope, or even sudden cardiac death. In addition, it has been shown that clinical characteristics in patients with VT are different from those with VF. In coronary artery disease, VF may be the first manifestation of hypoxemia. Patients with VT more often have a lower ejection fraction and left ventricular aneurysm, while patients suffering from VF generally have better left ventricular function. Thus, clinical observations suggest that in the general population, monomorphic VT may be a less common arrhythmia preceding sudden cardiac death.

To date, there is no medical antiarrhythmic management available with a recurrence rate of sudden cardiac death as low as that of the automatic implantable cardioverter/defibrillator (ICD). As a consequence, the use of ICDs has increased during the last 15 years, with more than 30 000 devices currently being implanted. Since the implantation of the first fixed-rate, nonprogrammable device in 1980 by Mirowski et al. (18), ICDs have evolved to become multiprogrammable units with more capabilities, such as antibradycardia pacing, antitachycardia pacing, and low- and high-energy cardioversion/defibrillation. In addition, third- and fourth-generation devices provide the possibility of storing the ECG and arrhythmia preceding the intervention. Thus, the onset of the malignant arrhythmias resulting in sudden cardiac death can be documented and analyzed more precisely.

In order to evaluate the arrhythmias preceding the intervention of the ICD, we analyzed stored ECG$_s$ in an ongoing, prospective study.

Patients and Methods

The study population consisted of 138 patients, 121 men and 17 women with a mean age of 63 years (11-84). The underlying cardiac disease was confirmed by cardiac

Table 1. Clinical characteristics of 29 patients who received ICD therapy and experienced discharges of the device

	Number	Percentage
25 Men, 4 women		
Age 11-84 years (mean 62)		
Underlying cardiac disease		
Coronary artery disease	16	55
Idiopathic dilated cardiomyopathy	11	38
No structural heart disease	2	7
Mean left ventricular ejection		
fraction 36 ±14% (9%-60%)		
Clinical arrhythmia prior to ICD implantation		
VF	8	28
Monomorphic sustained VT	11	38
Polymorphic sustained VT	5	17
Nonsustained VT (recurrent syncope)	5	17

ICD, implantable cardioverter defibrillator; VF, ventricular fibrillation; VT, ventricular tachycardia.

catheterization and coronary angiography and revealed coronary artery disease in 86 patients (62%), dilated cardiomyopathy in 38 (28%), congenital heart disease in four (3%), and valvular heart disease in two (1%), while eight patients (6%) had no evidence of structural heart disease. The mean left ventricular ejection fraction was 37% (range 9%-88%). All patients had a history of symptomatic VT or cardiac arrest. Before ICD implantation, they underwent invasive electrophysiologic investigation and were either noninducible or did not respond to medical antiarrhythmic management as confirmed by serial electrophysiologic testing and/or spontaneous recurrence of the arrhythmia. During a follow-up of 2-28 (mean 12) months, 29 of these patients (21%) experienced spontaneous episodes of ventricular tachyarrhythmia resulting in successful discharges of the device. No differences could be established between patients with and without discharges with respect to the underlying cardiac disease, age, sex, hemodynamic status and clinical arrhythmia (Table 1). Eleven of the patients (38%) had been treated in addition with antiarrhythmic drugs: amiodarone was administered to five patients, sotalol to three, propafenone to one, and mexiletine and sotalol to two patients.

Different third- and fourth-generation ICDs were implanted: CPI P2 in three patients, CPI P3 in one, CPI PRX II in 23, and CPI PRX III in two patients.

Stored ECG₅ of all episodes of ICD discharges were analyzed with respect to the spontaneous preceding rhythm, the incidence of ventricular extrasystoles, supraventricular extrasystoles and pauses, and the rate of the ventricular arrhythmia resulting in discharges of the device. In all patients, the rhythm analysis included the last ten beats before the occurrence of ventricular tachyarrhythmia. Furthermore, the stored ICD-ECGs were compared to the clinically documented arrhythmia and/or to the one that was inducible at programmed ventricular stimulation.

Results

Of the 29 patients, eight (28%) were survivors of cardiac arrest due to VF and 16 (55%) had recurrent monomorphic (n=11) or rapid polymorphic VT (n=5).

In the remaining five patients (17%) who had a history of recurrent syncope, only nonsustained VT was recorded electrocardiographically. During right ventricular stimulation in the absence of isoproterenol, VF could reproducibly be induced in six of the eight patients while two were noninducible. Sustained VT could be reproduced in all VT patients. Of the five patients with syncope, four had inducible, sustained VT at programmed stimulation while the other patient was noninducible. During the follow-up, stored ICD ECGs revealed recurrence of VF in all patients with clinical and inducible VF and in one patient with idiopathic dilated cardiomyopathy without inducible arrhythmia. In all VT patients, the clinically documented and induced VT recurred with the same rate at least once. However, it is noteworthy that in most patients, not only the documented and inducible arrhythmia could be observed but also other types of ventricular tachyarrhythmias. Differences of heart rate of up to 80 beats/min were observed in an individual patient.

In the 29 patients 129 episodes of malignant ventricular tachyarrhythmias were documented. Twenty-one patients had more than one episode (2-11) recorded during the follow-up. The mean rate of the arrhythmia was 198±42 (126-337) beats/min. In 39 episodes (30%) a rate of more than 220 beats/min (221-337) was recorded, in 19 (15%) a rate of more than 250 beats/min. Most of these 39 episodes could be classified as rapid polymorphic VT, ventricular flutter, and VF. In 85 of the remaining 90 episodes, monomorphic VT was documented.

Before the onset of the ventricular tachyarrhythmia, sinus rhythm was present in 22 patients, atrial fibrillation in three, while four patients required antibradycardia pacing. In all but one patient, the rhythm was stable with a rate of <100 beats/min. Only one episode was preceded by sinus tachycardia (120 beats/min). Furthermore, this episode was the only one that was preceded by ST segment depression (Fig. 1).

Sudden onset of the tachyarrhythmia was found in 10 patients (35%), while in 14 patients (48%) the arrhythmic event was preceded by different arrhythmias, and in the remaining five patients (17%), both sudden and nonsudden onset was documented. The analysis of the onset of ventricular arrhythmia of the 129 episodes revealed that 55 (43%) occurred spontaneously, that is, without any triggering arrhythmia (Fig. 2). In 29 cases (23%), singular ventricular extrasystoles preceded the event, in 12 cases (9%) ventricular pairs (Fig. 3), and in six cases (5%) nonsustained VT with three to six consecutive premature contractions were documented. Four episodes (3%) were preceded by an R-on-T phenomenon resulting in VF. In another case (1%), supraventricular extrasystoles were observed prior to the onset of the ventricular arrhythmia. The remaining 22 arrhythmic events (17%) were pause-dependent, due to various mechanisms (ventricular extrasystoles, pairs and nonsustained VT, supraventricular extrasystoles or a sinuatrial pause; Fig. 4; Table 2).

Analysis of the onset mechanism in the individual patient revealed that only two of the 21 patients with more than one episode of VT/VF always exhibited the same mechanism. In some patients, one type of arrhythmia was triggered by different mechanisms.

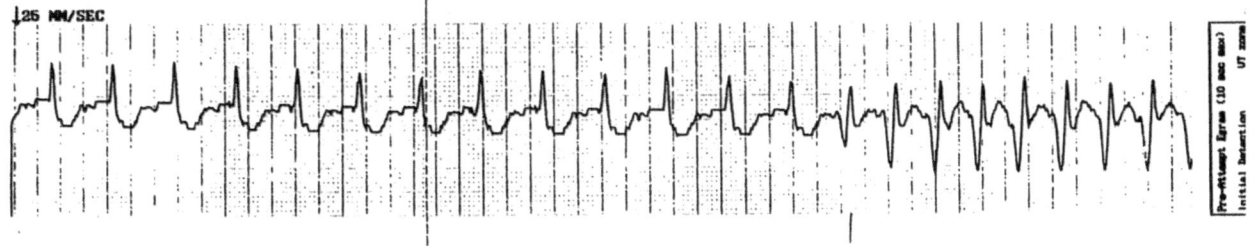

Fig. 1. Spontaneous onset of monomorphic VT with a rate of 170 beats/min in a patient with coronary artery disease. The preceding rhythm is sinus tachycardia (120 beats/min) and there are marked ST depressions possibly due to myocardial ischemia

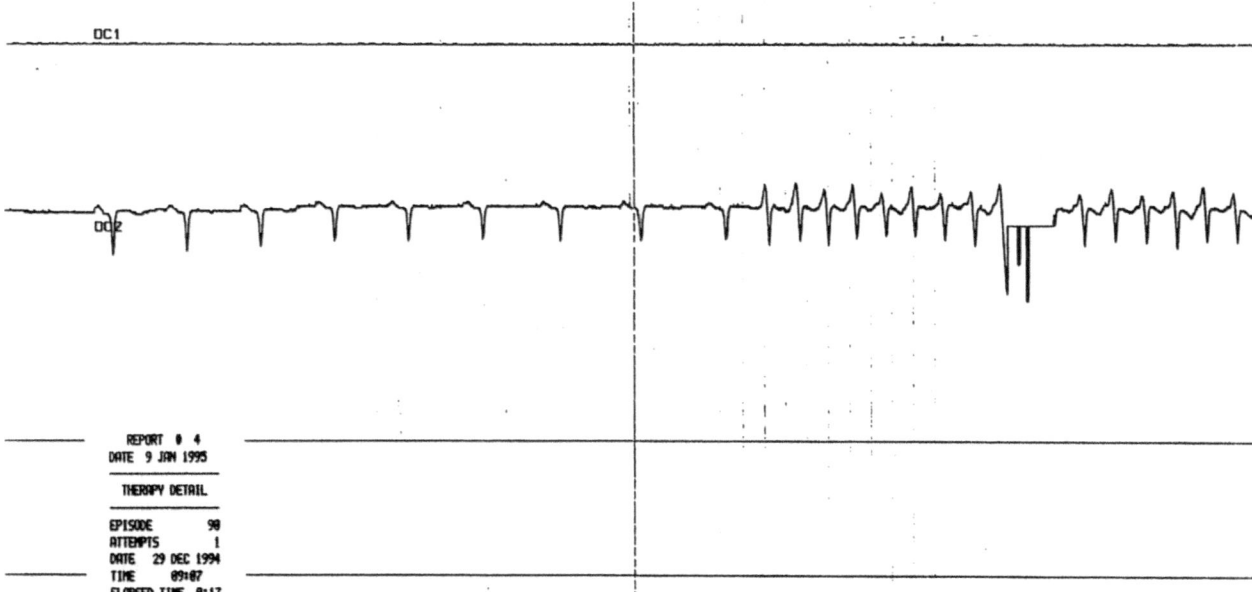

Fig. 2. Spontaneous onset of ventricular tachycardia with a rate of 210 beats/min. The preceding rhythm is normal sinus rhythm (85 beats/min)

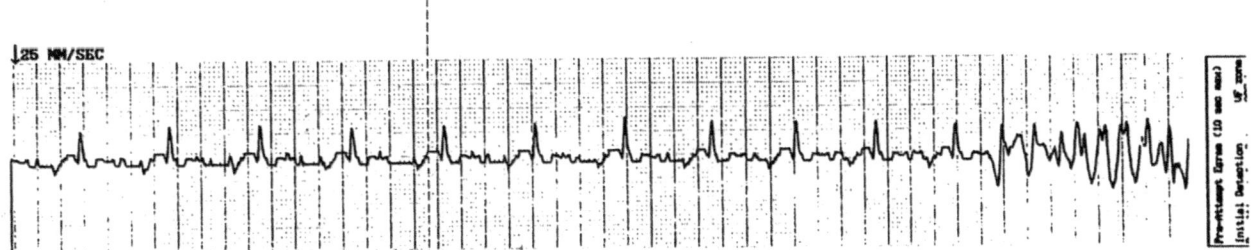

Fig. 3. During sinus rhythm (75 beats/min), a premature ventricular couplet induces ventricular fibrillation

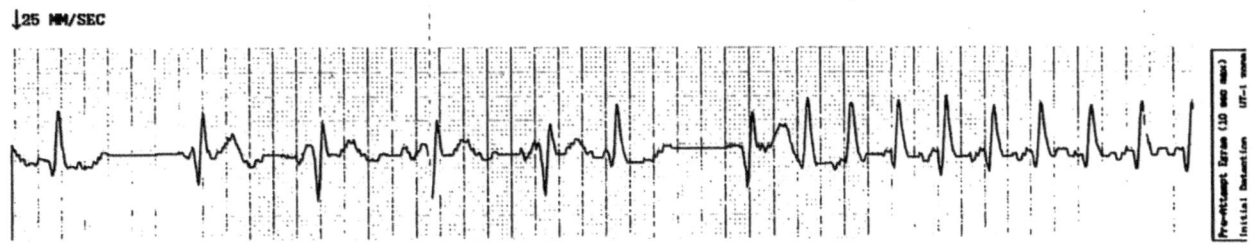

Fig. 4. Registration of a "short-long-short" phenomenon which induces monomorphic ventricular tachycardia with a rate of 190 beats/min

Table 2. Stored ventricular tachyarrhythmias requiring ICD intervention and onset mechanisms

	Number	Percentage
Arrhythmias during ICD therapy[a]		
VF	6	21
VT	17	58
VF and VT	6	21
Preceding arrhythmia		
of the 129 episodes of VT/VF[b]		
None	55	43
VES	29	23
VP	12	9
ns-VT	6	5
R-on-T-phenomenon	4	3
SVES	1	1
Pause-dependent	22	17
VES and pauses	13	10
VP/nsVT and pauses	4	3
SVES and pauses	4	3
Sinuatrial pause (1800 ms)	1	1

VES, ventricular extrasystole; VP, ventricular pair; ns, nonsustained; SVES, supraventricular extrasystole; ICD, implantable cardioverter defibrillator; VT, ventricular tachycardia; VF, ventricular fibrillation.
[a] Number and percentage of patients.
[b] Number and percentage of episodes.

Discussion

The mechanism of sudden cardiac death is still not completely understood. Factors such as ischemia, catecholamines, myocardial wall stress, drugs, and many others influence the onset of life-threatening ventricular tachyarrhythmias. In the last 20 years, great effort has been made to evaluate triggering factors that may induce these arrhythmias, such as premature ventricular contractions, ventricular pairs, and nonsustained VT. Ambulatory electrocardiographic studies have emphasized the role of triggering arrhythmias (19). However, the suppression of these arrhythmias by antiarrhythmic drugs generally did not result in a significant prevention of sudden cardiac death (20), while ß-blocking agents did even in the absence of significant reduction of single and complex ventricular arrhythmias (21-23). These results demonstrate that ventricular arrhythmias form only one aspect of the entity of sudden cardiac death and that these arrhythmias have to be seen in the context of the hemodynamic variables, altered myocardial structure, metabolic disorders, and the autonomic nervous system.

Stored ECGs in ICDs can provide further insights into the arrhythmogenic mechanisms. However, it has to be taken into consideration that this is a selected patient population with various cardiac diseases, different hemodynamic states, special arrhythmias, for example, those which are not reproducible by programmed stimulation or those which do not respond to medical antiarrhythmic management, and there are patients with and without pharmacological antiarrhythmic therapy. This population is not representative of the entity of patients who experience sudden cardiac death. Therefore the preliminary results of the present study have to be viewed with caution. These results are more comparable to those obtained from patients during ambulatory monitoring than to those from patients who suffer out-of-hospital cardiac arrest. Holter studies of sudden cardiac death have mainly included patients with coronary artery disease (on the average 70%), more than 50% being treated with antiarrhythmic drugs at the time of recording. The arrhythmia documented was monomorphic or polymorphic VT in about 70%, primary VF in only 5%-10%, and bradyarrhythmias in 15%-20% (11-17). These general results correspond to those in our patients.

The finding that 43% of the ventricular tachyarrhythmias occurred spontaneously, without preceding ventricular arrhythmias, demonstrates that there are other factors than rhythm abnormalities which trigger the onset of life-threatening ventricular tachyarrhythmias.

Concerning the onset mechanism of life-threatening ventricular tachyarrhythmias, it is widely believed that the phenomenon of R-on-T ventricular premature contractions is of major arrhythmogenic importance. Data based on ambulatory monitoring (16) showed that prematurity of ventricular extrasystoles initiating VT or VF is a common finding, preceding the arrhythmic event in about 20% of patients. However, only a minority of tachyarrhythmic episodes in the present study (3%) was preceded by this phenomenon, initiating VF in all cases. In several studies the phenomenon of pause-dependent ventricular premature beats and the "short-long-short" coupling interval have been identified as an initiating factor of VT and VF (11,13,14,24). Coumel et al. (25), also evaluating the data of ambulatory ECG recordings, felt that pause dependency is a critical prerequisite for the development of life-threatening ventricular tachyarrhythmia. If we extend this definition of the short-long-short interval to ventricular couplets, nonsustained VT, and supraventricular extrasystoles, 16% of the episodes in the present study had a pause-dependent onset. Bardy and Olsen (26) reported results from 41 patients with a history of cardiac arrest. Of these patients 14 exhibited VT or VF during the monitoring period. The onset of six of the 60 episodes of VT/VF (10%) recorded in these patients was classified as pause-dependent.

Only two of the 21 patients with more than one episode of VT/VF always demonstrated the same onset mechanism. This finding confirms the results of Bardy and Olsen (26) in the above-mentioned study. Of these 14 patients 10 had more than one arrhythmic event. Only one patient was found to have the same pattern of arrhythmia onset for each episode.

As in our study group, VT or VF in the Bardy and Olsen (26) study population was not preceded by an increase in heart rate. In Holter studies, increases in heart rate were reported by Kempf and Josephson (14) and von Olshausen et al. (17), while Panidis and Morganroth (12) and Pratt et al. (13) did not observe any major changes. However, imbalance of the autonomic nervous system cannot be ruled out from the absence of increased heart rate since we have to consider that this mechanism cannot be determined by standard monitoring techniques such as ambulatory monitoring or stored ICD-ECGs.

Our results demonstrate that different ventricular tachyarrhythmias can be observed in an individual patient. Thus, antitachycardia pacing modalities should be applied. Cross et al. (27) recently showed that anti-tachycardia pacing can lower the number of shocks required to terminate the arrhythmia significantly. Even nontested antitachycardia pacing is helpful for this purpose (28).

Stored ECG$_s$ do not only offer the opportunity to analyze the onset of the ventricular tachyarrhythmia which causes intervention of the device, but may also detect sensing failure of the ICD. Almeida and Buckingham (29) proved the additional value of stored ECG$_s$ for the documentation of sensing abnormalities that, in selected patients, may lead to VT initiation.

Conclusion

The present study has attempted to provide some insights into the onset mechanism of VF and VT in a study population which underwent implantation of an ICD because of spontaneous VF or VT either resistant to medical antiarrhythmic management or noninducible at programmed ventricular stimulation. Thus, these patients are highly selected and the onset mechanisms found cannot be extrapolated to the general population. Stored ICD-ECGs showed a wide variety of onset mechanisms. Four results are of interest:

1. Of the episodes of VT/VF 43% occurred spontaneously without preceding arrhythmia.

2. Different onset mechanisms could be found in an individual patient.

3. A pause-dependent onset of the arrhythmia was documented in 17%.

4. The R-on-T-phenomenon appears to be of minor importance for the initiation of VT.

Thus, stored ICD-ECGs may provide an additional tool for the understanding of the onset mechanisms of malignant ventricular arrhythmias. Further information about the mechanisms of initiation of ventricular arrhythmias is required in order to encourage the development of improved treatment modalities for preventing sudden cardiac death.

References

1. Myerburg RJ, Conde CA, Sung RJ, Mayora-Cortez A, Mallon SM, Sheps DS, Appel RA, Castellanos A (1980) Clinical, electrophysiological and hemodynamic profile of patients resuscitated from prehospital cardiac arrest. Am J Med 68:568-576
2. Gillum RF (1989) Sudden coronary death in the United States: 1980-1985. Circulation 79:756-765
3. MacWilliam JA (1889) Cardiac failure and sudden death. Br Med J 1:6-11
4. Lewis T (1915) Lectures on the heart. Paul B. Hoeber, New York
5. Weaver WD, Lorch GS, Alvarez HA, Cobb LA (1976) Angiographic findings and prognostic indicators in patients resuscitated from sudden cardiac death. Circulation 54:895-900
6. Kuller LH (1980) Sudden death: definition and epidemiologic consideration. Prog Cardiovasc Dis 23:1-12
7. Weaver WD, Hill D, Fahrenbruch CE, Copass MK, Martin JS, Cobb LA, Hallstrom AP (1988) Use of external defibrillator in the management of out-of-hospital cardiac arrest. N Engl J Med 319:661-666
8. Hallstrom AP, Eisenberg MS, Bergner L (1983) The persistence of ventricular fibrillation and its implication for evaluating EMS. Emerg Health Serv Q 1:41-47
9. Weaver WD, Cobb LA, Hallstrom AP, Copass MK, Ray R, Emery M, Fahrenbruch C (1986) Considerations for improving survival from out-of hospital cardiac arrest. Ann Emerg Med 15:1181-1186
10. Cobb LA, Weaver WD, Fahrenbruch CD, Hallstrom AP, Copass MK (1992) Community-based interventons for sudden cardiac death. Impact, limitations, and changes. Circulation 85 [Suppl. I]: I-98-I-102
11. Nicolic G, Bishop RL, Singh JB (1982) Sudden death recorded during Holter monitoring. Circulation 66:218-225
12. Panidis P, Morganroth J (1983) Sudden death in hospitalized patients: cardiac rhythm disturbances detected by ambulatory electrocardiographic monitoring. J Am Coll Cardiol 2:798-805
13. Pratt CM, Francis MJ, Luck JC, Wyndham CR, Miller RR, Quinones MA (1983) Analysis of ambulatory electrograms in 15 patients during spontaneous ventricular fibrillation with special reference to preceding arrhythmic events. J Am Coll Cardiol 2:789-797
14. Kempf FC, Josephson ME (1984) Cardiac arrest recorded on ambulatory electrocardiograms. Am J Cardiol 53:1577-1582
15. Milner PG, Platia EV, Reid PR, Griffith LSC (1985) Ambulatory electrocardiographic recordings at the time of fatal cardiac arrest. Am J Cardiol 56:588-592
16. Bayes de Luna A, Coumel P, Leclerq JF (1989) Ambulatory sudden cardiac death: mechanisms of production of fatal arrhythmia on the basis of data from 157 cases. Am Heart J 117:151-159
17. Olshausen K von, Witt T, Pop T, Treese, N, Bethge KP, Meyer J (1991) Sudden cardiac death while wearing a Holter monitor. Am J Cardiol 67:381-386
18. Mirowski M, Reid PR, Mower MM , Watkins L, Gott, VL, Schauble JF, Langer A, Heilman MS, Kolenik SA, Fischell RE, Weisfeldt ML (1980) Termination of malignant ventricular arrhythmias with implanted automatic defibrillators in human beings. N Engl J Med 303:322-324
19. Bigger JT Jr, Fleiss JL, Kleiger R, Miller JP, Rolnitzky LM (1984) The relationship among ventricular arrhythmias, left ventricular dysfunction, and mortality in the 2 years following acute myocadial infarction. Circulation 69:250-258
20. The Cardiac Arrhythmia Suppression Trial (CAST) Investigators (1989) Preliminary report: effect of encainide and flecainide on mortality in a randomized trial of arrhythmia suppression after myocardial infarction. N Engl J Med 327:227-233
21. Hjalmarson A, Elmfeldt D, Herlitz J, Holmberg S, Malek I, Nyberg G, Ryden L, Swedberg K, Vedin A, Waagstein F, Waldenström J, Wedel H, Wilhelmsen L, Wilhelmsen C (1981) Effects on mortality of metoprolol in acute myocardial infarction. A double-blind randomised trial. Lancet II:823-827
22. The Norwegian Multicenter Study Group (1981) Timolol-induced reduction of mortality and reinfarction in patients surviving acute myocardial infarction. N Engl J Med 304: 801-807
23. Beta-Blocker Heart Attack Trial Research Group (1982) A randomized trial of propranolol in patients with acute myocardial infarction. JAMA 147:1707-1714
24. Bisset, JK, Watson JW, Scovil JA, De Soyza N, Ohrt DW (1980) Sudden death in cardiomyopathy: role of bradycardia-dependent depolarization changes. Am Heart J 99:625-629
25. Coumel P, Leclerq JF, Zimmermann M, Funck-Brentano JL (1987) Antiarrhythmic therapy: non-invasive guided strategy versus empirical or invasive strategies. In: Brugada P, Wellens HJJ (eds) Cardiac arrhythmias: where to go from here? Futura, Mount Kisco, NY, pp 403-419
26. Bardy GH, Olsen WH (1990) Clinical characteristics of spontaneous-onset sustained ventricular tachycardia and ventricular fibrillation in survivors of cardiac arrest. In: Zipes DP, Jalife J (eds) Cardiac electrophysiology. From cell to bedside. Saunders, Philadelphia, pp 778-790
27. Gross JN, Sackstein RD, Song SL, Chang CJ, Kawinishi DT, Furman S (1993) The antitachycardia pacing ICD: impact on patient selection and outcome. PACE 16:165-173
28. Schaumann A, Gonska BD, zur Mühlen F von, Meyer O, Kreuzer H (1995) A prospective study of tested versus nontested antitachycardia pacing in implantable cardioverter defibrillators. J Am Coll Cardiol 25:212A
29. Almeida HF, Buckingham TA (1993) Inappropriate implantable cardioverter defibrillator shocks secondary to sensing lead failure: utility of stored electrograms. PACE 16:407-412

Implantable Cardioverter Defibrillator: A Therapy for Everyone or for Selected Patients?

F. Bellocci, G. Pelargonio, M.G. Bendini, A. Intini, V. Affinito, O. Sacchetti,
G. Bruni, A.S. Montenero, and P. Zecchi

Istituto di Cardiologia, Università Cattolica del Sacro Cuore,
Rome, Italy

The implantable cardioverter defibrillator (ICD) is an important and unique new method of potentially preventing recurrent sudden cardiac death (SCD) due to malignant ventricular arrhythmias (MVA).

Guidelines are essential for every new procedure and treatment, and many groups have therefore published guidelines for the use of the ICD. However, as suggested by Kappenberger (1), the main problem with guidelines that refer to a relatively new treatment is that, as all the components of guidelines undergo rapid changes, the basis of discussion is instable. These guidelines should help physicians to justify a therapeutic decision to financial authorities in view of commercial interests and can even be considered as the legal background for a given medical procedure; as such, they can be of great value if legal problems arise. However, two aspects have to be taken into account: on the one hand, indications should be defined in such a way as to leave space for individual judgment; on the other hand, they should be strict enough to prevent abuse and to provide credible documentation for the medical profession.

With this in mind, guidelines must define what is considered to be generally accepted and must, therefore, describe the candidates for whom ICD implantation is warranted.

Initially, the criteria for ICD implantation were very strict: ICD therapy was reserved only for patients with drug-refractory MVA, who had survived at least two episodes of documented cardiac arrest due to ventricular fibrillation (VF).

In 1985 the Food and Drug Administration (FDA) approved the device for commercial use and the indications were extended: ICD could be implanted only in patients with recurrent, symptomatic ventricular tachycardia (VT) that were not suppressed by drugs in the electrophysiologic laboratory (in fact, all patients in whom arrhythmias were not inducible in basal conditions were considered to have a relatively good prognosis).

Only 4 years ago, in 1991, two reports by the AHA/ACC (2) and the NASPE (3) established official guidelines for the implantation of ICD. In brief, an ICD could only be considered in patients with MVA that could not be controlled with appropriate treatment, i.e., in patients with drug-refractory VT/VF, in patients with MVA and intolerance to drugs, and in cardiac arrest victims with no inducible MVA. Although the etiology of MVA might have an important impact on prognosis, it was not clear whether the underlying heart disease had any relationship to the clinical decision to implant an ICD; therefore, the guidelines issued by both AHA/ACC and NASPE did not relate the results of electrophysiologic study to underlying organic heart disease.

Although the device was described as "last resort" therapy, the guidelines were defined fairly liberally by the authors (2-3) but the indications were considered evolutionary and controversial.

After the early demonstration that ICD reduced the incidence of SCD to approximally 2% or less per year, several investigators (4-6) called the ICD the "gold standard" of treatment for all patients with MVA and considered the device the appropriate first-line treatment.

Brugada (4), for example, considered that any patient with a calculated risk of SCD of 10% or more per year, in spite of alternatives, should receive an ICD and has formulated a very simple decision-making process: ICD therapy would be indicated for any patients who meets one of these criteria: (a) the patient has experienced VF or syncopal VT or (b) the patient has experienced MVA and is in NHYA (New York Heart Association) functional class III or has had multiple myocardial infarctions. Similarly, Henthorn (6) conservatively suggested that 1-year risk of SCD from MVA of more than 10% was the appropriate incidence for which ICD therapy should be considered; despite several shortcomings, ICD remained the standard for prevention of SCD.

Accordingly, since patients with MVA and an ejection fraction (EF) less than 30% have a high risk of SCD (more than 10% per year) irrespective of the results of programmed ventricular stimulation (PVS), several authors (3-7) have recommended ICD implantation as the therapy of first choice in all patients with

MVA and EF less than 30%, irrespective of the results of PVS.

The availability of transvenous lead systems further obviously broadened the indications for ICD implantation, and several investigators claimed that there were sufficient data to demonstrate that withholding ICD therapy in patients at high risk was ethically unacceptable and medically wrong (4).

However, several other investigators disagreed with these broad indications. In 1992, a Task Force of the European Society of Cardiology (8) published guidelines for the use of ICD; the indications were quite different from those accepted in the United States. In patients who have survived cardiac arrest, the decision is easy only in two extreme situations. Contrary to established beliefs, ICD would be most cost-effective in patients with no or minimal heart disease, since it can reasonably be presumed that patients who are likely to benefit the most from the periodic device therapy are those who have a good ventricular function. Paradoxically, however, many of these patients would be drug responders at electrophysiologic testing and would therefore be expected to have a good overall prognosis even without ICD. Conversely, ICD would be less cost-effective in patients whose prognosis is poor, based on irrecoverable and progressive myocardial damage (currently, until more data are available, the use of ICD as a bridge to transplantation should be regarded as investigational). The majority of potential ICD recipients are patients with some risk of MVA who have different types of heart disease and a broad spectrum of left ventricular dysfunction. Because patients with low EF are at the greatest risk for SCD, they would seem to be the most likely to benefit from an ICD implantation; however, this was not the case, probably because such patients have the highest incidence of nonsudden cardiac death. Therefore, the correct indication in these patients is complicated, and the presentation of arrhythmia, the hemodynamic toleration, the nature and the severity of the underlying heart disease, and the presence of modifying features (such as assessment of left ventricular dysfunction, age, autonomic factors, and ischemia) must be taken into consideration.

Therefore, although guidelines should define which patients at which moment benefit most from ICD, it is unclear whether such guidelines are helpful in establishing a treatment algorithm for patients with MVA. Curiously, despite the increasing use of extremely costly devices of increasing complexity and versatility, neither the magnitude of their impact on total mortality nor which patients are likely to benefit from such treatment is known with any measure of certainty. The main problem is that, as with many other new medical technologies, the dramatic explosion in the use of ICD has occurred before conclusive evidence of the efficacy of the treatment is available; this underlines the difficulties in assessing the impact of new therapies without the advantage of well-designed, prospective randomized studies.

The results of the initial studies (5-9) demonstrating the efficacy in preventing SCD have made the ethics of performing randomized controlled trials difficult. As a consequence, there are no results from randomized trials of ICD versus other modes of treatment, and there is no scientific evidence that ICD improves total mortality even in the short term. Several skeptics (10-12) have noted that treatment with ICD is not paralleled by a proportionate reduction in overall mortality and have seriously questioned the ability of ICD to improve survival, giving rise to a controversy described as the "ICD backlash." Although biases due to patient selection, longer time to treatment, and the use of ICD as an endpoint affect all available studies, SCD rates of 5% – 8% at 5 years are so low that it seems likely that ICD treatment does provide protection against SCD. However, even if SCD were totally eliminated by ICD, it might not have much impact on the overall occurrence of death, since patients dying of MVA usually have other risks as well as arrhythmic ones.

A critical review of the currently available randomized studies does not provide reliable evidence of the efficacy of the ICD to improve overall survival. As the methods of evaluation have become more rigorous and hence more reliable, the benefits of ICD on total mortality appear modest (10-12). Connolly and Yusuf (11) argued that the reduction by ICD implantation in overall mortality could not be larger than 33%. Mortality reductions in this range have been seen with at least two antiarrhythmic drugs in postmyocardial infarction survivors. An overview of the randomized trials using beta blockers in postmyocardial infarction patients reported a 26% reduction in mortality. A meta-analysis of randomized trials of amiodarone after myocardial infarction indicated a reduction in mortality of 34%. Recently, a randomized trial of amiodarone in patients with heart failure showed a reduction in mortality of 30% (13). In contrast, extensive meta-analytic data from randomized clinical trials of class I antiarrhythmic drugs in postmyocardial infarction survivors demonstrated that these drugs as a whole might increase the mortality as a class action (14). It is highly improbable that the effects of class I antiarrhythmic drugs could be different in another subset of patients (e.g., in patients with MVA) if Holter monitoring or PVS-guided therapy were used. In fact, the data from the ESVEM trial (15) demonstrate that there are no significant differences between the two technologies in predicting the long-term outcome in patients with MVA and that comparison of sotalol with six class I drugs, collectively or individually, shows a significant difference in favor of sotalol in terms of arrhythmia recurrences, SCD, or total cardiac mortality. The fact that PVS cannot be unreservedly accepted as the control arm of antiarrhythmic drug therapy has been confirmed by a recent randomized study by Steinbeck et al. (16), who demonstrated that, as compared with empiric metoprolol therapy, PVS-guided antiarrhythmic class I drug therapy does not improve the overall outcome in patients with MVA. This is further supported by the results of the CASCADE study (17), in which survival was significantly greater and cardiac mortality lower in the empiric amiodarone treatment arm than in the PVS-guided class I antiarrhythmic drugs arm.

These results indicate the superiority of the drug-specific responses over technique-specific responses and confirm that class I antiarrhythmic drugs, even guided by PVS, are inferior to therapy with empiric amiodarone or beta blockers and therapy with sotalol guided by Holter monitoring or PVS. Therefore, these data essentially limit the choice of antiarrhythmic drugs to class II or III agents in all patients with MVA.

On the other hand, there are now several lines of evidence from controlled clinical trials which indicate that neither the use of ICD nor the use of therapy guided by PVS or Holter monitoring may be the appropriate gold standard for judging therapy of MVA.

In a recent provocative editorial, Singh (18) reported data from Montefiore Hospital (19) demonstrating that ICD therapy in patients with MVA does not carry a dramatically better prognosis than PVS-guided therapy with class I antiarrhythmic drugs. Assuming that the Montefiore data are valid, Singh (18) suggested that, used empirically, amiodarone, as in the CASCADE study (17), beta blockers, as in the study of Steinbeck (16), or therapy guided by Holter monitoring or PVS using sotalol, as in the ESVEM study (15), as monotherapy is likely to be superior to the use of ICD alone in improving survival in comparable patients with MVA. There are theoretical considerations which also suggest that, in the absence of any controlled comparison, this is a reasonable presumption: ICD has no impact on the state of substrate or its modulating factors, the prime determinants of the nature and severity of electrical instability that give rise to MVA.

All these data indicate that the benefits of the ICD implantation should be demonstrated to be larger or equal to the best available medical management. Since comparison of ICD implantation with drug therapy as the first-line treatment has never been tested, it is possible that drug therapy could either be equivalent to, superior to, or worse than that with ICD. Therefore, controlled (sufficiently large) clinical trials comparing the best medical regimens (beta blockers, amiodarone, or sotalol) with ICD need to be performed to determine the comparative effects in MVA. Such trials should use randomization, analysis by intention to treat, and total mortality as the primary endpoint.

That such trials are not only ethically justified even in high-risk patients (considering the weak data supporting the overall clinical benefits from the ICD, its high cost, the significant morbidity associated with its implantation, and the availability of at least two relatively simple forms of therapy with substantial proof of efficacy), but also urgently needed is confirmed by several editorials published in recent cardiologic literature.

Saksena et al. (20) acknowledged the need for more clinical trials for current indications of ICD, since if drug therapy is demonstrated to be at least as effective in reducing total mortality as ICD and the side effects profile was not significantly worse, the higher cost of ICD may be counterbalanced in many patients.

Kim (21) correctly emphasized the importance of the total mortality rate as the primary endpoint in the much-needed multicenter trials comparing ICD with the best alternative therapies. Sweeney and Ruskin (22) confirmed that ICD implantation markedly reduces the risk for SCD in diverse populations; however-

er, the benefit is predictably limited in certain subsets of patients and more dramatic in others. Therefore, future randomized trials should permit a rational, complete, and unbiased assessment of the clinical benefit, addressing one fundamental question: which patients are most likely to derive a significant benefit in terms of survival from the ICD implantation. Obviously, patients must be followed up long enough to determine the real value of ICD. Adequate follow-up is important since in patients with preserved left ventricular function the relative benefit of ICD in terms of survival compared with drugs is likely to be a late one and may not be demonstrated for years after follow-up. Conversely, in patients with depressed left ventricular function, the relative survival benefit of ICD in terms of survival is likely to be early but may not be sustained, since over time the survival advantage will dissipate. The point at which this occurs cannot be determined without a randomized trial with adequate follow-up.

Similarly, Zipes (23) argued that several important questions must be answered: can ICD really be adequate as a gold standard? Does it reduce overall or total mortality compared with the best medical therapy? Indeed, is that the correct question to ask? Or should we accept the fact that ICD successfully terminates MVA and should we be implanting ICD in all patients who survive a cardiac arrest? Or are there subgroups in whom we can eliminate competing causes of death so that their risk of dying is from MVA alone, and should only they receive the ICD? Are patients with reduced left ventricular function more likely to suffer a nonarrhythmic death and therefore not profit from ICD implantation? Are patients with cardiac arrest resulting from VF more likely to have a cardiac arrest recurrence, and with that the possible need for an ICD, than the patients with stable but recurrent episodes of sustained-ventricular tachycardia (SVT)? Might patients with chronic, stable SVT benefit from the antitachycardia pacing (ATP) capabilities of ICD? Attempts to answer these and related issues about the use of ICD based on reports in the literature often fall short of completely satisfying careful scientific scrutiny. Until we directly randomize ICD against the best medical management, we will not know which therapy is best in general or for a specific patient group. To answer some of the questions raised above, prospective, randomized, multicenter trials are needed.

Although such trials have been called into question (24-26) we are fortunate that at least three large, randomized trials are now in progress: the CASH (Cardiac Arrest Study Hamburg), the CIDS (Canadian Implantable Defibrillator Study), and the AVID (Amiodarone Versus Implantable Defibrillator) trial. (On the other hand, the CAST – Cardiac Arrhythmia Suppression Trial – was similarly questioned, and in this study a therapy that was felt to be beneficial was proved to be harmful.)

In the CASH trial (29), patients with previous cardiac arrest and inducible MVA are randomized to the ICD group or to one of three drug treatment groups, each with a different mechanism of action: propafenone guided by PVS, empiric metoprolol, or empiric amiodarone.

In the CIDS trial (30), patients with cardiac arrest, VT with syncope, symptomatic VT, and EF less than 36% are randomized to empiric amiodarone or to the ICD group.

In the AVID trial (31), patients with cardiac arrest, VT, with syncope and symptomatic VT and EF less than 41% are randomized to the empiric amiodarone or guided sotalol and to the ICD group.

In all these trials the primary endpoint is total mortality, and the antiarrhythmic drug treatment is mostly empiric. Today, sufficient data exist from controlled and uncontrolled studies to make a good case for using empiric amiodarone (although it is not particularly effective in preventing electrically induced MVA, it does appear to have a favorable impact on spontaneous MVA and death: low specificity of PVS during amiodarone therapy). Therefore the Planning Committee of AVID felt that the evidence was sufficiently good to support the empiric use of amiodarone. Moreover, it feared inappropriate crossover of patients to the ICD arm of the study if patients were not suppressed, only partially suppressed, or had poor hemodynamic tolerance of induced MVA while receiving amiodarone. On the other hand, although PVS-guided therapy was well established as a standard practice, the efficacy of PVS-guided antiarrhythmic drug therapy was never established in controlled trials, since physicians were not willing to randomize patients with MVA to no therapy. (Similarly, we will probably never see a large scale randomized clinical trial that compares ICD with no therapy in patients with MVA. Thus, the magnitude of the improvement in the overall survival rate caused by ICD for patients with MVA will remain unknown.)

The Netherlands Cost-Effectiveness Study (32) was recently completed, the first to be published in which survivors of cardiac arrest due to late postmyocardial infarction MVA were randomized to an ICD implantation or conventional antiarrhythmic drug group, first guided by serial electrophysiologic testing. Although the number of patients was very small, this study demonstrated that ICD is superior to class I antiarrhythmic drugs for patients with postmyocardial infarction MVA. However, it is important to stress (33) that it has still not been shown whether ICD is better than class II or III antiarrhythmic drugs.

We must await the completion of the CASH, CIDS, and AVID trials for this information, from which we will learn how ICD and the best drug therapy compare with respect to survival, arrhythmic recurrences, quality of life, and cost-effectiveness.

Preliminary data from these trials are interesting. Regarding the CASH trial (33), the propafenone arm was stopped because of high mortality, but the other therapies are being continued because there appear to be no significant differences in total mortality among the three groups. It is important to emphasize that none of these trials can accurately estimate the magnitude of ICD benefits, because each has a positive control group, i.e., ICD treatment is being compared to drug therapy. The apparent advantage of ICD treatment over propafenone found in the CASH trial might represent a substantial benefit of ICD or a moderate or no benefit of ICD combined with substantial harm

from propafenone. It would not be surprising if propafenone doubled the overall mortality rate, since this was the magnitude of adverse effects on mortality seen with class I drugs in the CAST trial. If this is so, then the results indicate no benefit of ICD on overall mortality.

Regarding the CIDS trial (33), the Data Safety and Monitoring Board has found no reason to stop the study. In the AVID trial (33), the preliminary feasibility study that randomized 200 patients to the amiodarone (a small number received sotalol) or to the ICD group has been completed and another 150 patients have been randomized into the main portion of the study. To date, the number of crossovers between amiodarone and ICD has been small and equal in both directions.

Thus, these preliminary data from three large, randomized trials raise the possibility that, while ICD may reduce SCD mortality, there may be no difference in total mortality between amiodarone (and metoprolol in the CASH trial) and ICD. However, before making any conclusion, it must be emphasized that these studies are ongoing and, until the results are obtained, it appears prudent to exercise restraint in rapidly escalating the use of ICD in the treatment of MVA as the first-line therapy, especially the extension of its application to a patient population in which the benefit has not been convincingly demonstrated by controlled observations (18).

It is important to recognize, as suggested by Kappenberger (1), that all of us who implant ICD and elaborate guidelines will do and write what they believe, based on what they see in individual cases, but not yet backed up by scientific and statistically acceptable data that would irrefutably demonstrate the benefits and limitations of ICD.

The time has come for us (27) to show that the therapies we apply really are the best available rather than simply the ones that we think are the best available.

References

1. Kappenberger LJ (1995) Reflections on guidelines for the use of ICD. In: Camm J and Lindeman F (eds) Transvenous defibrillation and radiofrequency ablation. Futura, New York, pp 65-71
2 ACC/AHA Task Force Report (1991) Guidelines for implantation of cardiac pace-makers and antiarrhythmic devices. J Am Coll Cardiol 18: 1-8
3. Lehmann MH, Saksena S (1991) ICD in cardiovascular practice. Report of the policy conference of the Naspe. PACE 14: 969-979
4. Brugada P, Andries E (1991) The patient with malignant ventricular tachyarrhythmias can be offered optimal treatment on the basis of simple clinical variables. PACE 14: 1201-1204
5. Fogoros RN, Elson J et al (1990) Efficacy of AICD in prolonging survival in patients with severe heart failure. J Am Coll Cardiol 16: 381-386
6. Hentmorn RW (1991) Are the benefits of AICD overstimated by SCD rate? J Am Coll Cardiol 7: 1593-1595
7. Kocks M, Eggeling T et al (1993) Pharmacological therapy in coronary artery disease. Eur Heart J 14: 107-112
8. Task Force of the European Society of Cardiology (1992) Guidelines for the use of ICD. Eur Heart J 13: 1304-1310
9. Winkle RA, Mead RH et al (1989) Long-term outcome with the AICD. J Am Coll Cardiol 13: 1353-1361

10. Furman S (1989) AICD benefit. PACE 12: 399-400
11. Connolly S, Yusuf S (1992) Evaluation of ICD in survivors of cardiac arrest: the need for randomized trials. Am J Cardiol 89: 959-962
12. Kim SG (1993) ICD therapy . Am J Cardiol 71: 1212-1218
13. Doval H, Nul D et al (1994) Randomized trial of low dose Amiodarone in severe congestive heart failure. Lancet 344: 493-499
14. Teo K, Yusuf S et al (1993) Effect of prophylactic antiarrhythmic drug therapy in myocardial infarction. JAMA 270: 1598-1596
15. Mason JW (1993) A comparison of 7 antiarrhythmic drugs in patients with ventricular tachyarrhythmias. N Engl J Med 329: 452-457
16. Steinbeck G, Andresen D et al (1992) A comparison of EPS-guided antiarrhythmic drug therapy in patients with symptomatic sustained ventricular tachyarrhythmias. N Engl J Med 367: 987-993
17. The CASCADE investigators (1993) The CASCADE study. Am J Cardiol 72: 280-286
18. Singh BN (1994) ICD not the ultimate gold standard for gauging therapy of VT/VF. Am J Cardiol 73: 121-125
19. Chove W, Kim SG et al (1994) Comparison of defibrillator therapy and other therapeutic modalities of VT/VF associated with coronary artery disease. Am J Cardiol 73: 1075-1080
20. Saksena S (1992) Survavival of ICD recipients. Circulation 4: 1616-1620
21. Kim SG (1993) ICD therapy. Am J Cardiol 71: 1213-1216
22. Sweeney MO, Ruskin JN (1994) Mortality benefits and the ICD. Circulation 89: 1851-1857
23. Zipes DP (1994) ICD: lifesaver or a device looking for a disease? Circulation 89: 2933-2937
24. Mower MM (1994) Letter to editor. PACE 17: 260-261
25. Singer J (1994) Letter to editor. PACE 17: 261-263
26. Fogoros RN (1994) An AVID dissent. PACE 17: 1707-1710
27. Epstein AE (1994) Reply to Editor. PACE 17: 262-265
28. Connolly S (1994) An AVID dissent commentary. PACE 17: 1712-1715
29. Siebels J, Cappato R et al (1993) ICD versus drug in cardiac arrest survivors. PACE 72: 103-106
30. Connolly S, Gent M et al (1993) Canadian ICD study. Am J Cardiol 72: 103-106
31. The AVID investigators (1995) AVID: rationale, design and methods. Am J Cardiol 75: 470-474
32. Wever EF, Hauer RN et al (1995) Randomized study of ICD as first choice therapy versus conventional strategy in postinfarct sudden cardiac death survivors. Circulation 91: 2195-2203
33. Zipes DN (1995) Are ICD better than conventional antiarrhythmic drug for survivors of cardiac arrest? Circulation 91: 2115-2117

Implantable Cardioverter Defibrillator Technology in the Next 10 Years: What Can Be Expected?

M. Block and G. Breithardt

Medizinische Klinik und Poliklinik, Innere Medizin C,
Westfälische-Wilhelms-Universität,
Münster, Germany

Introduction

Fifteen years after the first implantation of an automatic defibrillator in humans (1), therapy with implantable cardioverter defibrillators (ICD) might become the therapy of first choice in patients with malignant ventricular tachyarrhythmias in the near future (2). The first ICD had no cardioversion and defibrillated the patient once a rhythm was observed above a fixed nonprogrammable heart rate (1). Defibrillation occurred after a fixed duration with a fixed energy. The ICD had to be implanted by a thoracotomy, as at least one defibrillation patch had to be positioned epicardially. Due to its volume of 145 ml, the device had to be implanted abdominally. Since 1980, major technical developments have been made which have improved ICD therapy and facilitated its widespread use (3).

• In 1988, programming of detection rate, energy (low energy cardioversion), and duration until defibrillation (so-called second generation ICD)
• Also in 1988, transvenous subcutaneous defibrillation leads, thus no need for thoracotomy
• In 1989, addition of pacing, especially antitachycardia pacing, to ICD functions and addition of multiple detection, redetection and therapy programming options (so-called third generation ICD)
• In 1990, biphasic defibrillation waveforms which improved defibrillation efficacy and practically abolished the need for thoracotomy due to high defibrillation thresholds with transvenous–subcutaneous defibrillation leads
• In 1993, reduction in size of ICD allowing for pectoral instead of abdominal implantation
ICDs can now (in 1995) be implanted with a very low perioperative mortality (less than 1%) in practically 100% of patients without thoracotomy using transvenous or transvenous–subcutaneous leads (4), and in most patients the device can be implanted pectorally similar to a pacemaker (5). However, the management of patients with ICDs is still troublesome and requires further improvements in ICD technology:
• The size of the device is about the same as that of a pack of cigarettes and causes cosmetic concerns in many patients, especially with pectoral implantations
• Battery longevity is only 3–5 years
• Leads show an unacceptably high failure rate of approximately 10% within 2 years (6, 7)
• Inappropriate ICD therapies are used in up to 30% of patients (3)
• Clusters of shocks occur in up to 40% of patients (8)
• Driving restrictions present a hardship for patients (9)
• Programming of ICD and handling of ICD memory data is too time-consuming and prone to failures

We will review how upcoming improvements of ICD technology might solve these clinical problems in the management of ICD patients.

Device Size

The volume of the ICD has declined (Fig. 1) from 145 ml (AID, Intec) to 60 ml (Sentinel model 2000, Angeion). Current ICDs are densely packed and a further size reduction can only be achieved by reducing the size of components. A reduction of ICD thickness might be most important to achieve better cosmetic results with pectoral implantations. The components

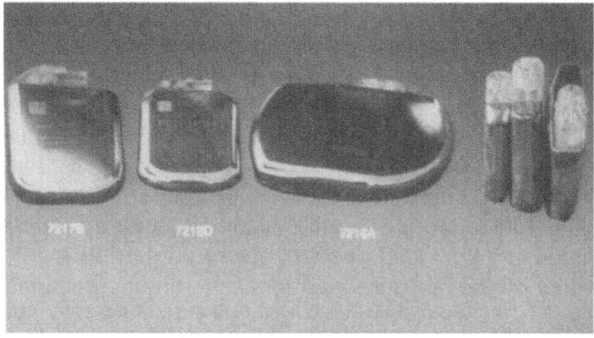

Fig. 1. Decline of implantable cardioverter defibrillator (ICD) size shown for the PCD (Medtronic). The original model 7216A of 1989 had a volume of 209 ml, the model 7217B of 1990 a volume of 113 ml and the model 7219D of 1993 a volume of 83 ml. Diameters were 27, 20, and 18 mm, respectively

which determine the thickness of the ICD are the cylindrical capacitors. A decrease can be achieved by using a new flat capacitor technology or using lower capacitances with current capacitor technology. While in 1995 no ICD with a flat capacitor technology have started to be clinically evaluated, the first implantations of an ICD with a lower capacitance have already occurred (Sentinel model 2000, Angeion). However, smaller capacitances are associated with lower maximum energy output (10) and can only be used in certain patients unless better waveforms or leads help to improve defibrillation efficacy (11). While the biphasic shape of the waveform seems to be optimal and cannot be improved by additional phases (12), ongoing research has to identify the ideal durations (or tilts) as a function of capacitance and defibrillation lead impedance (11). Based on this information, forthcoming ICDs might automatically alter their waveform based on the defibrillation impedances measured. Additionally, defibrillation might be achieved with less energy if the timing of energy delivery is optimized (14-16). Improvements of defibrillation efficacy by new leads and/or lead configurations might be achieved by adding a third defibrillation electrode to the right ventricular/active can configuration (17) to reduce defibrillation impedance and improve the defibrillation field. An additional defibrillation electrode placed subcutaneously at the left dorsolateral chest (13, 18; Fig. 2) or in the superior vena cava (19) might be used in the future.

Battery Longevity

Battery longevity of current ICDs (Fig. 3) is short in comparison to pacemakers (20). Assuming an average battery longevity of 4 years, at least 50% of all patients survive their first ICD and need device replacement. Device replacements are expensive and expose the patient to a significant risk of ICD infection (21). However, battery capacities cannot be increased if smaller devices are desired. Thus, energy consumption has to be minimized. Three different sources of energy consumption can be identified:
• Monitoring background current
• Bradycardia pacing current
• Energy used for cardioversion and defibrillation charging

In the future, monitoring circuits might use improved low current components. Furthermore, instead of running several monitoring circuits in parallel, monitoring functions have to be used in a hierarchical order to avoid high current drain from the battery. The rate of the ventricles and perhaps the atria as well as the electrograms from the sensing and perhaps defibrillation electrodes should not be continuously monitored in parallel. Only when the rate criterion is fulfilled by the ventricles additional monitoring functions should be started. In contrast, some devices (Fig. 4) currently continuously monitor the electrogram, thus allowing to store a few beats before the onset of the tachycardia. In the future, this function might be activated automatically and temporarily once a shock has occurred to collect information about the prearrhyth-

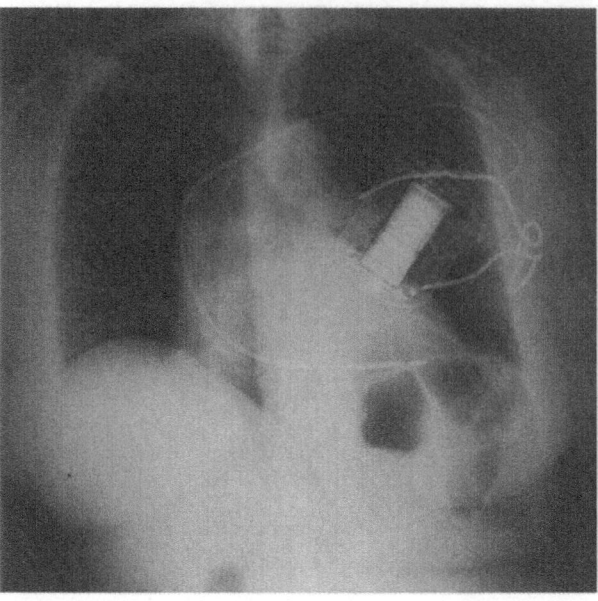

Fig. 2. Subpectorally implanted cardioverter defibrillator (PCD model 7218SP1) with an active shell used as defibrillation anode in combination with a two-finger array lead implanted subcutaneously at the left dorsolateral chest (Transvene model 13014). The multifunctional right ventricular lead serves as the defibrillation cathode (Transvene model 6936)

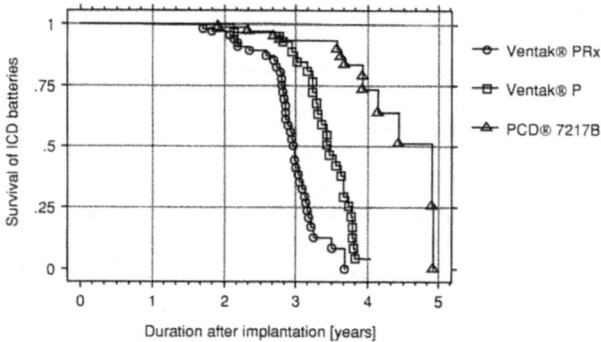

Fig. 3. Battery longevity of 227 second- and third-generation implantable cardioverter defibrillators (ICD) implanted at our institution. ICDs of patients who died or ICDs which were explanted due to other reasons were not included

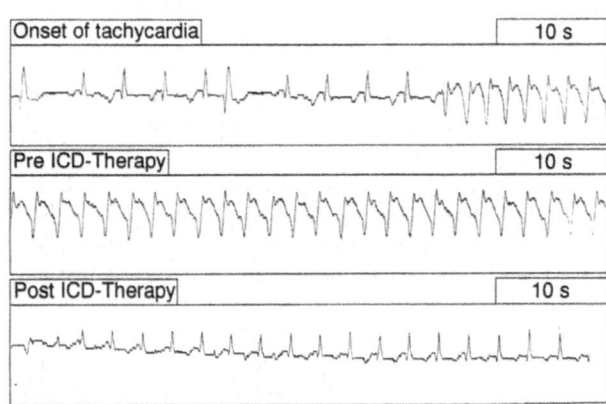

Fig. 4. Stored electrograms of a tachycardia treated by an implantable cardioverter defibrillator (PRx II, CPI) by cardioversion. The ICD has stored 10 s of electrograms before the detection criterion was fulfilled, showing a sinus rhythm of 90 beats per min with two premature beats and the onset of a ventricular tachycardia of 170 bpm. Another 10 s were stored while the capacitors were charged and the tachycardia was reconfirmed, showing a stable tachycardia. After termination by cardioversion further 10 s of electrograms were stored, showing a sinus tachycardia of 120 bpm

mia rhythm for subsequent episodes, especially if these occur in clusters.

Cadence model V110 ICD pacing significantly reduces battery longevity. Ventitrex predicts that the longevity of their Cadence V110 ICD will be shortened from 4.5 years to 3.8 years once pacing is used 100% instead of 0% and one shock per month is delivered. While few ICD patients are fully pacemaker dependent, many are using beta-blocking agents. Thus, some degree of VVI pacing cannot be avoided. In comparison to pacemakers, current ICD leads show a poor performance in terms of the acute and chronic pacing thresholds (22). Improved designs of the lead tip including steroid diluting tips will be evaluated in the next few years.

Frequent shocks might also significantly decrease battery longevity. Charging of capacitors decreases longevity by approximately 0.2-0.6 days for every 1 J (23). Energy consumption by shocks can be decreased by
• Decreasing the energy used for cardioversion/defibrillation
• Decreasing the number of inappropriate shocks
• Decreasing the number of appropriate shocks

The energy needed for a single shock can be decreased by improved waveforms and/or defibrillation leads, as discussed above. However, primary ventricular fibrillation (VF) is rare, and most patients receive shocks for ventricular tachycardia (VT). Energies needed for cardioversion might be substantially reduced if the ICD would distinguish between VF and VT (24) and deliver a different waveform for VT than for VF (25). Technological improvements which might decrease the number of inappropriate shocks will be discussed below.

Reduction of Failure Rate of Leads and Injuries Due to Leads

Recent reports on the long-term stability of transvenous(–subcutaneous) defibrillation leads have shown unacceptably high failure rates with the need for operative revisions (6, 7, 26). Additionally, significant rates of complications (perforation, thrombosis, infection, etc.) have been reported (3, 6). In one lead showing a high failure rate (Endotak 60 and 70 series), lead design changes have been made to reduce lead fractures and insulation failures (Endotak DSP). The diameter of leads has already been reduced to some degree (Endotak 60 and 70 series, 12 F; Endotak DSP, 10 F) (27) to avoid thrombosis and perforation due to stiff leads (3). Further reductions to diameters as low as 5 F are possible (28-30). Use of two separate right ventricular leads for defibrillation and sensing/pacing (28) might acutely yield better defibrillation and sensing/pacing results as both electrodes could be used in optimal positions. In addition, deterioration of sensing/pacing due to high defibrillation currents could be prevented.

Reduction of the Rate of Inappropriate Shocks

Approximately 10%-30% of all patients experience inappropriate ICD therapies (3). Inappropriate ICD shocks cause pain, consume energy, and might even induce ventricular tachyarrhythmias. Inappropriate ICD therapies due to sinus tachycardia or rapidly conducted atrial fibrillation might be avoided to a substantial degree using the onset and stability criteria of current devices (31, 32). However, fairly regular atrial tachycardias such as atrial flutter with a fixed conduction ratio to the ventricles cannot be distinguished from VT with current ICDs. Ideally, an atrial signal should be integrated into the algorithm to distinguish between atrial and ventricular tachyarrhythmias (33). After a great deal of research had been done in this area, an ICD has finally started to be clinically evaluated (Defender, Ela Medical) using a dual-chamber lead system introduced in 1993 (Enguard, Telectronics) (34). Other dual-chamber ICDs using new algorithms to classify tachycardias are being developed (35). However, lead positioning and stability problems inherent to bifocal pacing lead systems might limit these defibrillation lead systems to those ICD patients who require dual-chamber pacing. As in dual-chamber sensing ventricular pacing systems (VDD) (36, 37), a single pass lead system including an atrial sensor might be used in future ICDs instead. Another approach to differentiate atrial from ventricular tachyarrhythmias uses the width of the ventricular signal detected from the defibrillation leads. Although this approach was used without great success in early ICDs (Ventak P, CPI), a new device using a more sophisticated approach is currently being investigated (PCD Jewel model 7218, Medtronic). In this ICD, the width measurement is individualized in terms of the unique QRS complexes recorded in each patient during basic rhythm and ventricular tachycardia.

Reduction of the Rate of Appropriate Shocks

ICDs are implanted to terminate VT/VF by cardioversion/defibrillation. However, shocks are painful and consume energy. Cluster shocks might cause a state of anxiety (38). Antitachycardia pacing has reduced the number of shocks needed in many patients (3). However, a significant subgroup of patients still experiences frequent shocks which cannot be avoided by antitachycardia pacing. Thus, methods which might prevent ventricular tachyarrhythmias are being sought. Pacing algorithms which prevent inductions of ventricular tachyarrhythmias by short–long R-R interval sequences are currently being investigated and might be integrated into an investigational ICD in the near future (39). Other techniques of VT prevention such as high current pacing or ultrarapid subthreshold stimulation are feasible with epicardial electrodes (40-42). However, endocardial electrodes require detailed mapping and placement of the electrode close to a critical site of the VT circuit, which might not be achieved from the right ventricle. Theoretically, prevention of VT might also be achieved by continuous administration of antiarrhythmic drugs from the leads (43) or drug delivery (44) initiated once precursors of ventricular tachyarrhythmias like low heart rate variability, ventricular runs, or myocardial ischemia have been detected (45).

Avoiding Driving Restrictions for Implantable Cardioverter Defibrillator Patients

In addition to pain and anxiety caused by shocks, driving restrictions are the major hardship for ICD patients (9). Two reasons account for the driving restrictions:

- Presyncope and syncope despite ICD therapy (46, 47)
- Significant pain during shock delivery (38)

As driving restrictions have to consider the likelihood of an accident and should not prevent all conceivable possibilities, technological developments should be directed at reducing syncopes and uncontrolled reactions due to painful shocks. Reduction of the rate of appropriate and inappropriate shocks, as described above, is one way to reduce the risk. Syncopes during hemodynamically not tolerated ventricular tachycardias (VT) are correlated to the time needed to terminate VT. These VT might be terminated by antitachycardia pacing (ATP). However, the success, the number of sequences, and the duration needed for termination is not predictable and might differ between different VT episodes. Thus, ATP for VT that are not tolerated hemodynamically is not an ideal way to avoid syncope. A better approach would be an instant shock once the VT is detected. The detection usually takes 4-6 s for these fast VT, which is too short to cause syncope. However, maximum shock energies usually used for these fast VT have to be stored on the capacitors before the shock can be delivered. For a Ventak P3, this takes approximately 9 s, sufficient additional time to cause syncope in some patients. If the technical developments described above were able to improve the defibrillation efficacy, the time until successful termination of fast VT might be shortened significantly, e.g., if only 10 J were required for defibrillation, these 10 J would be available in a Ventak P3 within 2 s. Additionally, future ICD$_s$ might attempt to terminate fast VT by ATP and charge the capacitors in parallel to deliver a shock if ATP fails.

Simplifying Programming of Implantable Cardioverter Defibrillators

The present generation of ICD$_s$ has a high number of programmable variables, e.g., up to 106 variables in case of the Ventak PRx III. In addition, these programmable variables differ between different devices. Sometimes, the values programmable for the same parameters in different devices have a different meaning; e.g., the onset criterion of the PCD Jewel and the Ventak PRx III have to be programmed with opposing percentages. Therapy histories retrieved from the memory of the device might cover hundreds of episodes with hundreds of R-R intervals and more than 1 min of electrograms for the last few episodes. Thus, dealing with present ICD$_s$ is demanding and time-consuming.

Future ICD$_s$ will gradually develop into expert systems which will require information on the hemodynamic tolerance of VT and then decide which therapy to use based on this information after automatic classifi-

cation of the tachycardia. Rate criteria, additional detection criteria, and different zones of therapies will no longer have to be programmed, and any tachycardia will be classified as nonventricular or ventricular and hemodynamically tolerated or not tolerated. ATP will be programmed automatically in every patient for tachycardia rates which are hemodynamically tolerated (48). Based on success or acceleration rates, the therapies will be altered automatically, e.g., the PCD Jewel model 7218, currently under clinical investigation, can decide on the further use of an antitachycardia pacing mode based on previous success rates ("smart mode"). A hemodynamic sensor could further reduce the programming requirements and let the ICD decide when to use ATP or cardioversion/defibrillation. However, no stable sensor is foreseeable yet which would safely allow us to predict hemodynamic intolerance of a VT early after onset of the VT (29, 49).

Information on therapies retrieved from the ICD will be presented to the physician as a graphical presentation in different layers of details indicating how changes of the detection and therapy algorithm influenced the outcome, e.g., the 9874 software for the PCD Jewel model 7218 represents the R-R interval of an episode graphically instead of listing hundreds of R-R intervals.

Other Future Developments

In addition to new ICD technology aimed at improving performance of the devices in the treatment of ventricular tachyarrhythmias, other technologies might be added to ICD which are not covered by this aspect. These technologies include biventricular pacing to ameliorate congestive heart failure (50), antitachycardia pacing in the atria to terminate atrial flutter and atrial tachycardias (51), and cardioversion in the atria to terminate atrial fibrillation (52).

References

1. Mirowski M, Reid PR, Mower MM et al (1980) Termination of malignant ventricular arrhythmias with an implanted automatic defibrillator in human beings. N Engl J Med 303: 322-324
2. Wever E, Hauer R, van Capelle F et al (1995) Randomized study of implantable defibrillator as first-choice therapy versus conventional strategy in postinfarct sudden death survivors. Circulation 91: 2195-2203
3. Block M, Breithardt G (1995) Long-term follow-up and clinical results of implantable cardioverter-defibrillators. In: Zipes DP, Jalife J (eds) Cardiac electrophysiology: from cell to bedside. Saunders, Philadelphia, pp 1412-1425
4. Neuzner J for the European Ventak P2 Investigator Group (1994) Clinical experience with a new cardioverter defibrillator capable of biphasic waveform pulse and enhanced data storage: results of a prospective multicenter study. PACE 17: 1243-1255.
5. Hammel D, Block M, Geiger A et al (1994) Single-incision implantation of cardioverter defibrillators using nonthoracotomy lead systems. Ann Thorac Surg 58: 1614-1616
6. Block M, Hammel D, Bänsch D et al (1995) Prevention of ICD complications. In: Allessie M, Fromer M (eds) Atrial and ventricular fibrillation – mechanisms and device therapy. Futura, Armonk
7. Nunain SO, Roelke M, Trouton T et al (1995) Limitations and late complications of third-generation automatic cardioverter-defibrillators. Circulation 91: 2204-2213

8. Kluger J, Veronneau J, Fisher J (1995) Cluster shocks: a strong predictor of subsequent mortality in patients with internal cardioverter defibrillators. PACE 18: 845 (abstr)
9. Anderson MH, Camm AJ (1994) Legal and ethical aspects of driving and working in patients with an implantable cardioverter defibrillator. Am Heart J 127: 1185-1193
10. Block M, Hammel D, Böcker D et al (1995) Internal defibrillation with smaller capacitors – a prospective randomized crossover comparison of defibrillation efficacy obtained with 90 µF- and 125 µF-capacitors in humans. J Cardiovasc Electrophysiol 6: 333-342
11. Block M, Breithardt G (1995) Optimizing defibrillation through improved waveforms. PACE 18 (II): 526-538
12. Jung W, Manz M, Moosdorf R et al (1994) Comparative defibrillation efficacy of biphasic and triphasic shock waveforms. New Trends Arrhythmias 9: 765-772
13. Block M, Seidel K, Hammel D et al (1995) Active can versus subcutaneous array. Which lead configuration shows lower defibrillation thresholds? PACE 18 (II): 887 (abstr)
14. Hsia PW, Suresh G, Allen C et al (1995) Improved nonthoracotomy defibrillation based on ventricular fibrillation waveform characteristics. PACE 18: 803 (abstr)
15. Sweeney RJ, Gill RM, Reid PR (1995) Characteristics of multiple-shock defibrillation. J Cardiovasc Electrophysiol 6: 89-102
16. Zimmermann S, Alt E, Kressierer P et al (1995) Organized de- and repolarization during ventricular fibrillation as indicated by signals with large amplitude and low frequency PACE 18: 938 (abstr)
17. Bardy GH, Johnson G, Poole JE et al (1993) A simplified, single-lead unipolar transvenous cardioversion-defibrillation system. Circulation 88: 543-547
18. Saksena S, Kaushik RR, Varanasi S et al (1995) Optimal lead system(s) for reduced output implantable cardioverter-defibrillators for ventricular defibrillation. PACE 18: 807 (abstr)
19. Bardy GH, Dolack GL, Kudenchuk PJ et al (1994) Prospective comparison in humans of a unipolar defibrillation system with that using an additional superior vena cava electrode. Circulation 89: 1090-1093
20. Song SL (1994) Performance of implantable cardiac rhythm management devices. PACE 17: 692-708
21. Wietholt D, Block M, Isbruch F et al (1993) Therapy of ventricular tachyarrhythmias with implantable cardioverter-defibrillators – mortality and complications with epicardial lead systems. Z Kardiol 82: 150-161
22. Mönnich A, Block M, Hammel D et al (1995) Langzeitstabilität der Wahrnehmungs-, Stimulations- und Defibrillationsfunktion einer multifunktionellen transvenösen ICD-Elektrode. Z Kardiol 84 [Suppl.1]: 108 (abstr)
23. Keimel JG, Abeyratne A (1995) Graphical presentation of factors influencing implantable cardioverter defibrillator (ICD) longevity. PACE 18: 889 (abstr)
24. Throne RD, Windle JR, Easley AR et al (1994) Scatter diagram analysis: a new technique for discriminating ventricular tachyarrhythmias. PACE 17: 1267-1275
25. Brewer JE, Tvedt MA, Adams TP, Kroll MW (1994) Low voltage shocks have a significantly higher tilt of the internal electric field than do high voltage shocks. PACE 18: 214-220
26. Fahy GR, Kleman JM, Wilkoff BL et al (1995) Low incidence of lead related complications associated with nonthoracotomy implantable cardioverter defibrillator systems PACE 18: 172-178
27. Kühlkamp V, O´Connor S on behalf of the Endotak DSP™ European Investigator Group (1995) A new downsized transvenous combined rate sensing and defibrillating electrode, Endotak DSP. PACE 18: 886 (abstr)
28. Leonelli FM, Wright H, Latterell ST et al (1995) A long thin electrode is equivalent to a short thick electrode for defibrillation in the right ventricle. PACE 18: 221-224
29. Sharma AD, Bennet TD, Erickson M et al (1990) Right ventricular pressure during ventricular arrhythmias in humans: potential implications for implantable antitachycardia devices. J Am Coll Cardiol 15: 648-655
30. Singer I, Goldsmith J, Maldonado C (1995) Electrode surface area is an important variable for defibrillation. PACE 18: 233-236
31. Neuzner J, Pitschner HF, Schlepper M (1995) Programmable VT detection enhancements in implantable cardioverter defibrillator therapy. PACE 18 (II): 539-547
32. Swerdlow CD, Chen PS, Kass RM et al (1994) Discrimination of ventricular tachycardia from sinus tachycardia and atrial fibrillation in a tiered-therapy cardioverter-defibrillator. J Am Coll Cardiol 23: 1342-1355
33. Schugger CD, Jackson K, Steinman RT, Lehmann MH (1988) Atrial sensing to augment ventricular tachycardia detection by the automatic implantable cardioverter defibrillator: a utility study. PACE 11: 1456-1464
34. Luceri RM, Zilo P, and the United States and Canadian Enguard Investigators (1995) Initial clinical experience with a dual lead endocardial defibrillation system with atrial pace/sense capability. PACE 18: 163-167
35. Kaemmerer WF, Olson WH (1995) Dual chamber tachyarrhythmia detection using syntactic pattern recognition and contexial timing rules for rhythm classification. PACE 18: 872 (abstr)
36. Longo E, Catrini V (1990) Experience and implantation techniques with a new single-pass lead VDD pacing system. PACE 13: 927-936
37. Variale P, Pilla AG, Tekrival M (1990) Single-lead VDD pacing system. PACE 13: 757-766
38. Dunbar SB, Warner CD, Purcell JA (1993) Internal cardioverter defibrillator device discharge: experiences of patients and family members. Heart Lung J Crit Care 22: 494-501
39. Leclercq JF, Maisonblanche P, Cauchemez B, Coumel P (1988) Respective role of sympathetic tone and of cardiac pauses in the genesis of 62 cases of ventricular fibrillation recorded during Holter monitoring. Eur Heart J 9: 1276-1283
40. Marchlinski FE, Buxton AE, Miller JM et al (1987) Prevention of ventricular tachycardia induction during right ventricular programmed stimulation by high current strength pacing at the site of origin. Circulation 76: 332-342
41. Shenasa M, Fromer M, Borggrefe M, Breithardt G (1991) Subthreshold electrical stimulation for termination and prevention of reentrant tachycardias. J Electrocardiol 24: 25-31
42. Skale BT, Kallok MJ, Prystowski EN et al (1985) Inhibition of premature ventricular extrastimuli by subthreshold conditioning stimuli. J Am Coll Cardiol 6: 133-140
43. Labhasetwar V, Underwood T, Heil RW et al (1994) Epicardial administration of ibutilide from polyurethane matrices: effects on defibrillation threshold and electrophysiologic parameters. J Cardiovasc Pharmacol 24: 826-840
44. Cammilli L, Furlanello F, Perna AM et al (1991) Suppression of precursors of impending ventricular fibrillation by drugs retroinfusion in coronary sinus. Experimental investigation for a possible automatic implantable pharmacological cardioverter defibrillator (AIPhCD). New Trends Arrhyth 7: 855-863
45. Zehender M, Faber T, Grom A et al (1994) Continuous monitoring of myocardial ischemia by the implantable cardioverter defibrillator. Am Heart J 127: 1057-1063
46. Grimm W, Flores BF, Marchlinski FE (1993) Symptoms and electrocardiographically documented rhythm preceding spontaneous shocks in patients with implantable cardioverter-defibrillator. Am J Cardiol 71: 1415-1418
47. Schöls W, Sarasin C, Beyer T, Brachmann J (1995) Should patients with the implanted defibrillator resume car driving? PACE 18: 945
48. Schaumann A, Meyer O, Dorszewski A et al (1995) A prospective study of tested versus nontested antitachycardia pacing in implantable cardioverter-defibrillators. PACE 18: 898 (abstr)
49. Bardy GH, Olson WH, Fishbein DP et al (1985) Transvenous right ventricular impedance during spontaneous ventricular arrhythmias. Circulation 72: 474A (abstr)
50. Bakker PF, Meijburg H, de Jonge N et al (1994) Beneficial effects of biventricular pacing in congestive heart failure. PACE 17: 820 (abstr)
51. den Dulk K, Brugada P, Smeets JL, Wellens HJ (1990) Long-term antitachycardia pacing experience for supraventricular tachycardia. PACE 13: 1020-1030
52. Murgatroyd FD, Johnson EE, Cooper RA et al (1994) Safety of low energy transvenous atrial defibrillation - world experience. Circulation 90: I-14 (abstr)

SYNCOPE

Spontaneous Asystolic Pauses: How Frequent Is a Neuromediated Mechanism?

C. Menozzi[1] and M. Brignole[2]

[1] Ospedale S. Maria Nuova, Reggio Emilia, Italy
[2] Ospedali Riuniti, Sezione di Aritmologia, Lavagna, Genova, Italy

Introduction

In a patient evaluated for syncope, the recording of a symptomatic ventricular asystole during electrocardiographic monitoring is usually regarded as a sign of severe dysfunction of the sinoatrial node or of the atrioventricular node with an ominous outcome; therefore pacemaker therapy is usually initiated. Recent studies have shown that a neurocardiogenic mechanism is the hidden, real cause of syncope in most patients presenting with asystolic pauses, which mistakenly suggest another cause for syncope. The identification of the neurocardiogenic mechanism has important clinical implications for prognosis and therapy.

Prevalence of Asystolic Pauses During Electrocardiographic Monitoring

In patients affected by unexplained syncope, a pause >3 s (symptomatic or asymptomatic) was found in 47 (2.5%) out of 1895 patients during 24-h electrocardiographic monitoring (Table 1). The asystolic pause was due to sinus arrest or paroxysmal atrioventricular (AV) block or atrial fibrillation with prolonged ventricular asystole, roughly in similar percentages. The prevalence of asystolic pauses in patients with syncope was significantly higher than the 1.1% value observed in the total population (105 of 9090 recordings) and the 0.2% value observed in healthy subjects (1 out of 654 recordings) undergoing 24-h electrocardiographic monitoring (1-13).

Mechanisms of Syncope Caused by a Ventricular Asystole During Electrocardiographic Monitoring

Recently we have prospectively investigated a series of consecutive patients with fortuitous documentation of intermittent syncope due to ventricular asystole who subsequently presented with no evident abnormality in order to clarify the exact mechanism of the episode (14). The study group consisted of 25 patients, with a mean age 66±15 years. They accounted for 1.8% of the total of 1094 patients with syncope referred to our institutions. A prolonged ventricular asystole (5-20 s; mean 9.5±3.5) was documented during syncope in all patients. The asystolic episode was due to a sinus arrest in 13 patients, AV block in 7 patients, sinus arrest plus AV block in 3 patients, and asystolic pause during atrial fibrillation in 2 patients. All the patients underwent a full electrophysiologic study, carotid sinus massage and head-up tilt test, baseline and, if negative, potentiated with sublingual trinitrin. Electrophysiologic testing and vasovagal maneuvers were able to identify the mechanism responsible for spontaneous bradycardic syncope in 23 (92%) of 25 patients. Based on the results of these tests, the likely final diagnosis was: sinus-node dysfunction – both intrinsic and extrinsic – one patient (4%); infrahisian AV block, 5 patients (20%); neurally mediated syncope, 17 patients (68%); and unknown, two patients (8%; Fig. 1). A positive response to carotid sinus massage or head-up tilt test or both was found in 20 patients (80%). Abnormal responses to carotid sinus massage were found in 14 patients (56%). The mean length of the induced pause was 8.6±2.2 s (range 5.8 to 13.5); the pause was due to

Table 1. Prevalence of asystolic pauses >3 s during Holter monitoring

Reference	Disease	Asystole (n pts)	>3 s
(1)	Healthy	1/183	0.5%
(2)	Healthy	0/26	0.0%
(3)	Healthy	0/50	0.0%
(4)	Healthy	0/260	0.0%
(5)	Healthy	0/50	0.0%
(6)	Healthy	0/32	0.0%
(7)	Healthy	0/20	0.0%
(8)	Healthy	0/33	0.0%
(9)	Various	53/1350	0.2%
(10)	Various	52/6740	0.8%
(11)	Syncope	9/235	0.4%
(12)	Syncope	17/1512	0.1%
(13)	Syncope	21/148	.14%

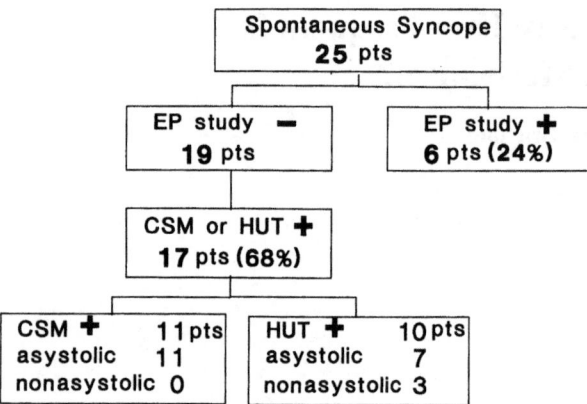

Fig. 1. Underlying mechanisms of asystolic syncope. *EP*, electrophysiologic; *CSM*, carotid sinus massage; *HUT*, head-up tilt test

sinus arrest in 11 cases, AV block in two cases, and AV block with marked sinus-rate slowing and sinus arrest in one case. The same type of responses in both spontaneous and induced asystole was found in 11 (79%) of 14 patients. Carotid sinus massage was positive in the patient with sick sinus syndrome; thus, in this case, two different mechanisms (one intrinsic and one extrinsic) were found to have caused syncope. Two patients who had spontaneous AV block and abnormal electrophysiologic study results had positive asystolic responses to carotid sinus massage, which therefore were probably unrelated to the spontaneous syncope. Abnormal responses to the head-up tilt test were found in ten (40%) of the patients: the test was positive in the baseline phase in eight cases and in the trinitrin phase in two cases. The response was asystolic in 7 cases (mean pause 14.3±8.3 s) and non-asystolic in 3 cases. The same type of response in both spontaneous and induced episodes was found in seven (70%) of the ten patients.

Thus, in patients who present with syncope due to intermittent ventricular arrest, the mechanism of syncope seems to be neurogenic in most cases and cardiogenic in only a minority of cases. This datum is not surprising if we consider that in the literature the neurogenic mechanism is considered to be the most frequent cause of syncope, while the cardiogenic mechanism accounts for 8%-29% of cases.

Adenosine-Mediated Asystolic Syncope ?

We have recently proposed a new mechanism for syncope in some patients in whom all conventional investigations, including vasovagal maneuvers and electrophysiologic study, were negative (15).

Adenosine, a ubiquitous biological compound with potent electrophysiologic activity on the AV node, is a potential cause of extrinsic paroxysmal AV block different from the neurally mediated mechanism, but clinical evidence of this is lacking (16). We have observed two patients who had a syncopal episode during electrocardiographic monitoring which showed a prolonged pause due to paroxysmal AV block at time of syncope. No other rhythm disturbance was observed. The first patient was a healthy female, 50 years old; during the previous 2 years, she had complained of six

syncopal episodes which had occurred without any prodromal symptoms or causative events; one of these was due to an AV block with an 8-s ventricular pause followed by immediate full return to normal heart rhythm. The second patient was a 68-year-old male, affected by Prinzmetal's angina and chronic atrial flutter; the thallium stress test results and coronary angiograms were normal. During the previous 6 months, he had complained of three syncopal episodes that always had occurred during anginal attacks. The electrocardiographic monitoring during a typical anginal attack revealed a marked elevation of the ST segment which lasted 3 min; 1 min after the beginning of the ischemic episode, a sudden 12-s ventricular pause occurred and the patient fainted; this was followed by irregular rhythm with ventricular premature beats for a few seconds. The spontaneous episodes could be reproduced by means of exogenous adenosine 5′-triphosphate (ATP) infusion (20 mg i.v. bolus, Striadyne, Wyeth). Within a few seconds after the end of the infusion, both patients developed sudden intranodal AV block with asystole of 11 s and 10 s, respectively, which caused syncope. This response was reproducible on different days, but not after administration of theophylline. In both patients the vasovagal maneuvers (carotid sinus massage, eyeball compression test, head-up tilt test, baseline and potentiated with nitrates) were negative; the electrophysiologic study showed normal AV conduction times baseline and after 1 mg/kg i.v. ajmaline infusion. The first patient was treated with oral theophylline 700 mg/day and the second with oral verapamil 240 mg/day; they both remained asymptomatic during the following 14 and 8 months, respectively.

ATP and its related nucleoside adenosine are ubiquitous biological compounds with potent electrophysiologic activity on the AV node. ATP and adenosine are released from myocardial cells under physiologic and pathological conditions (for example, in the case of myocardial oxygen supply-demand imbalance) and have similar effects. The negative dromotropic action of ATP is due to its rapid catabolism to adenosine and the subsequent action of adenosine at purinoceptor sites (17,18). Therefore, it is possible that an abnormal release of endogenous adenosine or an increased sensitivity of purinoceptors or both could cause AV block in the absence of an intrinsic disease of the AV conduction or of an abnormal neural reflex. In our two patients, exogenous ATP exactly reproduced syncope and spontaneous electrocardiographic pattern. No other known mechanism able to cause paroxysmal AV block seemed to be present, neither intrinsic (AV conduction disease) nor extrinsic (through an activation of neurally mediated cholinergic receptors). In one case the spontaneous AV block was clearly linked to a transient myocardial ischemic episode, a condition under which endogenous ATP and adenosine are likely to be released. In healthy subjects and in patients affected by neurally mediated syncope, ATP infusion is unable to cause ventricular pauses as prolonged as those observed in our cases, although minor conduction disturbances are frequent (16). The etiologic therapy with theophylline, an adenosine antagonist, and with verapamil, for the prevention of coronary spasm, seemed to be efficacious in preventing syncopal recurrences. Thus, an "adenosine-mediated syndrome" could be the underlying mechanism in some cases of unexplained syncope.

Practical Implications

A different therapeutic approach, other than back-up pacing therapy, may be considered for patients with syncope due to neurocardiogenic asystole. Indeed, from a theoretical point of view, therapy should first be aimed at preventing the onset of abnormal reflexes. Therefore, therapy able to prevent both cardioinhibitory and vasodepressor reflexes appears to be reasonable as an alternative to, or in association with, pacemaker therapy. At present, however, there are no drugs which are reliably effective in the prevention of vasovagal syncope. Moreover, the benign prognosis of neurocardiogenic syncope makes it reasonable to avoid or to delay pacing therapy in less severe cases.

Similarly, the etiologic therapy with theophylline, an adenosine-antagonist, and with verapamil, for the prevention of coronary spasm, seemed to be efficacious in patients affected by adenosine-mediated asystolic syncope.

References

1. Molgaard H, Sorensen E, Bjerregard P (1989) Minimal heart rates and longest pauses in healthy adult subjects on two occasions eight years apart. Eur Heart J 10: 758-764
2. Wajngarten M, Grupi C, Bellotti G, Lemos da Luz P, Azul L, Pileggi F (1990) Frequency and significance of cardiac rhythm disturbances in healthy elderly individuals. J Electrocardiol 23: 171-176
3. Kantelip JP, Sage E, Duchene-Marullaz P (1986) Findings on ambulatory electrocardiographic monitoring in subjects older than 80 years. Am J Cardiol 57: 398-401
4. Bjerregard P (1983) Mean 24 hour heart rate, minimal heart rate and pauses in healthy subjects 40-79 years of age. Eur Heart J 4: 44-51
5. Brodsky M, Wu D, Denes P, Kanakis C, Rosen KM (1977) Arrhythmias documented by 24 hour continuous electrocardiographic monitoring in 50 male medical students without apparent heart disease. Am J Cardiol 39: 390-395
6. Hanne-Paparo N, Kellermann JJ (1981) Long-term Holter ECG monitoring of athletes. Med Sci Sports Exercise 13: 294-298
7. Talan DA, Bauernfeind RE, Ashley WW, Kanakis C Jr, Rosen KM (1982) Twenty-four hour continuous ECG recordings in long-distance runners. Chest 82: 19-24
8. Viitasalo MT, Kala R, Eisalo A (1982) Ambulatory electrocardiographic recording in endurance athletes. Br Heart J 47: 213-220
9. Ector H, Rolies L, De Geest H (1983) Dynamic electrocardiographic and ventricular pauses of 3 seconds and more: etiology and therapeuthic implications. PACE 6: 548-551
10. Hilgard J, Ezri M, Denes P (1985) Significance of ventricular pauses of three seconds or more on twenty-four-hour Holter recordings. Am J Cardiol 55: 1005-1008
11. Kapoor W, Cha R, Peterson J, Wieand H, Karpf M (1987) Prolonged electrocardiographic monitoring in patients with syncope. Am J Med 82: 20-28
12. Gibson T, Heitzman M (1984) Diagnostic efficacy of 24-hour electrocardiographic monitoring for syncope. Am J Cardiol 53: 1013-1017
13. Aronow W, Mercando A, Epstein S (1992) Prevalence of arrhythmias detected by 24-hour ambulatory electrocardiography and value of antiarrhythmic therapy in elderly patients with unexplained syncope. Am J Cardiol 70: 408-410
14. Brignole M, Menozzi C, Bottoni N, Gianfranchi L, Lolli G, Oddone D, Gaggioli G (1995) The mechanism of syncopes caused by transient bradycardia and the diagnostic value of electrophysiologic testing and vasovagal maneuvers. Am J Cardiol 76: 273-278
15. Brignole M, Menozzi C, Gianfranchi L (1995) Syncope caused by adenosine-mediated paroxysmal atrioventricular block. (submitted)
16. Brignole M, Menozzi C, Alboni P, Oddone D, Gianfranchi L, Gaggioli G, Lolli G, Paparella N (1994) The effect of exogenous adenosine in patients with neurally-mediated syncope and sick sinus syndrome. PACE 17: 2211-2216
17. Pelleg A, Mitsuoka T, Michelson E, Menduke H (1987) Adenosine mediates the negative chronotropic action of adenosine 5' triphosphate in the canine sinus node. J Pharmacol Exp Ther 242: 791-795
18. Lerman B, Belardinelli L (1991) Cardiac electrophysiology of adenosine. Basic and clinical concept. Circulation 83: 1499-1507

Pathophysiology of Neurally Mediated Syncope: Peripheral and Central Mechanisms

D.G. Benditt, K.G. Lurie, and S.W. Adler

Cardiac Arrhythmia and Syncope Centers, Department of Medicine
(Cardiovascular Division), University of Minnesota Medical School,
Minneapolis, USA

Introduction

The neurally mediated syncopal syndromes (especially the "common" or vasovagal faint) have long been recognized as being among the most frequent causes of syncope in humans (Table 1; 1-7). Nonetheless, it is only recently (as the availability of tilt-table testing has increased physician awareness) that the pathophysiology and treatment of these syndromes have become the subject of widespread clinical interest (8-11).

The principal elements comprising the reflex arcs responsible for neurally mediated faints may be classified as being located peripherally (e.g., organ-based receptors which respond to pain, chemical changes, or mechanical distortion) or centrally (various central nervous system [CNS] regions or tracts) (Fig. 1).

The clearest example is in carotid sinus syndrome (12-14). In this case it is the interaction of afferent neural signals from "peripheral" carotid artery baroreceptors with the CNS that triggers the syncopal episodes. Whether it is the peripheral receptor which is "hypersensitive" or whether the fault lies centrally, or perhaps both, cannot be clearly identified in most cases. Similar arguments may also be made in both postmicturition syncope in which neural afferent signals arise from bladder wall receptors, and in posturally induced hypotension-bradycardia in which peripheral cardiopulmonary receptors have been implicated (15, 16). In both of these cases central processing of afferent signals may be crucial in determining whether a faint occurs. On the other hand, in the form of vasovagal faint induced by fear, anxiety, or emotional upset, the CNS component predominates as both the source of afferent signals to cardiovascular control areas in the medulla as well as the determinant of the efferent response. In these cases, the relevance of peripheral neural afferent signals is uncertain, yet they may still play an important feedback role in the efferent limb of the reflex arc.

It is the goal of this review to address current understanding of the roles played by central and peripheral elements in the genesis of the most common forms of neurally mediated syncopal spells. To this end, the apparent contribution of peripheral and central elements to neurally mediated syncope is first examined in general, following which we focus on the so-called spontaneous vasovagal faint as modeled by posturally induced, neurally mediated hypotension-bradycardia.

Table 1. Neurally mediated reflex syncopal syndromes

Vasovagal (emotional, common) faint

Carotid sinus syncope

Head-up tilt / gravitational / postural syncope

Increased intrathoracic pressure
    Cough syncope
    Sneeze syncope
    Trumpet player's
    Weight lifter's
    'Mess Trick'
    Valsalva-induced

Postmicturition syncope

Gastrointestinal stimulation
    Rectal examination
    Defecation syncope
    Gastrointestinal instrumentation

Esophageal / nasopharyngeal stimulation
    Swallow syncope
    Glossopharyngeal neuralgia
    Oropharyngel esophageal

Airway stimulation

'Diving' reflex

Drug-induced syncope
    Nitroglycerin
    Isoproterenol
    Sympatholytic agents, (e.g., bretylium, guanethidine)

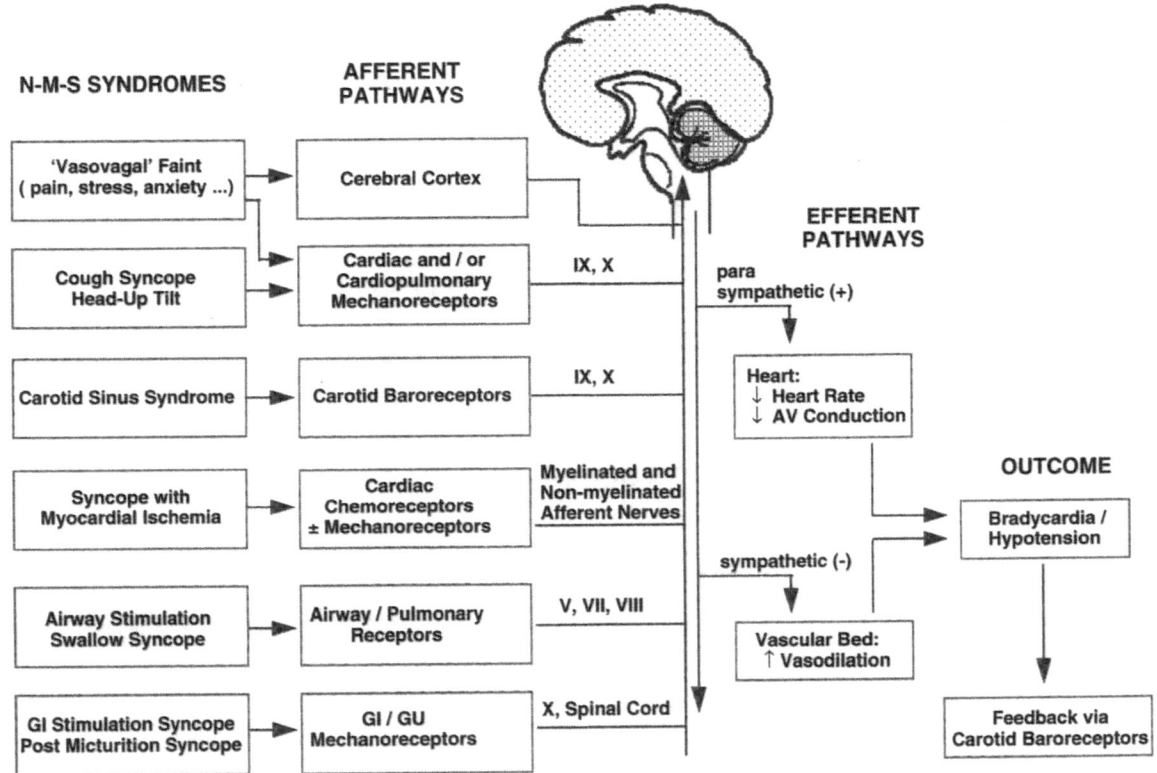

Fig. 1. The most common neurally mediated syncopal (*N-M-S*) syndromes and their principal afferent and efferent CNS connections. *GI*, gastrointestinal; *GU*, genitourinary

Overview of Peripheral and Central Aspects of the Neural Reflex in Neurally Mediated Syncopal Syndromes

Afferent Limb

Afferent neural signals in many of the neurally mediated syncopal syndromes originate from non-CNS peripheral receptors which respond to mechanical (e.g., increased or decreased wall stress) or chemical (e.g., ischemia-induced) stimuli, or pain (Fig. 1). The prototype is carotid sinus hypersensitivity. In this case, mechanical stimulation of the region now known to incorporate the carotid sinus baroreceptors results in afferent impulses within the carotid sinus nerve which itself travels primarily within the glossopharyngeal nerve. These impulses are transmitted to the nucleus solitarius in the medulla, a site closely related to the dorsal and ambiguous nuclei of the vagus nerve (2). The efferent response may incorporate slowing of heart rate, negative dromotropic effects at the level of the atrioventricular node, and vasodilatation.

From the clinical perspective, the various neurally mediated syndromes are distinguished from each other primarily by the site or nature of the initiating stimulus. Thus, the principal receptors (whether peripheral or central) which initiate neural afferent activity, and to some extent the afferent limb itself, differ among the syndromes. In certain cases the differences may seem readily apparent (e.g., carotid sinus syncope versus postmicturition syncope). However, it is probably uncommon for only one set of receptors to be at fault. For example, whereas stimulation of bladder mechanoreceptors is a crucial trigger in postmicturition syncope, arterial baroreceptors are also believed to play a critical role, possibly by failing to respond promptly to hemodynamic changes induced by bladder receptor afferent traffic as bladder wall decompression occurs. The common clinical association of postmicturition syncope with prior alcohol consumption also raises the possibility of a central effect modifying susceptibility. In the emotionally induced vasovagal faint central CNS trigger sites may be predominant. However, peripheral elements remain important considerations. The potential contribution of afferent trigger signals from peripheral receptors such as cardiac mechanoreceptors has been a source of continued interest and debate (so-called neurocardiogenic syncope; 9-11, 17-21). Furthermore, the inability of the carotid baroreceptors to stem the tide of evolving hypotension and bradycardia suggests another point at which important interaction of central and peripheral elements takes place (i.e., feedback stage).

Central Sites

The nucleus tractus solitarius (NTS) of the medulla is the region responsible for integrating afferent cardiovascular baro- and chemoreceptor nerve traffic arriving principally via the vagus and glossopharyngeal nerves (22-25). In addition, the NTS receives afferent impulses from other cranial nerves, the hypothalamus, the spinal cord, and brainstem. The NTS may also be influenced by circulating neurohumoral factors by virtue of its close vascular and neural relationship to the area postrema, which lacks an efficient blood-brain barrier. Signals from the NTS address the vagal preganglionic nuclei in the medulla, sympathetic preganglionic nuclei in the spinal cord, as well as other brain-

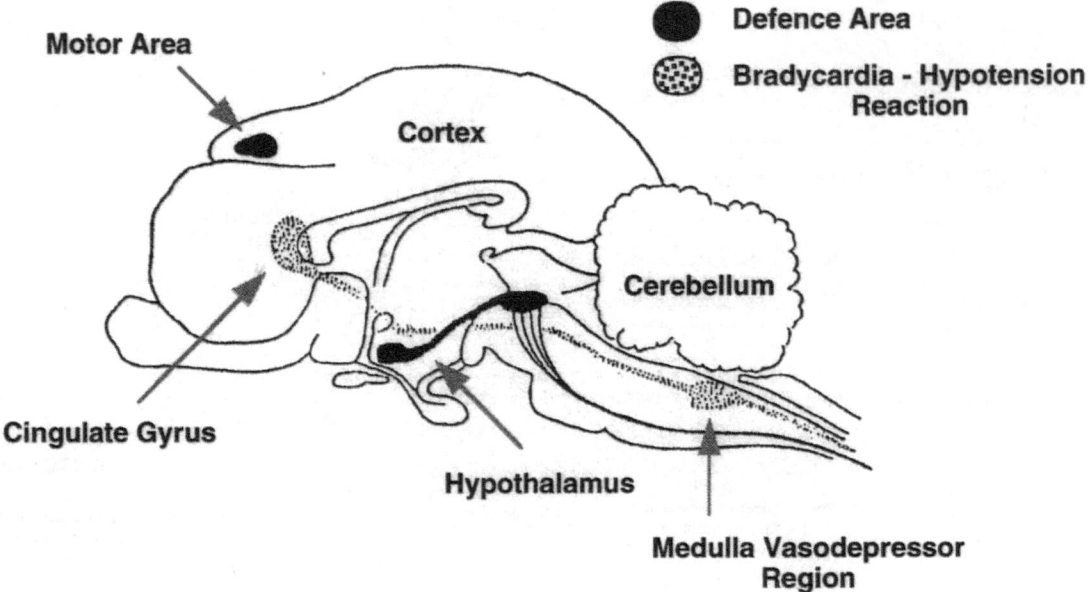

Fig. 2. The location of CNS pathways mediating the defense reaction (*solid zone*) and the vasodepressor reaction (*stippled zone*). Modified from Simone (26)

stem nuclei and higher central nervous system centers .

Among the least well understood aspects of CNS contribution to the neurally mediated syncopal syndromes is the interindividual differences in the manner in which afferent neural impulses are processed. The result of these differences is manifest as a range of hemodynamic and arrhythmic responses, with two extremes being well recognized (Fig. 2; 26).

One is the so-called defense reaction characterized by somatomotor and sympathetic neural activation. This response occurs in a various species, conforming to the fight or flight concept. At the opposite end of the spectrum, an alternative response (which may occur through activation of the anterior cingulate gyrus directly or via somatic and visceral afferent signals) results in vagally mediated bradycardia, sympathetic withdrawal, and diminished muscular tone. The outcome, often of sufficient severity to elicit cerebral hypoperfusion and syncope, may be a human parallel of the "playing dead" protective strategy employed by some animals. Little is known of the determinants of which response is to become manifest in a given individual. Furthermore, it

seems clear that the same individual may exhibit either, depending on the circumstances. Nonetheless, in terms of the tilt-induced neurally mediated syncope model, the more susceptible fainter appears to be differ from less susceptible individuals with respect to release of certain neurohumoral mediators and in regard to parasympathetic nervous system responses to upright posture. These findings are discussed in more detail below.

The interaction of peripheral and central factors also contributes to determining the manner in which a syncopal event becomes manifest. Thus, the efferent response to afferent neural signals appears to differ, depending upon the origin of the primary stimulus and presumably the principal site(s) at which afferent neural activity accesses the brain. For example, bradycardia is usually the initial manifestation in carotid sinus syndrome (14). The vasodepressor (vasodilation) response evolves moments later. Conversely, hypotension due to vasodilation is typically evident prior to marked bradycardia in posturally induced, neurally mediated syncope (10). The basis for such differences are currently unexplored.

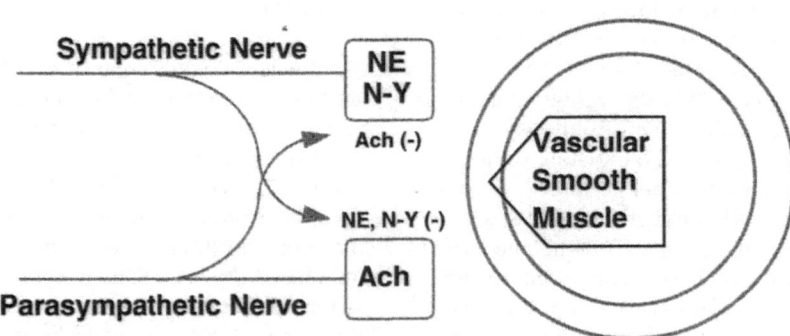

Fig. 3. Peripheral feedback interaction between sympathetic and parasympathetic neurotransmitters which may contribute to determining the magnitude of vasodilation observed during vasovagal syncope (see text for discussion). Abbreviations are as follows: *NE*, norepinephrine, *N-Y*, neuropeptide-Y; *Ach*, acetylcholine

Efferent Limb

An inappropriately slow heart rate and vasodilatation are characteristic features of the neurally mediated faint. The bradycardia, which may be dramatic in some cases but only relative with respect to the severity of hypotension in others, is primarily due to enhanced (or possibly unbalanced) efferent parasympathetic tone and is mediated by efferent signals transmitted via the vagus nerve. Vasodilatation, on the other hand, is thought to be primarily the result of diminished sympathetic vasoconstrictor tone (27-30).

An important aspect of the control of vascular tone is the interaction between peripheral elements of the sympathetic and parasympathetic nervous systems (Fig. 3). In this regard, release of acetylcholine by the parasympathetic nervous system is known to exert a feedback inhibitory effect on norepinephrine release from nearby sympathetic nerve endings. Conversely, release of both norepinephrine and neuropeptide-Y from sympathetic nerve terminals inhibits synaptic acetylcholine release (31-35). As a result, the temporal sequence as well as the magnitude of sympathetic or parasympathetic activation may have important consequences in terms of the severity of vasodilation or the degree of bradycardia associated with an evolving neurally mediated syncopal episode.

Intrinsic responsiveness of cardiac and vascular smooth muscle cells to neurohumoral mediators may differ in fainters and nonfainters, and such differences could affect both afferent and efferent neural reflex responses. In this regard, Perry et al. (36) suggested that increased ß-adrenergic sensitivity may be a characteristic finding in certain young individuals susceptible to posturally induced faints. Further study of this aspect of peripheral contribution to the vasovagal response is warranted.

Vasovagal Syncope: Peripheral and Central Factors

Peripheral Receptors and Afferent Neural Signals

The importance of the actions of various peripheral "receptors" in triggering spontaneous vasovagal spells is currently the center of debate. For example, it is widely accepted that peripheral pain receptors can initiate neurally mediated syncopal events. Similarly, unpleasant sights or even thoughts might trigger a spontaneous event in certain individuals. In such cases, the reflex arc incorporates corticohypothalamic centers and thereafter descends to the medullary cardiovascular control areas. Whether the individual susceptibility for such high level inputs to induce inappropriate hypotension-bradycardia resides solely within the CNS is unclear. It is possible that concomitant factors may be needed. For example, afferent signals from peripheral cardiopulmonary mechanoreceptors exposed to a transiently elevated catecholamine environment may be important. Similarly, an inadequate protective carotid baroreceptor response may be essential.

The significance of the contribution of peripheral cardiopulmonary mechanoreceptors in triggering vasovagal episodes is controversial. Apart from the carotid baroreceptors, other sites such as the aortic arch and the atrial and ventricular myocardium contain receptors which respond to changes in local distention or wall stress. In the case of the atria, neural afferents (predominantly myelinated) are derived from several types of receptors located primarily in the region of the atrial junctions with the vena cavae and the pulmonary veins. These receptors appear to be particularly sensitive to central volume changes and relatively insensitive to changes in myocardial contractile state (24). Atrial receptor distention increases heart rate and urinary output (the latter by both enhanced vasopressin release and via atrial peptides). Afferents from ventricular receptors are predominantly unmyelinated C fibers from both chemically and mechanically sensitive sites. The frequency of impulses generated by the ventricular mechanically sensitive receptors are directly related to contractile state and end-diastolic pressure. It appears that cardiac neural afferent activity participates in establishing the level of tonic sympathetic neural outflow to the renal and splanchnic beds in particular, with a smaller impact on skeletal muscle blood flow (24, 37). Additionally, these afferent signals also influence renin secretion and contribute to control of vasopressin release from hypothalamic sites (24,38-40). In situations where markedly increased wall tension occurs (e.g., due to excessive wall distention or enhanced inotropic state) there is increased frequency of afferent neural signals to the dorsal vagal nuclei (41); as the afferent traffic increases, sympathetic efferent stimulation decreases.

From the clinical perspective, the spontaneous vasovagal faint is most often associated with the upright posture. Normally, upon assumption of upright posture, circulating volume is displaced from intrathoracic to more dependent vascular spaces, with as much as 70% of the total blood volume being below the heart (42). As a consequence, central venous pressure, stroke volume, and systemic arterial pressure tend to fall. In health, the appropriate response is sympathetic activation (presumably activated via various cardiopulmonary baroreceptors) resulting in a series of compensatory responses including vasoconstriction, increased inotropic drive, tachycardia, and activation of the renin-angiotensin system in order to stabilize the circulation. However, under certain circumstances a different outcome may transpire. In these cases, for unknown reasons, the afferent neural activity triggers paradoxical bradycardia and vasodilation. It has been proposed that abrupt diminution of central volume results in a greater cardiac inotropic response in syncope-prone patients than in nonfainters. The result is activation of ventricular cardiac mechanoreceptors which are usually more sensitive to stretch than to contraction. The resulting afferent signals initiate the hypotension-bradycardia. A similar scenario may occur during abrupt hemorrhage, and is presumed to account for the second stage response in which marked bradycardia and vasodilatation develop (43-46). Once again, it is unknown whether the susceptibility to induction of inappropriate hypotension-bradycardia is solely determined within the CNS or in part resides in the nature of the afferent signal.

Plasma catecholamines measured prior to and during spontaneous and tilt-induced syncope exhibit important similarities. First, as has been noted earlier, premonitory increases in circulating catecholamines appear to characterize the spontaneous vasovagal faint (29,47,48). Chosy and Graham (49) observed an approximately 30% greater urinary epinephrine and norepinephrine concentrations in fainters prior to spontaneous vasovagal syncopal episodes compared to control subjects (49). Further, Vingerhoets (47) reported an increase of 60% or more in plasma epinephrine and norepinephrine concentrations in two patients just prior to a vasovagal faint, compared to control (sitting) values. Similar findings have been reported in tilt-induced syncope, with the increased catecholamine being primarily epinephrine. For instance, during 60° head-up tilt testing, Fitzpatrick et al. (50) observed both a more abrupt increase as well as higher overall levels of circulating epinephrine in 14 patients in whom syncope occurred compared to control subjects. Sander-Jensen et al. (51), have similarly observed a doubling of epinephrine levels in fainters when the episode was induced during 60° head-up tilt, while reporting no substantial change in norepinephrine levels. The latter is also consistent with findings reported by Abi-Samra et al. (52). In our laboratory, circulating epinephrine and norepinephrine concentrations have also been studied during head-up tilt procedures. In general, the most evident change has been a marked increase in circulating epinephrine concentration. Further, this increase antedates evident changes of heart rate or blood pressure, suggesting that it is not simply reactive, but may in fact be part of the triggering mechanism, possibly increasing receptor sensitivity (53).

The role of the carotid and aortic baroreceptors in the vasovagal faint may be important. Under normal conditions these receptors would be expected to counteract induction of inappropriate hypotension-bradycardia triggered by overly stressed ventricular mechanoreceptors or abruptly unloaded cardiopulmonary baroreceptors. However, for unclear reasons the usual protective actions of the carotid and aortic baroreceptors may be insufficient to fully reverse the course of events in certain circumstances. Thus, in the syncope patient it may be hypothesized that these receptors have inadequate intrinsic sensitivity to respond promptly and fully to the deteriorating hemodynamic state, or they may have inadequate efficacy to overcome the ventricular afferent signals. However, certain findings suggest that baroreceptor sensitivity may actually be greater in the syncope-prone subject. Thus, Fitzpatrick et al. (54) and Raviele et al. (55) have noted a relatively high frequency of positive carotid sinus massage among patients with positive tilt tests. If this proved to be the case in more detailed study of baroreceptor responsiveness, then it may be necessary to hypothesize that during evolving vasovagal faints, the normal response to carotid/aortic baroreceptor afferent signals is overridden for reasons as yet unexplained. On the other hand, in patients who exhibit oscillatory blood pressure and heart rate behavior (possibly fighting off the faint), the carotid and aortic baroreceptors may be exerting their protective function.

Central Centers and the Contribution of Certain Neurotransmitters

It is evident clinically that higher CNS centers are frequently involved in initiating spontaneous syncopal episodes. They probably also play an important role in facilitating development of symptoms in susceptible patients, thereby perhaps partially accounting for the variability in occurrence of syncopal events. Clearly, fear, pain, and unpleasant experiences or smells can instigate hypotension-bradycardia episodes. Stimulation of certain cortical and subcortical regions can elicit vasodepressor responses along with bradycardia and apnea, while other cortical regions have been associated with suppression of baroreceptor-induced bradycardia and hypotension (24) (Fig. 2).

Several lines of evidence suggest that certain central neurotransmitters may play a role in eliciting or facilitating reflex hypotension-bradycardia responses. For example ß-endorphin levels have been reported to be increased in both vasovagal syncope (56), and the analogous second stage of hemorrhagic shock (57,58). Further, in the experimental hemorrhage model, intracisternal administration of the opioid receptor blocker naloxone was more effective in preventing hypotension than when administered intravenously (59). On the other hand, even in very high doses, parenteral naloxone failed to prevent induction of hypotension-bradycardia during lower body negative pressure studies in humans (60). The latter finding suggests that naloxone-blocked ∂-opioid receptors may not be critical to the central neural processing in the neurally mediated syncopal syndromes. However, other opioid receptors which are less readily blocked by naloxone (e.g.,μ-opioid receptors) may be of importance.

Recently, there has been increasing interest in the role played by serotonin in modulating central nervous system sympathetic neural outflow and thereby participating in the vasovagal reflex (21,61,62). Intracerebroventricular serotonin has been reported to inhibit sympathetic neural outflow in general while increasing adrenal sympathetic stimulation. This finding is compatible with the occurrence in neurally mediated syncope of hypotension due to diminished vasoconstriction in conjunction with accentuation of adrenal epinephrine release. In an analogous setting, experimental studies reveal serotonin to play an important role as a mediator of the hyotension-bradycardia response during severe hemorrhage. The serotonin receptor blocker methysergide blocks this effect. Furthermore, clinical observations suggest that serotonin re-uptake blockers may diminish susceptibility to certain neurally mediated syncopal events, possibly by diminishing postsynaptic sensitivity to serotonin. Additional examination of the role played by serotonin, and the various serotonin receptor subtypes is needed.

Increased levels of a number of other centrally released vasoactive agents have been associated with neurally mediated syncope. Experimental studies suggest that nitric oxide release may be a regulator of sympathetic neural tone. Whether this agent plays any role in the vasovagal faint has yet to be determined. Similarly, pancreatic polypeptide and vasopressin have both been noted to increase in association with spontaneous and tilt-induced syncope (50, 51, 63). Pancreatic polypeptide is closely associated with and often considered a marker of parasympathetic efferent neural activity (63). Vasopressin release, on the other hand, is attributable to neural connections from the NTS which are presumably triggered by the afferent neural impulses from peripheral receptors as described above.

Peripheral Receptors and Efferent Neural Signals

As suggested above, vasodilatation in vasovagal syncope is thought to be primarily the result of diminished sympathetic vasoconstrictor tone (27-29). Similarly, bradycardia (which may be severe in some cases, yet only relative with respect to the severity of the hypotension in others) is predominantly due to enhanced efferent vagal tone. However, whether the severity of either vasodilation or bradycardia is solely related to the magnitude of centrally mediated parasympathetic influence, or possibly partly related to end-organ sensitivity has yet to be defined. In this regard several peripheral mechanisms may be contributory: (a) accentuated antagonism (a presumed interaction between parasympathetic and sympathetic mediators at the postsynaptic receptor site), (b) presynaptic feedback inhibition discussed above, and (c) action of noncatecholamine circulating neurohumoral agents.

In regard to accentuated antagonism, it has already been pointed out that both spontaneous and tilt-induced vasovagal faints are associated with increased circulating epinephrine and to a lesser extent norepinephrine concentrations. In this context, accentuation of parasympathetic effects by concomitant action of sympathetic mediators – in this case epinephrine – has been demonstrated experimentally (23, 24) and may play a role at the level of the heart in facilitating the bradycardic response. In general, individuals exhibiting greater tendency to accentuated antagonism at cardiac and peripheral vascular sites might be more susceptible to fainting due to the development of more severe bradycardia (sinus arrest, increased susceptibility to paroxysmal AV block, etc.) and/or greater degrees of vasodilatation.

The role of a direct cholinergic vasodilator mechanisms in eliciting the vasodepressor response remains controversial (42,64). Based on failure of muscarinic blockade with atropine to substantially affect hypotension in most patients, it is unlikely that this mechanism is of major importance. On the other hand, in a small subset of individuals in whom atropine appears to ameliorate the severity of hypotension, a cholinergic vasodilator mechanism may be relevant. It is most likely in such cases that presynaptic feedback inhibition of norepinephrine release by acetylcholine (as alluded to earlier) may be the key factor. In essence, acetylcholine may accentuate the magnitude of vasodilation associated with sympathetic neural withdrawal by further diminishing norepinephrine release from sympathetic nerve endings.

A final potential peripheral contributor to reflex vasodilatation is the effects of certain non-catecholamine neurohumors reported to be present in increased concentrations in association with vasovagal faints. Specifically, certain vasoactive peptides (e.g., vasoactive intestinal peptide, calcitonin gene related peptide), and purinergic agonists (e.g., adenosine) released from perivascular nerves may decrease norepinephrine release as well as contribute directly to vasodilatation (64-67).

Summary

The causes of hypotension and bradycardia in neurally mediated syncope are multifactorial, comprising inputs from both central and peripheral sites. In general, the tendency to faint is most often associated with the upright posture and displacement of circulating volume from intrathoracic to more dependent vascular spaces and may be facilitated by conditions such as moderate dehydration (e.g., hot environments, athletic competition) and sympathetic neural activation (e.g., emotional upset). In the case of the spontaneous vasovagal faint, afferent neural signals (whether arising in the periphery or within the CNS) that might have normally been expected to initiate a protective fight or flight response instead trigger reflex vasodilation and bradycardia. Perhaps excessive concentrations of certain CNS neurotransmitters, particularly endogenous opioid receptor agonists (e.g., endorphins) and / or serotonin are responsible. The outcome is a further fall in central venous pressure, stroke volume, and systemic arterial pressure. Meanwhile, centrally triggered adrenal activation results in increased circulating epinephrine levels. Presumably, the evolving hypotension in conjunction with increased sensitivity of peripheral receptors due to epinephrine exposure results in further activation of arterial and central cardiopulmonary mechanoreceptors. The end result is additional accentuation of neural afferent traffic and consequent aggravation of hemodynamic compromise. In the meantime, carotid baroreceptor signals are either inadequate to stem the tide or their signals are centrally over-ridden for unknown reasons in those individuals who ultimately go on to faint.

Why certain individuals appear to be more susceptible to the development of paradoxical hypotension and bradycardia than others, or why the event occurs at one time and not at others remains a mystery. The concept of susceptibility appears to be a real phenomenon clinically. Perhaps the baseline neuroendocrine state of the individual is a marker. Recent unconfirmed findings suggest that the level of heart rate and circulating epinephrine increment during onset of upright tilt testing may predict susceptibility to a positive test (50). Additionally, a hyperparasympathetic state in which upright posture is not associated with normal diminution of parasympathetic influence on heart rate may be a marker of increased susceptibility (68). The latter, perhaps compounded by accentuated antagonism in which parasympathetic effects are exaggerated in the presence of increased circulating catecholamine, may in part account for the occurrence of marked vagally induced bradycardia. Similarly, apart from a centrally mediated reflex inhibition of sympathetic efferent traffic to vascular beds, norepinephrine release may be further diminished due to pre-synaptic effects of acetylcholine and other neurohumors.

Although understanding of the potential contributions of central and peripheral elements to the pathophysiology of spontaneous vasovagal faints remains limited, the treatment implications have already been important. In particular, despite continued uncertainty regarding their efficacy, the rationale for use of ß-adrenergic blockers or serotonin re-uptake inhibitors in affected patients is based on the pathophysiologic concepts discussed above. However, much greater insight is needed before a satisfactory treatment strategy encompassing all individuals with these various syncopal disorders, can be developed.

Acknowledgment. The authors thank Wendy Markuson and Barry L.S. Detloff for valuable assistance in preparation of the manuscript.

References

1. Lewis T (1932) Vasovagal syncope and the carotid sinus mechanism. With comments on Gower's and Nothnagel's syndrome. Br Med J 1: 873-876
2. Ross RT (1988) Syncope. (1936) Saunders, London
3. Stults BM, Gandolfi RJ (1936) Diagnostic evaluation of syncope. West Med J 144: 234-236
4. Wayne HH (1961) Syncope: physiological considerations and an analysis of the clinical characteristics in 510 patients. Am J Med 30: 418-438
5. Ruetz PP, Johnson SA, Callahan R, Meade RC, Smith JJ (1967) Fainting: a review of its mechanisms and a study in blood donors. Medicine (Baltimore) 46: 363-384
6. Savage DD, Corwin L, McGee DL, Kannell WB, Wolf PA (1985) Epidemiologic features of isolated syncope: the Framingham Study. Stroke 16: 626-629
7. Kudenchuk PJ, McAnulty JH (1985) Syncope: evaluation and treatment. Mod Conc Cardiovasc Dis 54: 25-29
8. Almquist A, Goldenberg IF, Milstein S, Chen M-Y, Chen X, Hansen R, Gornick CC, Benditt DG (1989) Provocation of bradycardia and hypotension by isoproterenol and upright posture in patients with unexplained syncope. New Engl J Med 320: 346-351
9. Abboud FM (1989) Ventricular syncope. Is the heart a sensory organ? (editorial). New Engl J Med 320: 390-392
10. Chen M-Y, Goldenberg IF, Milstein S. Buetikofer J, Almquist A, Lesser J, Benditt DG (1989) Cardiac electrophysiologic and hemodynamic correlates of neurally-mediated syncope. Am J Cardiol 63: 66-72
11. Benditt DG, Sakaguchi S, Schultz JJ, Remole S, Adler S, Lurie KG (1993) Syncope. Diagnostic considerations and the role of tilt table testing. Cardiol Rev 1: 146-156
12. Weiss S, Baker JP (1933) The carotid sinus reflex in health and disease. Its role in the causation of fainting and convulsions. Medicine 12: 297-354
13. Thomas JE (1969) Hyperactive carotid sinus reflex and carotid sinus syncope. Mayo Clin Proc 44: 127-139
14. Almquist A, Gornick CC, Benson DW Jr, Dunnigan A, Benditt DG (1985) Carotid sinus hypersensitivity: evaluation of the vasodepressor component. Circulation 67: 927-936
17. Scherrer U, Vissing S, Morgan BJ, Hanson P, Victor RG (1990) Vasovagal syncope after infusion of a vasodilator in a heart-transplant recipient. New Engl J Med 322: 602-604
18. van Lieshout JJ, Wieling W, Karemaker JM, Eckberg DL (1991) The vasovagal response. Clin Sci 81:575-586
19. Abboud F (1993) Neurocardiogenic syncope. N Engl J Med 328: 1117-1120
20. Rea R, Thames MD (1993) Neural control mechanisms and vasovagal syncope. J Cardiovasc Electrophysiol 4:587-595
21. Kosinski D, Grubb B, Temesy-Armos P (1995) Pathophysiological aspects of neurocardiogenic syncope: current concepts and new perspectives. PACE 18:716-724

22. Pelletier CL, Shepherd JT (1973) Circulatory reflexes from mechanoreceptors in the cardio-aortic area. Circ Res 33: 131-138
23. Donald DE, Shepherd JT (1978) Reflexes from the heart and lungs: physiological curiosities or important regulatory mechanisms. Cardiovasc Res 12: 449-469
24. Abboud FM, Thames MD (1983) Interaction of cardiovascular reflexes in circulatory control. In: Shepherd JT, Abbond FM (eds) Peripheral circulation and organ blood flow. American Physiological Society, Bethesda, PA 675-753 (Handbook of physiology, section 2; The Cardiovascular System)
25. Benarroch EE (1993) The central autonomic network. Functional organization, dysfunction, and perspective. Mayo Clin Proc 68:988-1001
26. Simone F (1990) Vegetative nervous system and syncopes. Funct Neurol 5;187-192
27. Beiser GD, Zelis R, Epstein SE, Mason DT, Braunwald E (1970) The role of skin and muscle resistance vessels in reflexes mediated by the baroreceptor system. J Clin Invest 49: 225-231
28. Wallin BG, Sundlof G (1982) Sympathetic outflow in muscles during vasovagal syncope. J Autonom Nerv Syst 6: 287-291
29. Goldstein DS, Spanarkel M, Pitterman A, Toltzis R, Gratz E, Epstein S, Keiser HR (1982) Circulatory control mechanisms in vasodepressor syncope. Am Heart J 104: 1071-1075
30. Ziegler MG, Echon C, Wilner KD, Specho P, Lake CR McCutchen JA (1986) Sympathetic nervous withdrawal in the vasodepressor (vasovagal) reaction. J Autonom Nerv Syst 17: 273-278
31. Muscholl E (1980) Peripheral muscarinic control of norepinephrine release in the cardiovascular system. Am J Physiol 239:H713-720
32. Levy MN (1984) Cardiac sympathetic-parasympathetic interactions. Fed Proc 43:2598-2602
33. Potter EK (1985) Prolonged non-adrenergic inhibition of cardiac vagal action by sympathetic stimulation : neuromodulation by neuropeptide-Y? Neurosci Lett 54:117-121
34. Potter EK (1987) Presynaptic inhibition of cardiac vagal postganglionic nerves by neuropeptide-Y. Neurosci Lett 83:101-106
35. Revington ML, McCloskey DI (1990) Sympathetic-parasympathetic interactions at the heart, possibly involving neuropeptide Y, in anaesthetized dogs. J Physiol (Lond) 428:359-370
36. Perry JC, Garson A Jr (1991) The child with recurrent syncope: autonomic function testing and beta-adrenergic hypersensitivity. J Am Coll Cardiol 17:1168-1171
37. Mancia G, Donald DE (1975) Demonstration that atria, ventricles, and lung each are responsible for a tonic inhibition of the vasomotor center in the dog. Circ Res 36: 310-318
38. Share L (1976) Role of cardiovascular receptors in the control of ADH release. Cardiology 61 [Supp 1]: 51-64
39. Jarecki M, Thoren PN, Donald DE (1978) Release of renin by the carotid baroreflex in anesthetized dogs: role of cardiopulmonary vagal afferents and renal arterial pressure. Circ Res 42: 614-619
40. Schrier RW, Bichet DG (1981) Osmotic and nonosmotic control of vasopressin release and the pathogenesis of impaired water excretion in adrenal, thyroid, and edematous disorders. J Lab Clin Med 98: 1-15
41. Thoren P (1979) Role of cardiac vagal C-fibres in cardiovascular control. Rev Physiol Biochem Pharmacol 86:1-94
42. Rowell LB (1986) Human circulation. Regulation during physical stress. Oxford University Press, New York
43. Barcroft H, Edholm OG, McMichael J, Sharpey-Shafer EP (1944) Posthaemorrhagic fainting. Lancet i: 489-491
44. Barcroft H, Edholm OG (1945) On the vasodilatation in human skeletal muscle during posthemorrhagic fainting. J Physiol (Lond) 104: 161-175
45. Oberg B, White S (1970) The role of vagal cardiac nerves and arterial baroreceptors in the circulatory adjustments to hemorrhage in the cat. Acta Physiol Scand 80: 395-403
46. Secher NH, Sander-Jensen K, Werner C, Warberg J, Bie P (1984) Bradycardia, a severe but reversible hypovolemic shock in man. Circ Shock 14: 267-274
47. Vingerhoets AJJM (1984) Biochemical changes in two subjects succumbing to syncope. Psychosom Med 46: 95-103
48. Schlesinger Z (1973) Life-threatening "vagal reaction" to physical fitness test. JAMA 226: 1119
49. Chosy JJ, Graham DT (1965) Catecholamines in vasovagal fainting. J Psychosom Res 9: 189-194

50. Fitzpatrick A, Williams T, Jeffrey C, Lightman S, Sutton R (1990) Pathogenic role for arginine vasopressin (AVP) and catecholamines (EP & NEP) in vasovagal syncope (Abstract). J Am Coll Cardiol 15: 98

51. Sander-Jensen K, Secher NH, Astrup A, Christensen NJ, Giese J, Schwartz TW, Warberg J, Bie P (1986) Hypotension induced by passive head-up tilt: endocrine and circulatory mechanisms. Am J Physiol 251: R742-R748

52. Abi-Samra F, Maloney JD, Fouad-Tarazi FM, Castle L (1988) The usefulness of head-up tilt testing and hemodynamic investigations in the workup of syncope of unknown origin. PACE 11: 1202-1214

54. Fitzpatrick AP, Theodorakis G, Vardas P, Sutton R (1991) Methodology of head-up tilt testing in patients with unexplained syncope. J Am Coll Cardiol 17:125-130

55. Raviele A, Gasparini G, Di Pede F, Delise P, Bonso A, Piccolo E (1990) Usefulness of head-up tilt test in evaluating patients with syncope of unknown origin and negative electrophysiologic study. Am J Cardiol 65: 1322-1327

56. Perna GP, Ficola U, Salvatori MP, Stanislao M, Vigna C, Villella A, Russo A, Fernelli R Vittori PGP, Loperfido F (1990) Increase of plasma beta endorphins in vasodepressor syncope. Am J Cardiol 65: 929-930

57. Rutter PC, Potocnik SJ, Ludbrook J (1987) Sympathoadrenal mechanisms in cardiovascular responses to naloxone after hemorrhage. Am J Physiol 252: H40-H46

58. Morita H, Nishida Y, Motochigawa H, Uemura H, Hosomi, H, Vatner SF (1988) Opiate receptor mediated decrease in renal nerve activity during hypotensive hemorrhage in conscious rabbits. Circ Res 63: 165-172

59. Evans RG, Ludbrook J, Potocnik SJ (1989) Intracisternal naloxone and cardiac nerve blockade prevent vasodilatation during simulated hemorrhage in awake rabbits. J Physiol (Lond) 409: 1-14

60. Smith ML, Carlson MD, Thames MC (1993) Naloxone does not prevent vasovagal syncope during simulated orthostasis in humans. J Auton Nerv Syst 45:1-9

61. Kosinski D, Grubb BP, Temesy-Armos P (1994) The use of serotonin reuptake inhibitors in the treatment of neurally mediated cardiovascular disorders. J Serotonin Res 1:85-90

62. Morgan DA, Thoren P, Wilczynski EA, Victor RG, Mark AL (1988) Serotonergic mechanisms mediate renal sympathoinhibition during severe hemorrhage in rats. Am J Physiol 255: H496-H502

63. Brody MJ (1978) Histaminergic and cholinergic vasodilator systems. In: Vanhoutte PM, Leusen I (eds) Mechanisms of vasodilatation. Karger, Basel, pp 266-277

64. Kellogg DL, Johnson JM, Kosiba WA (1990) Baroreflex control of the cutaneous active vasodilator system in humans. Circ Res 66: 1420-1426

65. Burnstock G (1972) Purinergic nerves. Pharmacol Rev 24: 509-581

66. Bevan JA, Brayden JE (1987) Nonadrenergic neural vasodilator mechanisms. Circ Res 60: 309-326

67. Warner MR, Levy MN (1989) Inhibition of cardiac vagal effects by neurally released and exogenous neuropeptide Y. Circ Res 65: 1536-1546

68. Lippman L, Stein KM, Lerman BB (1995) Failure to decrease parasympathetic tone during upright tilt predicts a positive tilt table test. Am J Cardiol 75: 591-595

Syncope of Unknown Origin: First Head-Up Tilt Test or Electrophysiologic Study?*

P. Alboni**, A. Raviele, C. Vecchio, G. Andrioli,
M. Brignole, C. Menozzi, E. Piccolo, and A. Proclemer

**Divisione di Cardiologia, Ospedale Civile, Cento, Italy

Syncope is a nonspecific symptom of a wide variety of disorders. It is defined as the temporary loss of consciousness and postural tone, followed by spontaneous recovery without resuscitative measures. It is diagnosed in about 3% of the patients seen in the emergency room and in about 1% of the patients admitted to a hospital (1, 2). Syncope can be classified as cardiovascular, noncardiovascular, and unexplained.

Diagnostic Approaches

The choice of the examinations aimed at defining the cause of syncope is based on the clinical presentation, the different prevalence of the various types of syncope, and the diagnostic yield of the various examinations.

Old age, absence of prodromic symptoms, and presence of symptoms and signs of organic heart disease and/or of electrocardiographic alterations suggest a cardiac cause; in such cases, cardiologic examinations should be given priority. In contrast, young age, presence of symptoms of autonomic activity (pallor, nausea, sweating, mydriasis, etc), and absence of symptoms and signs of organic heart disease and/or of electrocardiographic alterations suggest a neuromediated syncope; here autonomic function tests should be given priority.

The most frequent type of syncope is the neuromediated one, followed, in order of prevalence, by the cardiac, neurologic (cerebrovascular and psychiatric), and metabolic types.

Some examinations, such as the head-up tilt test (HUT) and the electrophysiologic study, have a high probability of being positive; they should be given priority over other examinations, such as the hemodynamic-angiographic study, the electroencephalogram, and brain computer axial tomography, which have a low probability of being positive.

In Fig. 1, the steps involved in a systematic approach to the diagnosis of syncope is shown. In the presence of a pathologic result, the diagnostic procedures are interrupted. However, it must be pointed out that the cause of syncope is often not certain; in such cases caution is required and in some cases further investigation should be carried out before defining the cause of syncope. The first diagnostic steps are history, physical examination with evaluation of blood pressure in the supine and erect positions, standard electrocardiogram and conventional laboratory tests when a metabolic cause is suspected (Fig. 1). These simple examinations allow us to define the cause of the syncope: they are "diagnostic" in about 50% of cases (2-6). In the other half of cases these examinations do not identify of the cause of syncope: they are "negative" or only "suggestive" of a particular cause. Table 1 presents "diagnostic," "suggestive," and "negative" results obtained by the initial examinations. When the results are negative or only suggestive, other examinations are indicated, as shown in Fig. 1. The subsequent diagnostic procedures allow us to define the cause of the syncope in a further 35% of cases. Therefore, at the end of all the diagnostic procedures, the cause of syncope remains unexplained in about 15% of cases. When suggestive data for a cardiac cause emerge, noninvasive tests should first be performed, e.g., echocardiogram in order to disclose a mechanical cause of syncope and Holter recordings in order to disclose an arrhythmic cause. An effort test is indicated when syncope is exercise related. When pulmonary embolism is suspected, a lung scan is indicated. If, after these noninvasive examinations, the cause of syncope has not been defined, an electrophysiologic study or autonomic function tests such as the tilting test and carotid sinus massage should be carried out. The latter should be performed both in supine and erect positions. Whether to autonomic function tests or an electrophysiologic study should be carry out first must be evaluated case by case. Generally, if the patient is affected by ischemic heart disease, by dilated or hypertrophic cardiomyopathy, or if conduction disturbances and/or hypokinetic, or hyperkinetic arrhythmias are present in the standard electrocardiogram or Holter recording, the electrophysiologic study must be performed first. If the patient does not show signs

---

* This manuscript summarizes the ANMCO Task Force Report
"Orientamenti sulla valutazione diagnostica dei pazienti con sincope"

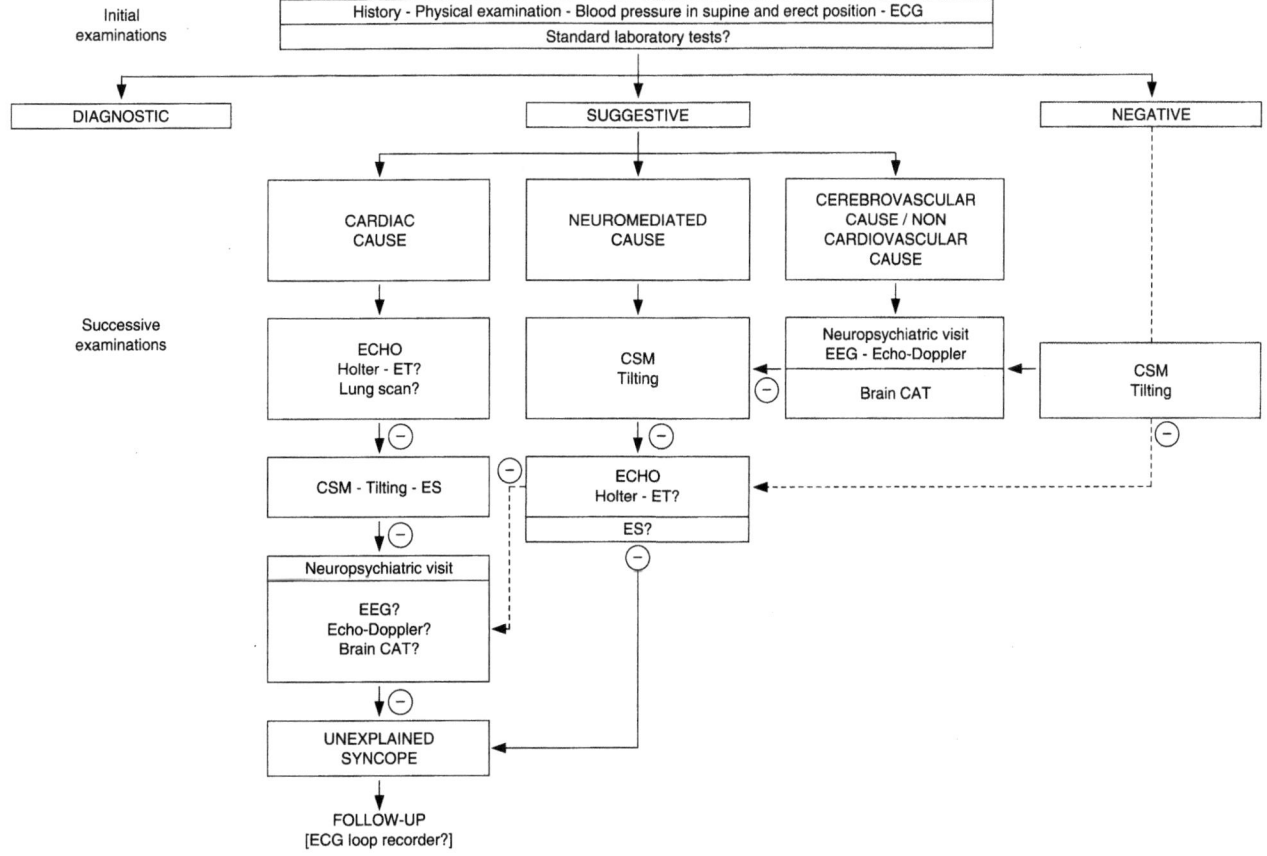

Fig. 1. Steps for a systematic approach to the diagnosis of syncope. *ET*, exercise text; *CSM*, carotid sinus massage; *ES*, endocavitary electrophysiologic study; *CAD*, computer axial tomography, ⊖ not a diagnostic examination; ?, indication to be evaluated case by case

of organic heart disease or is affected by hypertensive heart disease without relevant arrhythmias, autonomic function tests must be performed first. If the results of examinations carried out to show a cardiac or a neuromediated cause of syncope are negative, a neurologic or a psychiatric cause must be considered. The consultant neurologist may request an electroencephalogram, Doppler flow studies of the neck vessels, and/or brain computer axial tomography. If after neurologic investigations, the cause of the syncope does not become clear, the syncope remains unexplained and the patient must be followed up. In subjects with frequently recurring syncope, an intermittent loop recorder could be useful.

When suggestive data for neuromediated syncope emerge, the first examinations to be performed are carotid sinus massage and HUT. If the results of these investigations are negative, the presence of a cardiac cause must be considered; if the latter does not emerge, we should look for a neurologic or psychiatric cause.

When suggestive data for neurologic or psychiatric syncope emerge, the first evaluation to be carried out is a neurologic and psychiatric one; the consultant neurologist may request the above-mentioned examinations. If after these investigations the cause of syncope is not revealed, autonomic function tests must be performed. If the results of the latter are also negative, a cardiac cause must be considered (see above).

When the results of the initial examinations (history, physical examination, standard electrocardiogram)

are completely negative, autonomic function tests must be performed first, because the most frequent cause of syncope is the neuromediated one.

Diagnostic Yield of Examinations

Echocardiogram. This is very useful in order to evaluate the presence and the severity of organic heart disease, but it rarely reveals the cause of syncope (7).

Holter Recordings. These can reveal an arrhythmic event as the potential cause of syncope, in 12%-53% of cases (mean, 17%) (8-15). The main problem in attributing syncope to arrhythmias is that the vast majority of detected arrhythmias in patients with syncope are brief and do not result in symptoms. On the other hand, arrhythmias are commonly reported in asymptomatic individuals. One method of assessing the impact of Holter recording in syncope is to determine the presence or absence of arrhythmias in patients who develop symptoms during monitoring. Only in 4% of patients were symptoms consistent with an arrhythmia (8-15). In approximately 17% of patients, arrhythmias were not associated with symptoms, thus potentially excluding rhythm disturbance as an etiology for the syncope (8-15). The causal relationship between arrhythmias and syncope, therefore, is uncertain. Arrhythmias highly suggestive of an arrhythmic origin of

Table 1. Diagnostic, suggestive, and negative results obtained in the initial examinations (history, physical examination, blood pressure in the supine and erect positions, standard electrocardiogram and sometimes conventional laboratory tests)

Diagnostic criteria	Suggestive criteria	Negative criteria
Cardiac cause Symptoms and signs of acute myocardial ischemia with or without myocardial infarction Presence in standard electrocardiogram of: Sinus bradycardia < 30 beats/min or repetitive sinoatrial blocks or sinus pauses > 3 s; the possible coexistence of an abnormal neural reflex should be evaluated (49,63)· Mobitz II or advanced (2:1, 3:1, etc) second degree AV block or third degree AV block Rapid (> 180 beats/min) and/or hypotensive supraventricular tachycardia; in the absence of high heart rate and hypotension, the possible co-existence of an abnormal neural reflex should be evaluated (64, 65) Sustained ventricular tachycardia, torsade de pointes, ventricular fibrillation Neuromediated cause *Vasovagal* Predisposing factors such as fatigue, prolonged standing, venipuncture, blood donation, heat, and invasive examinations Syncope preceded by signs of autonomic activity such as pallor, nausea, sweating, and mydriasis Quick recovery of consciousness; pallor and asthenia may be long-lasting Absence of signs of organic heart disease *Situational* Syncope occurring during or immediately after urination, defecation, cough, swallowing Absence of signs of organic heart disease *Orthostatic* Syncope occurring upon assuming the upright position Decrease of systolic blood pressure (> 30 mmHg) upon assuming the upright position associated with dizziness Cerebrovascular cause *Transient ischemic attack* Syncope co-existing with focal neurological symptoms *Seizure* Prolonged loss of consciousness (> 5 min), convulsions lasting > 30 s, and sphincter incontinence in the presence of a reliable witness Slow resumption of consciousness, headache, retrograde amnesia Metabolic cause *Hyperventilation* Syncope occurring in young and anxious subjects, reproducible during prolonged hyperventilation Absence of signs of organic heart disease *Hypoglycemia* Syncope preceded by confusion, salivation, tremors, hunger, hyperadrenergic state Glycemia < 40 mg/dl	Cardiac cause Symptoms and/or physical signs and/or electrocardiographic signs of organic heart disease Old age (> 60 years) Syncope not preceded by prodromic symptoms Conduction disturbances less severe than the above-mentioned ones (sinus bradycardia with heart rate between 30 and 50 beats/min, isolated sinoatrial block, first-degree AV block, Mobitz I second-degree AV block, intraventricular conduction disturbances, frequent supraventricular or ventricular premature beats) Neuromediated cause Syncope preceded by light prodromic symptoms Uncertain causal relationship between syncope and predisposing factors Young age (<30 years) Absence of signs of organic heart disease Cerebrovascular cause *Transient ischemic attack* Very light focal neurologic symptoms *Seizure* Symptoms only suggestive of seizure Witness not reliable	History, physical examination, and standard electrocardiogram do not suggest any cause of syncope

syncope, even in the absence of neurologic symptoms during monitoring, include the following: second-degree atrioventricular (AV) block, particularly Mobitz II, third-degree AV block, rapid supraventricular arrhythmias (more than 180 beats/min), and unsustained and sustained ventricular tachycardias. Arrhythmias less suggestive of an arrhythmic cause of syncope include: frequent and repetitive premature ventricular beats, sinus bradycardia (heart rate between 30 and 50 beats/min), or sinus pauses (longer than 2 s) during diurnal hours. Extending the duration of monitoring to longer than 24 h does not seem to solve the problem of interpretating the abnormalities found (13).

Effort Test. This can be used to provoke syncope with exercise and to search for tachyarrhythmias occurring during or after abrupt termination of exercise. In a study of exercise and syncope, complex premature ventricular beats or supraventricular tachycardia were found in only three of 119 patients (2.5%) (8).

Electrophysiologic Study. The indications for this study in patients with syncope have not been systematically defined, but it is more likely to be positive in patients with heart disease who have an abnormal ventricular function, electrocardiogram, or Holter monitoring.

In studies of patients with syncope undergoing electrophysiologic testing, the percentage with positive findings has ranged between 18% and 75% (mean, 55%), (13, 16-33). Approximately 37% (range, 11%-60%) had conduction disturbances (abnormal sinus node, AV node, or His-Purkinje function), and 30% (range 0-68%) inducible supraventricular tachycardia. Several issues need to be considered when using electrophysiologic studies in the evaluation of syncope. First of all, in most instances arrhythmias during electrophysiologic study do not produce syncope in the laboratory; thus a causal relationship often has to be inferred. The marked variability of the diagnostic yield of electrophysiologic studies depends on several factors, in particular on the more or less restrictive criteria applied define "positive" results of the study (34, 35). In order to avoid a high number false positives and to avoid beginning useless, if not harmful treatments, it is preferable to apply restrictive criteria:
– Sinus node recovery time greater than 3000 ms
– Baseline HV of 100 ms or more or appearance of infra-hisian second or third degree AV block during atrial pacing or after ajmaline
– Induction of syncopal or symptomatic (low cardiac output) supraventricular tachyarrhythmias
– Induction of syncopal unsustained ventricular tachycardia
– Induction of sustained monomorphic ventricular tachycardia, polimorphic ventricular tachycardia or ventricular fibrillation, especially if a nonaggressive stimulation protocol is used (two extrastimuli).

Carotid Sinus Massage. The technique of carotid massage is not standardized. The massage is commonly performed in the supine position and is considered positive in the presence of ventricular asystole (greater than 3 s) or a decrease in systolic pressure of more than 50 mmHg. Using these criteria, a positive re-

sponse was found very frequently: in 26%-59% of subjects affected by unexplained syncope (9-11, 36) and in about 30% of asymptomatic elderly subjects with ischemic and/or hypertensive heart disease (37-39). This response, therefore, shows low specificity and it is practically useless from the clinical point of view. A more adequate endpoint appears to be the reproduction of a spontaneous syncope or presyncope in the presence of a ventricular asystole (greater than 3 s) or a decrease in systolic blood pressure of more than 50 mmHg. When performed using this method, carotid massage induced a syncope in 49% of subjects with unexplained syncope and in 4% of the controls (40).

Tilting Test. This is being increasingly used to establish vasovagal responses in patients with unexplained syncope. Several protocols have been proposed; some require the use of drugs (provocative tests). The baseline tilting test is generally performed, using the Westminster protocol (60°, 45 min) (41). A positive response to HUT is defined as the development of syncope or presyncope in association with hypotension, bradycardia, or both. The range of diagnostic results reported for the baseline HUT varied extensively from 32% to 74% (mean, 47%) (40-46). However, in more recent studies the positivity rate of the baseline HUT decreased to values of 23%-31% (47, 48), likely because of a different patient selection (patients who had not previously undergone other diagnostic procedures). The specificity of baseline HUT is about 90% (41-43, 49).

During the provocative tests, drugs favoring an abnormal reflex are administered, generally after a baseline tilting test of short duration. The most commonly used provocative tests are the isoproterenol test (50) and the nitroglycerin test (51).

The positivity rate of the isoproterenol test in patients with unexplained syncope is 71% (range, 50%-87%) and the specificity is 76% (range, 51%-100%) (3, 45, 50, 52-61).

The positivity rate of the nitroglycerin test in patients with unexplained syncope is 48%-53% and the specificity is 92%-94% (51).

The examinations for revealing a neurologic cause of syncope are of limited use in patients with unexplained syncope (62). Brain computer axial tomography and electroencephalogram can reveal the cause of unexplained syncope only in 3.5% of cases (31 of 901 patients) (2, 4-6) and should only be used in selected cases.

References

1. Feruglio GA, Perraro F (1987) Rilievi epidemiologici sulla sincope nella popolazione generale e come causa di ricovero. G Ital Cardiol [Suppl I] 17: 11-13
2. Day SC, Cook EF, Funckestein H, Goldman L (1982) Evaluation and outcome of emergency room patient with transient loss of consciousness. Am J Med 73: 15-23
3. Silverstein MD, Singer DE, Mulley AG, Thibault GE, Barnett GO (1982) Patients with syncope admitted to medical intensive care units. JAMA 248: 1185-89
4. Eagle KA, Black HR (1983) The impact of diagnostic tests in evaluating patients with syncope. Yale J Biol Med 56: 1-8
5. Kapoor WN, Karpf M, Wieand S, Peterson JR, Levey GS (1983) A prospective evaluation and follow-up of patients with syncope. N Engl J Med 309: 197-204

6. Martin GJ, Adams SL, Martin HG, Mathews J, Zull D, Scanlon PJ (1984) Prospective evaluation of syncope. Ann Emerg Med 13: 499-504

7. Recchia D (1994) Echocardiography has a low diagnostic yield in the evaluation of syncope of unclear etiology. J Am Coll Cardiol 23: 435A (abstr)

8. Boudoulas H, Schaael SF, Lewis RP, Robinson JL (1979) Superiority of 24-hour outpatient monitoring over multi-stage exercise testing for the evaluation of syncope. J Electrocardiol 12: 103-108

9. Zeldis SM, Levine BJ, Michelson EL, Morganroth J (1980) Cardiovascular complaints: correlation with cardiac arrhythmias on 24-hour electrocardiographic monitoring. Chest 78: 456-462

10. Clark PI, Glasser SP, Spoto E (1980) Arrhythmias detected by ambulatory monitoring. Lack of correlation with symptoms of dizziness and syncope. Chest 77: 722-728

11. Kala R, Viitasalo MT, Tiovenon L, Eisalo A (1982) Ambulatory ECG recording in patients referred because of syncope or dizziness. Acta Med Scand 668 [Suppl]: 13-19

12. Gibson TC, Heitzman MR (1984) Diagnostic efficacy of 24-hour electrocardiographic monitoring for syncope. Am J Cardiol 53: 1013-1018

13. Bass EB, Curtiss EI, Arena VC et al (1990) The duration of Holter monitoring in patients with syncope: is 24 hours enough? Arch Intern Med 50: 1073-1078

14. Kapoor W (1990) Evaluation and outcome of patients with syncope. Medicine 69:160-169

15. Moazez F, Peter T, Simonson J, Mandel WJ, Vaughn C, Gange E (1991) Syncope of unknown origin: clinical, non invasive and electrophysiologic determinants of arrhythmia induction and symptom recurrence during long-term follow-up. Am Heart J 121: 81-88

16. Brandenburg RO Jr, Holmes DR Jr, Hartzler GO (1981) The electrophysiologic assessment of patients with syncope. Am J Cardiol 47: 433 (abstr)

17. Di Marco JP, Garan H, Harthorone JW, Ruskin JN (1981) Intracardiac electrophysiologic techniques in recurrent syncope of unknown cause. Ann Intern Med 95: 542-548

18. Gulamhusein S, Naccarelli GV, Ko PT et al (1982) Value and limitations of clinical electrophysiologic study in assessment of patients with unexplained syncope. Am J Med 50: 1309-1315

19. Hess DA, Morady F, Scheinman MM (1982) Electrophysiologic testing in evaluation of patients with syncope of undetermined origin. Am J Cardiol 50: 1309-1315

20. Akhatar M, Shenasa M, Denker S, Gilbert CJ, Rizwi N (1983) Role of cardiac electrophysiologic studies in patients with unexplained recurrent syncope. PACE 6: 192-201

21. Morady F, Shen E, Schwartz A et al (1983) Long-term follow-up of patients with recurrent unexplained syncope evaluated by electrophysiologic testing. J Am Coll Cardiol 2: 1053-1059

22. Denes P, Ezri MD (1985) The role of electrophysiologic studies in the management of patients with unexplained syncope. PACE 8: 424-435

23. Doherty JU, Pembrook-Rogers D, Grogan EW et al (1985) Electrophysiologic evaluation and follow-up characteristics of patients with recurrent unexplained syncope and presyncope. Am J Cardiol 55: 73-78

24. Olshansky B, Mazuz M, Martins JB (1985) Significance of inducible tachycardia in patients with syncope of unknown origin: a long-term follow-up. J Am Coll Cardiol 5: 216-223

25. Teichman SL, Felder SD, Matos JA, Kim SG, Waspe LE, Fisher JD (1985) The value of electrophysiologic studies in syncope of undetermined origin: report of 150 cases. Am Heart J 110: 469-479

26. Krol RB, Morady F, Flaker GC et al (1987) Electrophysiologic testing in patients with unexplained syncope: clinical and non-invasive predictors of outcome. J Am Coll Cardiol 10: 385

27. Proclemer A, Gianfagna P, Fontanelli A, Bernardi G, Feruglio GA (1987) Utilità dello studio elettrofisiologico nella valutazione prognostica dei pazienti con sincopi di incerta origine. G Ital Cardiol 17: 402-407

28. Raviele A, Di Pede F, Delise P et al (1987) Quando e fino a che punto sono utili le indagini invasive per l'accertamento diagnostico delle sindromi sincopali. G Ital Cardiol 17 [suppl I]: 18-19

29. Sugrue DD, Holmes DR, Gersh BJ, Wood DL, Osborn MJ, Hammill SC (1987) Impact of electrophysiologic testing on the management of elderly patients with recurrent syncope or near syncope. J Am Geriatr Soc 35: 1079-1083

30. Lacroix D, Dubuc M, Kus T, Savard Shenasa M, Nadeau R (1991) Evaluation of arrhythmic causes of syncope: correlation between Holter monitoring, electrophysiologic testing and body surface potential mapping. Am Heart J 122: 1346-1354

31. Sra JS, Anderson AJ, Sheikh SH et al (1991) Unexplained syncope evaluated by electrophysiologic studies and head-up tilt testing. Ann Intern Med 114: 1013-1019

32. Denniss AR, Ross DL, Richards DA, Uther JB (1992) Electrophysiologic studies in patients with unexplained syncope. Int J Cardiol 35: 211-217

33. Middlekauff HR, Stevenson WG, Saxon LA (1993) Prognosis after syncope: impact of left ventricular function. Am Heart J 125: 121-127

34. Raviele A, Piccolo E (1987) La problematica dello studio elettrofisiologico nei pazienti con sincope di natura indeterminata. G Ital Cardiol 17: 411-413

35. Kapoor WN (1992) Hypotension and syncope. In: Braunwald E (ed) Heart disease. A textbook of cardiovascular medicine. Saunders, Philadelphia, pp 875-886

36. Brignole M, Menozzi C (1992) Carotid sinus syndrome: diagnosis, natural history and treatment. Eur J Cardiac Pacing Electrophysiol 4: 247-254

37. Walter PF, Crawley IS, Dorney ER (1978) Carotid sinus hypersensitivity and syncope. Am J Cardiol 42: 396-403

38. Brown KA, Maloney JD, Smith HC, Hartzler GO, Ilstrup DM (1980) Carotid sinus reflex in patients undergoing coronary angiography: relationship of degree and location of coronary artery disease to response to carotid sinus massage. Circulation 62: 697-703

39. Brignole M, Gigli G, Altomonte F et al (1985) Il riflesso cardioinibitore provocato dalla stimolazione del seno carotideo nei soggetti normali e con malattie cardiovascolari. G Ital Cardiol 15: 514-519

40. Brignole M, Menozzi C, Gianfranchi L, Oddone D, Lolli G, Bertulla A (1991) Carotid sinus massage, eyeball compression and head-up tilt test in patients with syncope of uncertain origin and in healthy control subjects. Am Heart J 122: 1644-1651

41. Fitzpatrick A, Theodorakis G, Ahmed R et al (1990) Methodology of head-up tilt testing in unexplained syncope. J Am Coll Cardiol 17: 125-130

42. Kenny RA, Ingram A, Bayliss J, Sutton R (1986) Head-up tilt: a useful tool for investigating unexplained syncope. Lancet 1: 1352-1355

43. Strasberg B, Rechavia E, Sagie A et al (1989) The head-up tilt table test in patients with syncope of unknown origin. Am Heart J 118: 923-927

44. Raviele A, Gasparini G, Di Pede F, Delise P, Bonso A, Piccolo E (1990) Usefulness of head-up tilt test in evaluating patients with syncope of unknown origin and negative electrophysiologic study. Am J Cardiol 65: 1322-1327

45. Cicogna R, Bonomi FG, Mascioli G et al (1992) Profilo emodinamico e neuroendocrino di due distinte risposte cardiovascolari nella sincope vasodepressiva indotta da head-up tilt test. G Ital Cardiol 22: 1367-1379

46. Sneddon JF, Counihan PJ, Bashir Y, Haywood GA, Ward DE, Camm AJ (1993) Impaired immediate vasoconstrictor responses in patients with recurrent neurally mediated syncope. Am J Cardiol 71: 72-76

47. Menozzi C, Brignole M, Raviele A et al (1993) The diagnostic value of head-up tilt test with sublingual glyceril trinitrate (Trinitrin head-up tilt test) in patients with unexplained syncope. New Trends Arrhyth 9: 219-224

48. Marangoni E, Zucchi A, Ferraris P et al (1993) A study on blood pressure and heart rate variations during head-up tilt testing supporting evidence for the two-phase model of postural syncope. New Trends Arrhyth 9:207-210

49. Brignole M, Menozzi C, Gianfranchi L, Oddone P, Lolli G, Bertulla A (1991) Neurally mediated syncope detected by carotid sinus massage and head-up tilt test in sick sinus syndrome. Am J Cardiol 68: 1032-1036

50. Almquist A, Goldberg IF, Milstein S et al (1989) Provocation of bradycardia and hypotension by isoproterenol and upright posture in patients with unexplained syncope. N Engl J Med 320: 346-351

51. Raviele A, Gasparini G, Di Pede F et al (1994) Nitroglycerin infusion during upright tilt: a new test for the diagnosis of vasovagal syncope. Am Heart J 127: 103-111
52. Waxman MB, Yao L, Cameron DA, Wald RW, Roseman J (1989) Isoproterenol induction of vasodepressor-type reaction in vasodepressor-prone persons. Am J Cardiol 63: 58-65
53. Pongiglione G, Fish FA, Strasburger JF, Benson DW (1990) Heart rate and blood pressure response to upright tilt in young patients with unexplained syncope. J Am Coll Cardiol 16: 165-170
54. Grubb BP, Temesy-Armos P, Hahn H, Elliott L (1991) Utility of upright tilt-table testing in the evaluation and management of syncope of unknown origin. Am J Med 90: 6-10
55. Raviele A, Gasparini G, Di Pede F, Piccolo E (1991) Head-up til test: a useful tool for evaluating unexplained syncope. Cardiol Board Rev 8: 86-93
56. Shalev Y, Gal R, Tchou PJ et al (1991) Echocardiographic demonstration of decreased left ventricular dimensions and vigorous myocardial contraction during syncope induced by head-up tilt. J Am Coll Cardiol 18: 746-751
57. Grubb BP, Temesy-Armos P, Moore J, Wolfe D, Hahn H, Elliott L (1992) The use of head-upright tilt table testing in the evaluation and management of syncope in children and adolescents. PACE 15: 742-748
58. Kapoor WN, Brant N (1992) Evaluation of syncope by upright tilt testing with isoproterenol. Ann Intern Med 116: 358-363
59. Sheldon R, Killam S (1992) Methodology of isoproterenol tilt table testing in patients with syncope. J Am Coll Cardiol 19: 773-779
60. Fouad FM, Sitthisook S, Vanerio G et al (1993) Sensitivity and specificity of the tilt table test in young patients with unexplained syncope. PACE 16: 394-400
61. Newman D, Lurie K, Rosenqvist M, Washington C, Schwartz J, Scheinman MM (1993) Head-up tilt testing with and without isoproterenol infusion in healthy subjects of different ages. PACE 16: 715-721
62. Manolis AS, Linzer M, Salem D, Estes III NAM (1990) Syncope: current diagnostic evaluation and management. Ann Intern Med 112: 850-863
63. Alboni P, Menozzi C, Brignole M et al (1993) An abnormal neural reflex plays a role in causing syncope in sinus bradycardia. J Am Coll Cardiol 22:1130-1134
64. Leitch JW, Klein GJ, Yee R, Leather RA, Kim YH (1992) Syncope associated with supraventricular tachycardia. An expression of tachycardia rate or vasomotor response? Circulation 85: 1064-1071
65. Brignole M, Gianfranchi L, Menozzi C et al (1993) Role of autonomic reflexes in syncope associated with paroxysmal atrial fibrillation. J Am Coll Cardiol 22: 1123-1129

Methodology of Head-Up Tilt Test: What is the Sensitivity and Specificity of the Different Protocols?

A. Raviele, S. Themistoclakis, and G. Gasparini

Divisione di Cardiologia, Ospedale Umberto I, Mestre-Venice, Italy

Transient hypotension and bradycardia of vasovagal origin are thought to be the most common cause of syncope (1). Substantiation of the diagnosis, however, is sometimes difficult when it is based solely on clinical history because of the possible absence of typical precipitating factors and prodromal symptoms, especially in older patients (2). A passive head-up tilt (HUT) for an extended time has proven to be a sufficiently strong gravitational stress to reproduce a vasovagal reaction in susceptible patients (3, 4). Thus, in recent years some investigators have proposed its use as a means of diagnosing vasovagal syncope in patients with otherwise unexplained loss of consciousness (5, 6). In normal individuals, assumption of passive upright posture produces a reduction in venous return and cardiac output with an immediate decrease in arterial pressure that is compensated for by a reflex arterial vasoconstriction and concomitant tachycardia essentially mediated by arterial baroreceptors (7). In patients prone to vasovagal reaction, instead of these compensatory adjustments, an abnormal reflex may develop which leads to paradoxical arterial vasodilatation and bradycardia with profound hypotension and syncope (8). Although the exact pathophysiological mechanism is not completely known (9, 10), it has been postulated that this reflex is caused by an inappropriate activation of the ventricular mechanoreceptors (C fibers) located in the base of both the left and right ventricles, as a consequence of a vigorous contraction of the adrenergically stimulated heart around a relatively empty ventricular cavity (4, 11, 12).

Despite the growing popularity of the HUT test as a diagnostic tool to unmask an individual's predisposition toward vasovagal events, the standardization of the test methodology remains an unresolved question (13). The HUT is generally performed in the morning, after overnight fasting, in a quiet slightly darkened room. All cardioactive and vasoactive drugs are commonly withdrawn for at least five half-lives before the study, preferably with the exclusion of those that patients had been taking at the time of symptom presentation. The HUT is carried out by means of an electronically controlled tilt table with a footboard for weight-bearing. Restraining belts are placed at chest and thigh levels. After an initial period of supine rest for 5-10 min, the subject is then tilted head-up to a variable angle (between 60° and 90°) for a variable time (10–90 min) with or without the administration of provocative drugs. Blood pressure, heart rate, and rhythm are continuously monitored during the tilt and recorded every 2–5 min (or more often if symptoms develop). Blood pressure is usually measured non-invasively by means of a cuff sphygmomanometer or the photoplethysmographic method. At the end of tilt protocol or as soon as syncope or presyncope occurs during the test, the patient is rapidly returned to the supine position.

Basically, there are two types of HUT test. The first type is the HUT without drug provocation, the so-called baseline, control, or unmedicated HUT test. According to its duration, this test may be further subdivided in two other types: long-duration (45-60 min) HUT and short-duration (10-30 min) HUT. The second type is HUT with drug provocation, the so-called provocative or pharmacologic HUT test. Essentially, two drugs have been employed for this test, isoproterenol and nitroglycerin, although other drugs have been proposed, such as epinephrine (14), edrophonium (15), and adenosine (16). Long-duration baseline HUT and nitroglycerin tests are fairly common in Europe, while short-duration HUT and isoproterenol tests are much more popular in the United States.

A prolonged HUT without drug provocation was first described by Kenny et al. in 1986 (5). A duration of 60 min was initially suggested. More recently, this time was reduced by Fitzpatrick et al. (17) to 45 min, which corresponds to the mean time to syncope (25 min) plus two standard deviations (10 min) in 53 patients with malignant vasovagal syncope. The mean literature data are listed in Tables 1 and 2 (5, 17-24).

A tilt angle of 60° has almost always been employed. Overall, a positive response with reproduction of syncope or presyncope in association with hypotension and/or bradycardia has been observed in 200 out of 420 patients with syncope of unknown origin (5, 17-24) and in six out of 118 asymptomatic control subjects

Table 1. Positivity of prolonged unmedicated head-up tilt (HUT) in patients with unexplained syncope

Reference	Duration (min)	Angle (°)	Total (n)	Posivitive responses (n)	Positive rate (%)
(5)	60	40	15	10	67
(18)	60	60	40	15	37
(19)	60	60	30	15	50
(20)	60	60	100	32	32
(17)	45-60	60	71	53	74
(22)	45	60	50	21	42
(23)	45	60	78	24	44
(24)	45	60	36	20	56
			420	200	48

Table 2. Positivity of prolonged unmedicated HUT in asymptomatic control subjects

Reference	Duration (min)	Angle (°)	Total (n)	Posivitive responses (n)	Positive rate (%)
(5)	60	40	10	1	10
(18)	60	60	10	0	0
(19)	60	60	11	0	0
(21)	60	60	25	1	4
(20)	60	60	35	2	6
(17)	45-60	60	27	2	7
			118	6	5

(5, 17-21), yielding a positive rate of 48% and a test specificity of 95%. Our recent data (unpublished) in a series of 591 consecutive patients, 279 men and 312 women with a mean age of 54 years, and 27 age-matched controls are quite different: a positive rate of 17% and a specificity of 93%. This is in agreement with other recent papers that report a much lower positive rate (24%-31%) for prolonged HUT (25-27). This is probably due to a less strict selection of the patients that now undergo HUT test (patients with a lower number of syncopal episodes in whom other diagnostic procedures, such as an intracavitary electrophysiologic study, were rarely performed before).

Regarding the type of positive response during prolonged unmedicated HUT, the mixed response (type I of the Vasis classification) (28) is the most frequent (up to 50% of cases and more), followed by the cardioinhibitory response (types IIA and IIB), and the vasodepressor response (type III) (29). A cardiac asystole greater than 3 s has been described in 18% of cases (30) and greater than 5 s in 9% of cases (31). The reported mean time to syncope is quite variable, ranging from 18 to 42 min (mean, 25 min) (5, 17-19, 22, 23). The reproducibility of positive results during long-duration HUT is acceptable (Table 3): overall 71% (range, 62% – 77%), with a trend toward a delayed and frequently attenuated response to repeat tilt (17, 32, 33; our unpublished results). The reproducibility of negative results is higher: 91% in 44 patients studied by Alboni et al (34).

The short-duration unmedicated HUT was first proposed by Abi-Samra et al. (35) in 1988 as an isolated procedure and was then employed by Almquist et al. (6) and many other investigators as the first phase (i.e., without drug intervention) of the isoproterenol test. The maximum duration of the shortened HUT ranges greatly from 10 to 30 min (most commonly 10 min; Tables 4 and 5) (6, 20, 35-46). The angle of tilting is also variable, from 60° to 90° (most commonly 80°;

Tables 4, 5) (6, 20, 35-46). This makes it quite difficult to compare the results from different centers. However, when combining the data of all published studies (Tables 4, 5) (6, 20, 35-46), a short-duration unmedicated HUT shows a positive rate of 30% (significantly lower than that of long-duration protocol: 47%) and a specificity of 92% (similar to that of long-duration protocol: 95%).

The isoproterenol test is widely used as a pharmacologic HUT test. The isoproterenol acts as a provocative agent by stimulating myocardial contractility, lowering arteriolar resistances, and reducing left ventricular volume, thus facilitating the activation of the ventricular mechanoreceptors (C fibers) during HUT (6, 36, 37, 39, 47, 48). Several different protocols have been proposed for the isoproterenol test. According to the original protocol used by Almquist et al. (6), after an initial period of 10 min of unmedicated HUT, intravenous isoproterenol infusion is initiated at a rate of 1 μg/min and is continued for 5 min with the patient or control subject supine. The HUT is then performed at 80° for 10 min. If the result of the test is negative, the subject is returned to the supine position and the entire sequence is repeated in successive stages (maximum of five) by progressively increasing the isoproterenol infusion by 1 μg/min at every stage. The endpoints of the test are the occurrence of syncope or presyncope, intolerance to isoproterenol (e.g., angina, life-threatening ventricular arrhythmias, severe headache, nausea, emotional lability, etc.), heart rate greater than 150 beats/min, and completion of the protocol. The numerous protocols employed for the isoproterenol test differ from Almquist's initial protocol and from each other in several aspects (Table 6) (6, 13, 20, 35-45, 49): presence or absence of a period of unmedicated HUT, duration of this period (from 5 to 30 min), angle of tilting (from 60° to 90°), number of stages (from one to five) and isoproterenol dosage and infusion rate (from 1 μg/min to 8 μg/min). Recently, however, for practical

Table 3. Reproducibility of prolonged unmedicated head-up tilt (HUT) in patients with unexplained syncope

Reference	1st HUT (n)	2nd HUT (n)	Reproducibility (%)	1st → 2nd HUT (days)
(17)[a]	31	24	77	?
(32)[a]	25	20	80	1
(33)[a]	13	8	62	7
(Raviele et al., unpublished)[a]	55	36	65 71[c]	3
(34)[b]	44	40	91	1-7

[a]Positive responses.
[b]Negative responses.
[c]Mean value of reproducibility of positive responses.

Table 4. Positivity of short-duration head-up tilt (HUT) (initial phase of isoproterenol test) in patients with unexplained syncope

Reference	Duration (min)	Angle (°)	Total (n)	Positive responses (n)	Positive rate (%)
(6)	10	80	15	4	27
(36)	10	80	14	0	0
(37)	10	60	8	0	0
(38)	15	90	20	4	20
(39)	15	70	18	9	50
(40)	15	70	57	22	39
(41)	30	80	25	6	24
(42)	30	80	30	6	20
(43)	15	80	20	2	10
(44)	10	80	85	5	6
			292	58	20
(35)[a]	20	60	154	63	42
(45)[a]	20	60	44	25	57
			490	146	30

[a]Only two papers in which short-duration HUT has been used as an isolated procedure and not as the initial phase of the isoproterenol test.

Table 5. Positivity of short-duration unmedicated HUT (initial phase of isoproterenol test) in asymptomatic control subjects

Reference	Duration (min)	Angle (°)	Total (n)	Positive responses (n)	Positive rate (%)
(6)	10	80	18	0	0
(20)	10	60	25	0	0
(41)	30	80	6	0	0
(43)	15	80	20	3	15
(43)	15	80	20	4	20
(46)	30	60	25	2	8
			114	9	8
(39)[a]	15	70	11	0	0
(35)[a]	20	60	15	0	0
(45)[a]	20	60	18	3	17
			158	12	8

[a]Only three papers in which short-duration HUT has been used as an isolated procedure and not as the initial phase of the isoproterenol test.

Table 6. Positivity of isoproterenol test (second phase, after drug administration) in patients with unexplained syncope

Reference	Stages (n)	Duration (min)	Dosage (μg/min)	Angle (°)	Total (n)	Posivitive responses (n)	Positive rate (%)
(6)	5	5+10	1 → 5	80	15	9	60
(36)	5	5+10	1 → 5	80	14	9	71
(37)	4	5+10	2 → 8	60	8	4	50
(38)	3	5+15	—	90	20	12	60
(39)	1	15	1 → 3	70	18	5	28
(40)	1	15	1 → 3	70	57	12	21
(41)	3	5+30	1 → 3	80	25	9	36
(42)	3	5+30	1 → 3	80	30	15	50
(43)	5	10	1 → 5	80	20	13	65
(44)	2	5+10	2 → 5	80	85	61	72
					292	149	51
(20)[a]	3	5+10	1 → 5	60	88	11	16
(49)[a]	1	5+10	5	80	40	22	52
					400	172	38

[a]Only two papers in which the administration of isoproterenol was not preceded by an initial period of unmedicated HUT.

reasons, there has been a tendency to prefer protocols of very short duration (49).

The positive rate of the isoproterenol test in patients with syncope of unknown origin (Table 6) ranges from 50% to 87% (mean, 71%; 20% for the initial unmedicated phase and 51% for the subsequent pharmacologic phase) (6, 13, 20, 35-45, 49). This is certainly a higher positive yield than that of prolonged HUT (48%). However, the percentage of positive results is significantly lower (15%-17%) when the isoproterenol test is performed in patients who have already undergone a long-duration (45-60 min) unmedicated HUT (20, 24, 50). Moreover, the isoproterenol test is usually performed at steeper angles than prolonged HUT (80° versus 60°) and, as shown in Table 6, the rate of positive responses increases (from 50% to 80%) by increasing the angle of tilting (from 60° to 90°) (37, 49). This may, at least in part, justify the difference in sensitivity found between the two methods. Indeed, if we compare the results of isoproterenol test at 60° (20, 37, 51) with those of prolonged HUT at the same angle, the rates of positive responses are similar (52% versus 48%). The specificity of isoproterenol test (Table 7) seems to be lower than that of prolonged HUT: 76% versus 95% (8% positive rate during control phase plus 16% positive rate during drug intervention) (6, 20, 41, 43, 46). In contrast, the reproducibility of the isoproterenol test (Table 8) is better: overall 84% for positive results and 88% for negative results (32, 42, 52-56). It is noteworthy that the specificity of the isoproterenol test increases in elderly patients and when protocols with low doses of isoproterenol are used (57-59).

The isoproterenol test has two important limitations: (1) the test is not feasible in about 10% of subjects due to the potentially dangerous effects of the drug which leads to the exclusion of patients with serious arterial hypertension, ischemic heart disease, congestive heart failure and ventricular arrhythmias; (2) the test may not be appropriately evaluated in another 16%-24% of subjects (20, 60) due to its early interruption because of the occurrence of intolerable side effects during isoproterenol infusion.

The nitroglycerin test is a pharmacologic HUT test which we recently proposed as an alternative test to isoproterenol challenge (25, 27, 61, 62). Nitroglycerin has been chosen as provocative agent because of its potent vasodilatatory effects on the capacity vessels (63) which may lead to a further increase in the venous pooling already caused by passive upright posture. We have employed two different types of nitroglycerin test

(25, 27, 61, 62). Initially, nitroglycerin, was administered intravenously, using a protocol similar to that of the isoproterenol test, the so-called intravenous nitroglycerin test (61). More recently, in order to simplify the test and to shorten its duration, nitroglycerin has been administered sublingually, the so-called oral nitroglycerin test (25, 27, 62).

The protocol of the intravenous nitroglycerin test (61) consists of a maximum of five consecutive stages of 5 min supine position plus 10 min 80° upright tilt at a progressively increasing infusion rate, starting from 1.72 µg/kg per hour and with successive increments of 0.86 µg/kg per hour every stage. We have tested (61) this protocol in a group of 40 patients with syncope of unknown origin at the end of a complete diagnostic work-up (including a prolonged unmedicated HUT) and in 25 age-matched control subjects. The results obtained with nitroglycerin test have been then compared with those obtained with the isoproterenol test. We considered three different types of responses during nitroglycerin or isoproterenol test: a positive response, an exaggerated response and a negative response. A positive response is defined as the reproduction of the clinical syncope or presyncope in association with sudden and marked hypotension and bradycardia, and an exaggerated response as the occurrence of minor symptoms in association with gradually increasing hypotension alone. The positive response is judged to be the expression of a neural reflex, and the exaggerated response the result of an excessive vasodilatation produced by the drugs. The main results found (61) are the following: during the nitroglycerin test, 21 of the 40 patients (53%) had a positive response, ten (25%) an exaggerated response, nine (22%) a negative response and none a drug intolerance. During the isoproterenol test, the results were as follows: ten patients (25%) showed a positive response, ten (25%) an exaggerated response, 13 (32%) a negative response and seven (18%) a drug intolerance. Only two (8%) of the control subjects had a positive response to the nitroglycerin test and two (8%) to the isoproterenol test. Thus the positive rate, the specificity, and the predictive accuracy of the intravenous nitroglycerin test were 53%, 92%, and 67%, respectively, and those of the isoproterenol test 25%, 92%, and 50%, respectively.

The oral nitroglycerin test is simpler and quicker than the intravenous one. We have recently evaluated two different protocols of this test (25, 27, 62). The first protocol (normal protocol) (25, 27) consists of giving nitroglycerin sublingually at a dosage of 0.30 mg following an initial period of 45 min of unmedicated

Table 7. Positivity of isoproterenol test in asymptomatic control subjects

Reference	Total (n)	Unmedicated phase		Pharmacologic phase	
		(n)	(%)	(n)	(%)
(6)	18	0	0	2	18
(20)	25	0	0	1	4
(41)	6	0	0	0	0
(43)	20	3	15	10	59
(43)	20	4	20	5	31
(46)	25	2	8	0	0
	114	9	8	18	16

Table 8. Reproducibility of isoproterenol test in patients with unexplained syncope

Reference	Positive responses (%)	Negative responses (%)
(42)	80	—
(52)	93	86
(53)	80	100
(54)	86	—
(55)	88	85
(32)	91	—
(56)	64	88
	84	88

upright tilting at 60 degrees. The HUT is then continued for other 20 min at the same angle. The second protocol (shortened protocol) (62) differs from the first one only in the duration of the initial period: 20 min instead of 45 min. The normal protocol has so far been tested in 290 patients with unexplained syncope and 52 asymptomatic control subjects and the shortened protocol in 27 patients and 14 controls. The results are encouraging (25, 62). The positive rate among the patients was 48% with the first protocol (24% during the control phase and 24% during drug administration) and 59% with the second protocol. The specificity was also good: 94% with the first protocol and 93% with the second protocol. An exaggerated response was observed in 16% and 7% of the cases using the first and second protocol, respectively. On the basis of this data, the shortened protocol seems to be superior to the normal protocol. However, the population studied is quite small and these results have to be confirmed in a larger number of a patients and controls before they are applied to clinical practice.

The oral nitroglycerin test (normal protocol) was also compared to the isoproterenol test in a group of 18 patients with syncope of unknown origin (64). The positive rate of the oral nitroglycerin test was 62% and that of the isoproterenol test 45%. However, the results obtained with the two tests were not infrequently discordant and the isoproterenol test was positive in a percentage (22%) of patients with a negative response to nitroglycerin test. This suggests the use of the isoproterenol test as an adjunctive means to diagnose vasovagal syncope in patients with a negative response to the initial HUT test with oral nitroglycerin (64). The reproducibility of the oral nitroglycerin test (normal protocol) was recently studied in 18 patients. It was 77% (ten out of 13) for positive responses and 80% (four out of five) for negative responses (our unpublished data).

In summary, on the basis of the literature and our personal data the following conclusions can be drawn: (a) when compared to prolonged unmedicated HUT, a short-duration, drug-free protocol seriously underestimates the number of positive results without increasing the specificity of the test; (b) the addition of drugs, especially isoproterenol, to HUT may enhance the positive rate of the test, but this is often at the expense of specificity. Moreover, it may provoke exaggerated responses, which are sometimes difficult to interpret and classify.

Thus, in our opinion, the prolonged (45 min) unmedicated HUT is, at the present time, the most accurate HUT protocol, and we recommend its use for the initial evaluation of patients with unexplained syncope. When the results of this test are negative and a strong suspicion remains about the vasovagal nature of the syncope, pharmacologic HUT tests may be used. Of these, the oral nitroglycerin test appears to be the most preferable: (a) because it is equally specific but more sensitive and feasible than the isoproterenol test and (b) because it is more practical and quicker than the intravenous nitroglycerin test and thus more suitable for routine clinical use.

References

1. Wayne HH (1961) Syncope: physiological considerations and an analysis of the clinical characteristics in 510 patients. Am J Med 30: 418-438
2. Fitzpatrick A, Theodorakis G, Travill C, Sutton R (1991) Incidence of malignant vasovagal syndrome in patients with recurrent syncope. Eur Heart J 12: 389-394
3. Weissler AM, Warren JV, Estes EH Jr, Mc Intosh HB, Leonard JJ (1957) Vasodepressor syncope: factors influencing cardiac output. Circulation 15: 875-882
4. Epstein SE, Stampfer M, Beiser GD (1968) Role of the capacitance and resistance vessels in vasovagal syncope. Circulation 37: 524-533
5. Kenny RA, Ingram A, Bayliss J, Sutton R (1986) Head-up tilt: a useful tool for investigating unexplained syncope. Lancet 1: 1352-1355
6. Almquist A, Goldberg IF, Milstein S et al. (1989) Provocation of bradycardia and hypotension by isoproterenol and upright posture in patients with unexplained syncope. N Engl J Med 320: 346-351
7. Abboud FM (1986) Pathophysiology of hypotension and syncope. In: Hurst JW, Logue RB, Rackley CE et al (eds) The heart. Mc Graw Hill, New York, pp 370-382
8. Sobel BE, Roberts R (1988) Hypotension and syncope. In: Braunwald E (ed) Heart disease. A textbook of cardiovascular medicine. Saunders, Philadelphia, pp 884-895
9. Sutton R, Petersen MEV (1993) Vasovagal syncope 1994. New Trends Arrhyth 9: 225-231
10. Raviele A, Alboni P (1994) Sincope: un aggiornamento sulla fisiopatologia, diagnosi e terapia. G Ital Cardiol 24: 1227-1260
11. Oberg B, Thoren P (1972) Increased activity in left ventricular receptors during hemorrhage or occlusion of caval veins in the cat – a possible cause of vasovagal reaction. Acta Physiol Scand 85: 164-173
12. Thoren P (1979) Role of cardiac vagal C fibers in cardiovascular control. Rev Physiol Biochem Pharmacol 86: 1-94
13. Kapoor WN, Smith MA, Miller NL (1994) Upright tilt testing in evaluating syncope: a comprehensive literature review. Am J Med 97: 78-88
14. Calkins H, Kadish A, Sousa J, Rosenheck S, Morady F (1991) Comparison of responses to isoproterenol and epinephrine during head-up tilt in suspected vasodepressor syncope. Am J Cardiol 67: 207-209
15. Lurie KG, Dutton J, Mangat R, Newman D, Eisemberg S, Scheinman MM (1993) Evaluation of edrophonium as a provocative agent for vasovagal syncope during head-up tilt-table testing. Am J Cardiol 72: 1286-1290
16. Shen WK, Hammill SC, Munger TM, Stanton MS, Packer DL, Gersh BJ (1993) Usefulness of adenosine in evaluating vasovagal syncope: comparison to tilt table and isoproterenol test. Circulation 88 [Suppl I]: 398 (abstr)
17. Fitzpatrick A, Theodorakis G, Ahmed R et al (1990) Methodology of head-up tilt testing in unexplained syncope. J Am Coll Cardiol 17: 125-130
18. Strasberg B, Rechavia E, Sagie A et al (1989) The head-up tilt table test in patients with syncope of unknown origin. Am Heart J 118: 923-927
19. Raviele A, Gasparini G, Di Pede F, Delise P, Bonso A, Piccolo E (1990) Usefulness of head-up tilt test in evaluating patients with syncope of unknown origin and negative electrophysiologic study. Am J Cardiol 65: 1322-1327
20. Brignole M, Menozzi C, Gianfranchi L, Oddone D, Lolli G, Bertulla A (1991) Carotid sinus massage, eyeball compression and head-up tilt test in patients with syncope of uncertain origin and in healthy control subjects. Am Heart J 122: 1644-1651
21. Brignole M, Menozzi C, Gianfranchi L, Oddone P, Lolli G, Bertulla A (1991) Neurally mediated syncope detected by carotid sinus massage and head-up tilt test in sick sinus syndrome. Am J Cardiol 68: 1032-1036
22. Cicogna R, Bonomi FG, Mascioli G et al (1992) Profilo emodinamico e neuroendocrino di due distinte risposte cardiovascolari nella sincope vasodepressiva indotta da head-up tilt test. G Ital Cardiol 22: 1367-1379
23. Sneddon JF, Counihan PJ, Bashir Y, Haywood GA, Ward DE, Camm AJ (1993) Impaired immediate vasoconstrictor respons-

es in patients with recurrent neurally mediated syncope. Am J Cardiol 71: 72-76

24. Ovadia M, Thoele D (1994) Esmolol tilt testing with esmolol withdrawal for the evaluation of syncope in the young. Circulation 89: 228-235

25. Menozzi C, Brignole M, Raviele A et al (1993) The diagnostic value of head-up tilt test with sublingual glyceril trinitrate (Trinitrin head-up tilt test) in patients with unexplained syncope. New Trends Arrhyth 9: 219-224

26. Marangoni E, Zucchi A, Ferraris P et al (1993) A study on blood pressure and heart rate variations during head-up tilt testing supporting evidence for the two-phase model of postural syncope. New Trends Arrhyth 9: 207-210

27. Raviele A, Menozzi C, Brignole M et al (1995) Value of head-up tilt testing potentiated with sublingual nitroglycerin to assess the origin of unexplained syncope. Am J Cardiol 77: 267-272

28. Sutton R, Petersen M, Brignole M, Raviele A, Menozzi C, Giani P (1992) Proposed classification for tilt induced vasovagal syncope. Eur J Cardiac Pacing Electrophysiol 3: 180-183

29. Morillo CA, Klein GJ, Zandri S, Yee R (1995) Neurally mediated syncope: long-term follow-up in patients with and without pharmacologic therapy and positive head-up tilt (submitted for publication)

30. Brignole M, Menozzi C, Gianfranchi L, Bottoni N, Lolli G (1992) The clinical and prognostic significance of the asystolic response during the head-up tilt test. Eur J Cardiac Pacing Electrophysiol 2: 109-113

31. Dhala A, Natale A, Sra J et al (1995) Relevance of asystole during head-up tilt testing. Am J Cardiol 75: 251-254

32. Brignole M, Menozzi C, Gianfranchi L, Lolli G, Bottoni N, Oddone D (1992) A controlled trial of acute and long-term medical therapy in tilt-induced neurally mediated syncope. Am J Cardiol 70: 339-342

33. Blanc JJ, Mansourati J, Maheu B, Boughaleb D, Genet L (1993) Reproducibility of a positive passive upright tilt test at a seven-day interval in patients with syncope. Am J Cardiol 72: 469-471

34. Alboni P, Raviele A et al (1995) Is a second unmedicated tilt test useful in patients with unexplained syncope? Am J Cardiol (submitted for publication)

35. Abi-Samra F, Maloney JD, Fouad-Tarazi FM, Castle LW (1988) The usefulness of head-up tilt testing and hemodynamic investigation in the work-up of syncope of unknown origin. PACE 11: 1202-1214

36. Chen MY, Goldenberg IF, Milstein S et al (1989) Cardiac electrophysiologic and hemodynamic correlates of neurally mediated syncope. Am J Cardiol 63: 66-72

37. Waxman MB; Yao L, Cameron DA, Wald RW, Roseman J (1989) Isoproterenol induction of vasodepressor-type reaction in vasodepressor-prone persons. Am J Cardiol 63: 58-65

38. Pongiglione G, Fish FA, Strasburger JF, Benson DW (1990) Heart rate and blood pressure response to upright tilt in young patients with unexplained syncope. J Am Coll Cardiol 16: 165-170

39. Shalev Y, Gal R, Tchou PJ et al (1991) Echocardiographic demonstration of decreased left ventricular dimensions and vigorous myocardial contraction during syncope induced by head-up tilt. J Am Coll Cardiol 18: 746-751

40. Sra JS, Anderson AJ, Sheikh SH et al (1991) Unexplained syncope evaluated by electrophysiologic studies and head-up tilt testing. Ann Intern Med 114: 1013-1019

41. Grubb BP, Temesy-Armos P, Hahn H, Elliott L (1991) Utility of upright tilt-table testing in the evaluation and management of syncope of unknown origin. Am J Med 90: 6-10

42. Grubb BP, Temesy-Armos P, Moore J, Wolfe D, Hahn H, Elliott L (1992) The use of head-upright tilt table testing in the evaluation and management of syncope in children and adolescents. PACE 15: 742-748

43. Kapoor WN, Brant N (1992) Evaluation of syncope by upright tilt testing with isoproterenol. Ann Intern Med 116: 358-363

44. Sheldon R, Killam S (1992) Methodology of isoproterenol tilt table testing in patients with syncope. J Am Coll Cardiol 19: 773-779

45. Fouad FM, Sitthisook S, Vanerio G et al (1993) Sensitivity and specificity of the tilt table test in young patients with unexplained syncope. PACE 16: 394-400

46. Newman D, Lurie K, Rosenqvist M, Washington C, Schwartz J, Scheinman MM (1993) Head-up tilt testing with and without isoproterenol infusion in healthy subjects of different ages. PACE 16: 715-721

47. Benditt DG, Remole S, Bailin S, Dunnigan A, Asso A, Milstein S (1991) Tilt table testing for evaluation of neurally mediated (cardioneurogenic) syncope: rationale and proposed protocols. PACE 14: 1528-1537

48. Raviele A, Gasparini G, Di Pede F (1993) Sincopi Vasovagali: utilità del tilting test nella valutazione della fisiopatologia, diagnosi e terapia. In: Disertori M, Marconi P (eds) La stimolazione cardiaca transesofagea e l'elettrocardiografia ad alta risoluzione. Centro Scientifico Editore, Torino, pp 185-198

49. Sheldon R (1993) Evaluation of a single-stage isoproterenol-tilt table test in patients with syncope. J Am Coll Cardiol 22: 114-118

50. Greenfield RA, Bacon ME, Barrington WW (1991) Duration of tilt test for neurally mediated syncope in adults. Circulation 84 [Suppl II]: 409 (abstr)

51. Thilenius OG, Quinones JA, Husayni TS, Novak J (1991) Tilt tests for diagnosis of unexplained syncope in pediatric patients. Pediatrics 87: 334-338

52. Grubb BP, Wolfe D, Temesy-Armos P, Hahn H, Elliott L (1992) Reproducibility of head upright tilt table test results in patients with syncope. PACE 15: 1477-1481

53. Chen XC, Chen MY, Remole S et al (1992) Reproducibility of head-up tilt-table testing for eliciting susceptibility to neurally mediated syncope in patients without structural heart disease. Am J Cardiol 69: 755-760

54. Fish FA, Strasburger JF, Woodrow Benson D Jr (1992) Reproducibility of a symptomatic response to upright tilt in young patients with unexplained syncope. Am J Cardiol 70: 605-609

55. Sheldon R, Splawinski J, Killam S (1992) Reproducibility of isoproterenol tilt-table tests in patients with syncope. Am J Cardiol 69: 1300-1305

56. De Buitleir M, Grogan EW, Picone MF, Casteen JA (1993) Immediate reproducibility of the tilt-table test in adults with unexplained syncope. Am J Cardiol 71: 304-307

57. Natale A, Sra J, Newby K et al (1995) Specificity of head-up tilt testing with different isoproterenol infusion rate in volunteers 60 years of age and older. PACE 18: 844 (abstr)

58. Natale A, Sra J, Dhala A et al (1995) Occurrence of syncope in normal volunteers with positive upright tilt test: protocol-dependent outcome. PACE 18: 950 (abstr)

59. Morillo CA, Klein GJ, Zandri S, Yee R (1995) Diagnostic accuracy of a low-dose head-up tilt protocol. Am Heart J (in press)

60. Mc Intosh S, Lawson J, Da Costa D, Kelly P, Kenny RA (1995) Use of sublingual glyceryl trinitrate during head-up tilt: a provocative test for reproduction of neurocardiogenic symptoms in unexplained syncope. (submitted)

61. Raviele A, Gasparini G, Di Pede F et al (1994) Nitroglycerin infusion during upright tilt: a new test for the diagnosis of vasovagal syncope. Am Heart J 127: 103-111

62. Gasparini G, Raviele A, Brignole M et al (1994) Head-up tilt test di breve durata potenziato con nitroglicerina sublinguale: utilità clinica. G Ital Cardiol 24 [Suppl I]: 494

63. Mason DT, Braunwald E (1971) The effects of nitroglycerin and amylnitrite on arteriolar and venous tone in the human forearm. Circulation 32: 756-766

64. Themistoclakis S, Gasparini G, Di Pede F et al (1995) Diagnosi di sincope vasovagale. Confronto tra tilting test con nitroglicerina sublinguale e tilting test con isoproterenolo (abstr). G Ital Cardiol (in press).

What Do We Know Today About the Outcome of Vasovagal Syncope?

R.S. Sheldon

Cardiovascular Research Group, University of Calgary

Division of Cardiology, Calgary General Hospital,
Calgary, Canada

Introduction

Sudden loss of consciousness is a dramatic and often very frightening event for both patients and their families. While syncope has a wide differential diagnosis, the development of tilt table tests over the past 10 years has shown us that most patients in the community with syncope probably faint because of one of several presentations of vasovagal syncope. A good grasp of the prognosis of the patient is necessary in order to determine whether therapy need be attempted, and whether it is successful. There are a number of variants of vasovagal syncope, and each may have their own prognosis. Before we consider the prognosis of vasovagal syncope, we will first review some of the variants of this disorder and also review our current diagnostic maneuvers.

The Variants of Vasovagal Syncope

Physicians have long recognized the classic vasovagal response to pain, severe emotional stress, or specific psychological stressors. Physicians and patients alike understand that this is a recurring but not life-threatening problem. However, there are other common forms of vasovagal syncope which have not been as easily recognized. Syncope in children and adolescents has now been shown to be due to vasovagal episodes in the large majority of patients who have structurally normal hearts (1-4). The reason for this characteristic appearance of syncope in adolescents is not known, but it appears to be self-limited. Most teenagers who faint stop doing so by the time they reach their third decade of life. Indeed, the Framingham study (5) showed that 90% of fainting adults do not faint before the age of 20. Thus although syncope in children may persist for a number of years and cause psychosocial stress and occasionally physical trauma, it usually does not appear to persist into adulthood.

Pregnancy is also associated with syncope, particularly in the second trimester. Although this has not been addressed systematically, anecdotal clinical experience amongst obstetricians and family practitioners suggests that this form of syncope is also self-limited. Few women who faint while pregnant continue to faint following delivery. During pregnancy, vasovagal syncope is rarely a cause of trauma or poor outcome. Thus, the outlook for vasovagal syncope associated with pregnancy is quite good.

In contrast, syncope associated with valvular aortic stenosis is a marker of poor outcome (6). Patients with valvular aortic stenosis usually have a long asymptomatic period, but when syncope ensues mortality is high over the next 3 years. Although this syncope may be due to ventricular arrhythmias or conduction block, it is thought that some patients who faint with aortic stenosis do so due to inappropriate activation of the left ventricular baroreceptor (7). Given the high risk which hypotension places on patients with critical aortic stenosis, it is not surprising that vasovagal episodes portend a poor prognosis.

The majority of patients with syncope do not present with such clearly defined historical characteristics. It is these patients who historically have been a cause of concern to many physicians, and whose etiology of syncope has been clarified with tilt table testing. Although a number of tilt test protocols exist (8), all involve orthostatic stress, and many include challenge during orthostatic stress with one of a number of provocative agents such as isoproterenol, nitroglycerin, adenosine triphosphate, or edrophonium. When patients with unexplained syncope (usually in the absence of demonstrable electrical or structural heart disease) undergo tilt table testing, most have syncopal or presyncopal responses associated with hypotension and/or bradycardia. The probability of a positive outcome to tilt table testing appears to depend upon the population of patients undergoing the test, as well as the nature of the test itself. However, between 25% and 80% of patients with undiagnosed syncope have a positive response to tilt table testing, and the symptoms they develop on tilt table testing closely resemble the symptoms which they have during their clinical syncope. Assuming that these patients are representative of patients who faint in the community, it appears that the majority of patients – perhaps at least 75% – have vasovagal syncope as the cause of their fainting. Since some of the largest studies of the outcome of patients with syncope predate the advent of tilt table testing, the majority of their patients with syncope of unexplained etiology may have vasovagal syncope.

Is Vasovagal Syncope a Threat to Life?

The bulk of the evidence suggests that vasovagal syncope is not a threat to life. The Framingham study (5) reported that syncope occurred in at least 3% of adults. The average age of onset was 51 years, and only 10% of adults had fainted before the age of 20. The investigators were unable to identify any obvious historical risk factor for syncope in 84% of the subjects who fainted. With the benefit of hindsight, we may assume that most of these subjects had vasovagal syncope. The age-adjusted risk of death was no different than that of the nonfainting subjects in all age groups, suggesting that vasovagal syncope does not pose a mortal risk to the large majority of patients.

In contrast to this community-based study, Kapoor et al. (9) assessed the mortality of 204 patients who presented with syncope to a large American tertiary care institution. In this study, which preceded the advent of tilt testing, 97 (48%) of patients had no diagnosed etiology of their syncope despite an aggressive series of diagnostic investigations. Another 26% of patients had a diagnosed cardiovascular cause of syncope such as sinus node dysfunction, complete heart block, or ventricular tachycardia. The actuarial risk of sudden death in 1 year in the latter group was 24%, while the risk of sudden death in patients without a diagnosed cause of syncope was only 3%. Only three of 16 sudden deaths did not have a clearly arrhythmic, ischemic, or mechanical cause. If we assume that the majority of the patients with undiagnosed syncope had vasovagal syncope, this study, too, suggests that patients with vasovagal syncope are at very low risk of sudden death.

In a similar study, Kushner et al. (10) determined the outcome of 99 consecutive patients with unexplained syncope and nondiagnostic findings in an electrophysiologic study who were assessed between 1984 and 1987. Structural heart disease was present in 47 patients and was absent in 52. The mean age of the patients was 56 years. Over a mean 20 months of follow-up, only two patients died suddenly. One of these patients was an elderly man with moderately severe left ventricular systolic dysfunction due to coronary artery disease, and one was a middle-aged chronic alcoholic who had sustained polymorphic ventricular tachycardia induced by programmed ventricular stimulation with triple extrastimuli. Although no patients underwent tilt table testing, the results of this study are consistent with an overall benign outcome of patients with vasovagal syncope. Thus all three studies, one of which was community-based and two of which were from tertiary care centers, indicate that the large majority of patients with vasovagal syncope are not at risk of sudden death.

Malignant Vasovagal Syncope

Are there specific subpopulations at higher risk of death? During headup tilt a variable minority of patients develop asystole in association with syncope. Some of these asystolic events last many seconds. Is this finding a marker of a mortal risk? Brignole et al. (11) prospectively addressed this question in a study of 56 patients with recurrent syncope and a positive tilt table test. Of these patients, 28 had an asystolic response of 7 ± 6 s (range 3-21 s) while the control group did not have asystole. Age, gender, and the history of syncopal symptoms were similar in the two groups. No patients died in either group over a 17 ± 14 month follow-up, although the actuarial risk of syncope at 40 months was about 40% in both groups. In a similar study, Dhala et al. (12) studied 19 patients who had asystole > 5 s on tilt testing. None of these patients died over a mean follow-up of 2.1 ± 1.4 years, despite a recurrence rate of syncope of 11%. Thus, an asystolic response on tilt table testing does not appear to be a risk for sudden death.

Finally, anecdotal reports have appeared about patients who have been resuscitated from sudden cardiac death, then found to have a positive tilt table test with no other abnormalities. This suggests that vasovagal syncope might cause death in isolated instances. However, one case involved a patient who fainted while swimming and was resuscitated from drowning, and several have reported the resuscitation of health care personnel at work, or the resuscitation of spouses of health care personnel. Given the alarming appearance of patients who faint, it is not unreasonable that an attempt at resuscitation would be made, but whether spontaneous recovery would have ensued without treatment is open to question.

The Chronic Nature of Vasovagal Syncope

Vasovagal syncope in many patients appears to be a chronic disorder. Several studies have reported the duration of symptoms of recurrent syncope among large populations of patients who have had a positive response to headup tilt table testing. For example, we reported (13) that in a population of 41 patients with syncope during headup tilt testing, the mean and median duration of symptoms was 49 and 18 months, respectively. Our longest suffering patient has fainted recurrently for over 60 years. Thus many patients who are referred for tilt table testing have been fainting for a considerable length of time. However, this may reflect a selection bias of patients who are referred for syncope. For example, it might be that the majority of patients with syncope faint only once or twice and are not referred for specialist assessment.

Few studies have specifically addressed the prognosis of patients with a positive tilt table test. However, recent randomized trials of the effectiveness of various treatments have included placebo arms (Table 1). Brignole et al. (14) reported the outcome of 15 placebo-treated patients who had had a positive tilt table test and a mean of seven historical syncopal spells. Over a mean follow-up of 10 months, syncope recurred

Table 1. Risk of a recurrence of syncope following a positive tilt test in five populations of drugfree patients.

Reference	Number of Patients	Follow-up period (years)	Risk of syncope (%)
(14)	15	1	30%
(15)	10	2.5	30%
(16)	51	1.3	29%
(17)	60	2.3	10%
(18)	101	1	28%

in four patients (27%) with an actuarial 1 year risk of syncope of about 30%. Morillo et al. (15) randomized 21 patients to treatment with disopyramide or placebo. They had had a mean of 11 ± 11 syncopal spells and all had had at least two positive tilt table tests. Over a mean follow-up time of 29 ± 8 months syncope recurred in 30% of the untreated patients. These trials, each with small numbers of patients, consistently showed that patients with small to moderate numbers of historical syncopal spells have a low risk of recurrence following tilt table testing.

In the past 2 years, several follow-up studies of larger numbers of patients who have had recurrent syncope and positive tilt table tests have been reported (Table 1). Natale et al. (16) studied 51 self-selected, drugfree patients with 10 ± 7 syncopal spells preceding a positive tilt table test. The risk of having at least one further syncopal spell was 29% in the 3.2 years following the positive tilt test, and no patients fainted beyond 16 months. Similarly, Morillo et al. (17) reported that 60 self-selected drugfree patients with recurrent syncope and a positive tilt table test had a 10% risk of syncope over a median 28 months following this test. We reported the results of a similar study of 101 patients (18) with syncope and a positive tilt table test who were followed without specific medical or pacing treatment. Although this population had a median pretest frequency of three syncopal spells per year, the actuarial risk of syncope-free survival was about 50% after 3 years of follow-up. The number of historical faints, frequency of historical faints, and duration of symptoms each predicted the risk of recurrent syncope. Unfortunately, none of these studies involved patients who were randomized to placebo, nor did they involve populations in which all patients were allocated to have no specific treatment.

Is asystole a risk for recurrent syncope? Menozzi et al. (19) followed 23 patients with syncope mainly due to carotid sinus hypersensitivity, and who had an asystolic response to carotid sinus massage, eyeball compression, or headup tilt. All patients received a pacemaker with a very long hysteresis lasting up to 6 s and a large memory for spontaneous bradycardic episodes. Over a mean 15 months of follow-up, frequent asystolic episodes occurred in 17/23 patients, including 47 episodes > 6 s. The actuarial risk of asystolic episodes > 3 s was 82% after 2 years of follow-up. Surprisingly, only 0.7% of episodes 3-6 s in duration and 43% of episodes > 6 s resulted in presyncope or syncope. Similarly, Dhala et al. (12) and Brignole et al. (11) both found that asystole on tilt testing did not predict a higher risk of recurrent syncope. Although an asystolic response to vasovagal maneuvers is associated with frequent spontaneous asystolic events during follow-up, these are rarely symptomatic unless they are > 6 s. Thus, although these studies involved relatively small numbers of patients over a brief duration of time, they did study patients with an asystolic response, and the results suggest that these patients are not at increased risk of syncope. All studies consistently demonstrated a relatively low risk of recurrence of syncope following a positive tilt test.

Does Treatment Prevent Recurrent Syncope?

Numerous studies have attempted to demonstrate that drug treatment improves the outcome in patients with recurrent syncope and a positive tilt table test. Generally, treatments have been directed at either correcting the bradycardia or hypotension seen during syncope, or intervening in the hypothesized pathophysiologic cascade which begins with orthostatic stress and possibly physical or emotional stress. Two types of studies have been reported (8). The first involves determining whether an intervention prevents syncope during a tilt test. The underlying assumption is that the pathophysiologic findings seen during tilt tests mimic those which occur clinically, and that therefore the demonstration that a treatment which prevents syncope on tilt testing will also prevent syncope during chronic follow-up. Treatments which have been shown to have some effect at preventing syncope during tilt testing include intracardiac pacing (20), ß-adrenergic blockers (21), α-adrenergic agonists (22), disopyramide (23), and specific serotonin reuptake inhibitors such as sertraline (24).

However, the hypothesis that the response to a drug on tilt testing predicts the eventual clinical outcome on that drug may not be true. In a randomized, placebo-controlled, parallel arm, prospective trial Morillo et al. (15) showed that the response to placebo or intravenous disopyramide during headup tilt did not predict the response of the patient to chronic oral therapy with the same agent. However, the study involved patients undergoing at least five sequential tilt tests in multiple crossovers and eventually most patients did not faint on tilt testing. Whether this protocol that included a high number of serial tilt tests resembles clinical reality, or confounds it, is unclear. Furthermore, only 30% of patients on either placebo (3/10) or disopyramide (3/11) fainted during follow-up. Therefore the study might have been underpowered to demonstrate a true difference or might have involved an agent which was truly ineffective. A second study by Brignole et al. (14) randomized patients to placebo or to drug therapy selected on the basis of serial tilt table tests. These authors were also unable to demonstrate that the outcome of treated patients was any better than untreated patients and therefore were unable to demonstrate the usefulness of using tilt table tests to guide medical therapy.

In contrast, several open label uncontrolled case report series have been published which have suggested the usefulness of various drugs. Strieper and Campbell (22) treated 16 pediatric patients (mean age 13 years) who had recurrent syncope and a positive tilt test with oral pseudoephedrine in a dosage of 60 mg twice daily for an average of 12 months. Fifteen of 16 patients had no recurrent syncope, and the risk of recurrent syncope was about 6%. Grubb et al. (23) administered sertraline 50 mg daily to 17 young patients (mean age 15 years). Nine patients subsequently had a negative tilt test and all were asymptomatic over 12 ± 5 months of follow-up. Similarly, Grubb et al. (25) chronically administered a variety of agents including ß-blockers, disopyramide, scopolamine, and hydrofluorocortisone to patients based upon their results to tilt tests, and all were reported well after a mean follow-up of 16 ± 2 months.

The effectiveness of drugs in preventing recurrent syncope is unproven. Previous studies either were not randomized or not placebo-controlled, and the patients who were in these studies often had a relatively small number of historic syncopal spells. They therefore might be predicted to do well regardless of whether or not they received treatment. The randomized, placebo-controlled studies were unable to demonstrate that either disopyramide or a combination of various treatments were effective in preventing syncope during the long-term follow-up. These studies in retrospect were probably underpowered. Given the relatively small risk of recurrence of syncope, studies will need to involve either larger numbers of patients, longer follow-up, or both.

Future Directions

Several important questions remain to be determined. First, what should an outcome be? Most authors have concentrated on syncope. It is a simple, quantifiable, binary, memorable event. However some believe that the total burden of syncope and presyncope determines the overall degree of affliction and have suggested the use of combined measures. In light of this uncertainty, we might determine which of these assumptions is correct by performing a study involving one or more quality of life measurement tools (26,27).

If syncope is to be used as an outcome measure, should we be determining the total number of syncopal spells over a fixed period of follow-up or using a simpler estimate such as the time to first syncopal spell following randomization to a treatment? The rationale for using time to first event has been well established with paroxysmal arrhythmias such as atrial fibrillation and supraventricular tachycardia (28). It depends upon a formal demonstration of a Poisson distribution of the probability of recurrence. No study has yet shown that

syncope recurs in a Poisson or Poisson-like probability distribution.

The second kind of study which is needed is an assessment of the outcome of a representative population of untreated patients with syncope and a positive tilt test. This information might be derived from the placebo arm of a randomized, controlled trial. From our preliminary data (18), we estimate that this kind of study would require at least 100 untreated patients. This will also help us understand which patients are at a sufficiently high risk of syncope that treatment is warranted. It would be difficult to demonstrate that medical therapy helps patients who only faint once or twice.

Large, randomized, controlled trials are required to evaluate whether treatment is effective. Given the relatively low risk of recurrent syncope following a positive tilt table test, such trials will need to involve either high numbers of patients with an average low to moderate risk, or smaller numbers of higher risk patients. Finally, a large, randomized, placebo-controlled, parallel design trial will need to be mounted to determine whether serial tilt tests are useful in selecting effective therapy.

Acknowledgment. This work was supported by grants from the Medical Research Council of Canada and the Calgary General Hospital Research and Development Committee.

References

1. Pongiglione G, Fish FA, Strasburger JF, Benson W (1990) Heart rate and blood pressure response to upright tilt in young patients with unexplained syncope. J Am Coll Cardiol 16:165-170
2. Perry JC, Garson A (1991) The child with recurrent syncope: autonomic function testing and beta-adrenergic hypersensitivity. J Am Coll Cardiol 17:1168-1171
3. Thilenius OG, Quinones JA, Husayni TS, Novak J (1991) Tilt test for diagnosis of unexplained syncope in pediatric patients. Pediatrics 87:334-338
4. Balaji S, Oslizlok PC, Allen MC, McKay CA, Gillette PC (1994) Neurocardiogenic syncope in children with a normal heart. J Am Coll Cardiol 23:779-785
5. Savage DD, Corwin L, McGee DL, Kannel WB, Wolf PA (1985) Epidemiologic features of isolated syncope: the Framingham study. Stroke 16:626-629
6. Schwartz LS, Goldfischer J, Sprague GJ, Schwartz SP (1969) Syncope and sudden death in aortic stenosis. Am J Cardiol 23:647-658
7. Grech ED, Ramsdale DR (1991) Exertional syncope in aortic stenosis: evidence to support inappropriate left ventricular baroreceptor response. Am Heart J 121:603-606
8. Sheldon R (1994) Tilt table testing in the diagnosis and treatment of syncope. Cardiovasc Rev Rep 8-28
9. Kapoor W, Karpf M, Wieand S, Peterson J, Levey G (1983) A prospective evaluation and follow-up of patients with syncope. N Engl J Med 309:197-204
10. Kushner JA, Kou WH, Kadish AH, Morady F (1989) Natural history of patients with unexplained syncope and a nondiagnostic electrophysiologic study. J Am Coll Cardiol 14:391-396
11. Brignole M, Menozzi C, Gianfranchi L, Bottoni N, Lolli G (1992) The clinical and prognostic significance of the asystolic response during the head-up tilt test. Eur J Cardiac Pacing Electrophysiol 2:109-113
12. Dhala A, Natale A, Sra J, Deshpande S, Blanck Z, Jazayeri MR, Akhtar M (1995) Relevance of asystole during head-up tilt testing. Am J Cardiol 75:251-254

13. Sheldon R, Killam S (1992) Methodology of isoproterenol-tilt table testing in patients with syncope. J Am Coll Cardiol 19:773-779
14. Brignole M, Menozzi C, Gianfranchi L, Lolli G, Bottoni N, Oddone D (1992) A controlled trial of acute and long-term medical therapy in tilt-induced neurally mediated syncope. Am J Cardiol 70:339-342
15. Morillo CA, Leitch JW, Yee R, Klein GJ (1993) A placebo-controlled trial of intravenous and oral disopyramide for prevention of neurally mediated syncope induced by head-up tilt. J Am Coll Cardiol 22:1843-1848
16. Natale A, Biehl M, Banks B, Maglio C, Krebs A, Budziszewski M, Koch K, Sra J (1994) Recurrence of neurocardiogenic syncope without therapeutic interventions. Circulation 90:I-54 (abstr)
17. Morillo CA, Zandri S, Klein GJ, Yee R (1994) Neurally mediated syncope: long-term follow-up of patients with and without pharmacological therapy. Circulation 90:I-54 (abstr)
18. Sheldon RS, Rose S, Flanagan P, Koshman ML, Killam S (1994) Multivariate predictors of syncope recurrence in drug-free patients following a positive tilt table test. Circulation 90:I-55 (abstr)
19. Menozzi C, Brignole M, Lolli G, Bottoni N, Oddone D, Gianfranchi L, Gaggioli G (1993) Follow-up of asystolic episodes in patients with cardioinhibitory, neurally mediated syncope and VVI pacemaker. Am J Cardiol 72:1152-1155
20. Benditt DG, Petersen M, Lurie KG, Grubb BP, Sutton R (1995) Cardiac pacing for prevention of recurrent vasovagal syncope. Ann Intern Med 122:204-209
21. Almquist A, Goldenberg IF, Milstein S et al. (1989) Provocation of bradycardia and hypotension by isoproterenol and upright posture in patients with unexplained syncope. N Engl J Med 320:346-351
22. Strieper MJ, Campbell RM (1993) Efficacy of alpha-adrenergic agonist therapy for prevention of pediatric neurocardiogenic syncope. J Am Coll Cardiol 22:594- 597
23. Milstein S, Buetikofer J, Dunnigan A, Benditt DG, Gornick C, Reyes WJ (1990) Usefulness of disopyramide for prevention of upright tilt-induced hypotension- bradycardia. Am J Cardiol 65:1339-1344
24. Grubb BP, Samoil D, Kosinski D, Kip K, Brewster P (1994) Use of sertraline hydrochloride in the treatment of refractory neurocardiogenic syncope in children and adolescents. J Am Coll Cardiol 24:490-494.
25. Grubb BP, Temesy-Armos P, Hahn H, Elliott L (1991) Utility of upright tilt-table testing in the evaluation and management of syncope of unknown origin. Am J Med 90:6-10
26. Linzer M, Pontinen M, Gold DT, Divine GW, Felder A, Brooks WB (1991) Impairment of physical and psychosocial function in recurrent syncope. J Clin Epidemiol 44:1037-1043
27. Linzer M, Gold DT, Pontinen M, Divine GW, Felder A, Brooks WB (1994) Recurrent syncope as a chronic disease: preliminary validation of a disease-specific measure of functional impairment. J Gen Intern Med 9:181-186
28. Pritchett ELC, Lee KL (1988) Designing clinical trials for paroxysmal atrial tachycardia and other paroxysmal arrhythmias. J Clin Epidemiol 41:851-858

Vasovagal Syncope with Asystolic Pause: Drugs, Pacemaker, or Both?

A. Moya, G. Permanyer-Miralda, and J. Sagristá-Sauleda

Servei de Cardiologia, Hospital General Universitari Vall d'Hebron,
Barcelona, Spain

Introduction

One of the problems in the assessment of syncope is that most clinical episodes are not witnessed. Therefore, features such as asystole during the attack must be assumed on the basis of indirect evidence such as its induction with provocative maneuvers. Head up tilt test (HUT) is the most widely used of such maneuvers, and most discussions on the management or significance of asystole during syncope are based on the development of asystole during HUT. Therefore, before addressing the particular issue of asystole in vasovagal syncope (VVS), a critical review of the reliability of HUT to draw conclusions about such a topic is justified.

In 1986, Kenny et al. (1) first described the use of HUT in patients with syncope of unknown origin (SUO). Since then HUT has been extensively used, mainly for the clinical diagnosis of VVS (2-6) in patients with SUO. During the past years HUT has been used not only for the diagnosis of VVS, but also to increase the knowledge of its pathophysiology (7-9), to characterize its different clinical patterns (10,11), and also to select and monitor the response to therapy (12-27).

Recently, a multicenter European Working Group has provided a classification of the type of responses observed during HUT (11). The responses are classified according to the contribution of hypotension or bradycardia to syncopal responses. Thus, three main types of responses are recognized: type I, defined as as mixed response, when both components, hypotension and bradycardia, are present; type 2, when there is a predominately cardioinhibitory response, defined as a bradycardia <40 beats per minute during more than 10 s or an asystole longer than 3 s; and type 3, when there is a predominately vasodepressor component. Type 2 is subdivided in two additional subtypes: 2A, when blood pressure decreases before the heart rate decreases, and 2B, when blood pressure decreases to hypotensive levels only after the time at which heart rate decreases. The therapeutic approach to patients in which type 2 response to HUT is observed are those which will be analyzed in this chapter.

In spite of the extensive use of HUT, some important aspects of the test remain to be established.

The presence of a positive response to HUT has been considered as diagnostic of vasovagal etiology in patients with SUO (1-4). Before using any test for diagnostic purposes, its sensitivity and specificity should be well known (28). Specificity of HUT has been studied by many authors (2,4,5,7,10,29-32), with figures that range between 55% and 100%. These variations in the specificity between different series can be, at least partially, explained by the lack of uniformity of the protocols, either in the degree of inclination, in the duration of the test, or using (versus not using) different provocative drugs such as isoproterenol (4,5,13,29,31) or nitroglycerine (32). Up to now, HUT has been performed in different groups of patients with SUO; however, for assessing the true sensitivity of the test, patients with proven VVS should be studied (28). The selection of a gold standard of VVS is a difficult matter. According to Kapoor (33) only those patients with a clear precipitating condition, such as pain, fear, or medical instrumentation, can be considered to have VVS, while the presence of premonitory symptoms alone is not enough for establishing the diagnosis of VVS. Accordingly, there are no series in which HUT has been performed in patients with proven VVS and, consequently, the true sensitivity of the test is not known (34).

The most widely accepted pathophysiologic mechanism of VVS is that central hypovolemia, usually secondary to orthostatism, dehydration, or other unknown causes, stimulates baroreceptors and leads to an increased sympathetic nerve tone that can be increased by other stressing factors such as pain or fear. In this situation there is an increased inotropism in a relatively empty left ventricle (7,35) which leads to a hyperstimulation of C receptors of the left ventricular wall (36,37). In susceptible patients, these hyperactivated C receptors can produce, via the tractus nucleus solitarius, a paradoxical sudden withdrawal of sympathetic nerve tone and an increased parasympathetic nerve tone which leads to hypotension and bradycardia (35-38).

Therapeutic Options in VVS

According to this pathophysiologic sequence of VVS, different drugs have been proposed: etilefrine (13,39), ß-blockers (7,23,40-43), disopyramide (17,44), fludrocortisone (23), transdermal scopolamine (23,41,45), and inhibitors of serotonin re-uptake (46). Cardiac pacing has been considered as a therapeutic alternative, alone or in combination with drugs, in patients with a severe cardioinhibitory response to HUT (type 2), to treat bradycardia (1,21-27).

Many articles have been published in which these drugs, or even pacemakers, have been used in patients with VVS. The efficacy of therapeutic interventions has been assessed either with sequential HUT or with follow-up of these patients, but most of the studies that have been published have some limitations and no definitive conclusions can be drawn. There are some unresolved issues regarding the use of HUT to select the appropriate therapy in patients with VVS. Although HUT has been used in most studies as a surrogate for clinical recurrences, its predictive value in the follow-up has not been demonstrated (43). In fact, it is not known to what extent the observed response to HUT reproduces the characteristics of spontaneous syncopal episodes (47). Many variables can influence the response of the patients to HUT. We have observed that the use of isoproterenol influences the heart rate during a positive response to HUT (48). Thus, heart rate is significantly higher when the response develops during isoproterenol infusion than when it develops without isoproterenol. Therefore, the rate of cardioinhibitory responses to HUT is significantly reduced when isoproterenol is used. For HUT to be of use in evaluating the beneficial effect of any therapeutic intervention, the test must be highly reproducible. The reproducubility of an initially negative response is high and has shown little variation between different series (6,49-53), ranging from 85% to 100%. However, the reproducibility of positive responses is lower and less uniform (6,30,49-54), ranging from 36% to 92%. There are few published data about the reproducibility of the type of response (53). In our experience, the observed positive response when sequential HUTs are performed can vary from a severe cardioinhibitory response to almost pure vasodepressor in the same patient. Thus, it has not been firmly established as to what extent the observation of asystole during HUT indicates that asystole is present in the spontaneous attacks. Additionally, most of the trials in which the efficacy of different drugs in patients with VVS has been assessed, either with HUT or with follow-up alone, have been uncontrolled (7,12,13,40,42,45,46). In those trials either the conversion from a positive to a negative response to HUT or the lack of recurrences during follow-up have been taken as evidence of efficacy of the admininistered therapy. Accordingly, all these studies have concluded that most of the tested drugs were effective in treating patients with VVS. However, the few controlled trials that have been published up

to now (17,20,39,43) have shown a high rate of negative responses to repeated HUT and a low rate of recurrences in the follow-up with placebo, and no beneficial effect of any tested drug when compared with placebo has been demonstrated. Although these results do not rule out the possibility that some of these drugs can be effective in some patients with VVS, up to now there is no convincing evidence of beneficial effect with any drug in patients with VVS.

Cardiac Pacing in VVS

It has been suggested that in patients with a severe cardioinhibitory response to HUT (that is, the type 2A and 2B) the implantation of a pacemaker can play a role in its treatment. The aims for implanting a pacemaker in patients with VVS and a cardioinhibitory response to HUT are different (27): to reduce the recurrence rate of syncopal episodes; to decrease the severity of syncopal episodes; to prevent severe long asystolic periods; and to decrease the possibility of sudden death secondary to severe cardioinhibitory response (55).

None of these possible benefits of pacing in patients with VVS has been convincingly demonstrated. The role of pacing either to prevent syncopal recurrences or to decrease its clinical severity has been assessed by many authors. Most of them have performed repeated HUT with pacemakers. It has been clearly shown that the use of ventricular pacing was ineffective in preventing a vasovagal response (21,25,56). Many authors have used dual-chamber pacemakers to prevent a syncopal response to HUT, with discordant results (22-26,47). Some have reported that the rate of positive responses to HUT was similar with dual-chamber pacemakers; however, the time interval from the beginning of symptoms to the occurrence of syncope was longer and the pattern of clinical presentation was diferent, changing from a sudden episode to a more progressive and less severe syncope (22). This would prevent injury as a consequence of sudden syncope. These results have not been confirmed by other authors, including our group (24,26), and even some have suggested that those patients can be treated with drug therapy (24). In any case, no one of those trials with pacemakers have been controlled, and thus, no definitive conclusion can be drawn. Some authors have suggested that VVS with a severe cardioinhibitory response can be associated with cardiac arrest in selected patients (55). In patients who have experienced a severe loss of consciousness and in whom cardiopulmonary resuscitation has been performed, a HUT conducted later showed a positive response. Accordingly, the authors have proposed that in some patients with a severe cardioinhibitory response to HUT a pacemaker should be implanted to prevent sudden death. In spite of the fact that the possibility that some patients with VVS might be at risk of cardiac arrest cannot be ruled out, up to now there has not been any clear evidence to support this contention. Additionally, some of those patients who "recovered" from severe episodes of cardiac arrest had a positive HUT without cardoinihibitory response, and therefore no clear markers of patients at risk of cardiac arrest have been identified. Brignole et al. (49) have shown that an asystolic response to HUT has no prognostic significance in the follow-up, neither for recurrences nor for the possible occurrence of cardiac arrest. So, the indication to implant a pacemaker to prevent sudden death in patients with VVS remains to be demonstrated.

Clinical Management of Patients with VVS and an Asystole to HUT

With all the available data in hand, we will try to answer the question that has been addressed in this communication: Vasovagal syncope with asystolic pause: drugs, pacemakers, or both? Indeed, the question should be "vasovagal syncope with asystolic pause: drugs, pacemakers, both or neither?" In fact, some studies have suggested that the recurrence of VVS is low (17,41,47). These data suggest that in most patients with a previous history of recurrent VVS, VVS will not recur after a complete diagnostic evaluation for SUO, including HUT, suggesting that HUT may play a role in reducing recurrences. In fact, the controlled studies that have been performed using HUT, have shown that in up to 50% of patients the test becomes negative with placebo (17,39), and that at clinical follow-up, 80% are free of recurrences, also with placebo (41,43). This suggests that mechanisms other than pharmacological effect may be responsible for the apparent remission of syncope.

As the prognosis of patients with VVS is good and there are not enough data to consider treatment for avoiding sudden death, the decision to treat patients with VVS is mainly for symptoms, to prevent recurrences. With all the available data, the use of HUT to monitor the effect of therapy is of limited value in individual patients; thus the selection of any treatment for patients with VVS is largely empirical. The natural history of syncope is not well defined, but it is well recognized that in some patients there are periods of clustered episodes followed by periods of remission that can be spontaneous or apparently induced by medical interventions. Thus, before initiating any treatment after complete diagnostic evaluation, even in patients with a recurrent history of syncope and an asystolic response to HUT, a period of follow-up without therapy can be recommended to evaluate the possibility of "spontaneous" remission of syncope.

Treatment can be recommended in those patients with asystolic response to HUT and recurrent episodes of VVS in the subsequent follow-up. Due to the lack of definite evidence of the beneficial effect of pacing in those patients, the initial treatment should be drug therapy. ß-Blockers are theoretically recommended to counteract hypersympathetic activity that triggers vasovagal response, thus helping to prevent it. In spite of that, the safety of ß-blockers in patients with VVS and severe cardioinhibitory response has not been fully demonstrated. The suggestion has been made that ß-blockers may facilitate the conversion of a pure vasodepressor response to a cardioinhibitory one (57). In agreement with these caveats, the first selected drug in patients with VVS and asystolic pause can be either of drugs, as proposed by different authors, such as etilefrine, fludrocortisone, scopolamine, or inhibitors of serotonin re-uptake. Due to the lack of criteria for using a specific drug in different groups of patients, the selection is empirical and must be made according to personal experience. The only valid parameter to assess the efficacy of the treatment is the presence of recurrences or the change in the severity of episodes. If in spite of drug therapy there are recurrences of syncope, cardiac pacing with a dual-chamber pacemaker can be considered. Before implanting a pacemaker it may be useful to repeat HUT with an external dual-chamber pacemaker to assess to what extent the pacemaker can modify the clinical presentation of syncope. A pacemaker can prevent syncopal recurrences, reduce the severity of its clinical presentation, or simply allow a safe use of ß-blockers in those patients. It has been suggested that the use of rate hysteresis in the pacing algorithm whereby pacing begins at 80 bpm when the heart rate falls below 40 bpm can be beneficial (27).

All previous considerations highlight the lack of consistent data concerning therapy in patients with VVS. This is especially true for patients with asystolic pauses, because the underlying question is whether to pace or not to pace, a decision with longer-lasting consequences than any drug therapy. This emphasizes the need of well-designed, prospective, controlled trials that address these questions. Due to the low rate of recurrences and to the low rate of observed cardioinhibitory responses to HUT, only multicenter trials that recruit a large number of patients can answer this question.

Conclusions

Up to now no definite data are available about the real efficacy of any drug or cardiac pacing in patients with VVS and a positive response to HUT. Accordingly, the selection of treatment is empirical. If after HUT, patients have recurrences, drug therapy can be recommended as a first option, and if in spite of drugs there are recurrences, implantation of a pacemaker can be considered. It seems that a pacing algorithm that includes rate hysteresis can be beneficial.

References

1. Kenny RA, Ingram A, Bayliss J, Sutton R (1986) Head-up tilt: a useful test for investigating unexplained syncope. Lancet 1:1352-1354
2. Almquist A, Goldenberg IF, Milstein S et al (1989) Provocation of bradycardia and hypotension by isoproterenol and upright tilt test in patients with unexplained syncope. N Engl J Med 320: 346-351
3. Milstein S, Reyes WJ, Benditt DG (1989) Upright body tilt for evaluation of patients with recurrent, unexplained syncope. PACE 12: 117-124
4. Strasberg B, Rechavia E, Sagie A et al (1989) The head-up tilt test in patients with syncope of unknown origin. Am Heart J 118: 923-927
5. Fitzpatrick AP, Theodorakis G, Vardas P, Sutton R (1991) Methodology of head-up tilt testing in patients with unex-

plained syncope. J Am Coll Cardiol 17: 125-30
6. Sheldon R, Killam S (1992) Methodology of isoproterenol-tilt table testing in patients with syncope. J Am Coll Cardiol 19: 773-779
7. Shalev Y, Gal R, Tchou P et al (1991) Echocardiographic demonstration of decreased left ventricular dimensions and vigorous myocardial contraction during syncope induced by head-up tilt test. J Am Coll Cardiol 1991; 18: 746-751
8. Grubb BP, Gerard G, Temesy-Armos P, Roush K, Hanhn H, Elliot L (1991) Cerebral vasoconstriction during upright tilt induced syncope. PACE 1991; 14: 662 (abstr)
9. Fitzpatrick A, Williams T, Ahmed R, Lightman S, Bloom SR, Sutton R (1992) Echocardiographic and endocrine changes during vasovagal syncope induced by prolonged head-up tilt. Eur J Cardiac Pacing Electrophysiol 2: 121-128
10. Moya A, Permanyer-Miralda G, Sagristá J, Mont L, Rius T, Soler-Soler J (1993) Análisis de las respuestas a la prueba en tabla basculante en función de las características clínicas de los episodios sincopales en pacientes sin cardiopatía aparente. Rev Esp Cardiol 46: 214-219
11. Sutton R, Petersen M, Brignole M, Raviele A, Menozzi C, Giani P (1992) Proposed classification for tilt induced vasovagal syncope. Eur J Cardiac Pacing Electrophysiol 2: 12.180-183
12. Milstein S, Buetikofer J, Dunnigan A, Benditt DG, Gornik C, Reyes WJ (1990) Usefulness of disopyramide for prevention of upright tilt-induced hypotension-bradycardia. Am J Cardiol 65: 1339-13344
13. Raviele A, Gasparini G, Di Pede F, Delise P, Bonso A, Piccolo E (1990) Usefulness of head-up tilt-test in evaluating patients with syncope of unknown origin and negative electrophysiologic study. Am J Cardiol 65: 1322-1327
14. Grubb BP, Wolfe DA, Samoil D, Temesy-Armos P, Hahn H, Elliott L (1993) Usefulness of fluoxetine for prevention of resistant upright tilt induced syncope. PACE 16: 458-464
15. Sra JS, Murthy VS, Jayazery M et al (1992) Use of intravenous esmolol to predict efficacy of oral beta-adrenergic blocker therapy in patients with neurocardiogenic syncope. J Am Coll Cardiol 402-408
16. Grubb BP, Temesy-Armos P, Hann H, Elliot L (1991) Utility of upright tilt-table testing in the evaluation and management of syncope of unknown origin. Am J Med 90: 6-10
17. Morillo CA, Leitch JW, Yee R, Klein GJ (1993) A placebo controlled trial of intravenous and oral disopyramide for prevention of neurally mediated syncope induced by head-up tilt. J Am Coll Cardiol 22: 1843-1848
18. Wolfe DA, Grubb BP, Temesy-Armos PN, Samoil D, Kosinski DJ, Brewster PS (1993) Usefulness of verapamil in preventing upright tilt induced (vasovagal-mediated) hypotension and bradycardia. J Am Coll Cardiol 21: 172A (abstr)
19. Natale A, Sra J, Dhala A et al (1993) Clinical follow-up in 327 patients with positive head-up tilt: how should appropriate therapy be chosen? Circulation 88: I-398 (abstr)
20. Fitzpatrick AP, Ahmed R, Williams S, Sutton R (1991) A randomised trial of medical therapy in "malignant vasovagal syndrome" or neurally-mediated bradycardia/hypotension syndrome". Eur J Cardiac Pacing Electrophysiol 2: 99-102
21. Fitzpatrick AP, Travill CM, Vardas PE et al (1990) Recurrent symptoms after ventricular pacing in unexplained syncope. PACE 13: 619-624
22. Fitzpatrick A, Theodorakis G, Ahmed R, Williams T, Sutton R (1991) Dual chamber pacing aborts vasovagal syncope induced by head-up 600 tilt. PACE 13: 13-19
23. Grubb BP, Temesy-Armos P, Moore J, Wolfe D, Hahn H, Elliot L (1992) Head-upright tilt-table testing in evaluation and management of the malignant vasovagal syndrome. Am J Cardiol 69: 904-908
24. Sra JS, Jayazery MR, Avitalli B et al (1993) Comparison of cardiac pacing with drug therapy in the treatment of neurocardiogenic (vasovagal) syncope with bradycardia or asystole. N Engl J Med 328: 1085-1090
25. Samoil D, Grubb BP, Brewster P, Moore J, Temesy-Armos P (1993) Comparison of single and dual chamber pacing techniques in prevention of upright tilt induced vasovagal syncope. Eur J Cardiac Pacing Electrophysiol 3: 36-41
26. Moya A, Permanyer-Miralda G, Sagristà J, Mont L, Rius T, Soler-Soler J (1993) Response to dual chamber pacing in pa-

tients with syncope and positive tilt test with cardioinhibitory response. PACE 16: 936 (abstr)
27. Benditt DG, Petersen M, Lurie KG, Giubb BP, Sutton R (1995) Cardiac pacing for prevention of recurrent vasovagal syncope. Ann Intern Med 122: 204-209
28. Kramer MS (1988) Diagnostic tests. In: Kramer MS (ed) Clinical epidemiology and biostatistics. Springer, Berlin Heidelberg New York, pp 201-219
29. Brignole M, Menozzi C, Gianfranchi L, Oddine D, Lollis G, Berttulla A (1991) Neurally mediated syncope detected by carotid sinus massage and head-up tilt test in sick sinus syndrome. Am J Cardiol 68: 1032-1036
30. Kapoor WN, Brant N (1992) Evaluation of syncope by upright tilt testing with isoproterenol. A nonspecific test. Ann Intern Med 116: 356-363
31. Ambrosi P, Djiane P, Durand JM et al (1992) Intérêt et limites du test d'inclinaison dans le diagnostic étiologique des malaises brefs. Arch Mal Coeur 85: 345-350
32. Raviele A, Gasparini G, Di Pede F et al (1994) Nitroglycerin infusion during upright tilt: a new test for the diagnosis of vasovagal syncope. Am Heart J 127: 103-111
33. Kapoor WN (1990) Evaluation and outcome of patients with syncope. Medicine 69: 160-175
34. Kapoor WN, Smith MA, Miller NL (1994) Upright tilt testing in evaluating syncope. A comprehensive literature review. Am J Med 97: 78-88
35. Glick G, Yu PN (1963) Hemodynamic changes during spontaneous vasovagal reaction. Am J Med 34: 42-51
36. Abboud FM (1989) Ventricular syncope: is the heart a sensory organ? N Engl J Med 320: 390-392
37. Thames MD, Kopfenstein HS, Abboud FM, Marck AL, Walker JL (1978) Preferential distribution of inhibitory cardiac receptors with vagal afferents to the inferoposterior wall of left ventricle during coronary occlusion in the dog. Circ Res 43: 521-529
38. García Civera R, Ruíz Granell R, Cosín Aguilar J, López Merino V (1989) Síncope vasovagal. In: García Civera R, Sanjuan Mañez R, Cosín Aguilar J, López Merino V (eds). Síncope. MCR, Barcelona, pp 177-198
39. Moya A, Permanyer-Miralda G, Sagristá-Sauleda J et al (1995) Limitations of head-up tilt test for evaluating the efficacy of therapeutic interventions in patients with vasovagal syncope: results of a controlled study of etilefrine versus placebo. J Am Coll Cardiol 25: 65-69
40. Sra JS, Murthy VS, Jayazery MR et al (1992) Use of intravenous esmolol to predict efficacy of oral beta-adrenergic blocker therapy in patients with neurocardiogenic syncope. J Am Coll Cardiol. 19: 402-408
41. Fitzpatrick AP, Travill CM, Vardas PE et al (1991) A randomised trial of medical therapy in "malignant vasovagal syndrome" or neurally-mediated bradycardia/hypotension syndrome". Eur J Cardiac Pacing Electrophysiol 2:99-102
42. Blanc JJ, Corber C, Mansourati J, Genet L (1991) Evaluation du traitement betabloquant dans les syncopes vasovagals reproduits par le test d'inclinaison. Arch Mal Coeur 84: 1453-1457
43. Brignole M, Menozzi C, Gianfranchi L, Lolli G, Bottoni N, Oddone D (1992) A controlled trial of acute and long-term medical therapy in tilt-induced neurally mediated syncope. Am J Cardiol 70: 339-342
44. Milstein S, Buetikofer J, Dunningan A, Benditt DG, Gornick C, Reyes WJ (1990) Usefulness of disopyramide for prevention of upright tilt-induced hypotension-bradycardia. Am J Cardiol 65: 1339-1344
45. López Candel J, Picó Aracil F, Sánchez Muñoz JJ et al (1993) Síncope vasovagal maligno. Diagnóstico y ensayo terapéutico basado en el test del ortostatismo (test del tilt). Rev Esp Cardiol 46: 28-33
46. Grubb BP, Wolfe DA, Samoil D, Temesy-Armos P, Hahn H, Elliot L (1991) Usefulness of fluoxetine for prevention of resistant upright tilt induced syncope. PACE 90: 6-10
47. Brignole M, Menozzi C, Gianfranchi L, Bottoni N, Lolli G (1992) The clinical and prognosis significance of asystolic response during the head-up tilt test. Eur J Cardiac Pacing Electrophysiol 2: 109-113
48. Moya A, Permanyer-Miralda G, Sagristá J, Rius T, Mont L, Soler-Soler J (1993) Influencia del uso del isoproterenol en la respuesta

a la exploración en tabla basculante en pacientes con síncope de causa desconocida. Rev Esp Cardiol 46 [Suppl I]: 11 (abstr)

49. de Buitleir M, Grogan EW, Picone MF, Casteen JA (1993) Immediate reproducibility of the tilt table test in adults with unexplained syncope. Am J Cardiol 71: 304-307

50. Chen XC, Chen MY, Remole S et al (1992) Reproducibility of head up tilt-table testing for eliciting susceptibility to neurally mediated syncope in patients without structural heart disease. Am J Cardiol 69: 755-760

51. Brooks R, Ruskin JN, Powell AC, Newell J, Garan H, McGovern BA (1993) Prospective evaluation of day-to-day reproducibility of upright tilt-table testing in unexplained syncope. Am J Cardiol 71: 1289-1292

52. Grubb BP, Wolfe D, Temesy-Armos P, Hahn H, Elliot L (1992) Reproducibility of head-up tilt table test results in patients with syncope. PACE 15: 1477-1481

53. Sheldon R, Splawinski J, Killiam S (1992) Reproducibility of isoproterenol tilt-table tests in patients with syncope. Am J Cardiol 69: 1300-1305

54. Fish FA, Strasburger JF, Benson DW (1992) Reproducibility of a symptomatic response to upright tilt in young patients with unexplained syncope. Am J Cardiol 70: 605-609

55. Milstein S, Buetikofer J, Lesser J et al (1991) Cardiac asystole: a manifestation of neurally mediated hypotension-bradycardia. J Am Coll Cardiol 14: 1622-1632

56. Rius T, Moya A, Sagristá J, Permanyer-Miralda G, Mont L, Soler-Soler J (1993) Valor de la prueba en tabla basculante en pacientes portadores de marcapasos VVI con síncopes recidivantes. Rev Esp Cardiol 46 [Suppl I]: 11 (abastract)

57. Dangovian MI, Jarandilla R, Frumin H (1992) Prolonged asystole during head-up tilt table testing after beta-blockade. PACE 15: 14-16

Invasive Tilt Testing:
The Search for a New Sensor To Permit Earlier Pacing Therapy in Vasovagal Syncope

R. Sutton and M.E.V. Petersen

Cardiology Departments, Royal Brompton and Chelsea and Westminster Hospitals,
London, United Kingdom

Introduction

Vasovagal syncope is the most common form of syncope. Few patients require any therapy but a small minority present with major symptoms which include complications of syncope, such as incontinence of urine and epileptiform seizures and, when studied, they show an important element of cardioinhibition. Older patients with this severe type, which has been called malignant vasovagal syncope (1) may experience little or no warning of the impending attack and, as a result, may be unable to avoid falling and receiving injuries. This group represents approximately 3% of patients for whom pacing is indicated (2).

The results of treatment are encouraging but 38% continue to experience some symptoms ranging from dizziness to delay in the onset of syncope permitting avoidance of injury. The mode of pacing chosen has been DDI with rate hysteresis typically programmed to a trigger rate of 45 and a pacing rate of 85 ppm (2). Thus, the application of the therapy depends on severe bradycardia at a time when the evolution of the attack may be too advanced for pacing to abort it. Higher trigger rates precipitate false introduction of pacing for bradycardias of rest and sleep. These episodes are often symptomatic and have to be circumvented by choice of a low trigger rate. Pacing, using the VDD mode, at the beginning of a tilt test has been shown to be ineffective in prevention of tilt-induced syncope in a group of patients rendered asymptomatic over a period of more than 3 years by the type of hysteresis pacing described above (3). These findings, however, should not be taken to imply that earlier pacing interventions during the evolution of an attack will also be ineffective. It is possible that intervention with a rapid rate pacing at a crucial, but as yet undefined moment of the development of a vasovagal attack could have such a dramatic effect on the neuroendocrine system so as to achieve reversal.

Vigorous left ventricular contraction has been reported in the early phase of vasovagal syncope, and it has been assumed that this reflects the high levels of circulating adrenaline which have been found (4, 5).

These phenomena might be expected to be associated with elevation of both left and right ventricular pressure rise times (dp/dt). Pacemaker technology has already been developed for use of right ventricular dp/dt as a sensor for rate modulation (6) using an endocardial catheter-based micromanometer. Investigations were therefore planned to monitor this parameter in tilt-induced vasovagal syncope.

Patients and Methods

Ten patients were studied during invasive tilt testing. The protocol, approved by the Hospital Ethical Committee, involved monitoring heart rate and arterial pressure (FINAPRES) non-invasively together with a right ventricular micromanometer catheter and temporary dual-chamber pacing. The patients underwent insertion of the necessary venous access and were then allowed to rest for at least 1 h before a series of tilts was performed, one without pacing and three with pacing, separately using DDI with standard 45-to 85-ppm hysteresis (actually DVI mode because this was readily available in the external pacing device used), DDI pacing triggered by Medtronic's rate drop response algorithm (7) in the first five patients and DDI at 100 ppm from the onset of upright tilt in the second group of five patients, and DDI with manually triggered hysteresis pacing at 120 ppm. In this latter mode of pacing, the triggering of the rapid pacing was prompted by the onset of symptoms combined with early blood pressure fall. Throughout all these tilt tests, right ventricular dp/dt was recorded.

All ten patients presented with severe symptoms and gave informed consent for the tilt test series. There were six women and four men, and the age range was 31-60 years.

Results

Syncope or severely symptomatic presyncope occurred in 35 of the 40 tilts performed with a reproducible pattern of haemodynamic collapse, but a variable time from tilt upward to onset of symptoms. DDI with standard rate hysteresis was effective in sufficiently ameliorating symptoms to permit a prodrome and an ability to abort an attack in two patients. Permanent pacing systems have subsequently been implanted in them. In the five tested with the rate drop response algorithm, amelioration of symptoms was demonstrated in all, and one received a permanent pacemaker, being one of the two previously mentioned. The manually triggered hysteresis with a rapid pacing rate was additionally effective in two other patients. These patients have not yet had pacemakers implanted, as an adequate trigger for this rapid pacing has not yet been identified.

Right ventricular dp/dt behaviour was found to be variable from one patient to another, there being no consistent finding of elevation in the early phase of onset of vasovagal syncope as had been expected from previous work. Combinations of right ventricular dp/dt maximum and minimum with heart rate and pressure in the right ventricle failed to yield any reliable pattern of change that could be utilised as a sensor to permit early pacing intervention in vasovagal syncope.

Discussion

From these studies of a highly symptomatic group of patients, we have shown that advanced pacing algorithms for the treatment of vasovagal syncope may have some value, but in such patients the standard DDI rate hysteresis system has limited applicability. The design of advanced algorithms depends on two major factors: determination of the ideal time of pacing intervention, which in turn depends on perfect sensor information and, secondly, the possibility, by programmability, of selecting a high interventional pacing rate. This latter facility now exists with the Medtronic rate drop reponse algorithm.

Evaluation of right ventricular dp/dt changes although promising has proved to be disappointing. This small experience has not shown any definite trend toward a dramatic rise in right ventricular dp/dt maximum as was expected from the adrenaline release data (4,5). It is likely, therefore, that this parameter will not fulfil the need for a specific haemodynamic change that can be sensed for this indication.

In contrast, we have found that, were a satisfactory parameter for sensing to be identified, the ability of pacemakers to combat the severe symptoms of an important minority of vasovagal syncope patients would be significantly increased. Additionally, we have shown that serial tilt testing is more reproducible in a group of very symptomatic patients than in those less symptomatic (8-10) and the pattern of haemodynamic collapse in these patients is quite consistent. However, the time from commencement of tilt to onset of syncope is variable. Finally, we have again shown in this study, as was the conclusion of the re-tilt study of asymptomatic paced vasovagal patients (3), that "premedication" by a form of dual-chamber pacing, in this case DDI or DVI, prior to the onset of vasovagal syncope is not only ineffective but cannot be the mechanism of benefit in those who have done well after pacemaker implantation for this indication.

Conclusions

The following conclusions may be drawn:

1. Right ventricular dp/dt is unlikely to prove to be an ideal sensed parameter for the introduction of dual-chamber pacing to combat vasovagal syncope.

2. If a suitable parameter can be identified, the benefits of pacing intervention in an evolving vasovagal attack may be expected to be enhanced, especially as the facility for programmable high pacing rates is now available.

3. Serial tilt testing in very symptomatic patients is associated with greater reproducibility than can be expected in a more heterogeneous group of vasovagal patients.

4. Continuous dual-chamber pacing is not the mechanism of benefit in patients with vasovagal syncope, and it is likely that critically timed pacing intervention is needed for its realisation.

References

1. Sutton R (1992) Vasovagal syndrome – could it be malignant? Eur J Cardiac Pacing Electrophysiol 2: 89
2. Petersen MEV, Chamberlain-Webber R, Fitzpatrick AP, Ingram A, Williams T, Sutton R (1994) Permanent pacing for cardioinhibitory malignant vasovagal syndrome. Br Heart J 71:274-281
3. Petersen MEV, Price D, Williams T et al (1994) Short AV delay VDD pacing does not prevent vasovagal syncope in patients with cardioinhibitory vasovagal syndrome. PACE 17: 882-891
4. Fitzpatrick A, Williams T, Ahmed R, Lightman S, Bloom SR, Sutton R (1992) Echocardiographic and endocrine changes during vasovagal syncope induced by prolonged head-up tilt. Eur J Cardiac Pacing Electrophysiol 2: 121-128
5. Sander-Jensen K, Secher NH, Astrup A et al (1986) Hypotension induced by passive head-up tilt: endocrine and circulatory mechanisms. Am J Physiol 251: R743-R749
6. Heynen H, Sharma A, Sutton R, Camm AJ, Ovsyshcher I, Naslund U, Gillis AM, Clarke M, Ruiter J, Brachmann J, Schallhorn R, Bennett T (1991) Clinical experience with VVIR pacing based on right ventricular dp/dt. Eur J Cardiac Pacing Electrophysiol 1: 138-146
7. Petersen M, Hess M, Markowitz T, Jensen N, Biallas R, van Bergen R, Sutton R (1995) Acute human investigation of an algorithm to treat vasovagal syncope using a computer based simulator. PACE 18: 825 (abstr)
8. Petersen M, Fitzpatrick A, Chamberlain-Webber R, Sutton R (1992) A clinical experience of the Westminster tilt test protocol. Eur J Card Pacing Electrophysiol 2 [Suppl 1A]: A135 (abstr)
9. Sheldon R, Splawinski J, Killam S (1992) Reproducibility of isoproterenol tilt-table tests in patients with syncope. Am J Cardiol 69: 1300-1305
10. Grubb BP, Wolfe DA, Temesy-Armos PN et al (1992) Reproducibility of head-upright tilt test results in patients with syncope. PACE 15: 1477-1481

CARDIAC PACING

Isolated First-Degree Atrioventricular Block: A New Indication for Dual-Chamber Pacing?

R. Cazzin, P. Golia, C. Bonanno, C. Lestuzzi, and V. Proietti

Servizio di Cardiologia, Ospedale di Portogruaro,
Portogruaro-Venice, Italy

Introduction

Since the importance of the atrioventricular (AV) interval in cardiac hemodynamics has been realized, first-degree atrioventricular AV block has been considered as one of the possible indications for permanent cardiac pacing.

Some authors (1,2) reported that patients (pts) with markedly prolonged PQ interval may complain of severe symptoms because of the hemodynamic impairment due to AV block. In these pts the application of a dual-chamber pacemaker with shorter AV delay induced an evident functional improvement.

The optimization of the AV interval can improve cardiac performance and may be particularly effective in some cardiac diseases, as recently reported in hypertrophic and dilated cardiomyopathy (3,4).

Optimal AV Interval

The assessment of the AV interval in cardiac pacing was introduced by Haskell (5), who demonstrated by echo-Doppler that the optimal hemodynamic result was obtained with a 150-ms AV delay. More recently, Ovsyshcher (6) evaluated cardiac output at different pacing rates, using impedance cardiography. In his study the best cardiac output was obtained with a mean AV delay of 120 ms.

The hemodynamic response to DDD pacing may vary whether the atrium is sensed or paced, and whether it is followed by a sensed or paced ventricle. Moreover, during right atrial and ventricular stimulation there are variable interventricular conduction delays, but the interval between right and left atrium activation is more prolonged and may vary from 30 to 100 ms (7,8). From the hemodynamic point of view, the more important aspect is to obtain the best synchronization between the left cardiac chambers.

Modern dual-chamber pacemakers can automatically vary the AV interval when ventricular pacing follows a sensed rather than a paced atrial activity or also reduce the AV interval proportionally to the increase in pacing rate (rate-adaptive AV delay), according to the physiologic behavior of the PR interval during heart rate variation.

Optimal AV Delay Versus Intrinsic Conduction

Ventricular activation through the normal His-Purkinje system differs from apical ventricular pacing; this difference can lead to significant hemodynamic changes. This problem may be relevant in pts with sick sinus syndrome and normal or slightly delayed AV conduction but mainly in those with first-degree and/or intermittent second-degree, LW type, AV block. In these particular pts it is possible to program the AV interval long enough to avoid ventricular stimulation, but this choice is not always hemodynamically advantageous.

When is ventricular stimulation with optimal AV interval preferable to normal ventricular activation with a long PR interval? Data in the literature are conflicting.

According to Mabo (1), a very long PR interval may facilitate a hemodynamic impairment mainly during physical activity. In five pts with a mean AV interval of 410 ms, without any shortening during effort, DDD pacing improved exercise duration by 72% and cardiac output by 19%.

Rosenqvist (9) studied by echo-Doppler and ventricular scintigraphy the systolic and the diastolic function of 12 pts during AAI, DDD, and VVI pacing. The mean AV interval was 248 ms during AAI and 140 ms during DDD pacing. The best output and ejection fraction were obtained with AAI rather than with DDD and VVI pacing. In this study no attempt was made to evaluate the optimal AV delay in dual-chamber pacing.

Jutzy (10) achieved similar results in the evaluation of nine pts by AAI pacing with a mean AV interval of 245 ms and DDD pacing with individual optimal AV delay and obtained the best cardiac output (+13%) during dual-chamber pacing. According to these results, in pts with first-degree AV block DDD pacing at rest leads to better hemodynamic performance than at normal cardiac activation, mainly in those pts with a PR interval > 220 ms

By and large, sequential AV pacing may improve the hemodynamic performance in pts with first-degree AV block. When the PR interval is particularly prolonged with no shortening during effort tachycardia, symptoms are usually present, even in the absence of heart disease. The greatest advantage of AV interval shortening is probably obtained in heart diseases with preponderant compliance impairment.

Crepaz (11), testing the hemodynamic response at various AV intervals in pts without organic heart disease, found little change in cardiac output. In contrast, in pts with left ventricular hypertrophy the optimal AV interval was identified at 150 ms.

Modena (12), in a study in seven pts with left ventricular hypertrophy and an abnormal left ventricular filling pattern, demonstrated that sequential pacing with an AV delay of 100 ms led to the normalization of the filling pattern and to the recovery of diastolic function.

Recently, a new way of pacing the right ventricle has been proposed. Instead of being placed at the ventricular apex, the tip of the catheter is fixed near to the pulmonary outflow tract. In this way it is possible to avoid or reduce the hemodynamic effects of altered contractility owing to right ventricular apex pacing (13).

Karpavich (14) evaluated the hemodynamic parameters in 17 pts with normal left ventricular function during sinus rhythm, AAI atrial pacing, and apical and septal ventricular stimulation. The hemodynamic data obtained during septal pacing are similar to those obtained during sinus rhythm and atrial pacing and significantly better than those at apical pacing. This noteworthy innovation seems to be mostly indicated in pts undergoing dual-chamber pacing when intraventricular conduction is normal.

First-Degree AV Block: Indication for Pacing

A delayed atrial emptying into the ventricle due to a functional obstacle, as occurs in hypertrophic or hypokinetic-dilated cardiomyopathy, leads to a prolongation of the pulmonary veins emptying time and atrial filling time. In pts with first-degree AV block, the longer the PR interval (and the shorter the RR interval), the earlier atrial systole is within diastole. In this setting atrial systole occurs before atrial filling is completed. As a result, the atrial systole contribution to ventricular filling is reduced and cardiac output is reduced as well. When the PR interval is extremely prolonged, atrial systole may occur when the mitral valve is still partially or completely closed. This leads to an increase in pulmonary venous pressure. Some authors (1,15) reported that cardiac output can be reduced at PR intervals longer than 300 ms even in pts without organic heart disease if the PR interval does not shorten with heart rate increase.

The first indication for permanent cardiac pacing is when pts with first-degree AV block complain of effort dyspnea or fatigue. Effort symptoms are often un-

derestimated by pts, who spontaneously reduce their physical activity as long as the functional impairment worsens. Pts with prolonged first-degree AV block should be evaluated with functional tests in order to assess exercise tolerance and PR interval behavior during heart rate increase.

Dual-chamber pacing can be recommended with the ventricular lead placed at the septal site in pts with an abnormal response to these tests, when the intraventricular conduction pattern is normal. In our preliminary experience with septal pacing in pts with first-degree AV block, echo-Doppler data are significantly better, as regards systodiastolic function, than those for apical pacing.

The presence of first-degree AV block in pts with heart failure and hypertrophic or dilated cardiomyopathy may be considered an indication for permanent dual-chamber pacing. In these cases the RR interval shortening due to heart failure-induced tachycardia makes the relationship between filling time and atrial contraction (both occurring in early diastole) extremely critical (16). If atrial systole is shifted to telediastole through AV interval shortening by dual-chamber pacing, more complete atrial filling and an increased atrial contribution to ventricular filling are possible. When mitral and/or tricuspidal regurgitation are present, the ventricular filling time is even shorter, mainly because of a long AV delay.

In some cases of severe cardiac failure, diastolic mitral regurgitation has been detected (17,18). Sequential pacing with a short AV delay (100 ms) reduces the diastolic regurgitation time. This is one of the possible mechanisms that can explain the improvement reported by Brecker and Hochleitner (3,19).

The improvement of diastolic function obtained by AV interval shortening led to hemodynamic improvement also in pts with nonobstructive hypertrophic cardiomyopathy (20,21). In the cases reported by Cannon (4), functional and symptomatic improvement was demonstrated by the increase of exercise time and the reduction of wedge pressure and effort ischemia.

Several studies in the literature (19-22) have been published with data suggesting favorable results of pacing therapy in cardiac failure due to various heart diseases, mostly as regards the improvement in quality of life. In presence of first-degree AV block, cardiac pacing is indicated when diastolic function assessment suggests normal atrial contractility, abnormal atrial and ventricular filling patterns, and abnormal timing within diastole of atrial and ventricular filling.

Conclusions

The observations on the relationship between prolonged AV interval in first-degree AV block and atrial and ventricular systole synchronization clearly show a relevant hemodynamic correlation within diastolic timing. In symptomatic pts with first-degree AV block, regardless of the presence of organic heart disease, sequential AV pacing is indicated and induces marked hemodynamic benefits, leading to an improvement in symptoms, hemodynamic balance, and quality of life.

References

1. Mabo P, Cazeau S, Forrer A, Varin C, De Place C, Paillard F, Daubert C (1992) Permanent DDD pacing for very long PR interval alone. PACE 15:509
2. Brinker JA (1989) Pursuing the perfect pacemaker. Mayo Clin Proc 64: 587
3. Hochleitner M, Hortnagl H, Hortnagl H, Fridrich L, Gschnitzer F (1992) Long-term efficacy of physiologic dual-chamber pacing in the treatment of end-stage idiopathic dilated cardiomyopathy. Am J Cardiol 70:1318-1325
4. Cannon RO III, Dilsiziam V, Bonow RO et al (1992) Symptom, hemodynamic and myocardial benefit of atrial synchronized ventricular pacing in non-obstructive hypertrophic cardiomyopathy. J Am Coll Cardiol 19: 120
5. Haskell RJ, French WJ (1986) Optimum AV interval in dual chamber pacemakers PACE 9:670-675
6. Ovsyshcher I, Zimlichman R, Katz A, Bondy C, Ferman S (1993) Measurements of cardiac output by impedance cardiography in pacemaker patients at rest: effects of various atrioventricular delays. J Am Coll Cardiol 21:761-767
7. Janosik DL, Pearson AC, Buckingham TA, Labovitz AJ, Redd RM (1989) The hemodynamic benefit of differential atrioventricular delay intervals for sensed and paced atrial events during physiologic pacing. J Am Coll Cardiol 14:499-507
8. Camous JP, Raybaud F, Dolisi C, Schenowitz A, Varenne A, Baudouy MA (1993) Interatrial conduction in patients undergoing AV stimulation: effects of increasing right atrial stimulation rate. PACE 16:2082-2086
9. Rosenqvist M, Isaaz K, Botvinik EH, Dae MW, Cockrell J, Abbott JA, Shiller NB, Griffin JC (1991) Relative importance of activation sequence compared to atrioventricular synchrony in left ventricular function. Am J Cardiol 67:148-156
10. Jutzy RV, Feenstra L, Pai R, Florio J, Bansal R, Aybar R, Levine PA ((1992) Comparison of intrinsic versus paced ventricular function. PACE 15:1919-1922
11. Crepaz R, Pitsheider W, Zammarchi A, Erlicher A, Mautone A, Braito E (1991) Role of echo-doppler in programming of sequential pacemakers. Evaluation of optimal atrioventricular delay in patients with normal or hypertrophic left ventricle. G Ital Cardiol 21:975-982
12. Modena MG, Rossi R, Mattiolo AV, Carcagni A, Mattioli G (1995) Short A-V delay interval improves filling in DDD pacing of patients with left ventricular hypertrophy and normal ejection fraction. J Am Coll Cardiol [Special issue]:152A
13. Cowell R, Paul V, Morris-Thurgood J, Ilsley C (1994) Septal short AV delay pacing: additional haemodynamic improvements in heart failure, Eur J Cardiac Pacing Electrophysiol 4:258
14. Karpawich PP, Seema M (1995) Septal pacing improves single chamber-paced left ventricular function: a comparative evaluation with atrial and apical pacing. J Am Coll Cardiol [Special issue] 151A
15. Mehta D, Gilmors S, Ward D et al (1989) Optimal atrioventricular delay at rest and during exercise with dual chamber pacemaker: a noninvasive assessment by continuous wave Doppler. Br Heart J 61:161-166
16. Antonini L, Montefoschi N, Greco S, Santini M (1994) Is prolonged 1st° AV block an indication for physiologic pacing? In: Santini M (ed) Progress in clinical pacing. Futura media services, Inc, Armonk, NY, pp 449-463
17. Ishikawa T, Kimura K, Miyazaki N, Tochikubo O, Usui T, Kashiwagi M, Ishii M (1992) Diastolic mitral regurgitation in patients with first-degree atrioventricular block. PACE 15:1927-1931
18. Ishikawa T, Kimura K, Nihei T, Usui T, Kashiwagi M, Ishii M (1991) Relationship between diastolic mitral regurgitation and PQ intervals or cardiac function in patients implanted with DDD pacemakers. PACE 14:1797-1802
19. Brecker SJD, Xiao H, Sparrow J, Gibson DG (1992) Effects of dual-chamber pacing with short atrioventricular delay in dilated cardiomyopathy. Lancet 342:1308-1312
20. Seidelin PH, Jones GA, Boon NA (1992) Effects of dual-chamber pacing in hypertrophic cardiomyopathy without obstruction. Lancet 340:369-373
21. Hochleitner M, Hortnagl H, Ng CK, Hortnagl H, Gsthnitzer F, Zechmann W (1990) Usefulness of physiologic dual-chamber pacing in drug-resistant idiopathic dilated cardiomyopathy. Am J Cardiol 66:198-202
22. Kataoka H (1991) Hemodynamic effect of dual chamber pacing in a patient with end-stage dilated cardiomyopathy: a case report. PACE 14: 1330-1333

Physiologic Dual-Chamber Pacing with Short Atrioventricular Delay in Dilated Cardiomyopathy: Which Hemodynamic Effects and Clinical Results?

S. Romano, M. Pagani, T. Forzani, P. Montanari, and G. Seveso

Divisione di Cardiologia, U.S.S.L. n. 34, Legnano (MI), Italy

Introduction

Congestive heart failure is one of the leading causes of morbidity and mortality in the western world. Therapy has been directed toward lowering preload, reducing afterload, improving contractility, and interfering with the detrimental neurohumoral mechanism activated in heart failure. Despite considerable improvement in the pharmacologic treatment of severe left ventricular dysfunction, the problem of treating drug-resistant, end-stage heart failure remains. In 1990 Hochleitner (1) introduced the use of physiologic dual-chamber (DDD) pacing with a shortened atrioventricular (AV) delay as an alternative, new approach in the treatment of patients with dilated cardiomyopathy and severe heart failure unresponsive to optimal medical therapy. The author demonstrated that left ventricular function and clinical symptoms improved considerably after stimulation. These results have been only partially confirmed (2-4), probably because they were derived from observational studies in a small, nonhomogeneous group of patients. The beneficial effects of this "electrical" therapy were explained by different hemodynamic mechanisms. Some authors considered the reduction of ventriculoatrial regurgitation obtained by shortening of AV delay to be the determining factor; others pointed out the modification of preload or the optimization of mechanical AV synchrony.

We have analyzed the main published studies, focusing our attention on the most important hemodynamic effects and clinical results obtained by DDD pacing with short AV delay in patients with severe heart failure.

Revision of literature

In 1990 Hochleitner studied a group of 16 critically ill patients with chronic heart failure due to idiopathic dilated cardiomyopathy. Drug therapy had ceased to maintain adequate cardiac function in each. Physiologic dual-chamber pacemakers were implanted, the programmed AV interval was 100 ms and the minimal and maximal rate were, respectively, 50 and 150 beats/min so that all patients had a ventricular paced rhythm guided by spontaneous sinus beats. During pacing cardiac function improved considerably. The characteristic clinical symptoms such as severe dyspnea at rest and pulmonary edema almost disappeared. The author observed a considerable increase in left ventricular ejection fraction and a significant decrease in New York Heart Association (NYHA) functional class evaluated 1 week before and 14 days after pacemaker implantation. During pacing, heart rate normalized and, in addition, systolic blood pressure increased significantly. The cardiothoracic ratio decreased from 0.60 ± 0.06 to 0.56 ± 0.05 ($p < 0.001$) and echocardiographic dimensions of both systolic and diastolic diameter decreased as well, from 62 ± 10 to 60 ± 10 mm ($p < 0.05$) and from 74 ± 11 to 72 ± 10 mm ($p < 0.05$), respectively. In contrast, no changes in fractional shortening were observed. Doppler color flow imaging performed in six patients demonstrated that mitral regurgitation was reduced during pacing. Hochleitner concluded that the improvement in symptoms observed was mainly due to a decrease in AV conduction delay (set by the pacer at 100 ms), which decreased mitral regurgitation and also preserved atrial systole, but this is only a speculative opinion because, in her study, there are no quantitative data of the degree of mitral and tricuspid regurgitation and there are no data on the importance of atrial contribution to left ventricular filling. A study by Brecker (5) 2 years later appeared in which mitral and tricuspid regurgitation and ventricular filling time during DDD pacing with shortened AV delay were evaluated. The author measured ventricular filling time and cardiac output with Doppler echocardiography and exercise capacity on a treadmill at baseline and with the best AV delay during pacing. Brecker evaluated 12 patients with dilated cardiomyopathy selected on the basis of Doppler echocardiography characteristics as having left ventricular or right ventricular filling time below 200 ms due to functional mitral or tricuspid regurgitation. Among the whole group of 12 patients, both mitral and tricuspid regurgitation times were shorter at the shorter AV interval; consequently, both left ventricular and right ventricular filling times were longer [mitral regurgitation time (MRT) at baseline AV interval: mean 420 ± 60 ms, MRT at the shortest AV interval: mean 335 ± 40 ms, $p < 0.001$; left ventricular filling time at baseline AV interval: mean 185 ± 90 ms; left ventricular filling time at the shortest AV interval: mean 225 ± 65 ms, $p < 0.001$). At the short AV interval, cardiac output was significantly greater than at baseline. The improvements in ventricular filling characteristics were associated with striking changes in exercise duration, maximum oxygen consumption, and perceived degree of breathlessness at peak exercise; there was a change in the nature of the symptom that limited exercise, from breathlessness to leg fatigue.

Brecker reported that it is possible to identify a subset of patients with severe ventricular disease in whom very short left ventricular and right ventricular filling times may limit stroke volume and who may benefit from short AV delay DDD pacing. According to the author if a short filling time on the right or left side of the heart, or both, is imposed on a severely diseased ventricle by extended functional AV regurgitation, correction of the abnormality might improve exercise tolerance. In all patients of this study, Brecker was able to eliminate the presystolic component as well as shortening the regurgitation itself with a short AV delay. In some cases, the time available for forward flow doubled and there were striking increases in stroke volume and cardiac output. Brecker concluded that the identification of individuals likely to benefit from this approach is important. Suitable patients have sinus tachycardia, jugular venous "A" wave, summation gallop, and functional mitral or tricuspid regurgitation. A long PR interval, presystolic regurgitation, and a single right or left ventricular filling pattern on Doppler echocardiography confirms suitability.

Recently, Nishimura (4) presented the results of an acute hemodynamic study in patients with acute, severe heart failure undergoing temporary DDD pacing at different AV intervals to determine: (a) the mechanisms by which DDD pacing may improve hemodynamic variables in such patients, and (b) whether all patients with severe left ventricular systolic dysfunction improve. The author measured left atrial pressure and the left ventricular pressure by transeptal cardiac catheterization, using a thermodilution balloon-tipped catheter to measure the cardiac output and the pulmonary artery pressure and a pigtail catheter placed in the ascending aorta to measure the systemic pressures. Continuous wave Doppler measurement of the mitral regurgitation signal was performed to determine the presence or absence of diastolic mitral regurgitation. Nishimura did not find any significant change in the mean left atrial pressure or cardiac output between the baseline state and AV sequential pacing at the shortest AV interval of 60 ms. He found a significant increase in the time constant of relaxation (tau) when the baseline state was compared with DDD pacing at an AV interval of 60 ms (64 ± 17 vs 73 ± 19 ms, $p<0.01$). The variables were then examined at the various AV intervals (60,100,120,140,180, and 240 ms) and no significant differences in mean left atrial pressure were found. There was a consistent increase in tau in all pacing modes compared with that at the baseline state. There was no significant difference in average cardiac output between the baseline state and the DDD pacing modes. However, the author found a wide variation in the cardiac output; some patients had a decrease and others an increase in this variable at different AV intervals. The patients were retrospectively classified into two groups on the basis of baseline PR interval (group 1, PR > 200 ms; group 2, PR < 200 ms). The optimal AV pacing interval in group 1 was selected as the interval when the increase in left ventricular pressure from left ventricular contraction began, after the peak of the increase in left ventricular pressure from atrial contraction but before atrial relaxation was complete. AV sequential pacing at this optimal AV interval lengthened the diastolic filling period. The optimal AV interval was 60 ms in one patient, 100 ms in three, 120 ms in two, and 180 ms in one. Pacing at the optimal AV interval produced a significant increase in left ventricular pressure just before ventricular contraction. Diastolic mitral regurgitation, present in the baseline state in five patients, was abolished and mean cardiac output was significantly increased during the optimal AV delay sequential pacing. Nishimura, in contrast to Brecker, found that pacing at too short an AV interval resulted in a decrease in cardiac output in the five group 1 patients. In group 2, there was no change from the baseline state in cardiac output at the different AV intervals of > 60 ms. For the AV interval of 60 ms, cardiac output decreased significantly (from 4.2 ± 1.8 to 3.4 ± 1.3 l/min, $p<0.01$) compared with the baseline state. There was no change in the diastolic filling period between the baseline state and any of the pacing states. Nishimura was the first to combine catheterization and Doppler methods to investigate the physiologic mechanisms by which DDD pacing may improve hemodynamic variables and to attempt to identify patients who would potentially receive the greatest benefit. According to the author, DDD pacing may improve hemodynamic variables in selected patients with dilated cardiomyopathy who have a prolonged PR interval, mainly by optimizing the timing of mechanical atrial and ventricular synchrony; the AV interval required to achieve this optimal AV synchrony varies from patient to patient and no universal AV interval can be used for all patients who receive a DDD pacemaker for hemodynamic purposes. Patients in whom there is already optimally timed mechanical atrial and ventricular synchrony may not benefit from sequential pacing; on the contrary, they may even experience hemodynamic deterioration.

Our experience

In our 2-year observational study, we had different conclusions than Nishimura. We implanted in 12 critically ill patients with end-stage heart failure a DDD pacemaker programmed as reported by Hochleitner (AV interval: 100 ms; lower rate: 50 beats/min; upper rate 150 beats/min). In our study group the mean PR baseline interval was 200 ms, and five patients (41%) had a PR interval ≤ 200 ms. In spite of this we observed during pacing a significant decrease in NYHA

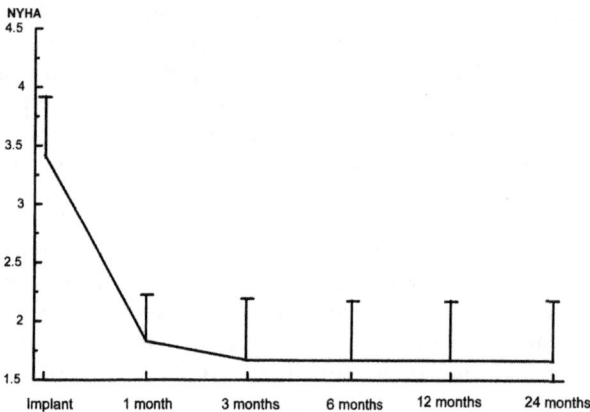

Fig. 1. Effect of 2-year electrophysiologic dual-camber pacing on New York Heart Association (NYHA) class in six surviving patients with end-stage heart failure

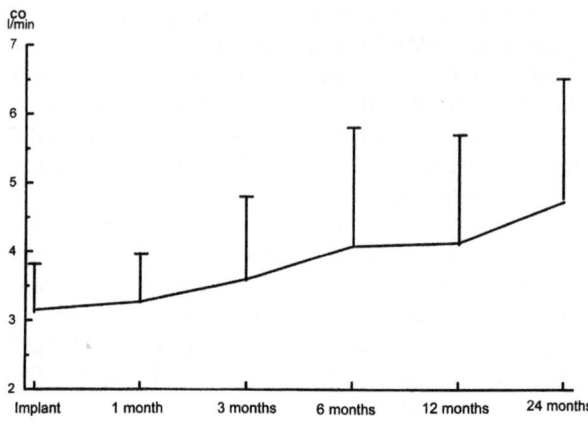

Fig. 3. Longitudinal changes in cardiac output (CO) in response to 2 years of electrophysiologic dual-chamber pacing in survivors. Mean ± SD at various time points

class just after the first month of follow-up and the improvement continued until the third month and, later on, remained unvaried during the 2 years of observation in the surviving patients (Fig. 1). Heart rate decreased from 93.7 ± 18.1 to 82.1 ± 12.4 beats/min ($p<0.006$) in the first month of follow-up and became stable at these values during the follow-up. Systolic blood pressure increased significantly from 106.6 ± 11.5 to 116.2 ± 11.5 mmHg ($p<0.00004$) 1 month after pacemaker implantation, and this improvement was important because most patients tolerated a higher dose of captopril than before pacemaker implantation. Echocardiographic data showed a progressive reduction in left ventricle diastolic and systolic diameters, but only the decrease in the systolic dimensions reached statistical significance (from 61.5 ± 7.5 to 60.2 ± 6.7 mm, $p<0.004$, in the group observed for 1 month, and from 59.3 ± 5.6 to 56.0 ± 5.9 mm, $p<0.03$, in the group that reached 2-year follow-up; Fig. 2). Cardiac output increased significantly just after the first month of observation and this improvement persisted during the 2-year follow-up (3.2 ± 1.3 vs 3.5 ± 1.2 l/min, $p<0.01$, at the first month; 3.2 ± 1.3 vs 3.7 ± 1.1 l/min, $p<0.05$, at the third month; 2.7 ± 1.0 vs 3.8 ± 1.5 l/min, $p<0.05$, at the sixth month; 2.8 ± 1.0 vs 4.0 ± 1.4 l/min,

$p<0.03$, at the first year; 3.1 ± 0.6 vs 4.7 ± 1.8 l/min $p<0.05$ at the end of second year) (Fig. 3). All our patients presented with mitral regurgitation before pacemaker implantation. MRT decreased immediately after pacing and this reduction persisted during the follow-up; moreover, in two patients, mitral regurgitation disappeared. Left ventricular filling time increased consequently, but not significantly (Fig. 4).

Ejection fraction, assessed by radionuclide scintigraphy, did not improve during the follow-up; on the contrary, the cardiothoracic ratio decreased from 0.59 ± 0.07 to 0.54 ± 0.05, $p< 0.04$, at 1-year follow-up and from 0.60 ± 0.08 to 0.54 ± 0.04, $p<0.05$, at 2 years.

In accordance with Nishimura, we did not observe any differences in improvement between the patients with severe heart failure due to coronary artery disease and the patients with idiopathic dilated cardiomyopathy. Within 2 years, six patients died (50%), but only one as a consequence of progressive heart failure. We did not observe any differences in baseline clinical and functional data between the patients who survived and those who died.

Guardigli and colleagues who observed their 10 patients for 2 months and Auricchio and collegues who observed their patients for 1 year confirmed the persis-

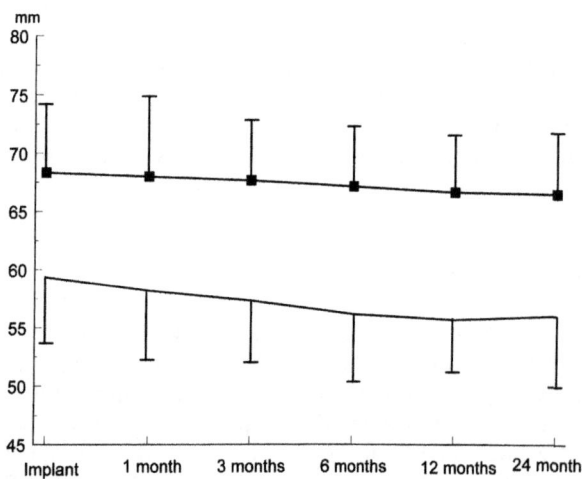

Fig. 2. Longitudinal changes in echocardiographic left ventricle systolic (—) and diastolic (-■-) diameter in response to 2 years of electrophysiologic dual-chamber pacing. Mean ± SD at various time points

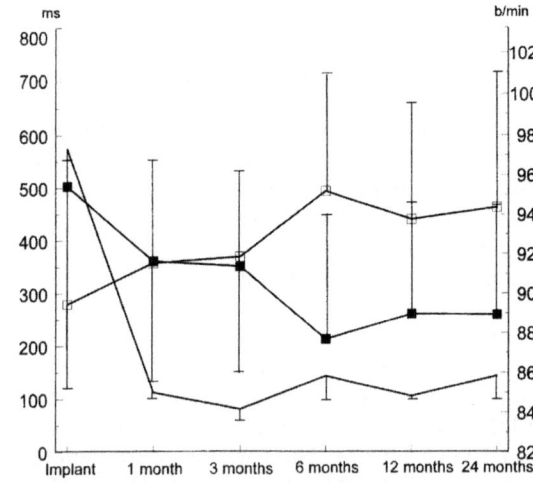

Fig. 4. Longitudinal changes in mitral regurgitation time (-■-), left ventricular filling time (-■-) and heart rate (—) in response to 2 years of electrophysiologic dual-chamber pacing in survivors. Mean ± SD at various time points

tence during the follow-up of the good results obtained in the short term.

Hochleitner's initial study group was observed for 5 years (6). The author did not observe reduction of cardiac function or progression of dilated cardiomyopathy at repeated routine, clinical control examinations (every 6-12 months). At the end of follow-up, three patients were still alive; of the remaining 14 subjects, nine had died suddenly, one died of noncardiac causes, and four received donor hearts. In the three surviving patients, the systolic and diastolic dimensions of the left ventricle decreased steadily (systolic from 59 ± 5 to 47 ± 5 mm and diastolic 72 ± 5 to 60 ± 3 mm, $p<0.001$), and the cardiothoracic ratio decreased, too (from 0.62 ± 0.02 to 0.52 ± 0.01, $p<0.001$). The left ventricular ejection fraction increased from $28\% \pm 1\%$ to $40\% \pm 2\%$, $p<0.05$.

Although these study results partially support the benefit of DDD pacing with short AV interval in patients with severe heart failure, other reports from the literature completely disagree with the above-mentioned one.

Innes (7) studied a consecutive series of 12 patients with dilated heart failure to determine the acute hemodynamic effect of atrial synchronous pacing with short nonphysiologic AV intervals. A balloon flotation catheter was positioned in the pulmonary artery for repeated measurements of cardiac output and wedge pressure during temporary VDD pacing. Three interventions were performed in random order: VDD pacing with an AV interval of 100 ms, VDD pacing at an AV interval of 60 ms, and a control period in sinus rhythm. Mitral valve flow and left ventricular filling time were assessed by Doppler echocardiography.

Despite an increase in ventricular filling time, Innes showed a decline in the stroke and cardiac indexes at the shortest AV interval (60 ms), but at an AV interval of 100 ms, the falls in stroke and cardiac index were not significantly different from those in controls. Blood pressure was also unaltered by pacing. The author did not observe a relationship between either PR interval or QRS duration and the hemodynamic effect of pacing. Mitral regurgitation was reduced in seven of 11 patients during pacing at the shortest AV interval (p=NS). The patient with the most substantial fall in mitral regurgitation was the only one to demonstrate an increase in stroke index with pacing.

In accordance with Innes other preliminary reports have appeared (8, 9). Feliciano (8) performed a randomized, double-blind, crossover trial of 12 patients with severe chronic heart failure refractory to medical therapy and with no accepted indication for pacing. Following pacemaker implantation, acute hemodynamic measurements were obtained during intrinsic sinus rhythm and during VDD pacing with a 100-ms AV delay. The author did not observe acutely an improvement in hemodynamic parameters during pacing; indeed, pulmonary capillary wedge pressure increased. Patients were then randomized to 1 month of VDD pacing with 100 ms AV delay or maintained in sinus rhythm, followed by a 1-month crossover period. Feliciano reported no differences in ejection fraction with chronic pacing between groups and no improvements in NYHA class with VDD in any patients.

Conclusions

All of these reports have many limitations. First of all, a lot of studies that reported benefits by pacing therapy are only observational studies with small numbers of patients and the mechanisms by which these good results were obtained have been speculative. Secondly, the study groups were nonhomogeneous in etiology and in severity of heart failure.

Fewer studies reported there not to be benefit by this kind of "electrical" therapy; however, in many cases they were only preliminary reports and only showed immediate results or results derived from short-term follow-up. In our experience, many of these studies were interrupted before the benefits from treatment could have become evident.

The authors who reported good results of pacing therapy do not agree in selection of patients: Brecker, like us, studied patients in whom mitral regurgitation was always present, so we ascribe more weight to this hemodynamic effect. Nishimura reported benefits in patients with long PR interval, and so he focused his attention on this electrical factor.

However, all the authors agree to identify in modification of preload, decrease of mitral regurgitation, optimization of the timing of mechanical atrial and ventricular synchrony, the main factors by which DDD pacing with short AV delay may improve hemodynamic vàriables.

Prospective, randomized studies are needed to further investigate the mechanisms by which hemodynamic benefits are obtained and to study the long-term clinical outcome of this new therapeutic modality for patients with severe end-stage heart failure.

References

1. Hochleitner M, Hortnagl H, Ng CK, Hortnagl H, Gschnitzer F, Zechmann W (1990) Usefulness of physiologic dual-chamber pacing in drug-resistant idiopathic dilated cardiomyopathy. Am J Cardiol 66: 198-202
2. Kataoka H (1991) Hemodynamic effect of physiological dual chamber pacing in a patient with end-stage dilated cardiomyopathy: a case report. PACE 14: 1330-1335
3. Guardigli G, Ansani L, Percoco GF et al (1994) AV delay optimization and management of DDD paced patients with dilated cardiomyopathy. PACE 17 (pt. II): 1984-1988
4. Nishimura RA Hayes DL, Holmes Jr DR, Tajik AJ (1995) Mechanism of hemodynamic improvement by dual-chamber pacing for severe left ventricular dysfunction: an acute doppler and catheterization hemodynamic study. J Am Coll Cardiol 25: 281-288
5. Brecker SJD, Xiao HB, Sparrow J, Gibson DG (1992) Effects of dual-chamber pacing with short atrioventricular delay in dilated cardiomyopathy. Lancet 340: 1308-1312
6. Hochleitner M, Hortnagl H, Hortnagl H, Fridrich L, Gschnitzer F (1992) Long-term efficacy of physiologic dual-chamber pacing in the treatment of end-stage idiopathic dilated cardiomyopathy. Am J Cardiol 70: 1320-1325
7. Innes D, Leitch JW, Fletcher PJ (1994) VDD pacing at short atrioventricular intervals does not improve cardiac output in patients with dilated heart failure. PACE 17 (pt II): 959-965
8. Feliciano Z, Fisher ML, Gottlieb SS, Gold MR (1993) Does short A-V delay pacing improve congestive heart failure? Circulation 88: 1-19 (abstr)
9. Linde C, Gadler F, Edner M, Nordlander R, Rosenqvist M, Ryden L (1994) Is DDD pacing with short AV delay a beneficial treatment in patients with severe heart failure? PACE 17 (pt II): 744

Dual-Chamber Pacing in Obstructive Hypertrophic Cardiomyopathy: Is There Evidence for a Real Benefit?

S.B. Betocchi, M.A. Losi, C. Pappone, and M. Chiariello

Dipartimento di Cardiologia e Cardiochirurgia, Università Federico II,
Naples, Italy

Introduction

Hypertrophic cardiomyopathy (HCM) is a primary myocardial disease whose typical pathophysiologic features include normal systolic dynamics, impaired diastolic function (1-7), and, in about one fourth of patients, left ventricular (LV) outflow tract obstruction (8-11).

Treatment for LV outflow tract obstruction has for decades rested upon the surgical resection of a septal wedge (myotomy-myectomy) (12). This approach has been shown to provide symptomatic benefit and improvement in prognosis, especially if associated with appropriate medical therapy (10). Recently, a new therapeutic tool for the treatment of LV outflow tract obstruction has drawn the attention of several investigators: sequential right atrioventricular (AV) pacing with short AV delay (i.e., apical pre-excitation) decreases the LV outflow tract gradient in patients with obstructive HCM (13-17). AV pacing diminishes the outflow gradient probably by inducing septal systolic asynchrony: qualitative analysis of motion of the upper septum shows that contraction is delayed and, consequently, the width of the outflow tract is increased, thereby reducing the outflow tract gradient (17).

Acute Hemodynamic Effects

Effects on LV Outflow Tract Obstruction

AV pacing reduces the degree of LV outflow tract gradient in most patients with obstructive HCM (up to 80%) (16).

The efficacy of AV pacing in reducing obstruction depends on the AV interval: Jeanrenaud and coworkers have shown that apical pre-excitation is necessary to that effect (17). Long AV intervals are ineffective, whereas too short intervals may interfere with filling, reduce cardiac output, and ultimately increase the gradient through a reduction in LV volume (17): AV intervals of 80-100 ms lower the degree of obstruction without altering the filling dynamics, as shown by the lack of decrease in aortic pressure both in studies of acute treatment with AV pacing and in studies after permanent pacemaker implant in atrial synchronized ventricular pacing mode (18,19).

Effects on LV Systolic Function and Hemodynamics

AV pacing minimally affects ejection fraction (20): the decrease in LV systolic pressure that occurs with AV pacing, however, should be associated with an increase in ejection fraction. This lack of an increase could then be interpreted as indirect evidence of a negative inotropic effect of AV pacing. In contrast, the reduction in the LV outflow tract gradient achieved by AV pacing is beneficial in that it increases aortic pressure and cardiac output (the latter at high heart rate only) (16).

Effects on LV Diastolic Function

It has been shown in experimental animal studies (21,22) and in patients with coronary artery disease (23,24) that asynchrony induced by AV pacing impairs active diastolic function (both isovolumetric relaxation and early filling).

If the same was true for patients with HCM, AV pacing would worsen diastolic function in a category of patients, those with obstructive HCM, in whom it is already jeopardized (1,7). We have shown that acute AV pacing impairs the time constant of isovolumetric relaxation despite a decrease in LV outflow tract gradient and, hence, of LV systolic pressure (20). Because the time constant of isovolumetric relaxation is inversely related to afterload (25), it should be shortened by a reduction in LV systolic pressure. In addition, maximal rate of LV filling decreased, despite an increase in the filling pressure (20), whereas in this setting filling should have been faster (26). These findings indicate that AV pacing damages the active part of diastole in an acute study. The elevation in the filling pressure, in addition, is potentially detrimental as it may induce symptoms of congestive heart failure.

Chronic Effects

Long-Term Hemodynamic Effects

LV outflow tract gradient decreases with permanent stimulation in atrial synchronized ventricular pacing mode (16) and it keeps decreasing over time (27); in addition, a decrease in provocable gradient is observed also in patients without significant obstruction at rest. The decrease in LV outflow tract gradient is associated with a progressive decrease in LV systolic pressure and an increase in aortic pulse pressure. Filling pressure and cardiac output do not change in the long term (27). Interestingly, such hemodynamic changes are also observed when the pace maker is turned off: although the degree of obstruction is lower in the long term with dual-chamber (DDD) pacing than in sinus rhythm, LV outflow tract gradient in sinus rhythm is less in the long term than it was in the acute study (27). The mechanism for this finding is unclear: a pacing-induced "plastic remodeling" of the LV has been advocated.

This hypothesis, however, has not been confirmed by analysis of LV anatomy: Fananapazir and coworkers (27) have observed a pacing-induced reduction in septal thickness in about one fourth of their patients, while Jeanrenaud and coworkers have seen no changes in LV anatomy (17).

In a subgroup of patients with angina, a reduction in septal ischemia has been observed by positron emission tomography 3 months following pacemaker implant (28). This may explain the effect of DDD pacing on angina pectoris.

Clinical Outcome

DDD pacing improves functional capacity in the majority of patients (16, 17, 27) as shown by a significant decrease in the New York Heart Association functional class. Symptomatic status is improved over the long term in approximately 90% of patients; angina pectoris, dyspnea, palpitation, and presyncope all decrease after DDD pacing and exhibit a further decrease in some patients at late follow-up (27). It is of note, however, that a few patients (about 10%) do not benefit from chronic DDD pacing for several reasons, including persistent obstruction and accelerated AV conduction (this latter precluding from pacing at long-enough AV intervals) (29). These data from the NIH group have been obtained in a large series of patients with drug-refractory symptoms who were treated with DDD pacing alone (i.e., they did not take any medication after pacemaker implant). Another group has had less favorable results in a similar population of patients with obstructive HCM (30): they saw no differences in the incidence of angina (it decreased in about as many patients as it worsened or developed with DDD pacing), whereas the occurrence of syncope decreased significantly; in one patient, however, syncope developed after pacemaker implant that was not present before. Older patients were more apt to improve with DDD pacing than younger ones (30). These results occurred although patients had been treated with conventional therapy (30).

Unanswered Questions

Mortality

The main goals of treatment for any diseases are reduction in mortality and improvement in quality of life. The efficacy of DDD pacing in lowering mortality (particularly sudden death, the leading cause of death in HCM) is still unknown: few studies have been published (most as abstracts) that include relatively small populations of patients followed up for too short time intervals. Because many patients with obstructive HCM are young and, if implanted, are likely to experience many years of DDD pacing, studies available so far appear inadequate in addressing this issue. To our knowledge, three multicenter studies have addressed the issue of the long-term effects of DDD pacing in controlled situations, having death as one of the endpoints; relative results, however, are far from being ready.

Symptoms

Although all previous studies have shown an improvement in New York Heart Association functional class, a placebo effect of pacemaker implant cannot be ruled out and objective evaluation of functional capacity is in order. A study aimed at evaluating whether DDD pacing has objective advantages in terms of functional capacity in patients with obstructive HCM has failed to show any changes in duration of exercise and VO_2max (31); the small number of patients and the short follow-up time, however, prevents any firm conclusions from being drawn from that study. Similarly, despite the observed reduction in palpitations, no controlled data are available on the incidence of arrhythmias in these patients: dispersion of LV electrical activation is a determinant of malignant ventricular arrhythmias in HCM and pacing has the potential for spreading LV electrical activation, therefore careful analysis of arrhythmias during chronic DDD pacing would be very helpful.

Acute AV pacing appears to be associated with a negative inotropic effect. If this effect persists in the long term, the possibility that DDD pacing leads to LV dilatation should be assessed in large, long-term studies.

Acute AV pacing impairs diastolic function. It is yet to be clarified whether long-term DDD pacing has the same unwanted effects: a negative lusitropic effect could be counterbalanced in the short term by the decrease in obstruction, and it may become evident again in the long term. In addition, even if diastolic dysfunction is detectable in the long term, as it is acutely, the impact of such dysfunction on symptoms and possibly survival will warrant further investigation.

A practical point that has to be defined is the necessity for medical treatment after pacemaker implant. The NIH group suggests no medical therapy, unless it is indicated to prolong the AV interval and, therefore, allow longer, paced AV delay. A role for calcium antagonists and ß-blockers as an adjunct therapy to reduce LV outflow tract obstruction and improve diastolic function is yet to be established.

References

1. Sanderson JE, Gibson DG, Brown DJ, Goodwin JF (1977) Left ventricular filling in hypertrophic cardiomyopathy. Br Heart J 39: 661-670
2. Hanrath P, Mathey DG, Siegert R, Bleifeld W (1980) Left ventricular relaxation and filling in different forms of left ventricular hypertrophy: an echocardiographic study. Am J Cardiol 45: 15-23
3. Bonow RO, Frederick TM, Bacharach SL, Green MV, Goose PW, Maron BJ, Rosing DR (1983) Atrial systole and left ventricular filling in patients with hypertrophic cardiomyopathy. Am J Cardiol 51: 1386-1991
4. Alvares RF, Shaver JA, Gamble WH, Goodwin JF (1984) Isovolumic relaxation period in hypertrophic cardiomyopathy. J Am Coll Cardiol 3: 71-81
5. Betocchi S, Bonow RO, Bacharach SL, Rosing DR, Maron BJ, Green MV (1986) Isovolumic relaxation period in hypertrophic cardiomyopathy: assessment by radionuclide angiography. J Am Coll Cardiol 7: 74-81
6. Hess OM, Murakami T, Krayenbuehl HP (1986) Does verapamil improve left ventricular relaxation in patients with myocardial hypertrophy? Circulation 74: 530-543
7. Hess OM, Grimm J, Krayenbuehl HP (1983) Diastolic function in hypertrophic cardiomyopathy: effects of propranolol and verapamil on diastolic stiffness. Eur Heart J 4 [Suppl F]: 47-56
8. Maron BJ, Gottdiener JS, Arce J, Rosing DR, Wesley YE, Epstein SE (1985) Dynamic subaortic obstruction in hypertrophic cardiomyopathy: analysis by pulsed Doppler echocardiography. J Am Coll Cardiol 6: 1-15
9. Maron BJ, Epstein SE (1986) Clinical significance and therapeutic implications of the left ventricular outflow tract pressure gradient in hypertrophic cardiomyopathy. Am J Cardiol 58: 1093-1096
10. Seiler C, Hess OM, Schoenbeck M, Turina J, Jenni R, Turina M, Krayenbuehl HP (1991) Long-term follow-up of medical versus surgical therapy for hypertrophic cardiomyopathy: a retrospective study. J Am Coll Cardiol 17: 634-642
11. Kaltenbach M, Hopf R, Kober G, Bussman WD, Keller M, Paterson Y (1979) Treatment of hypertrophic cardiomyopathy with verapamil. Br Heart J 42: 35-42
12. Morrow AG, Fogarty TJ, Hannah H III, Braunwald E (1968) Operative treatment in idiopathic hypertrophic subaortic stenosis: techniques and the results of preoperative and postoperative clinical and hemodynamic assessment. Circulation 37: 589-596
13. Hassenstein P, Walther H, Dittrich J (1975) Haemodynamische Veranderungen durch einfach und gekoppelte Stimulation bei Patienten mit obstruktiver Kardiomyopathie. Verh Dtsch Ges Inn Med 81: 170-173
14. Duck HJ, Hutschemeister W, Paneau H, Trenckmann H (1984) Atrio-ventricular stimulation with reduced AV-delay time as a therapeutic principle in hypertrophic obstructive cardiomyopathy. Z Ges Inn Med 39: 437-447
15. McDonald K, McWilliam E, O'Keeffe B, Maurer B (1988) Functional assessment of patients treated with permanent dual chamber pacing as a primary treatment for hypertrophic cardiomyopathy. Eur Heart J 9: 893-898
16. Fananapazir L, Cannon RO III, Tripodi D, Panza JA (1992) Impact of dual-chamber permanent pacing in patients with obstructive hypertrophic cardiomyopathy with symptoms refractory to verapamil and ß-adrenergic blocker therapy. Circulation 85: 2149-2161
17. Jeanrenaud X, Goy JJ, Kappenberger L (1992) Effects of dual-chamber pacing in hypertrophic obstructive cardiomyopathy. Lancet 339: 1318-1323
18. Betocchi S, Losi MA, Franculli F, Perrone-Filardi P, Russolillo E, Piscione F (1993) Dual chamber pacing in hypertrophic cardiomyopathy: impact of atrio-ventricular coupling on left ventricular obstruction. Circulation 88: I-210 (abstr)
19. Losi MA, Betocchi S, Briguori C, Manganelli F, Stabile G, Franculli F, Pappone C, Chiariello M (1995) Hypertrophic cardiomyopathy and dual chamber pacing: impact of atrio-ventricular delay on obstruction assessed by Doppler echocardiography. J Am Coll Cardiol 25: 234-A (abstr)
20. Betocchi S, Losi MA, Piscione F, Russolillo E, Perrone-Filardi P, Pace L, Boccalatte M, Salvatore M, Chiariello M (1994) Atrio-ventricular pacing relieves obstruction but impairs diastolic function in hypertrophic cardiomyopathy. J Am Coll Cardiol 23: 11-A (abstr)
21. Zile MR, Blaunstein AS, Shimizu G, Gaasch WH (1987) Right ventricular pacing reduces the rate of left ventricular relaxation and filling. J Am Coll Cardiol 10: 702-709
22. Aoyagy T, Iizuka M, Takahashi K, Ohya T, Serizawa T, Momomura S, Satoh H, Mochizuki T, Matsui H, Ikenouchi H, Shin I, Ma YX, Sugimoto T (1989) Wall motion asynchrony prolongs time-constant of left ventricular relaxation. Am J Physiol 257: H883-H890
23. Bedotto JB, Grayburn PA, Black WH, Raya TE, McBride W, Hsia HH (1990) Alteration in left ventricular relaxation during atrioventricular pacing in humans. J Am Coll Cardiol 15: 658-664
24. Betocchi S, Piscione F, Villari B, Pace L, Ciarmiello A, Perrone-Filardi P, Salvatore C, Salvatore M, Chiariello M (1993) Effects of induced asynchrony on left ventricular diastolic function in patients with coronary artery disease. J Am Coll Cardiol 21: 1124-1131
25. Gaasch WH, Blaunstein AS, Andrias CW, Donahue RP, Avitall B (1980) Myocardial relaxation. II. Hemodynamic determinants of rate of left ventricular isovolumic pressure decline. Am J Physiol 239: H1-H6
26. Ishida Y, Meisner JS, Tsujoka K, Gallo JI, Yoran C, Frater RWM, Yellin EL (1986) Left ventricular filling dynamics: influence of left ventricular relaxation and left atrial pressure. Circulation 74: 187-196
27. Fananapazir L, Epstein ND, Curiel RV, Panza J, Tripodi D, McAreavey D (1994) Long-term results of dual-chamber (DDD) pacing in obstructive hypertrophic cardiomyopathy. Evidence for progressive symptomatic and hemodynamic improvement and reduction of left ventricular hypertrophy. Circulation 90: 2731-2742
28. Posma JL, Blanksma PK, Haagen FDM, Vaalburg W, Lie KI (1995) Effects of dual chamber pacing on myocardial ischemia in hypertrophic cardiomyopathy studied with 13N ammonia and 18FDG positron emission tomography. J Am Coll Cardiol 25: 30-A (abstr)
29. Sadoul N, Slade AKB, Simon JP, Saumarez RC, Dodinot B, Allot E, McKenna WJ (1995) Dual chamber pacing in refractory hypertrophic obstructive cardiomyopathy: a two-center european experience in 34 consecutive patients. J Am Coll Cardiol 25: 233-A (abstr)
30. McAreavey D, Fananapazir L (1995) Long term results of dual chamber (DDD) pacing in 114 adult patients with obstructive hypertrophic cardiomyopathy and severe drug-refractory symptoms. J Am Coll Cardiol (abstr) 25: 233-A
31. Nishimura RA, Trusty JM, Hayes DL, Allison TG, Holmes DR, Hayes SH, Espinosa RE, Symanski JD, Tajik J (1995) Dual-chamber pacing for patients with hypertrophic obstructive cardiomyopathy: a prospective randomized, double-blind crossover trial. J Am Coll Cardiol 25: 10-A (abstr)

Automatic Mode Switching: How Useful Is It?

E. Adornato[1], P. Monea[1], and E.M. Adornato[2]

[1]Divisione di Cardiologia, Ospedale Regionale, Reggio Calabria, Italy
[2]Divisione di Medicina, Università degli Studi, Messina, Italy

Introduction

In patients with episodic or recurrent supraventricular arrhythmias (atrial fibrillation or flutter) dual-chamber pacemaker (DDD/DDDR) implantation might be rejected because of the possibility of irregular and rapid ventricular rhythm. Moreover, it has to be taken into consideration that in about 10%-15% of patients with dual-chamber pulse generators, episodes of supraventricular tachyarrhythmia may occur because of the atrial competition between spontaneous and electrical atrial rhythm.

Automatic mode switching (AMS) is a new function in DDD pacemakers to manage atrial arrhythmias by changing the pacing modality from atrial synchronous to a nontracking mode (DVI – DDI/DDIR – VVI/VVIR pacing modes according to the design or programmability) and stopping the atrial synchronization (1-4). It allows the use of the dual-chamber pacemaker to be extended to circumstances (i.e., bradycardia-tachycardia syndrome) that would previously not have been possible. Symptoms due to irregular and rapid ventricular rhythm and frequent, time-consuming pacemaker reprogramming can be avoided and patients should have the benefits of physiologic pacing as long as possible because the pacemaker reverts back to the previous pacing mode when the sinus rhythm is restored.

With conventional pulse generators the strategies to avoid tracking of rapid atrial rates during supraventricular tachyarrhythmias should consist in the selection of nontracking pacing modes (DVI, DDI/DDIR, VVI/VVIR) or in the programming of a low upper rate limit that permits the ventricular rate acceleration on sinus rhythm, i.e., during exercise, and limits the ventricular rate during atrial tachycardias. However, this variety of modes or responses is unsatisfactory because they often compromise the optimal pacemaker function and waste energy or cause arrhythmogenicity (5).

For the correct operation of AMS some problems have to be considered:
- Detection of atrial arrhythmias that must be constant and reliable
- Distinction of pathological atrial rhythm from sinus tachycardia
- Number of rapid atrial beats to be sensed for tachycardia identification before AMS
- Value of ventricular pacing rate during AMS
- Time for the ventricular rate to decline toward the lower rate.

The capability of the pacemaker to correctly detect the presence of atrial arrhythmias and to distinguish sinus tachycardia from supraventricular tachyarrhythmia is imperative for this function. The algorithms for atrial tachycardia detection used in the majority of pacemakers are based on the analysis of cardiac rhythm and its characteristics; pathological tachycardia is recognized when spontaneous cardiac events are faster than the programmed value of upper rate and are stable for the predetermined number of atrial events. These high rate-based criteria for tachycardia detection are very sensitive but not very specific because a sinus tachycardia with sudden onset, e.g., for exercises or intense emotions, or a sinus tachycardia at rest in heart failure may also be identified as pathological tachycardia and inappropriately activate the AMS. Moreover, the pacemaker sensing level must be programmed to constantly detect pathological endocardial A waves, considering that the amplitude of atrial events may significantly decrease during supraventricular tachyarrhythmias and render ineffective the detection of pathological rhythm even if the pacemaker detection setting is at the highest available.

For these instances different algorithms for the correct detection of atrial tachyarrhythmias have been implemented in some new pacemakers. The Elamedical Chorus II DDD pacemaker for tachycardia recognition utilizes a special algorithm based on the assumption that the onset of physiologic sinus tachycardia is usually gradual, whereas that of pathological tachycardia occurs suddenly. This algorithm analyzes the atrial acceleration thanks to a detection window, the window of atrial rate acceleration detection (WARAD), that is the interval after the last spontaneous sinus P wave where a sensed atrial event will be recognized as an atrial premature complex and corresponds to 75% of the average of the last eight sinus beats.

The Vitatron Diamond DDDR pacemaker analyzes beat-to-beat the sensed atrial rate to form a "physiologic band" that is set to 15 ppm above or below the physiologic rate. An atrial tachyarrhythmia is diagnosed if the atrial rate exceeds the upper limit of the physiologic band in a pathological manner, resulting in automatic switching of pacing mode to DDI/VVI if the pacemaker was programmed in DDD/VDD modes or to DDIR/VVIR if in DDDR/VDDR. The pacemaker switches back to the previous programmed mode when the sensed atrial rate decreases below the upper rate limit of physiologic band. Because atrial sense interpretation works on a beat-by-beat basis, single atrial ectopic beats may also be classified as pathological so that the pacemaker can immediately adapt its behavior, resulting in frequent inappropriate changes of pacing mode in cases of frequent atrial ectopic beats.

The Medtronic Thera DDD/DDDR pacemaker uses the patient's atrial electrogram to determine the presence or the absence of atrial tachycardia. Because P wave amplitude may change in supraventricular tachyarrhythmias, an amplifier with high sensitivity, wide frequency response and suitable timing windows is included and special circuit designs are used to reduce the possibility of detecting myopotentials or other interfering signals. The algorithm employed in this device for tachyarrhythmia detection is the mean atrial rate (MAR) or its inverse mean atrial interval (MAI). The Thera pacemaker monitors and measures each atrial cycle length and adjusts MAI, reducing it by 23 ms if the detected and measured P-P interval is less than the MAI and, conversevely, increasing it by 8 ms if the P-P interval is greater than the MAI. In this way the time for the detection of supraventricular tachyarrhythmia is slightly prolonged (about 10 s) in order to confirm the presence of tachycardia and to avoid the recognition of frequent atrial extrasystoles as tachycardia.

The pacemaker recognizes supraventricular tachycardia as occurring when the MAR reaches the "tachy detection rate" of 180 ppm. Upon detection the pacemaker automatically switches to nonatrial tracking mode (DDI/DDIR, VVI/VVIR according to the programming) and the ventricles are paced at the programmed lower rate if the pacemaker was in DDD mode or at the sensor-indicated rate if in DDDR mode. It switches back to DDD or DDDR modes after either five consecutive atrial paced beats or a substantial lowering of the detected atrial rate below the programmed maximum tracking rate. Either marks the termination of the atrial tachyarrhythmia.

Recently, sensors used to modulate the rate of antibradycardia pacemakers have been applied to tachycardia recognition so that an atrial rate higher than the programmed upper rate in the absence of body motion and of sensor activity is recognized as being pathological and not sinus tachycardia (6).

The Swing DR1 (Sorin Biomedica), a dual-chamber, rate-responsive pacer, uses a gravitational accelerometer sensor for rate adaption and even utilizes the sensor's data to distinguish pathological from sinus tachycardia. Pathological tachycardia is recognized when the spontaneous atrial rhythm is higher than the programmed upper rate and the sensor calculated rate is equal to or lower than the "confirmation rate" (= basic rate + 20 ppm), indicating the absence of sensor activity (7).

The Intermedics Relay, a dual-chamber, rate-modulated pacemaker sensitive to acceleration forces, utilizes the activity sensor for the arrhythmia detection and an algorithm called conditional ventricular tracking limit (CVTL) to limit the ventricular pacing rate in the presence of supraventricular tachyarrhythmia. The pacemaker recognizes supraventricular tachycardia as occurring when the sensed atrial rate exceeds the programmed maximum rate and the sensor-calculated rate is equal to or lower than the lower rate plus 20 ppm, indicating the absence of patient activity. In this situation the ventricular pacing rate becomes limited in a Wenckebach fashion to a CVTL rate, a value of 35 ppm above the programmed lower rate, without changing the pacing mode.

If the sensor-calculated rate exceeds the programmed lower rate by 20 ppm or more, indicating the presence of patient activity, the CVLT will be disregarded and 1:1 atrioventricular (AV) synchrony occurs up to the programmed upper rate. For sensed atrial rates exceeding the upper rate, the ventricular pacing rate is limited by a Wenckebach mechanism.

The Telectronics Meta DDDR 1250 model utilizes the information coming from the minute ventilation sensor to influence the postventricular atrial refractory period (PVARP), the duration of which is progressively reduced on the basis of the measurement of the transthoracic impedance correlate to minute ventilation variations. The pacemaker detects and monitors atrial events that are judged to be nonphysiologic when they fall into a PVARP immediately after a nonprogrammable 100-ms absolute refractory period. In this instance the AMS switches to VVIR when the pacemaker is programmed to DDDR, DDIR, or VDDR or to VVI mode, when programmed to non-rate-responsive mode (8). In practice a retrograde A wave or isolated premature atrial complexes can induce AMS. For this reason in the new version of the Meta DDDR device (Model 1254) the number of sensed atrial events for tachycardia detection are programmable from 5 to 11 and the atrial rate must be higher than 150, 175, or 200 ppm (programmable parameter) before the mode is switched.

Limitations of these sensor-derived criteria concern the inappropriate and nonphysiologic activation of AMS in case of sinus tachycardia arising at rest or persisting for long enough at the end of exercise and the nondetection of pathological tachycardias arising during physical activity.

For the correct activation of AMS it is important that the number of rapid atrial beats required for the arrhythmia identification is programmable and higher than one and that the intervals between the consecutive spontaneous atrial events are stable or lower than the programmed value of stability. These features offer the advantage of being able to confirm pathological tachycardias and to avoid the inappropriate and frequent activations of AMS in case of single or frequent atrial ectopic beats.

In the CPI Vigor DR mode switching may be programmed to take place between 10 and 2000 atrial cycles after the initial detection in order to obtain the tachycardia confirmation; during this time a Wenckebach mechanism may occur to permit a smooth transition to the lower-rate ventricular pacing, so minimizing hemodynamic disturbances. After eight atrial events occurring below the upper rate limit the pacemaker automatically switches back to DDD/DDDR pacing mode, synchronizing AV activity.

In the Elamedical Chorus II DDD Pacemaker AMS to the VDI mode occurs after 30 s of tachycardia analysis, during which the pulse generator may exhibit a 2:1 Wenckebach response.

The value of the ventricular pacing rate during AMS and the time for the ventricular pacing rate to decline toward the lower rate are also important to avoid an inadequate ventricular pacing rate, a sudden drop in the ventricular rate, and hemodynamic disturbances. These problems may be minimized or eliminated by appropriately programming the ventricular pacing rate, which should be different from the basic lower rate, and by using the rate smoothing or the fallback behavior to achieve a gradual decrease of the pacing rate during AMS.

In the sensor-modulated DDD pacemakers the AMS is to VVIR so that the pacing rate is controlled by the sensor activity at all times; in this way the hemodynamic benefits continue to be maintained during supraventricular tachyarrhythmias arising during physical activity or emotional stress, circumstances in which a ventricular rate higher than the programmed lower rate is needed.

At the end information about the occurrence of atrial tachyarrhythmias for retrospective diagnosis and telemetric ECG for the interpretation of pacemaker function is necessary.

DDD pacing may be considered appropriate in the majority of patients; however, in patients with paroxysmal or intermittent AV block, carotid sinus syndrome, or sick sinus syndrome without overt AV block, DDD pacing may be responsible for two adverse effects: high current drain due to frequent unnecessary ventricular pacing and alteration of ventricular function due to the desynchronization of ventricular contraction. In fact, during DVI and VVI compared with AAI pacing mode at the same pacing rate a higher myocardial oxygen consumption and many adverse hemodynamic effects, such as prolongation of the time constant of relaxation, fall in the lengthening speed and ventricular filling, have been demonstrated (9).

For this instance the ideal pacemaker would function in AAI mode in the presence of normal AV conduction and switch automatically to DDD mode whenever an AV block occurs or the A-V interval exceeds a programmable value. When the AV block disappears or the AV interval reverts to a shorter value, the pacemaker would automatically switch back to AAI mode, thereby reducing battery drain and optimizing left ventricular function because of normal ventricular activation.

The Elamedical Chorus II DDD pacemaker fulfills these criteria by a special algorithm. In presence of intact AV conduction the pacemaker initiates an atrial postatrial refractory period equal to 75% of the sinus cycle length to avoid the effects of atrial extrasystoles and a ventricular surveillance period equal to the average of the eight preceding spontaneous PR intervals plus an extension of 47 ms in order to detect the occurrence of a spontaneous ventricular depolarization. The device functions in DDD mode if a spontaneous ventricular depolarization does not occur at the end of the ventricular surveillance period and automatically resumes the AAI mode if the pacemaker detects, during 16 consecutive cycles, spontaneous R waves synchronous with atrial activity.

In conclusion, AMS is indicated in patients who have or could have recurrent paroxysmal atrial tachyarrhythmias; these are mainly patients with bradycardia-tachycardia syndrome, the form of sick sinus syndrome in which atrial tachyarrhythmias are common, patients with recurrent, drug-refractory atrial flutter/fibrillation episodes with iatrogenic complete AV block after His bundle ablation (10), and in patients with spontaneous AV block and recurrent, drug-refractory paroxysmal supraventricular tachyarrhythmias.

In fact, in these clinical scenarios the DDD pacemaker has traditionally constituted a limitation or a contraindication to avoid atrial tracking and correspondingly rapid ventricular pacing rate during atrial tachycardia. AMS is an intelligent solution to avoid frequent and time-consuming reprogramming of the pacing modalities in case of their appearance and to allow patients to have the benefits of physiologic DDD/DDDR pacing as long as possible because the pacemaker reverts back to the previous pacing mode when the sinus rhythm is restored.

It may be expected that all models of DDD/DDDR pacemakers will include this feature but improvements in the detection algorithms for the correct diagnosis of pathological tachycardias and additional therapeutic approaches (antitachycardia pacing, atrial defibrillation) are expected.

References

1. Ilvento J, Fee JA, Shewmaker AA (1990) Automatic mode switching from DDDR to VVIR. A management algorithm for atrial arrhythmias in patients with dual chamber pacemakers. PACE 13: 1199
2. Mond HG, Barold SS (1993) Dual chamber, rate adaptive pacing in patients with paroxysmal supraventricular tachyarrhythmias: protective measures for rate control. PACE 16: 2168
3. Sweesy M, Batey R, Forney R et al (1991) Automatic mode change in a DDDR pacemaker for supraventricular tachyarrhythmias. PACE 14: 737
4. Barold SS: (1991) Automatic switching of pacing mode. Cardiostimolazione 9: 121
5. Barold SS, Mond HA (1993) Optimal antibradycardia pacing in patients with paroxysmal supraventricular tachyarrhythmias: role of fallback and automatic mode switching mechanism. In: Barold SS, Mugica J (eds) New perspectives in cardiac pacing, vol 3. Futura, Mount Kisco, NY, p 483
6. Lee MT, Adkins A, Woodson D et al (1990) A new feature for control of inappropriate high tracking in DDDR pacemakers. PACE 13: 1852
7. Garberoglio B, Bernasconi A (1992) Evoluzione dei sensori per applicazioni su pacemaker R-R. In: Adornato E, Galassi A (eds) The '92 scenario on cardiac pacing. Luigi Pozzi, Rome, p 367

8. Lau CP, Tai YT, Fong PC et al (1992) Atrial arrhythmia management with sensor controlled atrial refractory period and automatic mode switching in patients with minute ventilation sensing dual chamber rate adaptive pacemakers. PACE 15: 1504
9. Baller D, Wolpers HG, Zipfel J et al (1988) Comparison of the effects of right atrial, right ventricular apex and atrioventricular sequential pacing on myocardial oxygen consumption and cardiac efficiency: a laboratory investigation. PACE 11: 394
10. Van Wyhe G, Sra J, Rovang K et al (1991) Maintenance of atrioventricular sequence after his bundle ablation for paroxysmal supraventricular rhythm disorders. A unique use of the fallback mode in dual chamber pacemakers. PACE 14: 410

Extraction of Chronically Implanted Pacemaker Leads: When and How?

M. G. Bongiorni, G. Arena, E. Soldati, G. Quirino, F. Vernazza, L. De Simone, and D. Levorato

Servizio di Elettrostimolazione ed Elettrofisiologia, Istituto di Fisiologia Clinica,
CNR-CREAS, Pisa, Italy

Introduction

The extraction of chronically implanted pacemaker leads is a challenging problem. Recently, the development of new extraction techniques has renewed the interest in this particular field.

The wide use of implanted cardiac pacemakers is associated with a variety of complications; among these, the retention of functionless pacing leads is becoming relatively common, especially in patients who have been paced for many years. Local infection of the pacing system is another possible complication, while septicemia is a rare, but life-threatening event.

The management of patients with retained functionless pacing leads is still controversial; some authors have reported a low complication rate associated with the abandonment of uninfected leads (1). On the other hand, fatal pulmonary artery embolization has been reported (2), as well as a significant incidence of (often asympomatic) venous obstruction in the presence of many leads, particularly if they come from opposite sides (3-5).

In contrast, most authors agree upon the fact that local infection of the pacing system can cause successive serious complications such as septicemia, superior vena cava syndrome, and venous obstruction, and it is associated with a high rate of reinterventions (6, 7). A conservative policy is often unsuccessful, and the total removal of leads is the most effective therapy. In the case of septicemia, which is doubtlessly a very dangerous condition, an aggressive treatment is necessary to eradicate the infection.

In the past, removal of chronic pacing leads has been performed by direct traction or by attaching weights via a pulley system (8, 9) and applying traction for several hours. The results have been discouraging and many complications have been reported, such as shock due to the invagination of the right ventricular wall, ventricular tachycardia, ventricular fibrillation (10), avulsion of a tricuspid valve leaflet (11), and lethal hemopericardium due to a tear in the right ventricular apex (12) or in the lateral right atrium wall (13) after too forceful a traction.

On the other hand, various surgical techniques have been efficaciously employed (14-16), but the associated high costs and the patients' discomfort have led most authors to agree upon the fact that only septicemic patients should be treated by this approach.

The availability of effective and relatively safe new systems allowing the transvenous extraction of the pacemaker electrodes is changing the management of these patients; more recently, in fact, intravascular countertraction techniques using locking stylets and sheaths via the implant vein, or sheaths, snares, and a retrieval basket via the femoral vein have been investigated, and many papers can be found on this subject in the literature (17-20).

Indications for Chronically Implanted Pacemaker Lead Extraction

The risks and morbidity of the extraction procedures strongly affect the indications for lead removal. While in the past only patients with septicemia were submitted to lead extraction procedures, at the present time the indications can be referred to as mandatory, necessary or discretionary (21) (Table 1).

Table 1. Indications for removal of leads

	Indication
Mandatory	Systemic infections
	Septicemia
	Endocarditis
	Myocarditis
	Recurrent fever without other explanations
	Migration of leads
Necessary	Pocket infection
	Chronic draining sinus
	Pacing system erosion
	Addition of a third lead
Discretionary	Noninfected functionless or abandoned leads

Mandatory Conditions. These are typically life-threatening conditions such as septicemia, endocarditis, and myocarditis or the presence of a fragmented lead with the possibility of a migration of the lead and of ventricular tachyarrhythmias.

Septicemia may result from a pocket infection, but it must also be suspected in the absence of external signs of infection. Despite intensive antibiotic therapy, septicemia persists until the pacemaker and, above all, the leads have been completely removed. Systemic infection must also be suspected in paced patients with a recurrent fever despite antibiotic therapy; if all causes of infection can be clearly excluded, the complete removal of the pacing system must be considered.

Necessary Conditions. These can become life-threatening. Examples include pocket infection, chronic draining sinus, and pacing system erosion with partial exposure of the pacemaker and/or the leads. All the situations with a chronic local infection are associated with a high number of reinterventions and if infected leads are not removed, the mortality rate can be as high as 66% (4). It is well known that too many leads in the venous system can produce a fibrous reaction with vein obliteration and, possibly, superior vena cava syndrome if the leads come from opposite sides; therefore, in the presence of a lead failure and if a third lead or more leads are needed, the extraction of the functionless ones may be indicated.

Discretionary Conditions. These include all the cases of noninfected functionless or abandoned leads. This is a controversial indication for lead removal and although abandoned leads do not cause any symptomatic abnormalities for many years, we must bear in mind the fact that the incidence of asymptomatic thrombosis has been reported to be as high as 44% (5, 22) and that removing the leads becomes more difficult with time. The discretionary conditions are probably influenced by other variables, such as the patient's age and his or her clinical condition or the implant duration of the leads.

Techniques of Lead Extraction

Lead extraction may be accomplished by traction, intravascular countertraction, or cardiac surgery.

Traction

Traction may be exerted on the exteriorized portion of the lead (external traction) or on devices that have grasped the lead inside the venous system. The traction force should be enough to feel the rhythmic movements of the lead without causing arrhythmias or cardiac wall invaginations. Traction methods may be successful with leads that have been implanted for only a few months. A more aggressive traction or the use of weights is discouraged because of possible serious and life-threatening complications; moreover, the lead may be damaged, making further extraction techniques impossible.

Intravascular Countertraction

Recently, new tools for extracting chronic leads have become available (23, 18).

Extensive worldwide experience has been reported with the system provided by Cook Pacemaker Corporation (Leechburg, PA, USA). This system is provided with locking stylets and dilator sheaths; they are used as a first choice when the proximal end of the lead is exposed (*superior approach*). A transvenous workstation with a tip-deflecting wire, a Dormier basket and a loop retriever is the tool of choice in the case of totally intravascular leads (*inferior approach*).

If the lead is exposed and free from the fibrotic tissue up to its insertion into the vein, the connector is removed using a surgical clipper and the conductor coil is expanded using a proper tool (coil expander) (superior approach, Fig. 1a). After checking the lumen patency with a normal stylet, the coil lumen is carefully sized with a proper gauge pin (Fig. 1b). The appropriate pin should exactly fit in the inner coil and an identical size locking stylet is chosen.

The locking stylet is a relatively stiff wire with a loop handle at the proximal end and a thin wire attached to its tip (Fig. 1c); it is inserted into the inner coil of the lead. When the locking stylet has reached the end of the lead, the loop handle is rotated in the opposite direction of the lead coil. The stylet tip is locked into the distal end of the lead. Consequently, the traction force is directly applied to the lead tip, avoiding coil lengthening (Fig. 1d). This alone may result in lead extraction, but frequently dilator sheaths are required. The dilator sheaths are advanced in order to overcome and disrupt the adherences to the vascular wall and to perform the countertraction, avoiding cardiac invagination.

In order to prevent complications due to tears in the venous system, it is very important to maintain the tension on the locking stylet while advancing the sheaths (Fig. 2a).

The inner sheath, which is more flexible, is advanced following the curvature of the lead in the venous system, and the outer sheath is advanced over the inner one to the myocardium, where it counters the traction applied to the locked stylet. Without the sheath, the traction could cause cardiac invagination with possible life-threatening complications (Fig. 2b).

In the case of intravascular leads, a 16-F sheath is introduced via the femoral vein as a workstation in which the tip-deflecting wire guide, the loop retriever, and the basket are successively inserted. The tip deflecting wire, externally maneuvered by a handle tool (Fig. 3a) or the loop retriever, is used to engage the lead (Fig. 3b, c); the Dormier basket is then closed over the lead allowing a firm traction. Countertraction is possible by advancing the long outer sheath.

In some cases, various tools are necessary in a combined approach for the complete removal of the lead.

Cardiac Surgery

The surgical approach may be reserved for mandatory conditions in which countertraction techniques have failed. However, some leads can only be removed via thoracotomy or median sternotomy because they cannot be reached by transvenous tools. Examples include in-

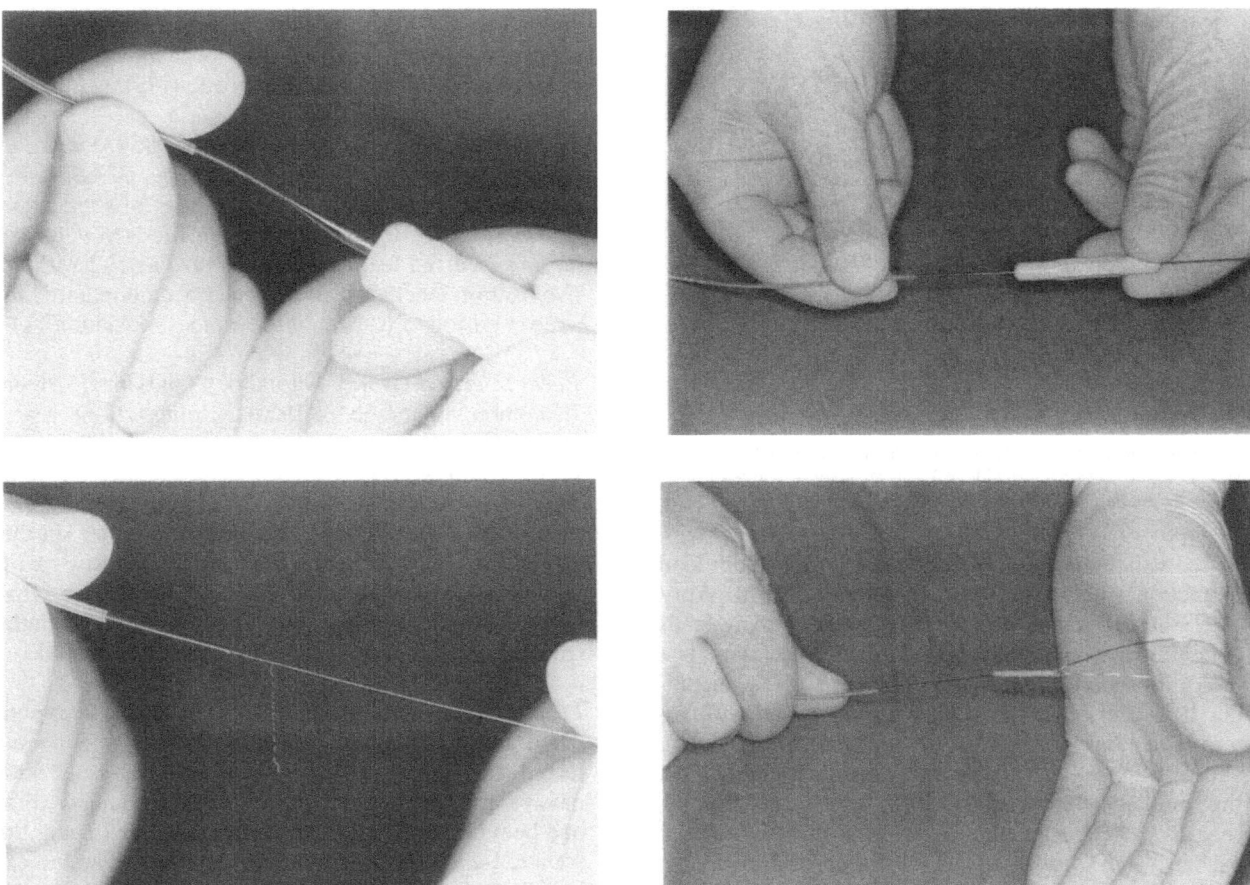

Fig.1a-d. Tools for the superior approach. **a** After having removed the connector, the coil is expanded. **b** The coil lumen is carefully sized with gauge pins. **c** The locking stylet is inserted. **d** After locking the stylet tip at the end of the lead, the traction force exerted by the loop handle is transmitted to the tip of the lead

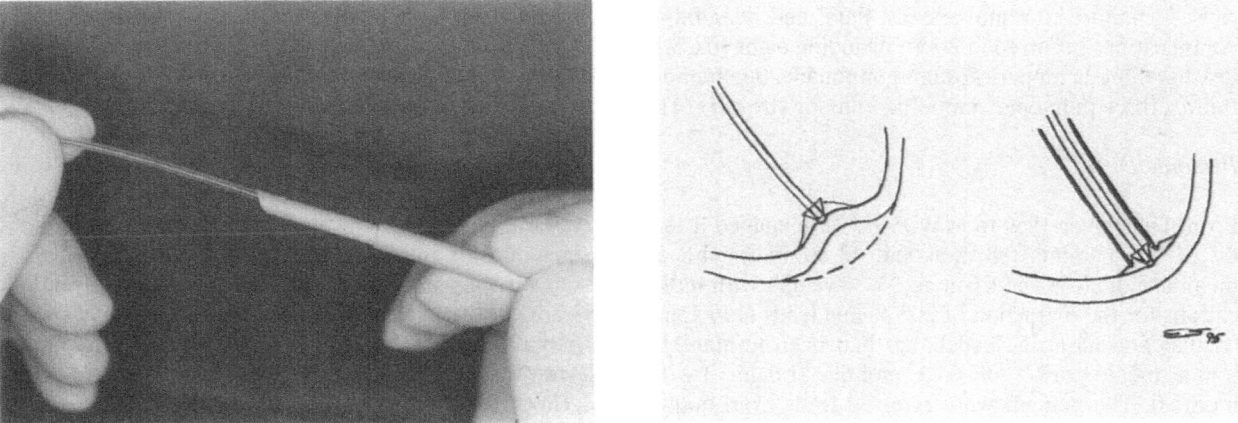

Fig. 2. a The inner and outer sheaths are advanced over the lead to overcome and disrupt adherences. **b** The outer sheath is advanced up to the wall in order to counter the traction applied to the locked stylet (countertraction)

fected lead segments impacted within the heart. Cardiac surgery is also indicated when vegetations are present on the tricuspid valve and/or attached to a pacing lead (demonstrated by transesophageal echocardiography) because of the high risks of septic pulmonary embolism.

A limited surgical approach, different from conventional approaches, must be mentioned (14). This approach eliminates the more extensive thoracotomy and median sternotomy. The procedure consists in resecting the right third or fourth costal cartilage, opening the pericardium, and placing an atrial purse-string

suture. Through an atriotomy incision, the lead is extracted, combining, if necessary, the countertraction technique. This approach is particularly indicated for patients whose veins are not usable.

Clinical Experience with Transvenous Techniques

USA Database

In the USA, a lead extraction database was established

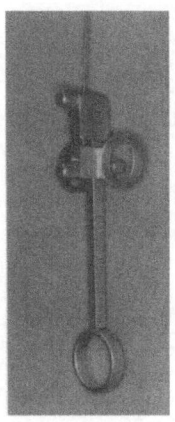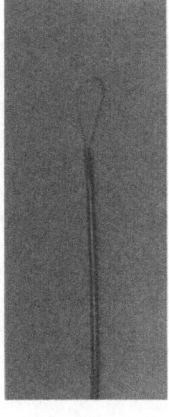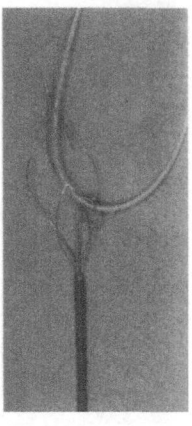

Fig. 3a-c. Tools for the inferior approach. **a** Handle tool to maneuver the tip deflecting wire guide. **b** Loop retriever. **c** The lead is engaged by the deflected tip and put into the basket

to allow the analysis of outcomes for intravascular lead extraction techniques. From December 1988 to April 1994, the extraction of 2195 intravascular pacing leads from 1299 patients was attempted at 193 centers. The indications were the following: infection (54%, including 10% septicemia), pacemaker reoperation with removal of nonfunctional or incompatible leads (40%), and other causes (6%). Extraction was attempted via the implant vein using locking stylets and dilator sheaths or via the femoral vein using snares, retrieval baskets, and sheaths, or via both approaches. Leads had been implanted for 0.2 months to 24 years (mean, 56 months). At the conclusion of the intravascular procedure, 86.8% of the leads were completely removed, 7.5% were partially removed, and 5.7% were not removed. Scar tissue increased in severity with implant duration, was a complicating factor, and was the main cause of failure to remove leads. Fatal and near fatal complications occurred in 2.5%, including eight (0.6%) deaths (three hemopericardium/tamponade, one hemothorax, three pulmonary embolus, and one stroke) (24).

Personal Data

From December 1989 to May 1995, we managed a total of 136 patients (88 men and 48 women) with a mean age of 68.51 years (range, 17-88 years), with indications for the extraction of 200 pacing leads (136 ventricular and 64 atrial leads) that had been implanted for a mean period of 63.2 months (range, 1-276 months). The patients were referred to us from many Italian cardiac pacing centers. The characteristics of the patients and the leads are shown in Table 2.

The population was divided in to three groups ac-

cording to the indications for the lead removal: (1) the septicemia group (SG); (2) the local infection group (LIG); and (3) the prophylaxis group (PG).

Septicemia Group. A total of 56 patients (35 men, 21 women; mean age, 69.24 years; range, 32-88 years) showed clinical and laboratory findings of septicemia. In this group, 89 leads had to be removed (61 ventricular and 28 atrial leads; 77 with passive and 12 with active fixation mechanism). They had been implanted for a mean period of 63.24 months (range, 1-245 months).

Local Infection Group. A total of 48 patients (32 men, 16 women; mean age, 68.19 years; range, 17-88 years) were referred to us because of pocket infection and/or skin erosion and/or chronic draining sinus. Most of these patients had previously undergone unsuccessful conservative procedures at the referring center. In this group, 73 leads (49 ventricular and 24 atrial; 69 with passive and 14 with active fixation mechanism) that had been implanted for a mean period of 63.52 months (range, 5-252 months) were considered for removal.

Prophylaxis Group. In 32 patients (21 men, 11 women; mean age, 67.38 years; range, 48-80 years) 38 noninfected leads (26 ventricular and 12 atrial leads; 33 with passive and five with active fixation mechanism) that had been implanted for a mean period of 63.1 months (range, 1-276 months) had to be removed. The indications were high pacing threshold (nine leads), sensing failure (two leads), both pacing and sensing failure (eight leads), intravascular leads (four leads), fracture (six leads), insulation failure (three leads), diaphragmatic contractions (one lead), lead tip dislodgment (three leads), and implant on the opposite side due to mastectomy for mammary cancer (two leads).

Methods and Patient Management

Before the removal procedure, the patient history was obtained regarding the implant, the insertion veins, previous complications, and treatments. The chest X-ray was examined to evaluate the lead's characteristics, including its integrity, and to look for adherences to the venous wall, cardiac structures, or among multiple leads. In the case of suspected venous obstruction, the patients were submitted to radioisotopic venography. Transthoracic and, when necessary, transesophageal echocardiography were used to exclude the presence of vegetation along the leads or on the valvular apparatus, which is considered to be a contraindication to the transvenous removal.

Table 2. Characteristics of patients and leads

				Age (years)			Paced chamber		Fixation		Pacing period (months)	
	Patients (*n*)	Men (*n*)	Women (*n*)	Mean	Range	Leads (*n*)	Ventricle (*n*)	Atrium (*n*)	Passive (*n*)	Active (*n*)	Mean	Range
Septicemia	56	35	21	69.42	32-38	89	61	28	77	12	63.24	1-245
Local infection	48	32	16	68.19	17-88	73	49	24	69	14	63.52	5-252
Prophylaxis	32	21	11	67.38	48-80	38	26	12	33	5	63.10	1-276
Total	136	88	48	68.51	17-88	200	136	64	169	31	63.20	1-276

After an initial experience, in which all the removal procedures were performed in the cardiosurgical room, a stepwise approach was developed (25). The first attempt was performed in the catheter laboratory; in the case of mandatory indications, if the procedure failed a second and more aggressive one was performed in the cardiosurgical room, and the patients were also prepared for emergency or elective thoracotomy.

The transvenous extraction procedures were performed under local anesthesia; external backup ventricular pacing, continuous electrocardiogram (ECG), and invasive blood pressure monitoring were always ensured. All the maneuvers of traction, countertraction, and sheath advancement were carried out under fluoroscopic monitoring. Echocardiographic equipment to diagnose possible complications was always readily available, e.g., as the possibility of performing pericardiocentesis and blood transfusion.

In all the procedures, we first attempted continuous manual traction for up to 5 min, avoiding irreversible damage deriving from excessive coil lengthening. If that proved ineffective, we performed the countertraction technique, with different grades of aggressiveness depending on the clinical indications, using the transvenous Cook Pacemaker Corporation (CPC) system.

Surgical extraction was reserved for septicemic patients when the manual and the countertraction technique had proved unsuccessful.

After the procedure, the patients were admitted to the intensive care unit for at least 24 h, under constant monitoring of their vital functions; blood samples, ECG, and echocardiogram were taken at the third and the 24th hour. If there were no complications, the patients were discharged between the fourth and the seventh day (Table 3).

In the patients with septicemia, the extraction was performed when fever had been absent for at least 10 days; the new implant was generally carried out after 48 h. Antibiotic therapy was continued for 1 week after the procedure. In case of a preexisting contralateral pacing apparatus not responsible for the infection, the lead was maintained.

Table 3. Transvenous removal procedures: patient management

Time	Management type
Before	Careful patient history
	Radiographic and echocardiographic evaluation of
	lead characteristics
	Patient typed for blood
During	Local anesthesia
	Transvenous backup pacing
	Invasive blood pressure monitoring
	Continuous electrocardiogram (ECG) monitoring
	Fluoroscopic monitoring
	Echocardiographic monitoring
	Rapidly available:
	Defibrillator
	Pericardiocentesis
	Blood products
After	Intensive care unit
	Radiographic and echocardiographic evaluation
	Follow-up

In patients with local infection, the new pacemaker was generally implanted on the other site at the end of the procedure, and antibiotic therapy was administered until discharge.

Results

Our results are first presented according to the different indications to pacing leads removal, followed by the overall results. Transvenous removal was defined as not applicable when a serious lead deterioration or previous attempts to repair or remove the lead had made it impossible to apply countertraction techniques.

Septicemia Group. Of 89 pacing leads, 11 leads were intravascular; seven of the 78 exposed pacing leads (7.86%) were removed by manual traction. The remaining 71 exposed and 11 intravascular leads were considered for the countertraction technique, which was not applicable in two cases (2.25%), while it was successfully carried out in 66 cases (74.16%). Because of the mandatory indication, 16 (17.98%) electrodes were removed by surgery. Therefore, 100% of the leads were removed, 82.02% by transvenous methods and 17.98% by surgical technique (Fig. 4).

Local Infection Group. All of the 73 pacing leads were exposed; manual traction was successfully performed on five (6.85%) electrodes. The countertraction technique was not applicable in two cases (2.74%), while it was effective in 57 (78.08%) and ineffective in nine (12.33%) pacing leads. In this group, the transvenous procedures could be used to remove 84.93% of the pacing leads (Fig. 5).

Prophylaxis Group. Of the 38 pacing leads, manual traction could be used to remove eight of the 34 exposed pacing leads (21.05%). The remaining 30 leads (26 exposed, four intravascular) were considered for the countertraction technique, which was not applicable in five cases (13.16%); 22 (57.90%) of the remaining 25 leads (65.79%) were extracted. Therefore, 78.95% of the leads were extracted (Fig. 6).

Of our entire population of 200 leads, we removed 90.5% pacing leads in total; of these, 82.5% were removed by the transvenous approach (Fig. 7) and 8% were surgically removed.

SEPTICEMIA GROUP

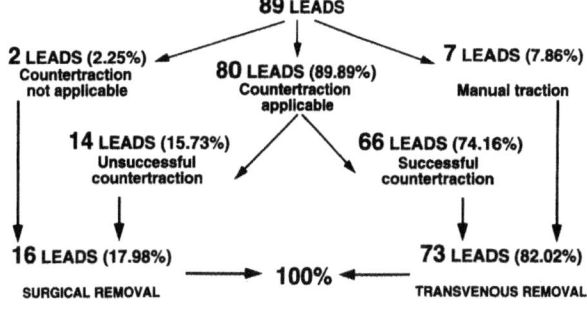

Fig. 4. Results of the removal procedure (including surgical technique) in the septicemia group

155

LOCAL INFECTION GROUP

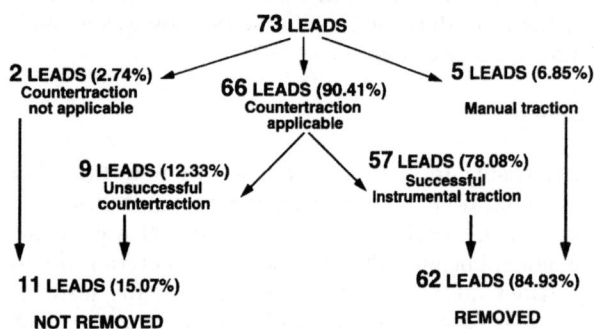

Fig. 5. Results of the transvenous removal procedure in the local infection group

PROPHYLAXIS GROUP

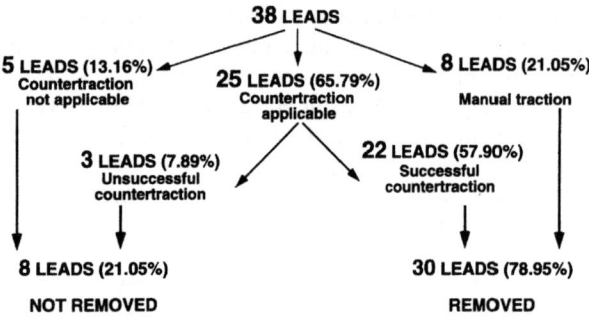

Fig. 6. Results of the transvenous removal procedure in the prophylaxis group

Complications. No lethal complications were observed during the procedures. In the septicemia group, there were two cardiac tamponades requiring emergency thoracotomy. In one case it was provoked by a tear in the lateral wall of the right atrium while using the Dormier basket to complete the removal of an intravascular ventricular electrode after the atrial lead had been removed. The other case occurred after the removal of a ventricular pacing lead where a very strong traction was performed with the locking stylet, while countertraction with the dilator sheaths could not be performed because of strong venous adherences.

Ventricular fibrillation was observed in one young patient affected by restrictive cardiomyopathy with lo-

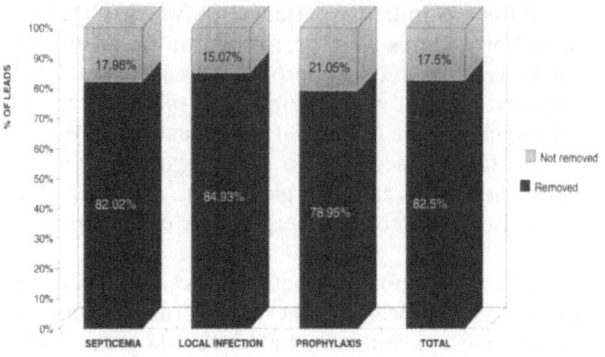

Fig. 7. Total results of our personal experience with the transvenous removal procedure (200 leads)

cal infection 2 h after the end of the effective removal procedure; the arrhythmia was due to a pulmonary septic embolism, which was solved by medical therapy.

The dislodgment of a chronic pacing lead not intended to be removed was observed in one patient from the local infection group.

During the traction on the leads, transient hypotension and bouts of nonsustained arrhythmias constantly occurred, but were promptly resolved by release of the traction. Hypotension requiring medical treatment was observed during the procedure in 13 patients with septicemia, nine patients with local infection, and five patients in the prophylaxis group; this mostly occurred while using the dilator sheaths, probably due to the stimulation of vagal termination.

During follow-up, two patients suffering from longstanding septicemia (from 4-6 months) died in hospital, 1 and 7 days after the removal procedure, respectively, because of intractable ventricular fibrillation followed by electromechanical dissociation. The previous morphologic examination had shown the absence of cardiac lesions related to the extraction; one of them had undergone a successful soft manual traction of one lead. The other patient had undergone three episodes of ventricular fibrillation before the extraction procedure. Such malignant arrhythmias were probably caused by myocarditis foci and were not related to the removal procedure.

One 84-year-old septicemic patient died in hospital 1 month after a successful transvenous procedure because of intercurrent pneumonia. One patient with local infection developed septicemia 4 months after an

Table 4. Complications related to transvenous procedures

Complications	Septicemia (n)	Local infection (n)	Prophylaxis (n)	Total (%)
Cardiac tamponade	2	—	—	1
Pulmonary embolism	1	1[b]	—	1
Dislodgment of chronic pacing lead not intended for removal	—	1	—	0.5
Hypotension	13	9	5	13.5
Septicemia[a]	—	1	—	0.5
Sublcavian trhombophlebitis[a]	1	2	—	1.5

[a]The connection with the removal procedure is suspected, but not definitively proved.
[b]Ventricular fibrillation was the first clinical presentation.

unsuccessful attempt to remove the lead; the lead extraction was performed by thoracotomy.

Clinical symptoms of subclavian thrombophlebitis occurring within 1 month were observed in three patients, two of them coming from the local infection group and one from the septicemia group. These cases were resolved using current medical treatment (anticoagulants, antibiotics, and anti-inflammatory drugs).

None of the patients with septicemia had fever during follow-up; late infective problems were not observed either in patients undergoing a new implant after the removal procedure or in patients with a preexisting pacing system.

The signs of local infection persisted in the patients (referred for local infection problems) with unsuccessful procedures. One patient personally chose surgical removal.

Discussion

The indications for pacing lead removal have been limited to cases of life-threatening permanent cardiac pacing complications, such as septicemia. In the last few years, a great interest has developed concerning the new techniques for transvenous removal, which have been shown to be highly effective and relatively safe (17-20).

Our experience confirms that manual traction is rarely effective, allowing the removal of only 6.9% of pacing leads, particularly those that have been implanted recently; better results could probably be obtained by applying a stronger traction force, but this is often associated with irreversible lead damage, making countertraction techniques impossible.

To optimize transvenous removal techniques, we have recently been using a dynamometer in order to graduate the traction force, depending on the type of approach and the clinical indications to pacing lead removal (25). Up to 82.5% of electrodes can be removed using the transvenous methods and countertraction techniques, allowing the surgical procedure to be reserved for a few unsuccessful cases when the indications are mandatory.

The results of the procedure did not depend on the indications for removal, ventricular or atrial placement, type of fixation mechanism, polarity of the leads, or age and gender of patients. Better results were observed in the last year of our experience, as indicated in Fig. 8 (total transvenous success rate of 92.2%), in-

dicating a learning curve that must be considered by the centers that are beginning this kind of experience. The results were worse for leads that had been implanted for a longer time, probably because of stronger adherences to venous and cardiac walls.

Complications, however, seemed to be strongly affected by the indications for extraction: the major complications (cardiac tamponades) directly related to the procedure were observed in patients with septicemia, because in one case a very aggressive procedure with a strong traction was applied in the presence of cardio-surgical standby, while in another case the complication was probably caused by maneuvering the basket. Remarkably, both cases were observed among the first 80 cases.

Septic pulmonary embolism was observed in one patient with septicemia and in another patient with local infection; although all patients had been submitted to echocardiography, this complication was probably caused by unrecognized vegetations.

The cases of septicemia and venous thrombophlebitis observed during follow-up are possibly procedure related, but all of them occurred in patients with infective long-standing problems; therefore, we cannot exclude the possibility that it is a complication of the underlying infection.

The three deaths reported in our experience were not related to the procedure but to septicemia, which must be considered as a very dangerous disease that requires an aggressive antibiotic therapy. Most importantly, it requires the total removal of the pacing apparatus as soon as possible. Two deaths were caused by malignant ventricular arrhythmias, probably due to an involvement of the cardiac muscle in the infective process. This is emphasized by the occurrence of a ventricular fibrillation in one of the two patients during hospitalization before the removal procedure. Another patient, who is not included in the present population, was affected by long-standing septicemia without documented cardiac disease and died suddenly the day before hospitalization. A third patient with septicemia was referred to us in a very bad clinical condition and, although the extraction was very easy and without complications, his clinical status worsened and the intercurrent pneumonia was fatal.

The complications observed in the septicemia group (not related to the removal procedure) and the well-established high risks of systemic infection occurring in patients with chronic local infection (7) suggest that local infection should also be considered an indication to transvenous lead removal if an attempt at a conservative treatment is unsuccessful.

In conclusion, the techniques now available for the transvenous removal of pacing leads are very effective in the treatment of serious complications of permanent cardiac pacing, and further improvements might extend the indications to most functionless abandoned leads.

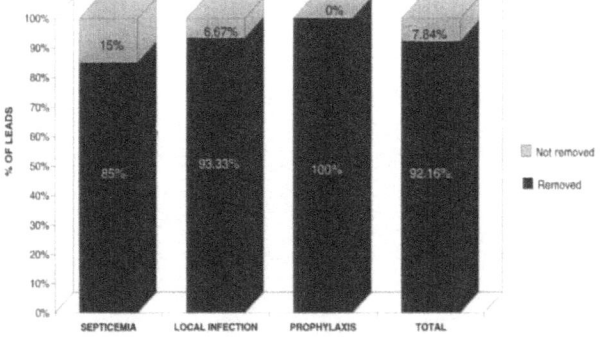

Fig. 8. Total results of the transvenous removal procedure in the last year (51 leads)

References

1. Furman S, Behrens M, Andrews C et al (1987) Retained pacemaker leads. J Thoracic Cardiovasc Surg 94: 770

2. Zerbe P, Ponizynski A, Dyszkiewicz W et al (1985) Functionless retained pacing leads in the cardiovascular system. Br Heart J 54: 76
3. Bongiorni MG, Berti S, Paperini L et al (1990) Should all paced patients be treated with anticoagulants in order to prevent thromboembolism? In: Santini M, Pistolese M, Alliegro A (ed) Progress in clinical pacing. Excerpta Medica, Amsterdam, pp 207-214
4. Pauletti M, Di Ricco G, Solfanelli S et al (1981) Venous obstruction in permanent pacemaker patients: an isotopic study. PACE 4: 36-42
5. Robboy SJ, Harthorne JW, Leinbach RC et al (1969) Autopsy findings with permanent pervenous pacemakers. Circulation 39: 495-501
6. Rettig G, Doenecke P, Sen S et al (1979) Complications with retained transvenous pacemaker electrodes. Am Heart J 98: 587
7. Parry G, Goudevenos J, Jameson S et al (1991) Complications associated with retained pacemakers leads. PACE 14:1251
8. Bilgutay AM, Jensen NK, Schmidt WR et al (1979) Incarceration of transvenous pacemaker electrode: removal by traction. Am Heart J 77: 377
9. Wallace HW, Sherafat M, Blakemore WS (1970) The stubborn pacemaker catheter. Surgery 68: 914
10. Imparato AM, Kim GE 1972 Electrode complications in patients with permanent cardiac pacemakers. Arch Surg 105: 705
11. Lee M, Chaux A, Matloff J (1977) Avulsion of a tricuspid valve leaflet during traction on an infected, entrapped endocardial pacemaker electrode. J Thorac Cardiovasc Surg 74: 433
12. Tallury VK, De Pasquale NP, Bruno MS et al (1972) Migration of retained transvenous electrode catheter. Arch Intern Med 130: 390
13. Garcia-Jimenez A, Botana Albà CM, Gutierrez Cortes JM, Galban Rodriguez C, Alvarez Dieguez I, Navarro Pellejero (1992) Myocardial rupture after pulling out a tined atrial electrode with continuous traction. PACE 15: 5
14. Byrd C, Schwartz S, Sivina M et al (1985) Technique for the surgical extraction of permanent pacing leads and electrodes. J Thorac Cardiovasc Surg 89: 142
15. Yarnoz MD, Attai LH, Furman S (1985) Infection of pacemaker electrode and removal with cardiopulmonary bypass. J Thorac Cardiovasc Surg 68: 43
16. Jarvinen A, Harjula A, Verkkala K (1986) Intrathoracic surgery for retained endocardial electrodes. Thorac Cardiovasc Surgeon 34: 94
17. Fearnot N, Smith H, Goode L et al (1990) Intravascular lead extraction using locking stylets, sheaths and other techniques. PACE 13 (II): 1864
18. Byrd CL, Schwartz SJ, Hedin NB et al (1990) Intravascular lead extraction using locking stylets and sheaths. PACE 13: 1871-1875
19. Byrd CL, Schwartz SJ, Hedin NB (1991) Intravascular techniques for extraction of permanent pacemakers leads. J Thoracic Cardiovasc Surg 101: 989
20. Bongiorni MG, Petz E, Levorato D et al (1991) Removal of chronic leads for permanent pacing. Clinical experience with transvenous extractors. In: Antonioli GE (ed) Pacemaker leads 1991. Elsevier, Amsterdam, pp 289-294
21. Byrd CL, Schwartz SJ, Hedin NB (1992) Lead extraction: indications and techniques. Cardiol Clin 10: 735-748
22. Lee ME, Chaux A (1980) Unusual complications of endocardial pacing. J Thorac Cardiovasc Surg 80: 934-940
23. Reinhardt J, Alt E, Neuzner J et al (1993) Clinic pacemaker lead removal-using a new method in 38 patients with 61 implanted leads. Multicenter experience. PACE 16: 1175 (abstr)
24. Heidi JM, Neal EF, Byrd CL, Wilkoff BL et al (1994) Five-years experience with intravascular lead extraction. PACE 17: 2016-2020
25. Bongiorni MG, Arena G, Soldati E, De Simone L (1994) A "step by step" protocol for leads extraction procedures: relation with success rate and complications. PACE 17/4 (II): 786 (abstr)

SUPRAVENTRICULAR TACHYCARDIAS

Transesophageal Pacing During Exercise: Is It Useful to Evaluate Palpitations of Unknown Origin?

A. Bonso, L. Corò, P. Delise, and A. Raviele

Divisione di Cardiologia, Ospedale Umberto I, Mestre - Venice, Italy

Transesophageal atrial pacing was first attempted by Shafiroff and Linder in 1957 (1). However, it could not be employed because of its low tolerance due to the high intensity necessary for the stimulation.This limitation was overcome by Gallagher in 1982 (2), who lengthened the distance between the electrodes while giving a longer electric pulse duration.

In this way the technique became useful not only to evaluate the passive monitoring of electric events recorded via the esophagus in the heart, but also to induce and interrupt different arrhythmias.

Because of the particular anatomic relationship between the heart and esophagus transesophageal stimulation is most frequently able to stimulate the left atrium. Thus the arrhythmias which can be studied using this technique are restricted almost exclusively to the supraventricular arrhythmias.

Transesophageal electrophysiologic study (TEPS) increasingly became a successful alternative to electrophysiologic endocavitary study (EPS) in evaluating the supraventricular arrhythmias because of the following advantages:
1. Noninvasive method
2. Use of X-ray not necessary
3. No important side effects
4. Higher flexibility of the technique, which can be employed both in the upright position and during exercise and can be repeated several times
5. Low costs

However, the technique is limited since it is difficult to continuously stimulate the ventricles, and it is impossible to perform an accurate mapping during arrhythmias.

In patients with documented supraventricular tachyarrhythmias, basal TEPS or TEPS performed during infusion of isoproterenol has a high sensitivity and specificity in reproducing documented supraventricular arrhythmias: about 100% (3) for reciprocating tachycardia and of about 80% for atrial flutter (AF) and atrial fibrillation (AF) (4).

Transesophageal Stimulation During Exercise

TEPS during exercise was employed for the first time to evaluate the arrhythmologic pattern in Wolf-Parkinson-White (WPW) patients (5), especially in young athletes. An assessment of the risk during exercise was necessary since very often the arrhythmias in these patients occur during effort. Therefore, transesophageal pacing was considered the most suitable method to reproduce the physiologic conditions needed to provoke arrhythmic events. For this reason, stimulation during infusion of isoproterenol or after atropine was preferred.

Usefulness of Transesophageal Study in the Diagnosis of Patients with Palpitations of Unknown Origin

Apparently normal subjects undergoing medical attention often report symptoms such as an unpleasant sensation of fast or intense heart beats lasting from some minutes to some hours. The sensation is sometimes associated with or is followed by atypical chest pain or neurovegetative alterations such as warmth or perspiration. A wide range of arrhythmias may be responsible for these symptoms. The most frequently occurring are Atrioventricular Node Reentrant Tachycardia (AVNRT), atrioventricular reentrant tachycardia (AVRT), atrial tachycardia (AT), AF, and aF (6-7). Occasionally, episodes of ventricular tachycardia (VT) can be observed.

Sometimes the diagnosis is easily made by through the description of the symptoms, but it is not always possible to make a diagnosis on the basis of the symptoms alone. This is true particularly when the electrocardiogram (ECG) is normal, the arrhythmias seem to be occasional or short, or the symptoms are atypical. Many patients suffer from palpitations induced by emotional stress or effort. The procedure is thus as follows: in addition to the routine examinations (complete blood test, thyroid hormone dosage, standard ECG, chest X-ray, M-mode and two-dimensional echocardiography) Holter monitoring and the stress test are performed.

Because of their low sensitivity, both Holter monitoring (8) and the stress test (9) are seldom helpful in identifying the arrhythmias. Echocardiogram is often normal or shows minimal alterations (light mitral valve prolapse).

Methods

In order to assess the clinical usefulness of TEPS during the exercise stress test in patients with palpitations of unknown origin, we studied 216 patients using basal TEPS (127 women and 89 men; mean age, 45 + 18 years; range, 12 - 77 years. All patients had episodes of paroxysmal palpitations occurring at different states (at rest, at night, during emotional stress, during effort) lasting from some minutes to some hours. All patients had more than two episodes of palpitations a year. Documented arrhythmias were not found in any patient.

All patients underwent standard ECG, M-mode and two-dimensional echocardiogram, and 24-h Holter monitoring, 156 patients (72%) underwent the effort test.

The exclusion criteria for this study were as follows: presence of major symptoms (syncope, angina, etc), heart disease (valvular, ischemic, myocardiopathy, WPW, etc), paroxysmal supraventricular tachycardia greater than 3 s or ventricular arrhythmias greater than Lown class I. In the study we included patients with slight hypertensive heart disease and hemodynamically nonsignificant mitral valve prolapse.

For 114 patients (53%) basal TEPS was negative or gave information only about the arrhythmogenic pattern without any sustained arrhythmia. All these patients underwent TEPS during effort.

Basal Transesophageal Study

A quadripolar catheter was inserted into the esophagus, where the highest atrial deflection with the distal poles was recorded. The distal poles were used to stimulate and the proximal ones to register atrial (A) and ventricular (V) deflections. Pulse duration was 9.9 ms. and output ranged from 10 to 18 mÅ. The stimulation protocol included single and double extrastimuli delivered every eight paced beats at a rate slightly faster than the sinus one at 100 and 150/m′ and ten per min incremental atrial pacing until the Wenckebach period of the AV node was reached. Atrial bursts (10″) were at 100 - 600/m′ and increasing rate bursts from 200 to 900 /m′.

Transesophageal Study During Supine Stress Test

The initial work load was 30 W. TEPS was begun after 2 min of exercise and included single and double extrastimuli delivered during atrial pacing at a rate slightly faster than the sinus one and incremental atrial pacing. Increasing rate bursts (10″) were from 200 to 900/m′. If no sustained arrhythmia (reciprocating tachycardia greater than 30 s, AT, AF, and aF greater than 1 m′) was induced, the work load was progressively increased by 30-W steps, repeating TEPS at every

step until more than 30″ reciprocating tachycardia was induced or 75% of maximal heart rate was achieved.

Definitions

Dual AV nodal pathways (DAVNP) were diagnosed in the presence of a sudden increase of more than 50 ms in P-R interval during atrial extrastimulation AVN-RT was defined as reciprocating tachycardia with a V-A interval of more than 70 ms. AVRT was defined as reciprocating tachycardia with a V-A interval of more than 70 ms, and AT as SVT with an A-V ratio of 1:1 spontaneously or as a result of vagal maneuvers or of drugs.

Results

Basal Transesophageal Study

After basal TEPS (Fig. 1) we documented a supraventricular tachyarrhythmias in 47% of patients (102 out of 216). Of this group (group I; Fig. 2) we observed AVNRT in 25% (26 of 102), AVRT in 14% (14 of 102), AT in 5% (five of 102), aF in 39% (40 of 102), AVNRT + aF in 11% (11 of 102), and AVRT + aF in 6% (six of 102). In 22% of the total patients (47 of 216), basal TEPS gave partial information, showing a possible arrhythmogenic pattern as a cause (group II; Fig. 3). In 49% (23 of 47) we documented a DAVNP (15 with atrial echo and eight without), in 19% (nine of 47) TEPS repeatedly showed the occurrence of single atrial echoes with a V-A internal greater than 70 ms suggesting a concealed Kent pathway. In 4% (two of

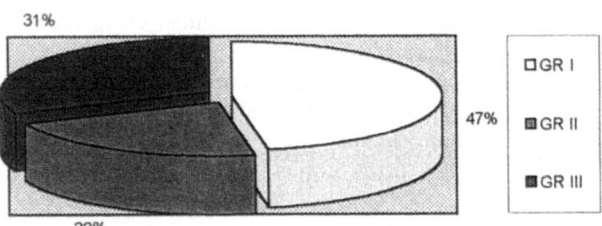

Fig. 1. Basal transesophageal study (TEPS) in 216 patients. *GR I*, patients with induced paroxysmal supraventricular tachycardia (PSVT) during rest TEPS (*n* = 102); *GR II*: patients with arrhythmic pattern without PSVT during rest TEPS (*n* = 47); *GR III*: patients with complete negative rest TEPS (*n* = 67)

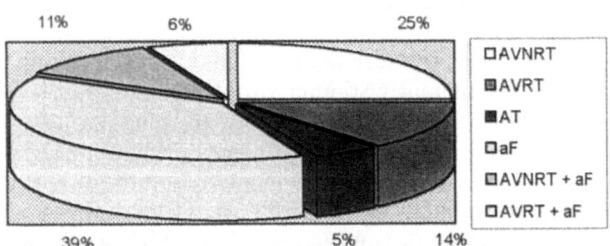

Fig. 2. Percentage of the different paroxysmal supraventricular tachycardia (PSVT) induced during rest transesophageal Study (TEPS) in 102 patients. *AVNRT*, atrioventricular node reentrant tachycardia (*n* = 26); *AVRT*, atrioventricular reentrant tachycardia (*n* = 14); *AT*, atrial tachycardia (*n* = 5); *aF*, atrial fibrillation (*n* = 40); *AVNRT + aF*, atrioventricular node reentrant tachycardia + atrial fibrillation (*n* = 11); *AVRT + aF*, atrioventricular reentrant tachycardia + atrial fibrillation (*n* = 6)

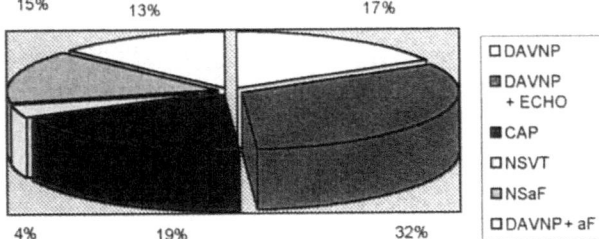

Fig. 3. Percentage of the different arrhythmia patterns found during rest transesophageal study (TEPS) in 47 patients. *DAVNP*, dual atrioventricular node pathway (*n* = 8); *DAVNP + ECHO*, dual atrioventricular node pathway + single atrial echo (*n* = 15); *CAP*, concealed atrioventricular pathway (*n* = 9); *NSVT*, nonsustained ventricular tachycardia (*n* = 2); *NSaF*, nonsustained atrial fibrillation (*n* = 7); *DAVNP + aF*, dual atrioventricular node pathway + atrial fibrillation (*n* = 6)

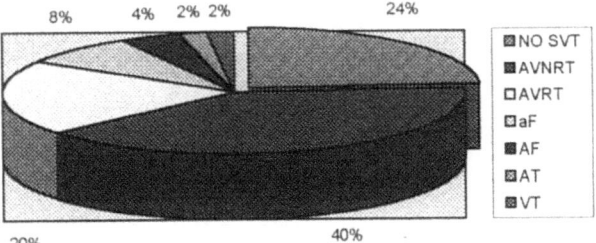

Fig. 4. Percentage of induced and noninduced arrhythmias during effort transesophageal study (TEPS) in 114 patients. *NO SVT*, patients with completely negative test (*n* = 28); *AVNRT*, atrioventricular node reentrant tachycardia (*n* = 46); *AVRT*, atrioventricular reentrant tachycardia (*n* = 22); *AT*, atrial tachycardia (*n* = 2); *AF*, atrial flutter (*n* = 5); *aF*, atrial fibrillation (*n* = 9); *VT*, ventricular tachycardia (*n* = 2)

47) episodes of nonsustained VT of maximum six beats, in 15% (seven of 47) episodes of nonsustained aF, and in 13% (six of 47) DAVNP + aF was observed. In 31% (67 of 216) basal TEPS gave no information (group III).

Transesophageal Study During Exercise

In 114 patients in whom basal TEPS was negative or had only given information about the arrhythmogenic pattern (groups II and III; Fig. 4), TEPS during exercise induced supraventricular and ventricular arrhythmias in 76% (86 of 114). The study was negative even after TEPS during exercise in 24% (28 of 114). We induced AVNRT in 53% (46 of 86), AVRT in 26% (22 of 86), aF in 11% (nine of 86), AF in 6% (five of 86), AT in 2% (two of 86) and VT in 2% (two of 86) (right bundle branch block, RBBB + LSBBB). Basal TEPS and effort TEPS were able to induce a sustained PSVT in 87% (188 of 216; Fig. 7). In the 47 patients in whom basal TEPS gave information only about the electrophysiologic pattern, TEPS during effort demonstrated the induction of PSVT in 66% (31 of 47; Fig. 6), compared to 34% (16 of 47) in which it was not possible to induce any arrhythmias. AVNRT was induced in 61% (19 of 31), AVRT in 29% (nine of 31), SVT in 6% (two of 31), aF in 4% (one of 31). In group II there was 100% correlation between the electrophysiologic pattern found at basal TEPS and the induction of arrhythmias by effort TEPS.

In 14% (one of seven) of nonsustained patients, a sustained aF was induced. In 100% of DAVNP + atrial echo with a V-A interval greater than 70 ms and in 38% (three of eight) of DAVNP patients, without atrial echo AVNRT was induced. In 100% of patients (nine of nine) with atrial echo and a V-A interval greater than 70 ms, AVRT was induced. In 100% of patients (two of two) with nonsustained VT, a sustained fascicular VT was induced. In only 14% of patients (one of seven) with DAVN + aF was induced an AVNRT.

In 67 patients (group III; Fig. 7) with negative basal TEPS, TEPS during effort demonstrated the induction of PSVT in 82% (55 of 67) compared to 18% (12 of 67) in which it was not induced. In group III, AVNRT was induced in 49% (27 of 55), of AVRT in 23% (13 of 55), aF in 15% (eight of 55), AF in 9% (five of 55), and AT in 4% (two of 55).

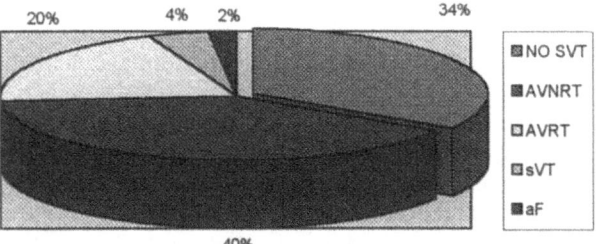

Fig. 5. Final data in the entire population (*n* = 216) studied during rest and effort transesophageal study (TEPS). *NO SVT*, patients with completely negative test (*n* = 28); *AVNRT*, atrioventricular node reentrant tachycardia (*n* = 72); *AVRT*, atrioventricular reentrant tachycardia (*n* = 36); *aF*, atrial fibrillation (*n* = 49); *AF*, atrial flutter (*n* = 5); *AT*, atrial tachycardia (*n* = 7); *VT*, ventricular tachycardia (*n* = 2); *AVNRT + aF*, atrioventricular node reentrant tachycardia + atrial fibrillation (*n* = 11); *AVRT + aF*, atrioventricular reentrant tachycardia + atrial fibrillation (*n* = 6)

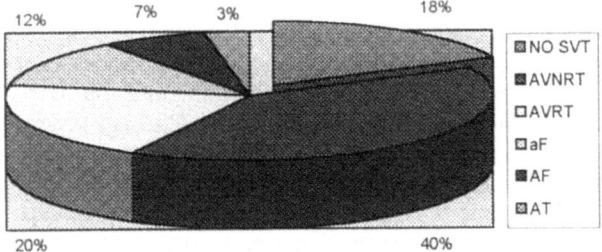

Fig. 6. Percentage of induced and noninduced arrhythmias during effort transesophageal study (TEPS) in 47 patients with only arrhythmia pattern at rest TEPS. *NO SVT*, patients with completely negative test (*n* = 16); *AVNRT*, atrioventricular node reentrant tachycardia (*n* = 19); *AVRT*, atrioventricular reentrant tachycardia (*n* = 9); *aF*, atrial fibrillation (*n* = 1); *SVT*, sustained ventricular tachycardia (*n* = 2)

Discussion

Basal TEPS gave both direct and indirect information about the cause of symptoms reported by patients with palpitations of unknown origin in 69% (149 of 216) of the group I and II patients.

In 70% (102 of 49; group I) it was possible to induce a supraventricular arrhythmia which was acknowledged by the patients as the origin of his or her symptoms. In the remaining 30% (47 of 149; group II) it was possible to discover the arrhythmogenic pattern. In the remaining 31% (67 of 216; group III), basal TEPS could not give any information.

In patients in group II and III, basal TEPS was not

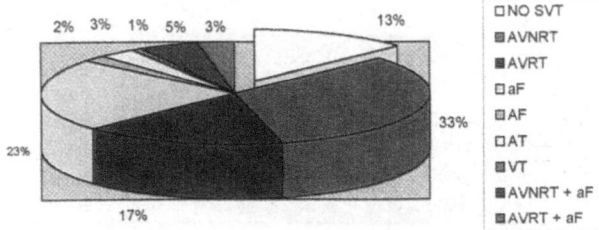

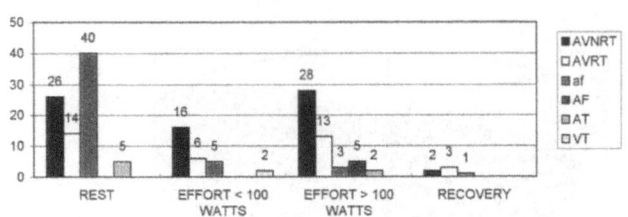

Fig. 7. Percentage of induced and not induced arrhythmias during effort Transesophageal Study (TEPS) in 67 patients with completely negative test at rest TEPS. *NO SVT*, patients still with completely negative test (*n* = 12); *AVNRT*, atrioventricular node reentrant tachycardia (*n* = 27); *AVRT*, atrioventricular reentrant tachycardia (*n* = 13); *aF*, atrial fibrillation (*n* = 8); *AF*, atrial flutter (*n* = 5); *AT*, atrial tachycardia (*n* = 2)

Fig. 8. Different percentage of arrhythmias induced through progressive study steps (rest, effort, and recovery transesophageal Study, TEPS). *AVNRT*, atrioventricular node reentrant tachycardia; *AVRT*, atrioventricular reentrant tachycardia; *aF*, atrial fibrillation; *AF*, atrial flutter; *AT*, atrial tachycardia; *VT*, ventricular tachycardia

the most adequate technique for reproducing the complex relationships between the electrophysiologic substrate and SNA which start the symptomatic arrhythmia.

Most of these patients actually reported arrhythmias at different moments of physical activity (effort peak, immediate recovery, during emotional stress, and in certain postures).

In many previous investigations it was found that the infusion of isoproterenol can be used to reproduce an adequate adrenergic tone (10, 11). Even if this technique has quite a high sensitivity it does have some limitations:
1. It is not a physiologic stimulus, and in the palpitations of unknown origin it is often not an adequate stimulus.
2. It can result in unpleasant side effects.
3. In evaluating palpitations of unknown origin the induction of AF, AT, and aF during the infusion of isoproterenol may not be clinically significant.

Some authors have suggested performing TEPS during exercise as an alternative to the infusion of isoproterenol to evaluate supraventricular paroxysmal tachycardias occurring during exercise or palpitations during exercise in athletes (12, 13). TEPS during effort is often able to reproduce the exact physiologic conditions to start arrhythmias not easily detachable otherwise.

TEPS during effort was able to discover the arrhythmia which is the origin of the symptoms in 76% of patients in group II and III. In our experience, all patients in group II presenting with atrial echoes blocked in the AV node (DAVNP and concealed Kent pathway) had a sustained supraventricular tachycardia induced by TEPS during exercise. In patients with reciprocating AVNT (RAVNT), arrhythmia was induced for a low stage of work (30 – 90 W) and showed a progressive increase of heart rate as the stages increased before slowing and being interrupted spontaneously after recovery.

In reciprocating tachycardias at higher work stages, frequencies higher than 250/m' can usually be induced. Low inducibility of RAVNT during effort in patients with nonsustained aF + DAVNP is probably due to the fact that the presence of DAVNP does not necessarily imply the presence of tachycardia. In fact, during electrophysiologic study, it is not rare to demonstrate the existence of DAVNP in subjects stud-

ied for other reasons and with no tachycardia. It is possible that in patients with nonsustained aF, the low inducibility of sustained arrhythmias during effort demonstrate that in this arrhythmia the action of catecholamine is not relevant.

As for patients in group III, TEPS during exercise can document the arrhythmias in a high percentage of patients (82%; 55 of 67). In this group, too, AVNRT i.e. were more frequently induced 49% (27 of 55) and 23% (13 of 55) respectively. It is interesting to note that 85% of subjects with AVNRT were athletes with a basal effective refractory period of the AV node greater than 320 ms.

In patients with AVNRT, the increased vagal tone at rest probably completely blocked the anterograde slow pathway conduction, which therefore could not be found during basal TEPS. As jump was not present, basal TEPS did not provide any information. Moreover, a sustained arrhythmia was induced with loads higher than in patients in group II (90 - 200 W; *p* < 0.01). These observations suggest that athletes have arrhythmias only during exercise, because training, by modifying neurovegetative conditions, protects patients at rest.

In patients with AVRT, TEPS during effort often induced arrhythmias at exercise peak or during recovery (Fig. 8). This confirms the fact that complex neurovegetative modifications are necessary to start the arrhythmias. It must be pointed out, however, that the diagnostic sensitivity of basal TEPS is lowered, as it is not possible to stimulate the ventricles and thus to disclose a concealed anomalous pathway. As for the inducibility of AF during effort, an interesting fact is apparent. This type of arrhythmia is characterized by the difficulty of induction, since it is induced with aggressive techniques, bursts, at exercise peak, or at immediate recovery. It is characterized by the high relationship of conduction to ventricles, sometimes with ventricles frequencies of more than beats/min and a of 300, wide QRS increasing during recovery. Interruption occurs spontaneously after several minutes, with a lowered ventricular response but an unchanged cycle of arrhythmias. Among the patients in whom arrhythmias were still not inducible at the end of the study, there are probably neurotic or anxious patients and patients for which the physiopathologic conditions required to start an arrhythmia can not be reproduced.

Conclusions

Owing to its feasibility, good tolerance, and absence of significant side effects, TEPS performed during effort is a technique that is suitable to integrate basal TEPS in apparently normal subjects presenting palpitations of unknown origin. This technique reproduces the complex modifications of the neurovegetative tone, through graded steps, stimulation at exercise peak, and immediate recovery. For this reason it is very flexible and useful for reproducing arrhythmias and related symptoms. The high sensitivity and specificity of the method are able to identity patients presenting with atypical symptoms probably due to anxiety.

References

1. Shafiroff BFP, Linder J (1957) Effects of external electrical pacemaker stimuli on the human heart. J Thorac Cardiovasc Surg 33: 544-550
2. Gallagher JJ, Smith WM, Kassel J et al (1982) Esophageal pacing: a diagnostic and therapeutic tool. Circulation 65:336-341
3. Brembilla-Perrot B, Spatz F, Khaldi E et al (1990) Value of esophageal pacing in evaluation of supraventricolar tachycardia. Am J Cardiol 65: 322-330
4. Delise P, Bonso A, Allibardi P et al (1990) Valore clinico e prognostico della valutazione della vulnerabilità atriale con lo studio elettrofisiologico endocavitario e transesofageo. G Ital cardiol 20: 533-542
5. Vergara G, Furlanello F, Disertori M et al (1988) Induction of supraventricular tachyarrhytmia at rest and during exercise with transesophageal atrial pacing in the electrophysiological evaluation of asymptomatic athletes with Wolf-Parkinson-White syndrome. Eur Heart J 9: 1119-1125
6. Bonso A, D'Este D, Delise P et al (1991) Palpitazioni di origine sconosciuta: qual'è l'utilità della stimolazione atriale transesofage? In: Piccolo E, Raviele A (eds) Proceedings of the International Workshop on Cardiac Arrhythmias, Venice, 24-26 October. Centro Scientifico Editore, Turin, pp 229-236
7. Pongiglione G, Saul JP, Dunnigam A et al (1988) Role of transesophageal pacing in evaluating of palpitations in children and adolescents. Am J Cardiol 62: 556-570
8. Brodsky M, Wu D, Denes P et al (1977) Arrhythmias documented by 24 hour continuous electrocardiographic monitoring in 50 male medical students without apparent heart disease. Am J Cardiol 39: 390
9. Coelho A, Palileo E, Ashlej W et al (1986) Tachyarrhythmias in young athletes. J Am coll Cardiol 7: 247-253
10. Huycke EC, Lai WT, Nguyen NX et al (1989) Role of intravenous isoproterenol in the electrophysiologic induction of atrioventricular node reentrant tachycardia in patients with dual atrioventricular node pathways. Am J Cardiol 64: 1131-1137
11. Rhodes LA, Walsh EP, Saul P (1994) Programmed atrial stimulation via the esophagus for the management of supraventricular arrhythmias in infants and children. Am J Cardiol 74: 353-356
12. Delise P, D'Este D, Bonso A et al (1989) Utilità dello studio elettrofisiologico transesofageo durante test ergometrico nella valutazione delle tachicardie parossistiche sopraventricolari insorgenti sotto sforzo. G Ital Cardiol 19: 1094-1104
13. Biffi A, Ammirati F, Caselli G et al (1993) Usefulness of transesophageal pacing during exercise for evaluating palpitations in top-level athletes. Am J Cardiol 72: 922-929

New Approaches to Treatment of Atrial Tachycardia

M. D. Lesh

Department of Medicine and the Cardiovascular Research Institute
University of California, San Francisco, USA

Introduction

Atrial tachyarrhythmias represent a great challenge to successful treatment. Therapy of ectopic atrial tachycardia may be approached with either medical management or, with increasing success, radiofrequency (RF) catheter ablation.

It is important to recall that atrial tachycardia may occur by one of several mechanisms, so that medical therapy will vary depending on the mechanism. Thus, those which require an enhanced catecholamine state for the production of tachycardia may respond to beta blockers. Those which are due to triggering and those due to micro-reentry involving decremental tissue (i.e., calcium-driven action potentials) may respond to calcium blockade. Class IA, IC, and III antiarrhythmic drugs have all been used, though success with any of these agents is no greater than 30%-40%.

Nonpharmacologic Therapy

Because of their poor response to medical therapy, atrial tachycardias are increasingly being approached with transcatheter ablation. RF catheter ablation has revolutionized treatment for patients with medically refractory paroxysmal supraventricular tachycardia involving either dual atrioventricular (AV) nodal pathways or an accessory AV connection. In these patients, catheter ablation is curative, and complications are rare. For patients in whom the substrate of the tachycardia is confined to the atrium and in whom the arrhythmia itself or the ventricular response cannot be controlled with drugs because of inefficacy or intolerable side effects, catheter ablation of the His bundle was an option (1-5). Unfortunately, while preventing rapid ventricular response, this procedure mandates the implantation of a permanent pacemaker and does nothing to restore normal hemodynamics to the atrium. While primary atrial arrhythmias, other than atrial fibrillation, are less common than other causes of supraventricular tachycardia, medical management can be particularly difficult and in the proper setting, such as following surgery for congenital heart disease, can themselves be the cause of significant morbidity and mortality (6-8).

For the purposes of ablative therapy, an updated classification schema is indicated (Table 1). Specifically, it must be determined whether the arrhythmia is due to a focal mechanism (automatic atrial tachycardia or micro-reentrant atrial tachycardia, for example); or to an intra-atrial macro-reentrant tachycardia involving anatomical and/or surgical barriers and a critical isthmus.

Development of Ablative Methods

The presence of either an isolated automatic focus or reentry with a protected zone of slow conduction implies that these forms of atrial tachycardia might be cured by targeting lesions at critical atrial tissue, without altering normal AV conduction. The earliest ablative approaches were surgical and were considered for the most severe cases (9). Intraoperative mapping was used to identify the focus and then either resection, cryoablation, or an isolation procedure was performed. A recent report (10) highlighted the long-term outcome in 15 consecutive patients with ectopic atrial

Table 1. Updated classification of atrial tachyarrhythmias

"Focal"
Automatic (or triggered) ectopic
Micro-reentrant
Sinus node
Crista terminalis
Other
Inappropriate sinus tachycardia
Macro-reentrant atrial tachycardia (involving a "critical isthmus")
Typical atrial flutter
Atypical atrial flutter
Clockwise "typical" flutter
Other atypical flutter
Left atrial
Right atrial – involving high right atrium/crista terminalis
Reentrant involving surgical scars/anatomical barriers
Atrial fibrillation

tachycardia. An effective drug regimen was found in only five (33%) of the 15 patients; the remaining ten patients were treated surgically. Focal ablation was performed in four patients and atrial isolation procedures in six. Atrial tachycardia recurred in one patient. There was a moderate rate of complications including need for permanent pacing but map-guided surgery did demonstrate long-term efficacy in abolishing symptoms in nine of the ten patients.

To avoid the morbidity and technical difficulties of surgery, several groups have reported results, albeit in small numbers of patients, using transcatheter direct current shock ablation (11-13). Because of the potential risks related to barotrauma associated with direct current shock ablation, the need for general anesthesia, and the difficulty in acutely assessing outcome, the search for a more appropriate form of ablative energy lead to the use of RF catheter ablation in the atrium. Recently, RF ablation has been reported to cure patients with atrial flutter (14-16) and automatic ectopic atrial tachycardia (17-22). In addition, recent clinical studies have detailed successful ablation in patients with repaired congenital heart disease.

Concern might be raised regarding the risk of perforation during ablation using RF energy in the thin-walled atrium. Based on the biophysics of RF lesion formation (23-25), it is to be expected that these lesions are transmural in the atrium. Indeed, in animal studies, we have found that the lesions are transmural in most instances (26). Yet atrial perforation has never occurred, to our knowledge, during atrial catheter ablation. This may be due to a favorable change in the viscoelastic properties of the myocardial wall when desiccation and protein denaturation occur.

General Aspects of Electrophysiology Testing and Ablation for Atrial Arrhythmias

The index arrhythmia(s) at which catheter ablation is to be directed should have been well-documented prior to invasive electrophysiologic testing, since aggressive atrial programmed stimulation will frequently induce nonclinical tachycardia as an artifact of electrophysiologic testing. Antiarrhythmic medication is discontinued at least five half-lives prior to the procedure whenever possible, though AV nodal blocking drugs (e.g., digoxin) should be continued if they do not inhibit tachycardia, since mapping is easiest when some degree of AV block is present during tachycardia. Sedation should be minimized, if possible, since many automatic and micro-reentrant atrial tachycardias are sensitive to the autonomic state, and sedation may suppress inducibility which cannot always be overcome with the infusion of isoproterenol.

Multipolar catheters are positioned throughout the atria, including the coronary sinus, high right atrium, and low septal right atrium. As a general principle, as many electrodes as possible should be deployed, depending on the constraints of the recording system. As described below, placing multipolar electrode catheters along regions of likely tachycardia origin, such as the crista terminalis (CT) in the right atrium may shorten the time required for mapping with a rov-

ing catheter. New multielectrode arrays, such as an atrial "basket" catheter, are being developed and should improve the efficiency of atrial mapping. When left atrial recordings are required other than those provided by a catheter in the coronary sinus, a transseptal puncture is generally performed using a Brockenbrough needle and Mullin's sheath (27, 28); alternatively, especially in children (29), a patent foramen ovale may be crossed. While a retrograde, transaortic, transmitral approach can be attempted for left atrial foci, catheter manipulation is more difficult and a transseptal approach is preferred.

Much of atrial mapping depends on determining the relationship of local activation to the surface P wave. However, unlike mapping for ventricular tachycardia (VT), the P wave is often difficult to see clearly. Nevertheless, an assiduous search for true surface P wave onset is absolutely essential, and time spent doing so is more than compensated by a shorter total mapping time. This point cannot be emphasized strongly enough. Recording should be made from as many simultaneous surface leads as possible during mapping. In our laboratory, a full 12-lead electrocardiogram (ECG) is simultaneously obtained, along with intracardiac electrograms filtered from 30 to 500 Hz and recorded using a computer-based digital amplifier/recorder system with optical disk storage. The gain of the ECG channels should be adjusted to visualize P waves, even if QRS complexes are clipped. It is mandatory that an isolated P wave be recorded during tachycardia, not obscured by QRS or T wave, even if only briefly. This can be carried out using such maneuvers as carotid massage or the infusion of adenosine. Caution should be used in interpreting the rhythm with adenosine, however, since it may terminate the tachycardia or cause atrial premature beats from sites other than the targeted tachycardia. Once a clear P wave is seen, a surrogate marker can be employed, such as a stable intracardiac electrogram in the coronary sinus or His bundle position. The activation time relative to accurate P wave onset at this surrogate marker location can then be subtracted from roving map sites to assure an accurate activation map.

If the target arrhythmia is not present spontaneously at the time of electrophysiology study (i.e., not an incessant arrhythmia), single and double programmed extrastimuli are delivered after an eight-beat drive of at least two cycle lengths and two atrial sites as well as atrial decremental burst pacing down to the cycle length at which two-to-one capture occurred. Since the atrium has a shorter refractory period than the ventricle, we chose basic drives of 400 and 300 ms, rather than 600 and 400 ms as is typical for VT induction. If tachycardia is not induced or is not sustained, isoproterenol is infused starting at a dose of 0.5 µg/minutes (or 0.025 ug/kg per min in children) with dose increases every 5 min until the heart rate increases by 40% or tachycardia becomes sustained either spontaneously or with pacing.

Ablation of Focal Atrial Tachycardia

Focal atrial tachycardia, regardless of whether it is due

to abnormal automaticity, triggering, or micro-reentry is best ablated by targeting the site of earliest atrial activation proceeding the *p* wave during tachycardia. Since those focal atrial tachycardias that are reentrant usually do not have a fully excitable reset gap (i.e., the shape of the reset curve is usually purely increasing without a flat portion) (30, 31), entrainment techniques are less useful than for those reentrant tachycardias involving large circuits and anatomical and/or postsurgical barriers and which can be entrained without decremental conduction. Pace mapping to match the surface *p* wave or the endocardial activation sequence (20) during tachycardia can be used adjunctively, but because of the difficulty in clearly discerning surface *p* wave morphology, activation mapping is more accurate.

After defining *p* wave onset and having identified a means for repeated tachycardia induction, activation mapping is undertaken. While mapping should be systematic, the vast majority of focal atrial tachycardias arise from a limited region of the right and left atria, and this knowledge allows a more directed search for the site of earliest local activation preceding the surface *p* wave. The site of origin of the majority of focal atrial tachycardias cluster at areas of change in fiber type and orientation. Specifically, most right atrial focal tachycardias arise from the crista terminalis at the junction of the trabeculated and smooth atrium. In the left atrium, the ostia of the pulmonary veins (usually upper) are favored. In our laboratory, we place a multipolar catheter directly on the crista terminalis using catheter-based intracardiac echocardiographic (ICE) guidance (32). This allows us to easily see the site of earliest activation along the crista terminalis. It also allows us to distinguish sinus rhythm from ectopic tachycardia, which may at times be difficult using surface *p* wave alone during catecholamine infusion when the ectopic tachycardia arises from high on the crista terminalis.

Left atrial tachycardias usually arise from near the pulmonary veins, but initial localization can at times be confusing, for several reasons. First, atrial activation times during tachycardia in the coronary sinus are usually late with respect to many times in the right atrium (right atrium appendage and His bundle electrogram, for example). This is because the coronary sinus is relatively inferior and anterior as compared to the pulmonary veins which enter the left atrium posteriorly. Second, it should be noted that the right pulmonary veins are actually *rightward* of substantial portions of the right atrium, especially the septum and the some of the appendage. When much of the posterosuperior right atrium has an equivalent activation time with respect to the *p* wave during tachycardia of -10 to -20 ms, it is most likely that the tachycardia has its origin at the ostium of the right upper pulmonary vein which enters directly behind the right atrium. Matters are further confounded by the unreliability of the surface *p* wave vector for indicating tachycardia origin. For example, tachycardias can arise from the most superomedial (i.e., leftward) portion of the crista terminalis and produce a negative *p* wave in lead aVl during tachycardia.

Ultimately, the site of earliest activation which precedes *p* wave onset by more than 30 ms must be identified. In a group of 20 patients with successful ablation of focal atrial tachycardia from our institution, the average activation time at successful sites was -48±8 ms before the surface *p* wave. Walsh et al. (22) also reported early activation at successful sites with atrial activation preceding the onset of surface P wave by 20-60 ms (median, 42 ms). Interestingly, low amplitude and fractionated electrograms are recorded from a small surrounding region before successful ablation in most patients, and this combined with early activation is the best site for targeting energy delivery. Atrial fractionation may be due to a region of more generally dysfunctional atrial tissue exhibiting abnormal automaticity in the midst of relatively poorly coupled fibers. Such relative uncoupling between normal surrounding atrium and a focus of automaticity may in fact be a requirement such that normal atrium is prevented from electrotonically inhibiting abnormal phase-4 depolarization. In other words, one beneficial outcome of normal cell-to-cell coupling is to *prevent* a few cells from becoming established as an ectopic automatic focus. The requirement of relative uncoupling for automatic cells to drive normal cells has been shown in computer modeling (33) and in vitro studies (34).

In general, energy application should be performed during tachycardia. At target sites, 20-50 W of unmodulated RF energy are delivered for 10-15 s between the tip of the ablation catheter and a large surface area skin patch. Acceleration of tachycardia is an excellent sign for impending success for automatic rhythms, presumably because the firing rate increases with heating. Once tachycardia terminates, energy application may be continued for 60-100 s. If a sudden rise in impedance occurs during energy application, energy delivery is discontinued, the catheter removed and adherent coagulum cleaned from its tip. New ablation systems employing thermistor-tipped catheters are particularly advantageous, since power can be titrated to achieve a tip–tissue interface temperature of 65°-70°C: high enough to ensure lesion formation, while avoiding boiling, coagulum formation and impedance rises (25, 35). Tip temperature monitoring should enhance the safety and efficacy of ablation in the atrium.

Ablation of Tachycardias Involving the Sinus Node

Tachycardias very near the sinus node can either be sinus node reentry, inappropriate sinus tachycardia, or a focal automatic atrial tachycardia at the superior aspect of the crista terminalis. Sinus node reentry can be viewed as a specific example of the more general focal reentrant atrial tachycardia which can occur anywhere along the crista terminalis. In patients with sinus node reentry, it appears that ablation can be successfully directed such that tachycardia is abolished without affecting sinus node function.

Focal automatic tachycardias near the sinus node are treated in the same fashion as those which occur anywhere else in the atrium.

For patients with inappropriate sinus tachycardia syndrome, RF energy can be used to modify sinus node function. The fundamental concept is that the sinus node is a distributed structure, with the most rapid (and most catecholamine-sensitive) portion at the most superomedial portion of the crista terminalis and progressively slower rates more inferiorly located. While the technique of sinus node modification is still in evolution, we have found that an essentially anatomical approach is effective. ICE is used in our laboratory to identify the most superomedial portion of the crista terminalis and to guide placement of the ablation electrode to the site where RF energy is applied. ICE is also able to confirm lesion formation. The goal is to obtain a reduction of 20-30 beat/min in the maximal heart rate after Isuprel (isoproterenol) and atropine infusion. In so doing, normal chronotropic responsiveness can be maintained without the excessive rates with minimal exertion so bothersome to these patients. It should be emphasized that this technique is difficult to effectively employ with fluoroscopic-guided catheter positioning alone. The ablation catheter tip must be firmly applied directly to the crista terminalis, and this endocardial feature cannot be visualized by X-ray. Indeed, with ICE it can be appreciated that a slight movement of the catheter, which is imperceptible with fluoroscopy, will take the tip well off the crista.

Approach to Catheter Ablation in Patients with Macro-Reentrant Atrial Tachycardia

Reentrant atrial tachycardia occurs most commonly in the setting of structural atrial defects, in particular prior to atrial surgery. Patients with atrial arrhythmias complicating the late postoperative course of surgery for congenital heart disease present a particular technical challenge because of distorted postsurgical anatomy and the presence of multiple arrhythmias in many. Nevertheless, arrhythmias are quite common following extensive atrial surgery (6, 8) and may be partially responsible for the occurrence of sudden death in such patients. Therapeutic options may be limited in these patients; sinus node disease and ventricular dysfunction may increase the risk of antiarrhythmic medication. Antibradycardia and antitachycardia pacing may be problematic in patients with residual intracardiac shunting. Finally, loss of AV synchrony, which may accompany AV node ablation, may not be well tolerated in such patients. Ablation of the substrate for atrial tachycardia avoids many or all of these problems and may be the preferred approach.

Successful ablation requires identification of a protected isthmus of conduction which is narrow enough for an RF lesion (or series of lesions) to be able to bridge constraining barriers. Unlike type I atrial flutter, however, the slow region is not in a constant anatomical location, but will vary from patient to patient depending on the operation which has been performed. Therefore, careful review of operative reports and echocardiograms is essential to plan mapping and ablation for patients with atrial tachycardia following atrial surgery. The critical isthmus can include the space between a Fontan conduit and the tricuspid annulus or superior vena cava (SVC), a corridor between a Mustard atrial baffle and the coronary sinus ostium,

or between an atrial septal patch and the tricuspid annulus (16, 36). The atriotomy scar on the lateral right atrium often plays an important role in the genesis of tachycardia in analogy to the animal models of atrial "flutter" (37-39), irrespective of the surgery performed, but particularly in the case of prior repair of atrial septal defects. The surgeon gains access to the interior of the right atrium and atrial septum via an oblique incision from the right atrial appendage down to the inferoposterolateral right atrial free wall. The incision typically stops short of the AV groove (and inferior vena cava) to avoid damaging coronary vasculature. However, this narrow isthmus between the inferolateral extent of the atriotomy and either the tricuspid annulus or the inferior vena cava can act as a protected isthmus, with the extensive atriotomy serving as an obstacle around which reentrant excitation can circulate. In some cases, the atriotomy scar can be palpated with the roving ablation catheter as a distinct "stepoff" or ridge. Markedly disparate activation times on either side of this ridge and the recording of double potentials in its vicinity further suggest the atriotomy as a line of block extending from the inferolateral to the anteromedial right atrial free wall. Extending the scar from the atriotomy to the inferior vena cava or tricuspid annulus using RF energy is curative in these patients. In some cases, extending the atriotomy superiorly using RF, making a lesion up to the SVC, has been curative.

Selecting target sites for ablation of reentrant atrial tachycardia requires careful electrophysiologic evaluation. The technique of entrainment with concealed fusion, developed initially for identification of successful ablation target sites in coronary disease VT (40), is quite useful for finding a protected isthmus in macro-reentrant atrial tachycardia.

Results of Ablation for Atrial Tachycardias

As shown in Table 2, acute success, defined by absence of tachycardia spontaneously, after the infusion of isoproterenol, or with aggressive programmed stimulation can be acheived in 80%-95% of cases (16, 18, 22). Recurrence is to be expected in approximately 5%-15% of apparently successfully treated individuals. In some cases this is due to the development of another focus.

Complications

Fortunately, it appears that complications of ablation in the atrium are unusual. The only complication in over 50 patients treated at our institution has been femoral venous thrombosis which developed the day after the procedure in a 77-year-old woman who had successful ablation of atrial flutter. We had not been routinely anticoagulating patients undergoing right-sided procedures, though this policy is now under review. There have not been complications from application of RF energy to the endocardium. Similar safety has been reported by others (14, 15, 18, 22, 26). However, no large series have been published and the follow-up has been brief. Therefore, atrial ablation must,

Table 2. Summary of the approach to ablation in patients with atrial arrhythmias, including the electrophysiologic method for chosing target sites and the commonest locations

Arrhythmia	Approach to targeting	Usual sites	Fragmented electrograms at successful sites?	Expected acute success rate[a] (%)	Expected recurrence rate[a] (%)
Focal automatic atrial tachycardia	Activation mapping; ± endocardial pace-mapping (20)	Crista terminalis, opening of pulmonary veins	++	80-95	10-20
Focal reentrant atrial tachycardia	Activation mapping; Endocardial pace-mapping or "concealed entrianment"	Crista terminalis, coronary sinus ostium	+++	80-95	10-20
Macro-reentrant atrial tachycardia	Activation mapping followed by concealed entrainment with PPI=TCL, and StP=AT	Near surgical scars and/or anatomical obstacles; esp. atriotomy; RF lesion must bridge critical isthmuis	+++	70-80	10
Sinus node reentry	Activation mapping	Between SVC and crista terminalis	++	80-95	5-10
Inappropriate sinus tachycardia	Anatomical approach guided by intracardiac echocardiography	Most superiomedial aspect of crista terminalis; multiple lesions over 1-1.5 cm may be required	–	95	??

AT, atrial tachycardia; RF, radiofrequency; SVC, superior vena cava; PPI, postpacing interval measured at the pacing catheter; TCL, tachycardia cycle length; S+P, interval from stimulus to P wave.
[a]Based on results reported from (10, 14-18, 20, 22, 41, 42).

at the time of this writing, still be considered to be under development and should only be performed by interventional electrophysiologists with adequate training and experience.

Conclusion

Chronic medical therapy, empirically chosen, is usually not totally effective for patients with atrial tachycardias. Table 2 summarizes the approach and expected results of curative catheter ablation for automatic and reentrant atrial arrhythmias. Results to date indicate that RF catheter ablation, by severing corridors of slow conduction or abolishing foci of abnormal automaticity, can safely treat atrial arrhythmias in humans. Recurrence is not uncommon in patients with structural heart disease, the reasons for which require further investigation. However, repeat ablation is usually successful. Tachycardia-related cardiomyopathy reverses after successful ablation of automatic atrial tachycardia, and it is quite important to recognize this disorder.

Long-term follow-up will be required to ascertain the incidence of recurrence or the emergence of new arrhythmias, given that many of these patients have progressive atrial disease. Nevertheless, RF catheter ablation offers the potential for curing patients with atrial arrhythmias who cannot be treated by other means. Time will tell whether the most common atrial arrhythmia, atrial fibrillation, will ever be curable using catheter ablative techniques.

References

1. Langberg JJ, Chin M, Schamp DJ, Lee MA, Goldberger J, Pederson DN, Oeff M, Lesh MD, Griffin JC, Scheinman MM (1991) Ablation of the atrioventricular junction with radiofrequency energy using a new electrode catheter. Am J Cardiol 67 (2): 142-147
2. Huang SK, Bharati S, Graham AR, Lev M, Marcus FI, Odell RC (1987) Closed chest catheter desiccation of the atrioventricular junction using radiofrequency energy-a new method of catheter ablation. J Am Coll Cardiol 9: 349-358
3. Jackman WM, Wang XZ, Friday KJ, Fitzgerald DM, Roman C, Moulton K, Margolis PD, Bowman AJ, Kuck KH, Naccarelli GV (1991) Catheter ablation of atrioventricular junction using radiofrequency current in 17 patients. Comparison of standard and large-tip catheter electrodes. Circulation 83 (5): 1562-1576
4. Gonzalez R, Scheinman M, Margaretten W, Rubinstein M (1981) Closed-chest electrode-catheter technique for His bundle ablation in dogs. Am J Physiol (Heart Circ Physiol 10) 241: H283-H287
5. Sousa J, el Atassi R, Rosenheck S, Calkins H, Langberg J, Morady F (1991) Radiofrequency catheter ablation of the atrioventricular junction from the left ventricle. Circulation 84 (2): 567-571
6. Garson A, Bink-Boelkens M, Hesslein PS, Hordof AJ, Keane JF, Neches WH, Porter CJ (1985) Atrial flutter in the young: a collaborative study of 380 cases. J Am Coll Cardiol 6: 871-878
7. Garson AJ, Moak JP, Friedman RA, Perry JC, Ott DA (1989) Surgical treatment of arrhythmias in children. Cardiol Clin 7 (2): 319-329
8. Bink-Boelkens M, Velvis H, Homan van der Heide J, Eygelaar A, Hardjowijono R (1983) Dysrhythmias after atrial surgery in children. Am Heart J 106 (1): 125-130
9. Josephson M, Spear J, Harken A, Horowitz L, Dorio R (1982) Surgical excision of automatic atrial tachycardia: anatomic and electrophysiologic correlates. Am Heart J 104 (5): 1076-1085
10. Prager NA, Cox JL, Lindsay BD, Ferguson TJ, Osborn JL, Cain ME (1993) Long-term effectiveness of surgical treatment of ectopic atrial tachycardia [see comments]. J Am Coll Cardiol 22: 85-92
11. Gillette PC, Wampler DG, Garson AJ, Zinner A, Ott D, Cooley D (1985) Treatment of atrial automatic tachcyardia by ablation procedures. J Am Coll Cardiol 6: 405-409
12. O'Nunain S, Linker NJ, Sneddon JF, Debbas NM, Camm AJ, Ward DE (1992) Catheter ablation by low energy DC shocks for successful management of atrial flutter. Br Heart J 67 (1): 67-71
13. Saoudi N, Atallah G, Kirkorian G, Touboul P (1990) Catheter

ablation of the atrial myocardium in human type I atrial flutter. Circulation 81 (3): 762-771

14. Cosio FG, Lopez GM, Goicolea A, Arribas F, Barroso JL (1993) Radiofrequency ablation of the inferior vena cava-tricuspid valve isthmus in common atrial flutter. Am J Cardiol 71 (8): 705-709

15. Feld GK, Fleck RP, Chen PS, Boyce K, Bahnson TD, Stein JB, Calisi CM, Ibarra M (1992) Radiofrequency catheter ablation for the treatment of human type 1 atrial flutter. Identification of a critical zone in the reentrant circuit by endocardial mapping techniques. Circulation 86 (4): 1233-1240

16. Lesh MD, Van Hare GF, Epstein LM, Fitzpatrick AP, Scheinman MM, Lee RJ, Kwasman MA, Grogin HR, Griffin JC (1994) Radiofrequency catheter ablation of atrial arrhythmias. Results and mechanisms. Circulation 89 (3): 1074-1089

17. Kall JG, Wilber DJ (1992) Radiofrequency catheter ablation of an automatic atrial tachycardia in an adult. Pace Pacing Clin Electrophysiol 15 (3): 281-287

18. Kay GN, Chong F, Epstein AE, Dailey SM, Plumb VJ (1993) Radiofrequency ablation for treatment of primary atrial tachycardias. J Am Coll Cardiol 21 (4): 901-909

19. Lau YR, Gillette PC, Wienecke MM, Case CL (1992) Successful radiofrequency catheter ablation of an atrial ectopic tachycardia in an adolescent. Am Heart J 123 (5): 1384-1386

20. Tracy CM, Swartz JF, Fletcher RD, Hoops HG, Solomon AJ, Karasik PE, Mukherjee D (1993) Radiofrequency catheter ablation of ectopic atrial tachycardia using paced activation sequence mapping. J Am Coll Cardiol 21 (4): 910-917

21. Van Hare GF, Velvis H, Langberg JJ (1990) Successful transcatheter ablation of congenital junctional ectopic tachycardia in a ten-month-old infant using radiofrequency energy. PACE 13: 730-735

22. Walsh EP, Saul JP, Hulse JE, Rhodes LA, Hordof AJ, Mayer JE, Lock JE (1992) Transcatheter ablation of ectopic atrial tachycardia in young using radiofrequency current. Circulation 86 (4): 1138-1146

23. Haverkamp W, Hindricks G, Gulker H, Rissel U, Pfennings W, Borggrefe M, Breithardt G (1989) Coagulation of ventricular myocardium using radiofrequency alternating current: biophysical aspects and experimental findings. Pace 14: 187-195

24. Haines DE, Watson DD, Verow AF (1990) Electrode radius predicts lesion radius during radiofrequency energy heating. Validation of a proposed thermodynamic model. Circ Res 67 (1): 124-129

25. Haines DE (1993) The biophysics of radiofrequency catheter ablation in the heart: the importance of temperature monitoring. Pace Pacing Clin Electrophysiol 23: 586-591

26. Chu E, Chin M, Fitzgerald P, Sudhir K, Heidenreich P, Schiller N, Yock P, Lesh M (1993) Intra-cardiac echocardiography during radio-frequency ablation: a new and accurate method of anatomic localization. J Am Coll Cardiol 21 (2): 417A

27. Brockenbrough E, Braunwald E (1960) A new technique for left ventricular angiocardiography and transseptal left heart catheterization. Am J Cardiol 6: 1062-1067

28. Neches W, Mullins C, RL W (1972) Percutaneous sheat cardiac catheterization. Am J Cardiol 30: 378-384

29. Van Hare GF, Silverman NH (1989) Contrast two-dimensional echocardiography in congenital heart disease: techniques, indications and clinical utility. J Am Coll Cardiol 13: 673-686

30. Chen SA, Chiang CE, Yang CJ, Cheng CC, Wu TJ, Wang SP, Chiang BN, Chang MS (1994) Sustained atrial tachycardia in adult patients. Electrophysiological characteristics, pharmacological response, possible mechanisms, and effects of radiofrequency ablation. Circulation 90 (3): 1262-1278

31. Chen SA, Chiang CE, Yang CJ, Cheng CC, Wu TJ, Wang SP, Chiang BN, Chang MS (1993) Radiofrequency catheter ablation of sustained intra-atrial reentrant tachycardia in adult patients. Identification of electrophysiological characteristics and endocardial mapping techniques. Circulation 88 (2): 578-587

32. Chu E, Kalman JM, Kwasman MA, Jue JC, Fitzgerald PJ, Epstein LM, Schiller NB, Yock PG, Lesh MD (1994) Intracardiac echocardiography during radiofrequency catheter ablation of cardiac arrhythmias in humans. J Am Coll Cardiol 24 (5): 1351-1357

33. Joyner R, Van Capelle F (1986) Propagation through electrically coupled cells. How a small SA node drives a large atrium. Biophys J 50: 1157-1164

34. Joyner R, Overholt E (1985) Effects of octanol on canine subendocardial Purkinje-ventricular transmission. Am J Physiol 249: H1228-H1231

35. Langberg JJ, Calkins H, el Atassi R, Borganelli M, Leon A, Kalbfleisch SJ, Morady F (1992) Temperature monitoring during radiofrequency catheter ablation of accessory pathways. Circulation 86 (5): 1469-1474

36. Van Hare GF, Lesh MD, Stanger P (1993) Radiofrequency catheter ablation of supraventricular arrhythmias in patients with congenital heart disease: results and technical considerations. J Am Coll Cardiol 22 (3): 883-890

37. Feld GK, Shahandeh RF (1992) Activation patterns in experimental canine atrial flutter produced by right atrial crush injury. J Am Coll Cardiol 20: 441-451

38. Boyden PA, Frame LH, Hoffman BF (1989) Activation mapping of reentry around an anatomic barrier in the canine atrium. Observations during entrainment and termination. Circulation 79 (2): 406-416

39. Rosenbluth A, Garcia-Ramos J (1947) Studies on flutter and fibrillation. Am Heart J 33: 577-584

40. Stevenson WG, Sager P, Nademanee K, Hassan H, Middlekauff HR, Saxon LA, Wiener I (1992) Identifying sites for catheter ablation of ventricular tachycardia. Herz 17 (3): 158-170

41. Zipes DP (1993) Arrhythmias on the endangered list (editorial). J Am Coll Cardiol 21 (4): 918-919

42. Gillette PC (1992) Successful transcatheter ablation of ectopic atrial tachycardia in patients using radiofrequency current (editorial). Circulation 86 (4): 1339-1340

Atrioventricular Node Anatomy and Physiology: What Have We Learned from Catheter Ablation?

F. Gaita, R. Riccardi, F. Lamberti, M. Scaglione,
L. Garberoglio, and M. Alciati

Divisione di Cardiologia, Ospedale Civile di Asti, Italy

Atrioventricular (AV) nodal reentrant tachycardia (AVNRT) is the most frequent form of supraventricular tachycardia. Its electrophysiologic mechanism has been known for many years. In 1913 Mines (1) first performed experiments on the AV connections of the heart and explained the mechanism of this arrhythmia as follows:

"A slight difference in the rate of recovery of two divisions of the AV connexion might determine that an extrasystole of the ventricle, provoked by a stimulus applied to the ventricle shortly after activity of the AV connexion, should spread up to the auricle by that part of the AV connexion having the quicker recovery process and not by the other part. In such a case, when the auricle became excited by this impulse, the other portion of the AV connexion would be ready to take up the transmission again back to the ventricle. Provided the transmission in each direction was slow, the chamber at either end would be ready to respond and thus the condition once established would tend to continue."

In the years that followed, several studies showed that this first genial explanation was correct, but they better defined the reentrant circuit responsible for the arrhythmia, which is constituted by two different pathways inside the AV node; one was called alpha and the other beta, showing different refractoriness and different conduction velocity.

This assumption was accepted for many years, until recent advances in surgical and catheter ablation techniques showed new findings. In 1985, Ross (2) showed that it was possible to cure AVNRT with surgical dissection or cryolesion of the atrium near the AV node without affecting the normal AV conduction. This suggests that part of the reentrant circuit is outside the AV node and that it also includes atrial fibers.

However, as early as 1981 Sung (3) was the first to show that during ventricular pacing two different zones of earliest atrial activation could be present at different cycle lengths in the same patients: one in the anterior part of the septum near the His bundle with a short VA interval (fast pathway) and the second near the coronary sinus os that was characterized by long VA conduction times (slow pathway).

In view of the fact that, in the common form of AVNRT, retrograde conduction occurs via the fast pathway localized in the anterior part of the septum, the first attempts at catheter ablation were performed in this zone (4,5). These papers showed that a selective catheter ablation via the fast pathway with DC shock was possible in about 80%-90% of patients; similar or better results were obtained using radiofrequency (RF) current. Unfortunately, due to the proximity of the fast pathway to the compact AV node and the His bundle a risk of complete AV block was present and occurred in about 2%-10% of patients. This is, however, too high a price for a generally well tolerated and non-life-threatening arrhythmia In 1990, Jackman (6) showed that selective ablation of the slow pathway in the posteroseptal region, far from the His bundle, was possible using retrograde mapping during atypical AVNRT or retrograde conduction through the slow pathway. However, this approach is applicable in only a small percentage of patients in whom retrograde slow conduction is demonstrable.

From April to June 1992, three different approaches for the slow pathway ablation in AVNRT were proposed. These approaches can be used in all patients with AVNRT. The anatomical approach was proposed by Jazayery (7) and is characterized by a stepwise movement of the catheter from the posterior zone of Koch's triangle to the midseptal and anteroseptal zone, using only the recording of a small AV ratio as an endocardial guide.

In the same period two other approaches were proposed, one by Haissaguerre and us (8-10) and the second by Jackman (11) both using endocardial potentials to guide the use of RF energy. These two potentials are often considered to be similar, which creates some confusion. However, these two potentials are different not only morphologically, but also in the sites at which they are recorded and in their electrophysiologic behavior and significance.

The potential described by Jackman (11) is sharp and it is the latest atrial electrogram following a low-amplitude atrial electrogram during sinus rhythm while during atypical AVNRT the sequence is inverted and the sharp potential precedes the atrial electrogram.

The region where it is usually recorded is less than 5 mm in diameter, but its location varies among patients. It can be recorded around the coronary sinus ostium, sometimes above it, sometimes inside it, but usually below it.

The potential described by Michel Haissaguerre and us (8, 9) is generally recorded at the mid- or posterior septum, anterior to the coronary sinus, but not inside or posterior to it. The site of a more vivid slow potential is usually projected at two thirds anterior one third posterior of the area between the His bundle and the coronary sinus ostium. The potential can change from patient to patient. Sometimes it is slow and sometimes it is slightly sharp, and the AV ratio may be different. However, the most common AV ratio ranges from 0.5 to 0.7.

Although the morphology of the slow potential may be different, it can be identified on the basis of its electrophysiologic behavior. In fact, it is characterized by a progressive reduction in amplitude until it disappears with atrial incremental pacing (Fig. 1).

This potential may be generally recorded in the posterior third of the septum, but it can sometimes also be recorded more anteriorly, up to the His bundle region. In order to minimize the risk of AV block, RF energy should be delivered in the most posterior region, in which the earliest slow potential is recorded.

When the potential is recorded more posteriorly it is sometimes sharper and very close to the atrial electrogram and thus difficult to recognize. Its true identity must be established using atrial pacing. With atrial pacing the potential is delayed and well separated from the atrium; with a further increase in the atrial pacing rate, the amplitude of the potential decreases.

The two potentials can be recorded simultaneously in the same patient in the posterior part of the septum: one, the sharp potential, more posteriorly and the other, the slow potential, slightly more anteriorly (Fig. 2). Sometimes, near the coronary sinus ostium, an overlapping zone where both the potentials can be recorded is present. This overlap zone has been well demonstrated by McGuire (12) using high-resolution mapping of Koch's triangle with 60 electrodes during open heart surgery in humans with AVNRT.

The origin and the significance of these two potentials is not completely clear, and investigations have been performed by experimenter electrophysiologists. Several hypotheses have been suggested. Racker (13, 14), using isolated canine heart preparation, suggested the presence of an atrionodal bundle, forming a sinoventricular conduction system with anterior and posterior AV nodal inputs. The posterior is formed by the medial and lateral internodal bundle converging in the proximal AV bundle. At the level of the proximal AV bundle, it was also possible to record a slow potential, which Racker called the P potential. In her paper published in 1993 (14), she proposed that the slow potential recorded in humans may represent the activation of the proximal AV bundle recorded in dogs, while the sharp potential may be the expression of the

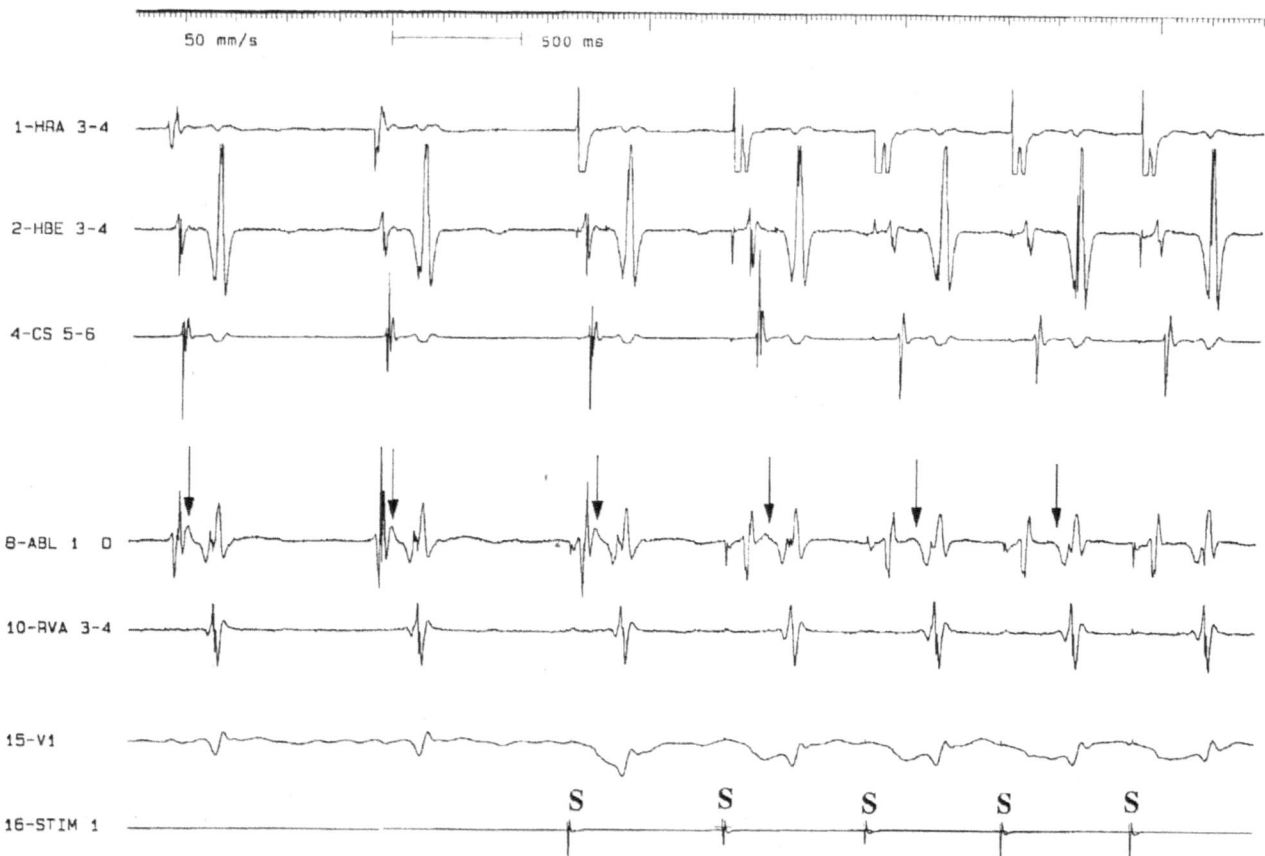

Fig. 1. The slow potential (*arrow*) is recorded close to the atrial electrogram during sinus rhythm. During incremental atrial pacing the slow potential progressively decreases in amplitude, and it moves later in the atrioventricular (AV) interval until it disappears

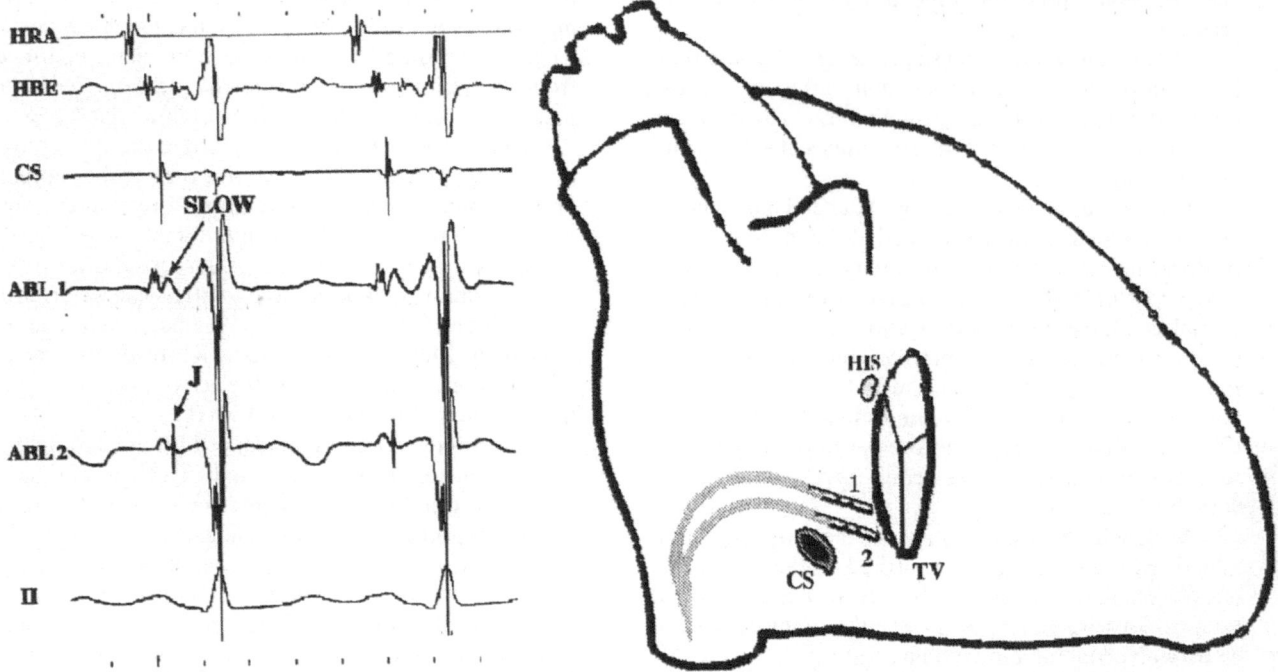

Fig. 2. Simultaneous recordings of the two different slow-pathway potentials using two catheters in a patient. *ABL1* records the slow potential (*slow*) described by Haissaguerre et al. (8), while the *ABL2* catheter shows the sharp potential (*J*) following a low-amplitude atrium described by Jackman et al. (11). *HRA*, high right atrium; *HBE*, his bundle electrogram; *CS*, coronary sinus. On the *right*, a schematic view in 30° degree right anterior oblique (*RAO*) projection of the sites where the slow pathway potentials were recorded. *I*, the catheter position recording the "slow potential" (*ABL1*); *2*, the catheter recording the "sharp potential" (*ABL2*). *CS*, coronary sinus ostium; *TV*, tricuspid valve

lateral atrionodal bundle lying in the low posterior septum. However, a recent study (15) showed that the concept of insulated atrionodal tracts has no morphologic basis in humans.

A different explanation was proposed by De Bakker (16). He showed that it was possible to record a slow potential between the atrium and the ventricle in the midseptal zone in human and in pig hearts and stated that slow potentials arise from transitional cells and have action potentials similar to nodal cells.

In a more recent paper, McGuire (17) showed that it was possible to record potentials such as the slow potential in the midseptal and posterior zones, while potentials such as the sharp potential were recorded more posteriorly. Intracellular recordings in the area where slow potentials were recorded showed an activation potential similar to that recorded in the AV nodal cells. In contrast, intracellular recordings in the zone where the sharp potentials were recorded showed an activation potential similar to that recorded in common atrial fibers.

McGuire explained the different significance of the two potentials, suggesting that the slow potential is due to a band of nodal-type cells close to the tricuspid annulus and not belonging to the compact AV node. These cells may represent the substrate of the slow AV nodal pathway; in contrast, the sharp potential may be caused by asynchronous activation of muscle bundles above and below the coronary sinus ostium.

Whatever their significance, the use of slow or sharp potentials as markers for slow pathway ablation in clinical practice allows us to obtain a high success rate with few RF pulses and a very low risk of complete AV block.

We performed 253 slow-pathway catheter abla-

tions in AVNRT using the slow potential as guide for locating the ablation site; the success rate was 99%, and there was only one case of complete AV block (0.4%). No other complications occurred. Similar results were obtained both by Haissaguerre, using the slow-potential technique, and by Jackman, using the sharp potential as a guide for RF energy delivery.

Only one RF pulse was delivered in about 60% of the AVNRT RF catheter ablations performed by these authors and ourselves, using an electrophysiologic marker (either the slow or sharp potential) for slow pathway ablation. It is important to remember that an RF pulse creates a lesion 4-5 mm wide and 3-4 mm deep; therefore, it is obvious that the fewer the lesions are, the less the damage.

Conclusions

The advent of catheter ablation of AVNRT has showed that the reentrant circuit of AVNRT is not completely located inside the compact AV node, but part of it also involves perinodal atrial myocardium. Selective catheter ablation of either the slow or fast pathway can be performed. The ablation of the slow pathway is associated with a lower risk of AV block than the fast pathway ablation, since the RF is applied in the posterior zone of the septum, which is more distant from the His bundle and the compact AV node than the ablation site for fast pathway ablation.

In Koch's triangle, two different potentials were recorded and used as guides in slow-pathway RF ablation. They differ in their anatomical location, morphology, and electrophysiologic characteristics and significance. These two potentials are recorded in the posterior part of Koch's triangle. The sharp potential is more posterior and the slow potential slightly more anterior. However, an overlap zone may be present. The sharp potential is a high-frequency deflection following a low-amplitude atrium, while the slow potential is a slow deflection following a large atrium. The slow potential changes with atrial pacing, while the sharp potential is not influenced by the pacing rate. The slow potential may be the expression of transitional cell activation, while the sharp potential may be the expression of the atrial insertion of the slow pathway.

Using electrogram-guided approaches in slow-pathway RF ablation for the treatment of AV junctional reciprocating tachycardia, it is possible to achieve a high success rate with few AV blocks, fewer RF pulses, and therefore less myocardial damage than using a purely anatomical approach. Accurate knowledge of the anatomical region where these potentials can be found and of the validation techniques is mandatory in order to achieve good results.

References

1. Mines GR (1913) On dynamic equilibrium of the heart. J Physiol 46: 349-382
2. Ross DL, Johnson DC, Denniss AR, Cooper MJ, Richards DA, Uther JB (1985) Curative surgery for atrioventricular junctional ("AV nodal") reentrant tachycardia. J Am Coll Cardiol 6: 1383-1392
3. Sung RJ Waxman HL, Saksena S, Juma Z (1981) Sequence of retrograde atrial activation in patients with dual atrioventricular nodal pathways. Circulation 64: 1059-1067
4. Haissaguerre M, Warin JF, Lemetayer P, Saoudi N, Guikkem JP, Blanchot P (1989) Closed chest ablation of retrograde conduction in patients with atrioventricular nodal reentrant tachycardia. N Engl J Med 320: 426-433
5. Lee MA, Morady F, Kadish A, Schamp DJ, Chin MC, Scheinman MM, Griffin JC, Lesh MD, Pederson D, Goldberg J, Calkins H, deBuitler M, Kou WH, Rosennheck S, Sousa J, Langberg JJ (1991) Catheter modification of the atrioventricular junction with radiofrequency energy for control of atrioventricular nodal reentry tachycardia. Circulation 83: 827-835
6. Roman CA, Wang X, Friday HJ, Moulton KP, Margolis PD, Klonis D, Calame J, Lazzara R Jackman WM (1990) Catheter technique for selective ablation of slow pathway in AV nodal reentrant tachycardia. PACE 13: 498 (abstr)
7. Jazayeri MH, Hempe SL, Sra JS, Dhala AA, Blanck Z, Desphande SS, Avital B, Krum DP, Gilbert CJ, Akhtar M (1992) Selective transcatheter ablation of the fast and slow pathways using radiofrequency energy in patients with atrioventricular nodal reentrant tachycardia. Circulation 85: 1318-1328
8. Haissaguerre M, Gaita F, Fisher B, Commenges D, Montserrat P, d'Ivernois C, Lemetayer P, Warin JF (1992) Elimination of atrioventricular nodal reentrant tachycardia using discrete slow potentials to guide application of radiofrequency energy. Circulation 85: 2162-2175
9. Gaita F, Haissaguerre M, Di Donna P, Scaglione M, Riccardi R, Bocchiardo M, Richiardi E, Warin JF (1993) Tachicardia da rientro nodale: efficacia e sicurezza a breve e lungo termine di una tecnica di ablazione selettiva della via lenta. G Ital Cardiol 23: 563-574
10. Gaita F, Sacchi R (1994) L'ablazione transcatetere mediante radiofrequenza nelle tachicardie da rientro nel nodo atrioventricolare è sempre una abolizione senza complicanze delle recidive tachicardiche. G Ital Cardiol 24: 931-938
11. Jackman WM, Beckman KJ, McClelland JH, Wang X, Friday KJ, Roman CA, Moulton KP, Twidale N, Hazlitt A, Prior MI, Oren J, Ovrholt E, Lazzara R (1992) Treatment of supraventricular tachycardia due to atrioventricular nodal reentry by radiofrequency catheter ablation of slow pathway conduction. N Engl J Med 327: 313-318
12. McGuire MA, Bourke JP, Robotin MC, Johnson DC, Meldrum-Hanna W, Nunn GR, Uther JB, Ross DL (1993) High resolution mapping of Koch's triangle using sixty electrodes in humans with atrioventricular junctional ("AV nodal") reentrant tachycardia. Circulation 88: 2315-2328
13. Racker DK (1991) Sinoventricular transmission in 10 mM K+ by canine atrioventricular nodal inputs, superior atrionodal bundle and proximal atrioventricular bundle. Circulation 83: 1738-1753
14. Racker DK (1993) Transmission and reentrant activity in the sinoventricular conducting system and in the circumferential lamina of the tricuspid valve. J Cardiovasc Electrophysiol 4: 513-522
15. Ho SY, Kilpatrick L, Kanai T, Germorth PG, Thompson RP, Anderson RH (1995) The architecture of the atrioventricular conduction axis in dog compared to man. J Cardiovasc Electrophysiol 6: 26-39
16. de Bakker JMT, Coronel L, McGuire MA, Vermeulen JT, Opthof T, Tasseron S, van Hemel NM, Defauw JJAM (1994) Slow potentials in the atrioventricular junctional area of patients operated for atrioventricular nodal tachycardias and in isolated porcine hearts. J Am Coll Cardiol 23:709-715
17. Mc Guire MA, de Bakker JMT, Vermeulen JT, Opthof T, Becker AE, Janse MJ (1994) Origin and significance of double potentials near the atrioventricular node. Correlation of extracellular potentials, intracellular potentials and histology. Circulation 89: 2351-2360

Radiofrequency Ablation of Atrioventricular Node Reentrant Tachycardias: Which Results and Predictors of Success and Recurrence?

P. Delise, S. Themistoclakis, L. Corò, R. Mantovan,
A. Bonso, A. Vaglio, A. Raviele, and G. Gasparini

Divisione di Cardiologia, Ospedale Umberto I,
Mestre-Venice, Italy

Atrioventricular (AV) node reentrant tachycardia (AVNRT) is the most common cause of paroxysmal supraventricular tachycardia (1). Many electrophysiologic data suggest that the reentry circuit in AVNRT contains, as its critical components, a "fast" AV nodal pathway connecting the atrium to the His bundle and a "slow" pathway with a longer conduction time (1, 2). In the common variety (slow–fast), AVNRT the slow pathway provides the anterograde limb of the circuit and the fast pathway the retrograde limb. In the uncommon variety (fast-slow) the fast pathway provides the anterograde limb of the circuit and the slow pathway the retrograde limb.

AVNRT can be eliminated by radiofrequency catheter ablation damaging both the "fast" and the "slow" pathways (3-18).

Fast pathway ablation can be performed in the anterior septum by withdrawing the catheter about 1 cm from the His bundle position. Slow pathway ablation can be performed in the posterior aspect of Koch's triangle along the septal insertion of tricuspid valve. Two main approaches are described. In the anatomical approach, energy is serially delivered along the tricuspid annulus starting at the posterior/inferior aspect of the right interatrial septum adjacent to the coronary sinus ostium. In the electrogram mapping approach, energy delivery is guided by the recording of sharp (Jackman) or slow (Haissaguerre) potentials. Jackman potentials are generally recorded in a more posterior and inferior position than Haissaguerre potentials.

The results obtained using these techniques are impressive, with a high success rate and a low incidence of complications and recurrences. Results are slightly better in the slow pathway ablation than in the fast pathway ablation. In a meta-analysis we calculated (14, 15) a success rate of 95% versus 83%, a recurrence rate of 4% versus 16%, and an incidence of permanent AV block of 0.7% versus 8% in slow-pathway and fast-pathway ablation, respectively.

In this report we will discuss the results of ablation of both the fast and slow pathway and the predictors of acute and late success. The discussion will be based on our personal experience and on published data.

Personal Experience

From April 1990 to April 1995, we treated 110 patients; 108 of them had the common and two had the uncommon variety of AVNRT. Patients had suffered from palpitations for 20 ± 12 years, had 20 ± 20 episodes per year, and had tried 2 ± 2 drug trials. In the majority of patients, AVNRT was documented with standard electrocardiogram. Seven patients also had electrocardiographic documentation of clinical atrial fibrillation.

Thirty-two patients underwent fast- and 82 patients slow-pathway ablation. Four patients had slow-pathway ablation after an unsuccessful (two cases) or only transiently successful (two cases) attempt at fast-pathway ablation.

Fast pathway ablation was performed on the basis of an anatomical approach. Distal electrodes of the ablation catheter were initially positioned at the His bundle region to obtain a bipolar recording of His bundle deflection. The catheter was then withdrawn until it recorded an atrial (A) deflection that was at least as large as the ventricular (V) deflection (A/V greater than 1) along with the smallest (less than 0.1 mV) or no His bundle potential. During applications of radiofrequency energy, the surface electrocardiogram was continuously monitored for the P-R interval prolongation and/or occurrence of AV block. During each ablation attempt, the application of radiofrequency current was immediately terminated if blocked P waves or impedance rise were noted.

Slow pathway ablation was performed on the basis of a combined anatomical and electrogram mapping approach. Using the right anterior oblique fluoroscopic view, the ablation catheter was initially positioned in the His bundle region. The catheter was then slowly withdrawn along the tricuspid septal leaflet down to the most posterior/inferior aspect of interatrial septum adjacent to the coronary sinus ostium (site P) in a site where the A to V electrogram ratio was 0.1 – 0.5 (7, 16). At such a site, Jackman or Haissaguerre potentials were carefully sought by slightly moving the catheter tip. Energy was delivered where Jackman or Haissaguerre potentials were recorded. If such potentials could not be identified, energy was nevertheless still delivered. After every energy delivery the inducibility of AVNRT was tested. In the case of repeated failure (generally after two to three attempts) to the P-site, the catheter tip was progressively moved along the septal leaflet of the tricuspid valve (A to V ratio of 0.1–0.5) to more anterior sites up to the midseptum (M-site).

Acute success was defined when AVNRT was no longer inducible. For fast pathway ablation, the abolition of fast retrograde conduction was also required. Acute success was obtained in 87.5% of patients (28 of 32) undergoing fast pathway ablation (Table 1) and in 98% of patients (81 of 82) undergoing slow-pathway ablation. The cumulative success rate was 97% (107 of 110).

Transient II-III degree AV block was observed in 28% of fast pathway ablations (9 of 32) and in 0% of slow-pathway ablations (0 of 82). In all cases AV conduction was spontaneously restored within 1 min and 1:1 conduction was present at the end of the procedure. One patient had an hemopericardium related to the perforation of the right ventricle provoked by a catheter positioned in the right ventricle. The hemopericardium was percutaneously drained.

Patients were followed up for 26 ± 18 months (range, 1-60 months). During follow up, AVNRT recurred in 32% of patients (nine of 28) who had an acute successful fast-pathway ablation and in 9% of patients (eight of 81) who had an acute successful slow-pathway ablation. All recurrences occurred in patients treated before February 1994. A second procedure was performed in ten out of 17 patients (in five patients on the fast pathway and in five patients on the slow pathway). In all cases the second procedure was successful. At the end of follow-up, 92% of patients (101 of 110) are asymptomtic without drugs; 8% (nine of 110) are asymptomatic with drugs or continue to have symptoms. All patients who previously had both AVNRT and atrial fibrillation were successfully ablated and became asymptomatic without drugs.

One patient who underwent the fast-pathway ablation developed a complete AV block 3 days after the procedure; this required a pacemaker implantation.

Table 1. Ablation of the fast pathway; early results in 28 patients successfully treated

		Baseline (ms)	After radiofrequency (ms)	
SCL		700 ± 87	617 ± 67	NS
AH		60 ± 20	120 ± 55	p<0.002
AVN-WCL		311 ± 46	330 ± 38	NS
Dual AVN	Yes	93%	33%	
	No	7%	67%	
HV		44 ± 4	44 ± 4	NS
Fast V-A conduction				
	No	0%	59%	
	Yes	100%	41%	
RAVN-WCL		285 ± 38	444 ± 102	

SCL, sinus cycle length; AH, atrial-His interval; AVN-WCL, AVN Wenckebach cycle length; Dual AVN, dual AVN physiology; HV, His-ventricle interval; RAVN-WCL, retrograde AVN-Wenckeback cycle length.

Fast-Pathway Ablation: Predictors of Acute and Late Success

Fast-pathway ablation is generally performed on the basis of an anatomical approach, as previously described. Some authors (6) prefer to map the Koch triangle during AVNRT and to deliver the energy to the site where the earliest atrial activation during AVNRT occurs. No particular potential is generally sought to identify target sites. We analyzed the endocardial electrogram recorded at the site where energy was delivered in 25 patients. A total of 137 electrograms were analyzed: 25 were recorded at sites where ablation was successful (both acute and late; S sites), 46 were recorded at sites where ablation was transiently successful (TS sites) and 66 were recorded at sites where ablation was unsuccessful (U sites). A slow potential following the sharp atrial potential was observed in 84% of S sites (21 of 25), in 85% of TS sites (41 of 46), and in 45.5% of U sites (30 of 66) (S sites versus U sites, $p < 0.01$).

The occurrence of an active junctional rhythm and the prolongation of the P-R interval are generally considered good predictors of a successful ablation. In our series, an active junctional rhythm during radiofrequency delivery was observed in 72% of S sites (18 of 25), in 54% of TS sites (25 of 46), and in 25% of U sites (17 of 66), (S sites versus U sites, $p < 0.001$). The increase of atrial-His (AH) interval occurred both in patients with definite success (S patients) and in patients with transient acute success (TS patients) or with unsuccessful ablation (U patients). However, the increase in the AH interval (delta AH) was more pronounced in S patients than in TS patients (83 ± 58 ms versus 52 ± 32 ms) or U patients (83 ± 58 ms versus 25 ± 23 ms, $p < 0.05$). Retrograde fast conduction was abolished by ablation both in S patients and in TS patients, while it remained in U patients. During follow-up P-R and AH intervals frequently decreased. In 24 patients we repeated the electrophysiologic study (EPS) 2-4 months after the procedure. Three groups were identified: group I (12 S patients), group II (seven TS patients), and group III (five U patients). In the three groups, the number of radiofrequency pulses were 4.4 ± 5, 6 ± 5, and 17 ± 7, respectively (group I versus group II, p = NS; group III versus group I and II, $p < 0.001$), while the total time duration of energy delivery was 120 ± 154s, 174 ± 100s, and 510 ± 358s, respectively (group I versus group II, p = NS; group III versus group I and II, $p < 0.01$). The main electrophysiologic parameters obtained during EPS I (basal), EPS II (soon after ablation), and EPS III (follow-up) in each group are listed in Table 2. In particular, the following data are worth emphasizing:

1. In most cases AH interval decreased during follow up, but in four cases in group I, in two cases in group II, and in two cases in group III the AH interval increased. Furthermore, one patient in group I developed a complete AV block.

2. The majority of patients in groups I and II lost the dual AVN physiology soon after ablation. During follow up six out of seven patients in group II resumed a dual AVN physiology.

3. Fast retrograde conduction was abolished soon after

Table 2. Main electrophysiologic data before ablation (EPS I), soon after ablation (EPS II) and during follow-up (EPS III) in three groups: I (successful ablation; $n = 12$), II (transiently successful ablation; $n = 7$), and III (unsuccessful ablation; $n = 5$).

Group		SR CL[a]	AVNRT CL	AVNRT VA	AH[a]	DUAL AVN[a] (n)	AWp[a]	RWp[a]
I	EPS I	760 ± 160*	380 ± 61	20 ± 25	64 ± 26***	10	176 ± 37**	187 ± 43*
	EPS II	707 ± 155*	—	—	147 ± 62**	2	164 ± 34**	118 ± 32**
	EPS III	800 ± 130	—	—	140 ± 72	3	173 ± 43	108 ± 25
II	EPS I	790 ± 153*	398 ± 77	13 ± 24	60 ± 17****	7	174 ± 52**	175 ± 43**
	EPS II	710 ± 125*	—	—	112 ± 34**	1	160 ± 33**	127 ± 39**
	EPS III	830 ± 130	408 ± 72	17 ± 28	104 ± 38	6	170 ± 45	170 ± 33
III	EPS I	795 ± 130**	380 ± 48**	24 ± 31**	55 ± 13**	4	176 ± 27**	200 ± 37**
	EPS II	770 ± 120*	381 ± 51**	28 ± 35**	80 ± 25**	4	162 ± 27**	176 ± 34**
	EPS III	905 ± 120	374 ± 39	24 ± 31	80 ± 23	4	170 ± 45	184 ± 27

SR CL, sinus rhythm cycle length; AVNRT, atrioventricular node reentrant tachycardia; AVNRT CL, cycle length of the AVN RT; AVNRT VA, V-A interval during AVNRT; Dual AVN, dual AVN physiology; AWp., anterograde Wenckebach period; R.Wp., lowest ventricular pacing rate at which interruption of VA 1:1 conduction occurred; AH, atrial-His interval.
[a] Mean values in group I are calculated in 11 cases, excluding the patient who developed a complete atrioventricular (AV) block during follow-up.
* $p < 0.01$
** Not significant
*** $p < 0.001$
**** $p < 0.005$

ablation in groups I and II. During follow-up in group I, seven out of 12 patients had no modifications of AV node retrograde conduction properties; three had a worsening of retrograde conduction (two of them lost the retrograde conduction which was present soon after ablation along a slow pathway); two patients in whom a complete ventriculoatrial (VA) block was documented soon after ablation had a recovery of the retrograde conduction over a slow pathway. In all patients with transiently effective success (group II), the fast pathway retrograde conduction recovered during follow-up. In patients with ineffective ablation (group III), no modification was observed.

All these data suggest a series of considerations. First, the increase in the P-R (AH) interval following the fast pathway ablation cannot be explained only on the basis of a shifting of the anterograde conduction from a fast to a slow pathway. It depends also on transient or permanent damage of the AV node. In fact, the increase in the AH interval was observed both in patients with effective fast-pathway ablation and with ineffective fast-pathway ablation. Furthermore, in patients with successful ablation, the increase in the AH interval ranged from a few milliseconds to more than 200 ms. Finally, during follow-up the behavior of anterograde and retrograde conduction properties could be different: in patients with effective ablation, while retrograde fast pathway conduction remained abolished, the AH interval frequently decreased. In contrast, in patients with transiently effective ablation despite the full recovery of the retrograde conduction over the fast pathway the AH interval remained significantly prolonged with respect to the basal state. An alternative explanation to damage of the AV node provoked by radiofrequency could be the existence of more than one fast pathway and/or of distinct fast fibers used for anterograde and retrograde conduction. Transient edema is the most likely cause of electrophysiologic modifications recovering during follow-up. The possible progressive worsening of anterograde and/or retrograde conduction properties (leading in one case to a complete total AV block) can be explained with healing.

From a practical point of view, our data suggest that the recording of a slow atrial potential is useful to identify the target site of ablation. The occurrence of a junctional rhythm is a good marker of definite or transient success. The success of ablation cannot be predicted, either soon after the delivery of energy or during follow-up, by the prolongation of the P-R and the AH interval. As anterograde conduction can worsen over time, a careful monitoring of the P-R interval during follow-up is recommended.

Slow-Pathway Ablation: Predictors of Acute and Late Success

Two approaches for ablating the slow pathway of AVNRT have been described. In one approach, the intracardiac electrogram configuration is used to identify target sites for ablation of the slow AV node pathway; in the other approach, target sites are identified primarily on an anatomical basis. Many studies have shown that both approaches for ablating the slow AV node pathway are safe and effective. Furthermore, some authors comparing the two methods in a random fashion suggest that the two approaches are comparable in efficacy and duration.

We use a combined anatomical and electrogram mapping approach, as previously described. We serially deliver the energy along the tricuspid anulus, starting at the posterior/inferior aspect of the right interatrial septum adjacent to the coronary sinus ostium. We carefully search for Jackman or Haissaguerre potentials by slightly moving the catheter tip. We prefer to deliver the energy where Jackman or Haissaguerre potentials are recorded. However, if their recognition is not possible a simple anatomical approach is employed.

In 59 patients we analyzed 369 electrograms recorded in 59 successful sites (S sites), 53 transiently successful sites (TS sites), and in 257 unsuccessful sites (U sites). A Jackman potential was recorded in 49% of S sites (29 of 59), in 45% of TS sites (24 of 53), and in

34% of U sites (88 of 257) (p = NS). A Haissaguerre potential was recorded in 35% of S sites (21 of 59), in 37% of TS sites (20 of 53), and in 24% of U sites (61 of 257) (p = NS). An active junctional rhythm was observed during energy delivery in 75% of S sites (44 of 59), in 51% of TS sites (27 of 53), and in 14% of U sites (35 of 257) (S and TS sites versus U sites, p < 0.0001). The positive predictive value of Jackman potentials regarding definite or transient success was 37.5% (53 of 141). The positive predictive value of Haissaguerre potential was 40% (41 of 102). The positive predictive value of active junctional rhythm regarding definite or transient success was 67% (71 of 106).

According to some authors (8, 13, 17) our own data suggest that the recording of a slow-pathway potential (Jackman or Haissaguerre potential) can be helpful in identifying a successful target site, but that its presence is not required for successful ablation of the slow pathway. Furthermore, the recording of such a potential is not a certain predictor of successful ablation. In contrast, the occurrence of an active junctional rhythm seems to have a good predictive value regarding definite or transient success of the procedure.

The modifications of AV node electrophysiologic properties after an acute successful ablation of the slow pathway are less impressive than ablation of the fast pathway. In particular, after ablation of the slow pathway anterograde AV intervals do not change and retrograde conduction properties are not modified. The discontinuous AV conduction curve (typical of dual AV nodal pathways) is frequently no longer observed after ablation of the slow pathway. In many cases, however, despite AVNRT no longer being inducible, the discontinuous AV conduction curve persists and echo beats are observed. Some authors (14) suggest that recurrence of AVNRT is more frequent in patients in whom AV node duality persists after ablation. We analyzed the AV node conduction curves (A1A2 versus A2H2) before and after acute successful ablation of the slow pathway in 48 patients. Three types of behavior were identified (Table 3). In 27 patients (56%) AV node duality was no longer observed after ablation (type 1); in 13 patients (27%) before and after ablation AV node conduction curves were similar (type 2); in five patients (10%) a discontinuous AV node conduction curve was present after ablation but the second part of the curve showed a significant increase (60-200 ms) of A2H2 intervals with respect to the basal curve (type 3). Three patients were not classified. The AVN ERP significantly increased in type 1, while it did not change in types 2 and 3. The AVN an-

Table 3. Ablation of the slow pathway. Early results

Type	Ablation (%)	(n)	Total (n)	Result
Type 1	56	27	48	Abolition of the anterograde conduction over the slow pathway
Type 2	27	13	48	Persistence of the anterograde conduction over the slow pathway
Type 3	10	5	48	Appearance after ablation of a "very slow pathway" anterogradely conducting

Table 4. Electrophysiologic modifications after the ablation of the slow pathway

	Type 1	Type 2	Type 3
Dual AV node	0%	100%	100%
Delta "jump" (ms)	—	−9 ± 27	+76 ± 76*
Delta AH (ms)	0	0	0
Delta AVN ERP (ms)	+52 ± 51*	+5 ± 17	+2 ± 20
Delta anterograde WP (beats/min)	−25 ± 29*	−18 ±19	−40 ± 18*
Delta retrograde WP (beats/min)	0	0	0

* p < 0.01
AV, atrioventricular; AVN, AV node; ERP, effective refractory period; WP, Wenckebach period

terograde Wenckebach period significantly decreased in types 1 and 3 (Table 4). Type 1 is easily explained by the abolition of the anterograde conduction over the slow pathway. Type 2 is consistent with the persistence of the anterograde conduction over the slow pathway, while the noninducibility of AVNRT is probably related to lesions of atrial muscle surrounding the AV node. Type 3 suggests the appearance after ablation of a "very slow pathway." The latter can be the result of damage to the slow pathway or of the disclosure of a third very slow pathway which was concealed by the slow pathway.

The three different types of behaviors in our series were not associated with significantly different recurrence rates (three of 27, one of 13, and one of five respectively, p = NS).

Conclusions

Radiofrequency ablation of both the fast and slow pathway is effective in curing patients with AVNRT. Slow-pathway ablation appears to be slightly more effective than fast-pathway ablation. The risk of permanent AV block is low but it is significantly higher during fast-pathway ablation. For all these reasons, slow-pathway ablation seems to be preferable at the present time.

On the basis of available data slow pathway ablation should be performed using a combined anatomical and electrogram mapping approach. The target of ablation is the noninducibility of AVNRT. As recurrence seems to be more frequent in patients in whom residual slow-pathway conduction persists after ablation, the slow-pathway conduction should be abolished if possible . However, tenacity in pursuing this end point by delivering energy in many different atrial sites should be tempered by the increasing risk of inadvertent AV block and by our ignorance about the long-term effects of radiofrequency current on the late development of AV block.

References

1. Wu D, Denes P, Amat-Y-Leon F, Dhingra R, Wyndham C, Bauerfeind R, Latif P, Rosen KM (1978) Clinical, electrocardiographic and electrophysiologic observations in patients with paroxysmal supraventricular tachycardia. Am J Cardiol 41: 1045-1051

2. Lee M, Morady F, Kadish A, Schamp D, Chin M, Scheinman M, Griffin JC, Lesh MD, Pederson D, Goldberger J, Calkins H, deBuitler M, Kou WH, Rosenheck S, Sousa J, Langberg J (1991) Catheter modification of the atrio-ventricular junction with radiofrequency energy for control of atrioventricular nodal reentry tachycardia. Circulation 83:827-835

3. Goy J, Fromer M, Schlaeper J, Kappenberger L (1990) Clinical efficacy of radiofrequency current in the treatment of patients with atrioventricular node reentrant tachycardia. J Am Coll Cardiol 16: 418-423

4. Chen S, Chiang C, Tsang W et al (1993) Selective radiofrequency catheter ablation of fast and slow pathways in 100 patients with atrioventricular nodal reentrant tachycardia. Am Heart J 125: 1-10

5. Delise P, Bonso A, Raviele A (1990) Tachicardia reciprocante idionodale insensibile alla profilassi farmacologica. Descrizione di un caso trattato con successo con la radiofrequenza. G Ital Cardiol 20: 1168-1173

6. Salerno JA, De Pieri G, De Ponti R et al (1991) Transcatheter ablation of the A-V junctional area by radiofrequency in cases with so called nodal tachycardia. Short and long term observations. Eur Heart J 12: 294

7. Jackman WM, Beckman KJ, McClelland J, Wang X, Friday K, Roman C, Moulton K, Twidale N, Hazlitt A, Prior M, Oren J, Overholt E, Lazzara R (1992) Treatment of supraventricular tachycardia due to atrioventricular nodal reentry by radiofrequency catheter ablation of slow-pathway conduction. N Engl J Med 327: 313-318

8. Jazayeri M, Hempe S, Sra J, Dhala A, Blank Z, Deshpande S, Avitall B, Krum D, Gilbert C, Akhtar M (1992) Selective transcatheter ablation of the fast and slow pathways using radiofrequency energy in patients with atrioventricular nodal reentrant tachycardia. Circulation 85: 1318-1328

9. Haissaguerre M, Gaita F, Fischer B, Commenges D, Montserrat P, d'Ivernois C, Lemetayer P, Warin J (1992) Elimination of atrioventricular nodal reentrant tachycardia using discrete slow potentials to guide application of radiofrequency energy. Circulation 85: 2162-2175

10. Wathen M, Natale A, Wolfe K, Yee R, Newman D, Klein G (1992) An anatomically guided approach to atrioventricular node slow pathway ablation. Am J Cardiol 70: 886-889

11. Kay G, Epstein A, Dailey S, Plumb V (1992) Selective radiofrequency ablation of the slow pathway for the treatment of atrioventricular nodal reentrant tachycardia. Evidence for involvement of perinodal myocardium within the reentrant circuit. Circulation 85: 1318-1328

12. Mitrani R, Klein LS, Hackett K, Zipes D, Miles W (1993) Radiofrequency ablation for atrioventricular node reentrant tachycardia: comparison between fast (anterior) and slow (posterior) pathway ablation. J Am Coll Cardiol 21: 432-441

13. Wu D, Yeh S, Wang C, Wen M, Lin F (1993) A simple technique for selective radiofrequency ablation of the slow pathway in atrioventricular node reentrant tachycardia. J Am Coll Cardiol 21: 1612-1621

14. Li H, Klein G, Stites W et al (1993) Elimination of slow pathway conduction: an accurate indicator of clinical success after radiofrequency atrioventricular node modification. J Am Coll Cardiol 22: 1849-1853

15. Delise P, Corò L, Bonso A et al (1993) L'ablazione della tachicardia da rientro nodale. Le confessioni sincere di un praticante. G Ital Cardiol 23 [Suppl I]: 112-115

16. Delise P, Coluccia S, Themistoclakis S et al (1994) I risultati a lungo termine dell'ablazione transcatetere della tachicardia parossistica sopraventricolare da rientro nodale sono così buoni come i risultati a breve termine? In: Alboni P (ed) Proceedings of "Giornate Cardiologiche Centesi," Cento (Ferrara) 20-21 October, pp 41-45

17. Kalbfleisch S, Strickberger A, Williamson B et al (1994) Randomized comparison of anatomic and electrogram mapping approaches to ablation of the slow pathway of atrioventricular node reentrant tachycardia. J Am Coll Cardiol 23: 716-723

18. Sra J, Jazayeri M, Blank Z, Deshpande S, Dhala A, Akhtar M (1994) Slow pathway ablation in patients with atrioventricular node reentrant tachycardia and a prolonged PR interval. J Am Coll Cardiol 24: 1064-1068

Surface Electrocardiogram in Ventricular Pre-excitation: How Reliable Is It To Locate the Site of Accessory Pathway?

E. Piccolo, P. Delise, and S. Themistoclakis

Divisione di Cardiologia, Ospedale Umberto I,
Mestre-Venice, Italy

It is estimated that about 3-4/1000 individuals are born with accessory pathway. These patients may have anterograde manifest conduction and hence show ventricular pre-excitation with short PR interval and delta waves (WPW electrocardiographic pattern). In some cases the accessory pathway may be concealed, manifesting only retrograde conduction over this tract. If so, the electrocardiogram is normal. In 5%-10% of series, multiple accessory pathways have been described.

Approximately 65% of accessory pathways are found on the left free wall, approximately 25% are septal and the remainder are on the right free wall. Left free wall accessory pathways may be located all around the mitral annulus anteriorly, laterally, or posteriorly. Septal accessory pathways may be located posteriorly near the ostium of coronary sinus or within the os of the coronary sinus (posteroseptal accessory pathways), anteriorly near the His bundle (anteroseptal accessory pathways) or between the His bundle and the os of coronary sinus (midseptal accessory pathways). Right free wall accessory pathways may be located all around the tricuspid annulus anteriorly, laterally, or posteriorly.

Ventricular pre-excitation is similar to a premature ventricular beat that originates in the area where Kent's bundle is connected to the ventricle, but has the features of the summation beat, whereby the earlier the pre-excitation of Kent's bundle occurs in comparison with the normal atrio-ventricular node activation the greater the initial anomalous ventricular activation will be. The analysis of anomalous activation becomes more complicated if multiple pre-excitation pathways are involved simultaneously.

The semiology of electrocardiographic and vectorcardiographic localization of Kent's bundle was initially based on the analysis of autopsy findings, and later on surgical findings in patients undergoing section of the anomalous pathway. More recently, it has been based on the electrophysiologic mapping performed in patients undergoing catheter ablation.

The first attempt at classifying Wolff-Parkinson-White (WPW) syndrome was made in 1945 (1) by Rosenbaum et al. of Wilson's group on the basis of the morphology of the QRS in the right precordial leads. They classified WPW as type A when the QRS in V_1-V_2 derivations was predominantly positive, and as type B when it was predominantly negative. The merit of this classification lies not only in the fact that it was the first and that it broadly distinguished between pre-excitation from the two ventricles, but also in the realization that the first precordial derivations consituted the main analytical key. Rosenbaum's classification was of course limited in that it indicated only an approximate location in one of the two ventricles. More importantly, it failed to pick out anomalous septal and paraseptal pathways.

Modern electrocardiographic (ECG) classifications are based on the results of electrophysiologic mapping, performed prior to surgical or transcatheter ablation, or on the results of ablation itself. These classifications now no longer have a merely semantic purpose; they also serve to guide the operator with regard to mapping techinque and the possible difficulties that may be encountered if ablation is undertaken.

The classification suggested by Milstcin and colleagues (2), which is based on intraoperative mapping, is commonly used, as it is very simple. According to this classification, the anomalous pathways are divided into four types: left lateral (free wall of the left ventricle), posterior paraseptal (right or left lower intraventricular septum), anteroseptal (node-His bundle region), and right lateral (free wall of the right ventricle). Initial analysis is based especially on the peripheral leads:

1. If the delta wave is negative or isoelectric in D_1 a V_L or V_6, Kent's bundle is left lateral. There is one exception to this: if the QRS has the appearance of left-branch block. Kent's bundle is right anteroseptal.

2. If delta wave is positive in D_2 a V_L or V_6, analysis of D_2, D_3, and V_F must be performed. If the delta wave is negative or isoelectric in at least two of these derivations, there are two possibilities: either posterior paraseptal Kent's bundle if at least one of the first three precordial derivations has an RS or RS morphology (e.g., QS in V_1 and RS in V_2) or right lateral Kent's bundle if the QRS is predominantly negative from V_1

to V_3. If a diagnosis has not yet been reached after this step, it should be ascertained whether the QRS is left-branch-block type. If so, Kent's bundle is right anteroseptal when the âQRS is greater than +30°; if it is not left-branch-block type, but V_1 or V_2 is predominantly positive, Kent's bundle is left lateral. If even this information is lacking, the location of the anomalous pathway will remain undetermined.

Milstein's classification has limits in that it does not indicate midseptal pathways, does not distinguish between left and right posteroseptal pathways, and fails to provide precise indications about other locations. Attempts to overcome these limitations were made by Fitzpatrick and colleagues (3) and by Rodriguez and colleagues (4) on the basis of the results of radiofrequency ablation. Returning to Rosenbaum's analysis, these authors reexamined the first precordial leads and concluded that: (a) if the transition of the QRS is in V_1 or to the right of V_1, thus with predominantly positive complexes on the first precordial leads, Kent's bundle is on the left; (b) if the transition is beyond V_2, thus with QRS predominantly negative on the first precordials, Kent's bundle is on the right; (c) if the transition is in V_2 or between V_1 and V_2, the D_1 lead opens to two possibilities: Kent's bundle is on the left if, in the latter lead, R is less than S or greater than S by no more than 1 mV; otherwise, Kent's bundle is on the right.

In this way, the left or right location becomes definitive; more precise indications can then be obtained from further analysis of the surface ECG. Regarding Kent's bundles on the left, when the âQRS is directed downward and the sum of polarities of the QRS in D_2, D_3 and a V_F is $\geq +2$, or if the S wave is greater than R wave in a V_L, the location is anterolateral; if, however, this is not the case, and if R wave is greater than S wave in D_1 by more than 0.8 mV and the sum of delta wave polarities in D_2, D_3, and a V_F is negative, Kent's bundle is posteroseptal. If even this combination is absent, the location of the Kent's bundle on the left is posterolateral. Regarding Kent's bundle on the right, if the transition does not go beyond V_3, or between V_3

and V_4 and has a delta wave in D_2 of 1 mV, the location is septal. In this case, if the sum of polarities in D_2, D_3 and a V_F is $\geq +2$, the location is anteroseptal; if it is ≤ -2, the location is posteroseptal; if the sum of polarities is between -1 and +1, the location is midseptal.

If the transition is further to the left (at least in V_4), or between V_3 and V_4 with a delta wave in D_2 of 1 mV, the location is in the right lateral wall. Here, an anterolateral position can be determined if the delta wave frontal axis is $\geq 0°$ or if an R wave in lead D_3 is present; if, however, the delta wave frontal axis is less than 0° or if the delta wave in D_3 is isoelectric or negative, a posterolateral location can be determined.

The algorithm of Fitzpatrick and Rodriguez offers the advantage of being very detailed, but also the disadvantage of being rather complex and difficult to memorize. Depending on the location, the sensitivity of the criteria ranges from 71.4% to 100% and the specificity from 71% to 100%. The most difficult differential diagnoses are reported to be those between right posteroseptal and right midseptal pathways (sensitivity, 76.5%; specificity, 71%) and those between left posterior and left posterolateral paraseptal pathways (sensitivity, 71.4%; specificity, 100%).

References

1. Rosenbaum F, Hect H, Wilson F, Johnston F (1945) The potential variation of the thorax and the oesophagus in anomalous atrioventricular excitation (Wolff-Parkinson-White Syndrome). Am Heart J 29: 281-288
2. Milstein S, Sharma AD, Guiraudon GM, Klein GJ (1987) An algorithm for the electrocardiographic localization of accessory pathways in the Wolff-Parkinson-White Syndrome. Pace 10: 555-563
3. Fitzpatrick AP, Gonzales RP, Lesh MD, Modin GW, Lee RJ, Scheinman MM (1994) New algorithm for localization of accessory atrioventricular connections using a baseline electrocardiogram. J Am Coll Cardiol 23: 107-116
4. Rodriguez L, Smeet J, De Chillou C et al (1993). The 12-lead electrocardiogram in midseptal, anteroseptal, posteroseptal and right free wall accessory pathways. Am J Cardiol 72: 1274-1280

Radiofrequency Ablation in the Wolff-Parkinson-White Syndrome: Do the Results Justify a Widespread Application?

R. Cappato

Division of Cardiology, University Hospital Eppendorf,
Hamburg, Germany

Introduction

In 1968, successful surgical division of an accessory atrioventricular (AV) connection in a patient with Wolff-Parkinson-White syndrome was first reported (1). This ushered in the era of ablative therapy for arrhythmias. The rationale of ablation is that irreversible alteration can be brought on to a discrete anatomical substrate responsible for arrhythmia generation and/or perpetuation.

The next technique using the same rationale was high-voltage direct current catheter ablation (2,3). This closed-chest technique overcame the significant morbidity associated with open thoracotomy; however, due to the relatively uncontrolled nature of this energy form, which produced thermal, electrical, and physical injury (barotrauma), concerns were raised about trauma to thin-walled structures in the heart such as the atrial free wall and the coronary sinus. Alternative modalities were therefore pursued, including intracoronary ethanol infusion (4), laser irradiation (5), cryothermy (6), microwave (7), ultrasound (8), and radiofrequency (RF) (9-16) ablation.

With evolving understanding of anatomical-electrophysiologic relationships, improvement of mapping techniques, and the introduction of RF ablation catheters with large (4-mm) distal electrode tips, the success rate by this technique improved significantly compared to that reported in initial experience. Currently, the use of RF current catheter ablation has increased dramatically in patients with supraventricular tachycardia, including AV nodal reentrant tachycardia and AV reciprocating tachycardia with or without pre-excitation, as well as in new subsets of patients, such as those with atrial flutter, ectopic atrial tachycardia, and ventricular tachycardia.

Mechanisms of RF Energy-Induced Myocardial Injury and Effects on Myocardial Tissue

The presumed mechanism of myocardial injury in response to RF current delivery is a thermal one. In addition, it has been suggested that the oscillating electromotive force may exert a direct effect on the myocyte sarcolemmal membrane. Thermal coagulation of about 100 mm^3 of the target tissue occurs in response to electrode tissue interface temperatures of about 50°C or more; when temperatures at the electrode tissue interface reach or exceed 100°C, the plasma boils at the electrode surface and an insulating film of coagulated plasma and desiccated tissue forms on the conductive surface. Reduction of the effective electrode surface area leads to increased current density, more tissue heating, more coagulum formation, and finally "breakdown" of delivered energy. In clinical practice, early recognition of this phenomenon is made possible by impedance monitoring; in case a sudden increase of impedance is observed during pulse delivery, immediate pulse discontinuation is mandatory to reduce the risk of thrombus formation. Anticoagulation with intravenous heparin is also performed in most centers to minimize the risk of thrombus formation and its complications.

Four to 5 days after ablation, the center of the lesion shows complete coagulation necrosis and early fatty changes, whereas a discrete border between living and dead tissue replaces the inflammatory transition zone observed acutely. It is likely that changes occurring in the transition zone are, at least in part, responsible for late success or late recurrence, depending on the evolution during this phase. By 8 weeks, the chronic lesion has been replaced by fibrosis and shows evidence of contraction and marked volume loss. The border zone of the lesion is well defined without any patchy necrosis or islands of viable myocardium. The uniform nature and the small volume of the lesion likely accounts for the low rate of reported late arrhythmic and nonarrhythmic complications from RF current catheter ablation.

Efficacy of RF Current Ablation in Patients with Accessory Pathways

Currently, success rates well exceeding 90% are being reported by experienced centers for RF current ablation of supraventricular tachycardias secondary to an accessory AV pathway. Two prerequisites must be fulfilled to make this strategy successful: first, the precise localization of the accessory pathway; recently developed catheter techniques allow, if properly searched for, direct recording of accessory pathway activation from the distal electrode pair at the tip of the mapping/ablation catheter (17). RF current delivery to sites of accessory pathway activation potential recording, expecially if associated with other local electrogram parameters suggestive of early local activation (18), almost always results in immediate conduction block within the accessory pathway. Often, very few RF current pulses are required to produce accessory pathway interruption. This underlines the importance of precise mapping technique, as compared to surgical approach (1) where extended areas along the AV annuli are frequently excised to minimize recurrence.

Second, the introduction of specially designed catheters with steerable tips that can be freely maneuvered from the outside has allowed easier and more precise positioning at any site along the AV annuli. The large-tip electrode of these catheters also allows delivery of higher energies to the myocardial tissue, thus resulting in a significantly higher success rate than that reported with small (2-mm) distal electrode tips (12).

Catheter maneuvering under fluoroscopic guidance also has important implications for optimizing catheter tissue contact and stability over time during RF current pulses; this is crucial to maximizing the probability of success (19-21). Several techniques have been proposed to optimize catheter tissue contact at the AV annuli. For left-sided accessory pathways, either the transaortic retrograde or the transseptal approach can be safely used with similarly reported efficacy (22); in principle, these approaches aim at interrupting accessory pathway conduction at the ventricular and atrial insertion site, respectively. Right-sided accessory pathways can at times present a challenge to the interventional electrophysiologist. A long-term success rate for RF current catheter ablation in this set of pathways may also exceed 90%, but multiple sessions may be required because of a lower success rate during the first procedure and a relatively high recurrence rate.

Anatomical differences of the tricuspid as opposed to the mitral annulus likely account for the difficulties encountered in RF current ablation of right-sided accessory pathways; they include a larger mappable circumference (ca. 12 cm of the tricuspid annulus versus ca. 10 cm of the mitral annulus in the normal adult), an annular development less pronounced with discontinuities of the fibrous skeleton, a more acute angle between the endocardium and the valve leaflet, the presence of Ebstein's anomaly or of Mahaim-like fibers accounting for about 10% of all right-sided accessory pathways, and, most importantly, the absence along the annulus of a conveniently accessible venous structure for mapping. In selected cases, the right coronary artery may be used to advance properly designed catheter electrodes and map along the epicardial right AV groove in search of the accessory pathway.

Once the accessory pathway has been localized, several techniques may be used to maximize catheter tissue contact and stability, depending on the target site along the tricuspid annulus. In our center, anterospetal, anterior, and anterolateral accessory pathways are most easily accessed using an approach from the superior vena cava (entrance either from the internal jugular vein or right subclavian vein); accessory pathways in the right lateral, posterolateral, posterior, posteroseptal, and midseptal positions are initially approached using a catheter inserted through the right femoral vein and into the inferior vena cava. Additional techniques can be used in selected cases, including the support of a long sheath embedding the mapping catheter from the entry site to the inferior vena cava opening and a looping technique allowing the catheter tip to approach the accessory pathway from the subannular site.

After successful ablation of an accessory pathway, careful monitoring is required before discharge to control the patient's clinical conditions and exclude pericardial reaction. During follow-up, recurrence is observed in about 5% of patients; repeat procedures are generally recommended in such cases and result in definitive abolition of the accessory pathway.

Complication of RF Current Ablation Techniques

General Complications

The complication rate of RF catheter ablation procedures is about 5%; this includes complications related to catheter manipulation and to RF current delivery. Among these are inadvertent complete AV nodal block, pericardial effusion, cardiac tamponade, coronary artery spasm or thrombosis, intracavitary thrombus formation, thromboembolism, pneumothorax, aortic wall dissection, local hematoma, and arterovenous fistulae. In cooperative reports, the incidence of complications was 3.8% in a large American collective (23) and 4.4% in the European MERFS survey (24). In the latter study, life-threatening complications such as tamponade and embolism have been reported in 0.7% and 0.6% of cases, respectively. A procedure-related death has been occasionally reported in patients undergoing RF current ablation.

Complications Related to the Location of the Accessory Pathway

Inadvertent complete AV nodal block has been reported in patients undergoing ablation of accessory pathways located in the septal space. Some precautions can be used to minimize this risk whenever RF current must be delivered in the midseptal or anteroseptal region; these include (a) selection of the venous access associated with the greatest catheter stability at these sites, (b) use of a temperature-controlled mode with initial preset values not exceeding 55°-60°C, (c) careful monitoring of atrial retrograde conduction if junctional ectopic rhythm ensues during RF current applications, with immediate discontinuation of pulse delivery in case of a retrograde (ventriculoatrial) block, and d) early discontinuation of energy delivery for pulses which fail to produce an early accessory pathway conduction block.

Accessory pathways ablated from within the coronary sinus or its tributary veins are referred to as epicardial accessory pathways; they account for about 5% of all left-sided accessory pathways. RF current pulses delivered inside the cardiac venous system should be titrated at low power (not exceeding 15 W/s) or low preset temperature (not exceeding 55°-60°C). In case of a sudden impedance rise during pulse delivery, which may not infrequently be observed due to a less pronounced cooling effect by the circulating blood in this region, immediate pulse discontinuation is mandatory to minimize the risk of thrombus formation and catheter adhesion to the venous wall. Despite these safety measures, thrombosis may nevertheless develop, leading occasionally to occlusion of the coronary sinus. In our experience, this event was never associated with clinical complications and complete recanalization could be documented a few days after the procedure. Thus far, there are no reports of perforation produced by RF current delivered within the cardiac veins leading to pericardial effusion or tamponade.

Potential Hazards of RF Current Catheter Ablation

A potential source of risk to the patient and the investigators performing RF current catheter ablation procedures is the radiation exposure from fluoroscopic imaging which is required to guide catheter manipulation. The estimated absorbed dose per RF ablation procedure in a high volume American center was 2.5 rem in the breast, 2.0 rem in the active bone marrow, and 7.5 rem in the lungs (25). These figures represent a lifetime risk of excess malignancies per 1 million patients undergoing 60 minutes fluoroscopy of 150 (only females), 120, and 710, respectively (a 0.07% lifetime risk of developing a fatal malignancy due to radiation exposure). In addition, the risk estimation for autosomal dominant abnormalities in the first generation is 5-35 cases per 1 million liveborn per absorbed rem, and the risk for all genetic disorders less than 50 cases per million liveborn per absorbed rem. Although difficult to be translated to the clinical practice, these estimates outline the necessity of minimizing fluoroscopy time during RF current catheter ablation procedures without reducing efficacy and safety; also, the volume of exposed body weight and the lifetime expectancy with respect to the effective clinical benefit should be taken into account at the time of patient selection.

In patients in whom RF current delivery in the proximity of the AV node is performed to ablate an accessory pathway, long term follow-up is recommended to evaluate the potential impact of fibrotic lesions on AV conduction.

Indications for RF Current Catheter Ablation of Accessory Pathways

RF energy is currently the source of choice for ablation of accessory AV pathways. It is highly effective

and carries a low risk. Owing to these properties, it has been proposed as a therapy in patients with incessant or drug-refractory tachycardias mediated by an accessory pathway and in symptomatic patients who refuse lifelong drug therapy (23). In asymptomatic patients with Wolff-Parkinson-White syndrome, the decision to ablate the accessory pathway should be an individual one, based on electrophysiologic data, type of occupation or physical activities of the patient, and the patient's personal motivation. In children, the benefits of this therapy should be carefully counterbalanced with the risks related to complications and fluoroscopy exposure, taking into account the not infrequent disappearance of the accessory pathway during growth (26); at our center, patients younger than 4 years of age or with a body weight lower than 50 kg are candidates for accessory pathway ablation only in case of incessant or drug refractory tachycardias in the presence of left ventricular dysfunction, or impaired growth.

RF Current Catheter Ablation as the Therapy of Choice in Patients with Reciprocating AV Tachycardia?

It has been estimated that the risk of sudden death in asymptomatic patients with Wolff-Parkinson-White syndrome is about 0.1% per patient-year (27); this figure may increase to 0.56% per patient-year in patients with an accessory pathway capable of rapid conduction during atrial fibrillation. Sudden death may be the first manifestation of Wolff-Parkinson-White syndrome in 25% of cases (28). In addition, in about 10% of sudden arrhythmic deaths in young people with an apparently normal heart who have never undergone a clinical investigation, histologic examination may disclose a substrate consistent with pre-excitation (29). An electrophysiologic investigation helps to identify those patients at low risk of ventricular fibrillation and should be performed routinely in patients with Wolff-Parkinson-White syndrome. This procedure carries an inherent risk of complication and in experienced centers the possibility of concomitant cure by means of RF current ablation is offered to the patient during the same session. Transesophageal electrophysiologic study is used as a surrogate of the intracavitary diagnostic procedure in some centers.

Antiarrhythmic drug therapy has long been used in the chronic treatment of patients with reciprocating AV tachycardia. The clinical efficacy of these agents in highly symptomatic patients ranges between 70% and 100%, although only about 50% of them become asymptomatic (30). In addition, antiarrhythmic drug therapy is associated with a 3%-34% risk of proarrhythmia, which at times may be fatal (31-34). Also, the use of these drugs does not necessarily prevent sudden death in patients with Wolff-Parkinson-White syndrome (28). Additional organ toxicity is seen with all antiarrhythmic agents and has an incidence as high as 26% in the case of amiodarone (35). Not infrequently, Wolff-Parkinson-White syndrome or reciprocating AV tachycardias is seen in women of childbearing age; in such cases, the risk of congenital defects resulting from pregnancy occurring in the presence of an antiarrhythmic agent must also be taken into account.

From these data, it is evident that RF current catheter ablation is an optimal tool to cure patients with an accessory pathway. It is mandatory to identify individuals with Wolff-Parkinson-White syndrome at risk of developing ventricular fibrillation by means of an electrophysiologic study. At this time, ablation of any accessory pathway is, in experienced hands, easily feasible in more than 90% of cases and should be offered to the patient as an option, provided that he/she has been correctly informed about the pathophysiology and the risk of his/her disease, as well as the risks of the therapeutic procedure.

References

1. Cobb RF, Blumenschein SD, Sealy WC et al (1968) Successful surgical interruption of the bundle of Kent in a patient with Wolff-Parkinson-White syndrome. Circulation 38: 1018-1029
2. Scheinman MM, Morady F, Hess DS et al (1982) Catheter-induced ablation of the atrioventricular junction to control refractory supraventricular arrhythmias. JAMA 248: 851-855
3. Haissaguerre M, Warin JF, Lemetayer P et al (1989) Closed-chest ablation of retrograde conduction in patients with atrioventricular nodal reentrant tachycardia. N Engl J Med 320: 851-855
4. Brugada P, de Swart H, Smeets JL, Wellens HJ (1989) Transcoronary chemical ablation of ventricular tachycardia. Circulation 79: 475-482
5. Littman L, Svenson RH, Tomcsanyi et al (1991) Modification of atrioventricular nodal transmission properties by intraoperative neodymium-YAG laser photocoagulation in dogs. J Am Coll Cardiol 17: 797-804
6. Gillette PC, Swindle MM, Thompson RF, Case CL (1991) Transvenous cryoablation of the bundle of His. PACE 14: 504-510
7. Haines DE, Whayne JG (1992) What is the radial temperature profile achieved during microwave catheter ablation with a helical coil antenna in canine myocardium? J Am Coll Cardiol 19: 99A
8. He D, Zimmer JE, Hynynen KH et al (1992) Application of ultrasound energy for intracardiac ablation of arrhythmias. Circulation 86: I-783
9. Borggrefe M, Buddle T, Podzeck A, Breithardt (1987) High frequency alternating current ablation of an accessory pathway in humans. J Am Coll Cardiol 10 576-582
10. Kuck KH, Kunze KP, Schlüter M, Geiger M, Jackman WM, Naccarelli GV (1988) Modification of a left-sided accessory atrioventricular pathway by radiofrequency current using a bipolar epicardial-endocardial electrode configuration. Eur Heart J 9: 927-932
11. Jackman WM, Wang X, Friday KJ, Roman CA, Moulton KP, Beckman KJ, McClelland JH, Twidale N, Hazlitt A, Prior MI, Margolis PD, Calame JD, Overholt ED, Lazzara R (1991) Catheter ablation of accessory atrioventricular pathways (Wolff-Parkinson-White syndrome) by radiofrequency current. N Engl J Med 324: 1605-1611
12. Kuck KH, Schlüter M, Geiger M, Siebels J, Duckeck W (1991) Radiofrequency current catheter ablation of accessory atrioventricular pathways. Lancet 337: 1557-1561
13. Calkins H, Sousa J, Rosenheck S, de Buitleir M, Kou WH, Kadish AH, Langberg JJ, Morady F (1991) Diagnosis and cure of the Wolff-Parkinson-White syndrome or paroxysmal supraventricular tachycardias during a single electrophysiologic test. N Engl J Med 324: 1612-1618
14. Schlüter M, Geiger M, Siebels J, Duckeck W, Kuck KH (1991) Catheter ablation using radiofrequency current to cure symptomatic patients with tachyarrhythmias related to an accessory atrioventricular pathway. Circulation 84: 1644-1661
15. Leather RA, Leitch JW, Klein GJ, Guiraudon GM, Yee R, Kim YH (1991) Radiofrequency catheter ablation of accessory pathways: a learning experience. Am J Cardiol 68: 1651-1655
16. Lesh MD, Van Hare GF, Schamp DJ, Chien W, Lee MA, Griffin JC, Langberg JJ, Cohen TJ, Lurie KG, Scheinman MM (1992) Curative percutaneous catheter ablation using radiofrequency energy for accessory pathways in all locations: results in 100 consecutive patients. J Am Coll Cardiol 19: 1303-1309
17. Jackman WM, Friday KJ, Yeung-Lai-Wah JA, Fitzgerald DM, Beck B, Bowman AJ, Stelzer P, Harrison L, Lazzara R (1988) New catheter technique for recording left free-wall accessory atrioventricular pathway activation. Identification of pathway fiber orientation. Circulation 78: 598-610
18. Cappato R, Schlüter M, Mont L, Kuck KH (1994) Anatomic, electrical, and mechanical factors affecting bipolar endocardial electrograms: impact on catheter ablation of manifest left free-wall accessory pathways. Circulation 90: 884-894
19. Calkins H, Kim YN, Schmaltz S, Sousa J, el-Atassi R, Leon A, Kadish A, Langberg JJ, Morady F (1992) Electrogram criteria for identification of appropriate target sites for radiofrequency catheter ablation of accessory atrioventricular connections. Circulation 85: 565-573
20. Chen X, Borggrefe M, Shenasa M, Haverkamp W, Hindricks G, Breithardt G (1992) Characteristics of local electrogram predicting successful transcatheter radiofrequency ablation of left-sided accessory pathways. J Am Coll Cardiol 20: 656-665
21. Silka MJ, Kron J, Halperin BD, Griffith K, Crandall B, Oliver RP, Walance CG, McAnulty JH (1992) Analysis of local electrogram characteristics correlated with successful radiofrequency catheter ablation of accessory atrioventricular pathways. PACE 15: 1000-1007
22. Ma C, Dong J, Yang X, Shang L, Iiu X, Sun Y, Hu D (1995) A randomized comparison between retrograde and transseptal approach for radiofrequency ablation of left-sided accessory pathways. PACE 18: 915II
23. Scheinman MM (1992) Catheter ablation for cardiac arrhythmias, personnel and facilities. PACE 15: 715-721
24. Hindricks G (1993) The multicentre European radiofrequency survey. Complications of radiofrequency catheter ablation of arrhythmias. Eur Heart J 14: 256-262
25. Calkins H, Niklason L, Sousa J, El-Atassi R, Langberg J, Morady F (1991) Radiation exposure during radiofrequency ablation of accessory atrioventricular connections. Circulation 84: 2376-2382
26. Perry JC, Garson A (1990) Supraventricular tachycardia due to the Wolff-Parkinson-White syndrome in children: early disappearance and late recurrence. J Am Coll Cardiol 16: 1215-1220
27. Klein GJ, Prystowski EN, Sharma AD, Laupacis A (1989) Asymptomatic Wolff-Parkinson-White syndrome: should we intervene? Circulation 80: 1902-1905
28. Torner Montoya P, Brugada P Smeets J, Talajic M, Della Bella P, Lezaun R, Dool A, Wellens HJJ, Bayes de Luna A, Oter R, Breitardt G, Borggrefe M, Klein H, Kuck KH, Kunze KP, Coumel P, Leclercq JF, Chouty F, Frank R, Fontaine G (1991) Ventricular fibrillation in the Wolff-Parkinson-White syndrome. Eur Heart J 12: 144-150
29. Corrado D, Basso C, Angelini A, Thiene G (1995) Sudden "arrhythmic" death in young people with apparently normal heart. J Am Coll Cardiol 188A
30. Henthorn RW, Waldo AL, Anderson JL, Gilbert EM, Alpert BL, Bhandari AK, Hawkinson AW, Pritchett EL (1991) Flecainide acetate prevents recurrence of symptomatic paroxysmal supraventricular tachycardia. The flecainide supraventricular tachycardia study group. Circulation 83: 119-125
31. Creamer JE, Nathan AW, Camm AJ (1987) The proarrhythmic effects of antiarrhythmic drugs. Am Heart J 2: 397-406
32. Velebit V, Podrid P, Lown B, Cohen BH. Graboys TB (1982) Aggravation and provocation of ventricular arrhythmias by antiarrhythmic drugs. Circulation 65: 886-894
33. Coplen SE, Antman EM, Berlin JA, Hewitt P, Chalmers TC (1990) Efficacy and safety of quinidine therapy for maintenance of sinus rhythm after cardioversion: meta-analysis of randomized control trials. Circulation 82: 1106-1116
34. The Cardiac Arrhythmia Suppression Trial (CAST) Investigators (1989) Preliminary report. Effect of encainide and flecainide on mortality in a randomized trial of arrhythmia suppression after myocardial infarction. N Engl J Med 321: 406-412
35. Mason JW (1987) Amiodarone. N Engl J Med 316: 455-466

Recurrent Palpitations After Successful Radiofrequency Ablation of Supraventricular Tachycardias: Which Significance?

M. Lunati, M. Gasparini, G. Maccabelli, G. Magenta, G. Cattafi, and G. Gadaleta

Servizio di Elettrofisiologia ed Elettrostimolazione
Dipartimento Cardiologico "A. De Gasperis" Ospedale Ca' Granda,
Milano-Niguarda, Milan, Italy

Introduction

Radiofrequency catheter ablation (RFCA) has become the treatment of choice in patients with recurrent, symptomatic, medical-refractory supraventricular tachycardias (SVT) due to an accessory anomalous pathway (AP) or a reentry in the region of the atrioventricular node (AVN; 1-7).

The reasons for the high popularity of the technique are: high success rate of the procedure (*efficacy*), low rate of procedure related complications (*safety*), favorable cost-effectiveness ratio (*cost*), (probable) low risk of long-term adverse consequences (*reliability*).

A well-known feature in the follow-up of the patients who underwent RFCA for AP and AVN SVT is the recurrence of "arrhythmic"or "pseudoarrhythmic" symptoms in the first months (1-4, 8-10) after a successful procedure. Following the reports of different centers and our experience (300 consecutive patients with a wide variety of SVT treated with RFCA at our own center) we address this problem.

Incidence and Clinical Features of Accessory Pathway-Mediated and AVN Reentrant Tachycardias After Initially Successful Radiofrequency Catheter Ablation

Owing to the differences among the series reported it is sensible to state what is now considered a successful ablation procedure: a successful procedure has rendered SVT noninducible and abolished all evidence of AP conduction (antegrade and retrograde) in the basal state and after infusion of isoproterenol, immediately and 30 min after the ablation.

The risk of true arrhythmia recurrence after a successful procedure appears to be quite low in adults, varying between 3% and 12% of patients (1-4,6,8-10). Differences in patient characteristics, duration of an adequate follow-up, and the fact that recurrences accounted for 45% of the failures overall in the series of the Pediatric Electrophysiologic Society [RFCA for tachyarrhythmias (11) in children and adolescents] should be kept in mind, however.

The recurrences may be early, before hospital discharge (between 1 and 12 h after RFCA) or late (between 1 and 100 days). In the series of Langberg et al. (8) failure after initial success for RFCA of AP SVT was 12% (early recurrence = 50%, mean time = 6±5 h, late recurrence = 50%, mean time = 53±39 days); in the studies of Chen et al. (12,13) the early recurrences were 70% and the late 30% (failure = 9%).

The factors that may predispose to this unfavorable early or late outcome have not yet been completely defined but some predictors of recurrences are known (1-3,6,8,12,13). Right-sided APs, ablated from the tricuspid anulus, show a much higher rate of recurrence than left-sided APs (this is probably due to anatomical reasons and to less contact pressure of the catheter over the right AV anulus). There is a higher recurrence rate for multiple APs than for single ones. Other determinants of failure in the follow-up are: longer initial ablation session, absence of recordable Kent potential, concealed APs, and site of energy delivery in ablation of left-sided APs (V>>A). The high efficacy rate of a second ablation session has been noted in all the series published.

Predictive Values of the Different Methods of Evaluation of Late Outcome of Radiofrequency Ablation

It should be stressed that:

1. Immediate results of RFA may be misleading (transient edema, catheter-induced mechanical trauma) → *pseudosuccess*

2. The extension over time of the lesion(s) may lead to delayed complete cure → *pseudofailure*.

The actual percentage of pseudosuccess is not known but it may account for 3% in all the series (12-15).

The methods of evaluation of the outcome of a successful RFCA are serial electrocardiogram (ECG), Holter monitoring, evaluation of symptoms, and electrophysiologic study (8,12,13,16).

Serial ECG. ECG is useless in evaluation of results of RFCA of SVT due to concealed APs and to AVN reentry. It is also useless in detection of new arrhythmic circuits and in determining the properties of residual APs (13).

In the series of Chen et al. (408 patients who received RFCA for SVT) serial ECG$_s$ had a good specificity but a very low sensitivity (15%).

Holter Monitoring. Holter monitoring is unrealistic and also expensive in this setting (only monitoring over weeks and months would be required). Probably event recording with transtelephonic transmission would be useful but experience with this is scarce at the moment (16).

Evaluation of Symptoms. It is extremely doutbtful to rely on the evaluation of symptoms to judge the real outcome of a RFCA procedure. In the reports of Chen et al. (12,13) the review of symptoms had a high specificity but a very low sensitivity. Indeed, the abolition of significant symptoms should be the major aim of the RFCA session (the "gold standard "of the outcome); we will see later on in detail how the patient's own assessment is probably an inaccurate way of evaluating the results of RFCA since most patients feel palpitations of some sort after ablation, and many patients are reluctant to disappoint themselves and their physicians by admitting to recurrence of palpitations.

Electrophysiologic Study. The value of electrophysiologic study is uncertain. The opinion of some authors is that routine follow-up electrophysiologic study is not warranted (8) due to the low yield of the test. In other studies (9,10,12,13) conclusions are quite different: Chen et al. perform immediate (20-30 min after RFCA), early (4-7 days after RFCA), and late (3-6 months after RFCA) electophysiologic study. They found that late electrophysiologic study had high predictive value in the outcome of both ablation for AP SVT and AVN SVT (sensitivity 100%, specificity 100%, predictive accuracy 100%). Probably the late test has a higher predictive value due to Bayes theory (lower pretest prevalence of recurrence in the first month after a successful ablation). Moreover, the test characterizes the properties of the residual arrhythmia circuits (recurrence of retrograde conduction only in a bidirectional AP previously ablated), detects new arrhythmia (17) circuits, helps in ruling out arrhythmogenicity of RF lesions, and helps relieve anxiety in this particular subset of patients.

Significance of Palpitations After Successful Ablation

The great majority of patients report some sort of palpitation after RFCA. Mann et al. (9) interviewed 77 patients in whom at least 4 weeks had passed since successful RFCA and found that in 45/77 (58%) extrabeats and the feeling that tachycardia was going to start up were present; moreover, 28/77 (36%) reported major palpitations similar to symptoms that occurred prior to ablation. The restudy in 53 patients showed that: eight patients (9%) had recurrence of AP conduction (six had major palpitations; two were symptomless), in one patient another SV tachyarrhythmia was inducible, and 15/22 patients with major symptoms had no AP recurrence or showed inducibility of other arrhythmic circuits. The absence of symptoms was highly predictive of a negative restudy (negative predictive study=94%) but judging the ablation failure on the basis of palpitations can be misleading (positive predictive value of AP recurrence=21%).

Grossman et al. (10) confirm a high incidence of recurrent palpitations in patients after successful RFCA (12/32, 37.5%), but most were pseudorecurrence as demonstrated by a negative electrophysiologic study. According to the authors these patients are more sensitive to other benign arrhythmias due to a heightened awareness from their preablation problem: there were significantly higher anxiety scores (Burns anxiety inventory score=26±6) in patients with than in patients without pseudorecurrence (9±3).

There are many real causes of palpitations:

1. True arrhythmia recurrence (up to 12%, see above).

2. Premature beats (5%-10%).

3. Sinus tachycardia due to anxiety (5%-10%).

4. Inappropriate sinus tachycardia, frequently observed in ablation of slow AVN pathway and posteroseptal APs (10%-15%). To shed light on the mechanism of this complication Kocovic et al. (18), in an excellent study using heart rate variability analysis (time and frequency domain), clearly demonstrated a significant increase in mean heart rate and significant reduction in heart rate variability in patients who had undergone successful ablation in the posterior regions of low interatrial septum, marked attenuation of high frequency components in this subset of patients, indicating parasympathetic denervation of fibers destined to innervate the sinus node (or reflexogenically mediated parasympathetic withdrawal ?), no acute changes in patients who underwent diagnostic study and in patients with ablation of left lateral APs, and resolution of abnormalities 1-6 months after RFCA (reinnervation ?). Moreover, the authors suggest the possibility that this complication could render these patients more susceptible to developing atrial arrhythmias in the months necessary to establish reinnervation.

5. Transient AV block, not rare (up to 3%) in modification of AV nodal conduction.

6. Unmasking of new arrhythmic circuits (3%) and development of new arrhythmogenic foci, perhaps due to lesions .

7. Runs of atrial fibrillation and atrial flutter (see above).

Conclusions

Palpitations after successful RFCA for AP-mediated and AV SVT are extremely common and the causes of complaints are heterogeneous (8-10,12,13) (true arrhythmic symptoms and nonarrhythmic symptoms). Electrophysiologists should be well aware of this problem so that every effort can be made to identify true recurrences and/or true arrhythmic hazards and to reassure symptomatic patients.

We can offer some recommandations from our analysis.

1. Many data suggest that only 1 day of inpatient monitoring is inadequate to detect problems after the procedure: pseudosuccess, pseudofailure, peculiar arrhythmias of RFCA for AVN SVT, etc. We hospitalize patients for at least 48 h after RFCA. An electrophysiologic restudy (transesophageal technique) is usually conducted 24-48 h after ablation; the need for prolonged monitoring and/or Holter recording is decided on the basis of emerging problems.

2. Some authors have questioned the need for routine electrophysiologic study 3 months after the procedure (the test is expensive and the yield is low). On the grounds of the reports and our experience we think that judging the absence and/or the return of pathway conduction by symptoms can be misleading on many occasions. Moreover, electrophysiologic study with tranesophageal technique is available (19) which is low in cost, adequate to predict freedom from SVT, and does not require hospitalization.

Consequently in our current practice a thorough examination, on an outpatient basis, is scheduled for every subject who has undergone RFCA at 3 months:

- In absence of palpitations (+ normal resting ECG, + history of "easy "ablation) we do not think that electrophysiologic study is warranted.

- In presence of palpitations (± abnormal ECG, + history of "complicated "ablation) we think that electrophysiologic restudy is mandatory.

References

1. Jackman WM, Wang X, Friday KJ et al (1991) Catheter ablation of accessory atrioventricular pathways (Wolff-Parkinson-White syndrome) by radiofrequency current. N Engl J Med 324, 1605-1611

2. Calkins H, Sousa J, El-Atassi R et al (1991) Diagnosis and cure of the Wolff-Parkinson-White syndrome or paroxysmal supraventricular tachycardias during a single electrophysiologic test. N Engl J Med 1991, 324, 1612-18

3. Schluter M, Geiger M, Siebels J et al (1991) Catheter ablation using radiofrequency current to cure symptomatic patients with tachyarrhythmias related to an accessory atrioventricular pathways. Circulation 84: 1644-1661

4. Jackman WM, Beckman KJ, McClelland JH et al (1992) Treatment of supraventricular tachycardia due to atrioventricular nodal reentry by radiofrequency catheter ablation of slow pathway conduction N Engl J Med 327: 313-318

5. Hogenhuis W, Stevens SK, Wang P et al (1993) Cost-effectiveness of radiofrequency ablation with other strategies in Wolff-Parkinson-White syndrome. Circulation 88-II: 437-446

6. Kay GN, Epstein AE, Dailey SM et al (1993) Role of radiofrequency ablation in the management of supraventricular arrhythmias: experience in 760 consecutive patients. J Cardiovasc Electrophysiol 4, 371-89

7. Lunati M, Montenero AS, Musto B (1994) L'ablazione transcatetere a radiofrequenza nelle tachicardie sopraventricolari e nel flutter atriale. Proceedings of the Djerba Consensus Conference Cardiologi e Aritmie-Strategie a Confronto. Tekne, Rome (in press)

8. Langberg JJ, Calkins H, Kim Y et al (1992) Recurrence of conduction in accessory atrioventricular connections after initially successful radiofrequency catheter ablation. J Am Coll Cardiol 19: 1588-1592

9. Mann DE, Kelly PA, Adler SW et al (1993) Palpitations occur frequently following radiofrequency catheter ablation for supraventricular tachycardia, but do not predict pathway recurrence. PACE, 1645-1649

10. Grossman DS, Cohen TJ, Goldner B et al (1994) Pseudorecurrence of paroxysmal supraventricular tachycardia after radiofrequency catheter ablation. Am Heart J 128: 516-519

11. Kugler JD, Danford DA, Deal BJ et al (1994) Radiofrequency catheter ablation for tachyarrhythmias in children and adolescents. N Engl J Med 330; 1481-1487

12. Chen SA, Chiang CE, Chiou CW et al (1993) Serial electrophysiologic studies in the late outcome of radiofrequency ablation for accessory atrioventricular pathway-mediated tachyarrhythmias. Eur Heart J 14: 734-743

13. Chen SA, Chiang CE, Yang CJ et al (1993) Usefulness of serial follow up electrophysiologic studies in predicting late outcome of radiofrequency ablation for accessory pathways and atrioventricular nodal reentrant tachycardia. Am Heart J 126: 619-625

14. Langberg JJ, Borganelli SM, Kalbfleisch SJ et al (1993) Delayed effects of radiofrequency energy on accessory atrioventricular connections. PACE 16: 1001-1006

15. Chiang CE, Chen SA, Wu TJ et al (1994) Incidence, significance and pharmacological responses of catheter-induced mechanical trauma in patients receiving radiofrequency ablation for supraventricualr tachycardia. Circulation, 90 1847-1854

16. Jordaens L, Vertongen P, Verstraeten T (1994) Prolonged monitoring for detection of symptomatic arrhythmias after slow pathway ablation in AV nodal tachycardia. Int J Cardiol 44: 57-63

17. Chiang CE, Chen SA, Wang DC et al (1993) Arrhythmogenicity of catheter ablation in supraventricular tachycardia. Am Heart J 125: 388-395

18. Kocovic DZ, Harada T, Shea JB et al (1993) Alterations of heart rate and of heart rate variability after radiofrequency catheter ablation of supraventricular tachycardia. Circulation 88: 1671-1681

19. Rhodes LA, Walsh EP, Saul JP (1994) Programmed atrial stimulation via the esophagus for management of supraventricular arrhythmias in infants and children. Am J Cardiol 74: 353-356

Antiarrhythmic Therapy of Supraventricular Tachyarrhythmias: Which Role for the Drugs Today?

G. Vergara

Divisione di Cardiologia, Ospedale S. Chiara, Trento, Italy

Introduction

The technological improvements and the high success rate of catheter ablation in the management of patients with supraventricular arrhythmias as well as the physicians' attraction to a "true therapeutic" approach may lead to an excessively interventional philosophy in which other therapeutic options, mainly pharmacologic treatment, is considered obsolete. In effect, catheter ablation presents some pitfalls that must be considered: there are complications, X-ray exposure, and studies of long-term follow-up are lacking. Thus this procedure cannot be considered a panacea for all patients with supraventricular arrhythmias.

In fact, according to the ACC guidelines (1) catheter ablation is generally indicated for drug-refractory supraventricular arrhythmias: thus pharmacologic treatment still has an important role in the management of these arrhythmias, even in the ablation era.

If we consider the pros and cons of the two therapeutic options, i.e., drugs and ablation, as well as the natural history of the arrhythmia in the individual patient we will get the best idea of which therapeutic option is most suitable.

Atrial Fibrillation

In treating a patient with atrial fibrillation there are two possible goals (1) to restore and to maintain the sinus rhythm and (2) to reduce the ventricular rate. If the first goal is the problem, the pharmacologic treatment (I C, III, and I A antiarrhythmic drugs) faces with nonpharmacologic treatment that is a surgical treatment (maze operation, left atrial insulation, corridor operation): in fact, there is no reliable alternative to pharmacologic in the majority of the patients. If the problem is to reduce the ventricular rate, drug treatment (verapamil, gallopamil, diltiazem, ß-blockers, digitalis) can be matched with atrioventricular (AV) node catheter ablation. The pros and cons of the two therapeutic options are summarized in Table 1.

No doubt the pros/cons ratio of the drug treatment is better than the pros/cons ratio of the catheter ablation in some patients, thus indicating pharmacologic treatment.

Atrial Flutter

Catheter ablation of the atrial flutter circuit may be considered as an investigational tool. The clinical results are unsatisfactory in some patients regarding clinical recurrences, new arrhythmias, and side effects. Thus I A, I C and III class drugs may be used: the clinical results are not excellent but fortunately the clinical trend of the recurrences is favorable in the majority of the patients.

AV Node Reentrant Tachycardia

An effective drug treatment with IC, II, III, and IV class drugs may be easily selected using a transesophageal electropharmacologic test and can be matched with the AV node radiofrequency catheter modification. The pros and cons of the two options are reported in Table 1.

The incidence of complete AV block is 5.1% in the Multicenter European Radiofrequency Survey (2); in addition, because of the lack of long-term follow-up, the late results of the procedure remain unclear in terms of late clinical recurrences of the ablated or of new arrhythmias as well as in terms of late side effects, including late occurrence of AV block. Thus catheter ablation is now indicated in highly symptomatic patients; patients with fewer symptoms can be correctly and satisfactorily managed by drug treatment.

Pre-excitation Syndrome

Both drug treatment (I C and III and combination of drugs) and catheter ablation of the anomalous pathway are suitable in the clinical management of pre-excitation syndrome. The pros and cons of the two options are listed in Table 1.

Table 1. Pros and cons of drug therapy and catheter ablation in supraventricular tachyarrhythmias

Drugs			Catheter ablation	
Pros	**Cons**		**Pros**	**Cons**
Effective No risk	↓ Compliance Side effects	**Atrial fibrillation**	Effective No risk	Pacemaker implantation Costs?
Effective Easy to select Easy to charge Discontinuation Therapy on occurrence Long-term follow-up	No curative Side effects ↓ Compliance	**AVN reentrant tachycardia**	Curative Effective	Unintended AV block (2) Lack of long-term follow-up
Effective Easy to select Easy to change Discontinuation Therapy on occurrence Long-term follow-up	No curative drug Side effects ↓ compliance	**WPW**	Curative Effective	Complications (5-12) Lack of long-term follow-up X-ray exposure

AV, atrioventricular; AVN, atrioventricular node; WPW, Wolff-Parkinson-White

The disadvantages of drug treatment are currently emphasized, but in our experience pharmacologic therapy is highly effective with a low incidence of side effects (3,4). In contrast, the disadvantages of catheter ablation are often grossly underemphasized. If we carefully examine the literature the procedure-related complication rates range from 2% to 18% (5-12) and there is no doubt that even an incidence of 2% of serious procedure-related complications acquires a relevant weight considering the benign natural history of the majority of WPW patients.

A correct evaluation of the pros and cons of the two options in the individual patients and a complete picture of the problem, including symptoms, risks, and patient acceptance, should provide us with the best therapeutic option (13). In our opinion, the two options are not very well matched in patients with pre-excitation syndrome "at risk": in these patients the pros/cons ratio for catheter ablation is better than the pros/cons ratio for drug treatment. In the other patients, i.e., those without an electrophysiologic pattern of risk, drug treatment can be matched against catheter ablation: in fact there are several patients in this group in whom the pros/cons ratio for drug treatment is better than pros/cons ratio for catheter ablation.

Conclusions

Although catheter ablation represents the most important therapeutic advance of the last decade in the treatment of supraventricular tachyarrhythmias, drug treatment cannot be considered an obsolete therapeutic option. Only with an objective assessment of the pros and cons of the two options in the individual patient can the best treatment be delivered. There are patients who are better treated with catheter ablation and patients who are more suitably managed with drugs. Accurate patient information regarding clinical condition and therapeutic options, unbiased evaluation of the pros and cons of the possible options together with the patient's wish will aid us in making the best choice.

References

1. American College of Cardiology Cardiovascular Technology Assessment Committee (1994) Catheter ablation for cardiac arrhythmias: clinical applications, personnel and facilities. J Am Coll Cardiol 24: 828-833
2. Hindricks G on behalf of the Multicenter European Radiofrequency Survey (MERFS) Investigators (1993) Incidence of complete atrioventricular block in 808 patients after radiofrequency modification of the atrioventricular node. Eur Heart J 14: (Suppl): 257 (abstr)
3. Vergara G, Visonà L, Inama G, Guarneiro M, Accardi R, Furlanello F (1990) Flecainide after the CAST: long-term follow-up (3 years) in patients with WPW syndrome responders to electropharmacological test. New Trends Arrhyth 6:241-244
4. Inama G, Furlanello, F Vergara G, Guarnerio M, Braito G, Nassivera E (1992) Il sotalolo nella sindrome di Wolff-Parkinson-White: studio elettrofisiologico e clinico. G Ital Cardiol 22: 701-714
5. Catheter ablation of arrhythmias. A teaching workshop. Organizzato da Nethan AW, Borggrefe M, Kuck KH, Camm AJ, Londra 28-29 ottobre 1992
6. Hindricks G, Haverkamp W on behalf of the Multicentric European Radiofrequency Survey (MERFS) Investigators (1993) The Multicenter European Radiofrequency Survey: summary of the results - complications of radiofrequency catheter ablation of cardiac arrhythmias in 4372 Patients. Eur Heart 14: (Suppl): 256 (abstr)
7. Mittleman RS, Huang SKS, Gillette P et al (1994) Comparison of the trans-septal vs retrograde aortic approach for left sided accessory pathway radiofrequency ablation: a prospective multi-center study PACE 17: 833 (abstr)
8. Khanedani A, Schlüter M, Cappato R, Kuck KH (1994) Serial echocardiography to assess the incidence and clinical course of pericardial effusion following radiofrequency catheter ablation of accessory pathways. J Am Coll Cardiol (Special issue): 82 (abstr)
9. Scheinman MM (1994) Patterns of catheter ablation practice in the United States: results of the 1992 NASPE Survey. PACE 17: 873-875
10. Minich LL, Snider R, MacDonald D II (1992) Doppler detection of valvular regurgitation after radiofrequency ablation of accessory connections. Am J Cardiol 70: 116-117
11. Greene TO, Huang SKS, Wagshal AB et al (1994) Cardiovascular complications after radiofrequency catheter ablation of supraventricular tachyarrhythmias. Am, J Cardiol 74: 615-617
12. Thakur RK, Klein GJ, Yee R, Zardini M (1994) Embolic complications after radiofrequency catheter ablation. Am J Cardiol 74: 278-279
13. Vergara G (1992) Ablazione transcatetere con radiofrequenza nel trattamento dei pazienti con WPW Ruolo attuale tra tanti entusiasmi e qualche riserva. G Ital Cardiol 22: 1267-1271

Radiofrequency Ablation of Supraventricular Tachycardias in Infants and Children: When Is It Really Indicated?

A.S. Montenero[1], F. Drago[2], F. Crea[1], R. Schiavello[4], A. Cipriani[3], G. Pelargonio[1], A. Intini[1], M.G. Bendini[1], M.C. Varano[4], S. Guarneri[4], F. Bellocci[1], P. Zecchi[1], and P. Ragonese[2]

[1]Istituto di Cardiologia, Università Cattolica del Sacro Cuore,
Rome, Italy
[2]Divisione di Cardiologia, Ospedale Pediatrico del Bambin Gesù,
Rome, Italy
[3]Istituto di Pediatria, Università Cattolica del Sacro Cuore,
Rome, Italy
[4]Istituto di Anestesia e Rianimazione, Università Cattolica del Sacro Cuore,
Rome, Italy

Introduction

Supraventricular tachycardia (SVT) is the most common sustained cardiac arrhythmia in children and adolescents, approximately 85% being due to reentrant circuits (1). Pharmacologic treatment has been proposed as the first-line therapy for frequent, sustained episodes of SVT associated with significant symptoms. However, patients refractory to medical therapy often require surgical intervention (2), which has recently been replaced by the procedure of transcatheter ablation (3).

Direct current catheter ablation creates a dispersive shock lesion in the targeted area of the myocardium and, in most instances, the resulting combination of heat and barotrauma made the exact energy delivery and lesion size difficult to control (4). In contrast, the more recent use of rapidly alternating electrical current [radiofrequency (RF) current] produces adequate heating to achieve small focal lesions in a much more regulated fashion. It has been employed in the treatment of most cardiac arrhythmias in adults and, in some cases, has become the most effective therapy.

In children and adolescents RF catheter ablation has been used with success as an effective and definitive technique for ablating the accessory atrioventricular (AV) connections (5-10). In contrast, only limited experience has been reported on RF ablation for AV nodal reentrant tachycardia in children (8).

The purpose of this study was to evaluate the efficacy and safety of RF ablation in young patients suffering from SVT due to a reentrant circuit.

Methods

Patients

Between February 1993 and October 1994, 45 patients (mean age 12.6 years, range 3-18 years) underwent RF catheter ablation. The majority of patients suffered from documented or doubtful SVT due to a reentry circuit. Only five patients also had paroxysmal atrial fibrillation.

Clinical evaluation, chest X-ray, surface electrocardiogram (ECG), 24-h Holter monitoring, and two-dimensional echocardiographic assessment showed no signs of structural heart disease in any patient. All patients underwent electrophysiologic transesophageal atrial study (TEAS), apart from one with permanent junctional reciprocating tachycardia (PJRT).

According to criteria proposed by Cox et al. (2), a macro-reentrant orthodromic tachycardia through AV accessory pathways was induced in 39 patients, but in five cases this evolved subsequently into atrial fibrillation. In six patients an atrioventricular nodal reentrant tachycardia (AVNRT) was induced.

Invasive electrophysiologic study and RF catheter ablation were indicated according to the following criteria:

1. Severe symptoms at high risk (syncope and presyncope)
2. Inefficacy of medical treatment
3. Drug intolerance
4. The wishes of the patient and family

Electrophysiologic Testing and Catheter Ablation

General anesthesia was performed in patients under 12 years of age. Electrophysiologic testing was performed in patients with AVNRT using two quadripolar catheters (USCI Bard, Bellerica, MA, USA), one inserted into the right atrium and the other on the His bundle. A 7-Fr quadripolar ablation catheter (EPTechnology Inc, Mountain View, CA, USA Mod: Blazer) was used for mapping the septal area and the tricuspidal annulus and for the ablation.

In patients with accessory pathways different approaches were used for different locations, while mapping was performed using the same technique: three quadripolar catheters (USCI) were positioned, one in the right atrium, one on the His bundle, and a third in the right ventricle.

A decapolar 6-Fr catheter (USCI special) was positioned in the coronary sinus to map the mitral valve annulus. A retrograde transaortic approach was used for the left accessory pathways in the first part of the study (ten ablations); in the second part, a transseptal approach was used (18 ablations).

Transseptal catheterization was performed using a 0.032-in. guide wire, an 8-Fr Mullins catheter (USCI), and a Brockenbrough needle (USCI). The ablation catheter was then advanced into the left atrium through the sheath of the Mullins catheter (USCI), which was withdrawn into the right atrium in order to improve the maneuvrability of the deflecting tip of the ablation catheter.

A right atrial approach was used in a patient with right, anteroseptal, and posteroseptal pathways. In the patient with PJRT, the right atrial approach was impossible because of a right and left femoral vein thrombosis; in this case the ablation catheter was introduced through the left subclavian vein.

ECG leads and intracardiac electrograms were recorded on a Bard Electrophysiology Lab System version 2.51 C and then 2.55 C. In all patients the electrograms were filtered between 30 and 250 Hz, amplified at a gain of 0.5 mV/cm, and recorded at a paper speed of 100 mm/s. Electrograms obtained from the coronary sinus and from the ablation catheter were recorded in unipolar configuration.

Programmed stimulation was performed with a programmable stimulator (Medtronic model 5328, Minneapolis, MN, USA) at a pulse width of 1.5 ms and at an intensity of twice the diastolic threshold. Pacing was performed in the right atrium or ventricle using bipolar stimulation while unipolar stimulation was performed in the coronary sinus. The energy was delivered between the distal electrode of the ablation catheter and a large adhesive skin electrode placed on the back of the patient.

In patients with an accessory pathway, both the mitral and tricuspidal valve annulus were mapped carefully during sinus rhythm in order to identify the shortest A-V interval and to record a possible accessory pathway potential (K) and the shortest A-K and delta-K intervals as previously described (11). Confirmation that the area of interest had been correctly located was made by measuring the shortest V-A interval, either during ventricular pacing or during induced or spontaneus reciprocating tachycardia. Once the area of interest was defined, a 7-Fr ablation catheter (EPTechnology, Inc. Mountain View, Mod: Blazer) was advanced from the femoral vein to the right atrium and then to the left atrium using the transseptal approach in 18 patients and from the femoral artery to the left ventricle using the retrograde approach in ten patients.

In patients with overt pre-excitation, a local atrial electrogram was recorded systematically during sinus rhythm and was considered stable when minimal variations in the amplitude of recorded potential were observed for at least 5 consecutive beats. When the recording was stable and continuous, the morphologic features of the local atrial electrogram were evaluated in order to identify the presence of the K potential. The K potential was defined as a stable deflection in the local electrogram distinct from the atrial and ventricular components, which preceded the onset of the QRS complex and were related to the delta wave on the surface ECG.

In addition the A-V, A-K, delta-K, and K-V intervals were measured carefully on the electrograms obtained from the ablation catheter, prior to the RF energy discharge as recently described by our group (12). A quadripolar 7-Fr electrode catheter (EPT) with a deflectable shaft and a large distal electrode (4 mm in length) was used for the ablation.

RF energy was produced by a power generator which delivered a continuous unmodulated wave output at 500-750 kHz (Liz 88, American Cardiac Ablation Corporation, Foxboro, MA, USA) and measured and displayed impedance and power. After recording the local electrogram, 30 V were delivered for 10 s to test the impedance, catheter stability, and effect on the accessory pathway conduction. If the delta wave disappeared, 50 V were given for 40 s at the same site.

If the conduction of the accessory pathway was not lost during the initial 10-s delivery at 30 V, the catheter was repositioned around the target area and a new electrogram was recorded before the ablation procedure was repeated using the same sequence.

If the impedance increased suddenly during the procedure, the delivery of energy was stopped and the ablation catheter removed, cleaned, and then readvanced into the atrium through the sheath.

In patients with AVNRT, RF ablation was performed on the slow pathway after an accurate mapping of the posteroseptal area. A slow pathway potential as described by Jackman et al. (13) was mapped in the majority of patients.

Anterograde and retrograde conduction were measured 30 min after ablation of the accessory pathways under basal conditions and following the i.v. administration of a bolus of propanolol (2.5 mg) and verapamil (5 mg).

The inducibility of reciprocating tachycardia was evaluated after the ablation of the slow pathway under basal conditions and following the i.v. administration of atropine (0.02 mg/kg).

Heparin (10 000 I.U.) was given intravenously during the procedure and then for the following 24 h (10 000 I.U.). Aspirin (100 mg once a day) was prescribed for the 3 months following the procedure.

Statistical Analysis

Student's *t*-test was used to compare the registered time of fluoroscopy in ablation of left accessory pathways carried out via the retrograde transaortic and transseptal approaches. A value of $p < 0.05$ was considered significant.

Follow-up

At 1 month and 1 year after ablation (successful or not) surface ECG, 24-h Holter monitoring, and TEAS were carried out. In the patients in whom the procedure demonstrated early or late unsuccess, an examination was also carried out at 6 months postablation.

The parents of the patients were also in constant contact with our institution.

Successful outcome of the procedure was defined as the disappearance of (a) symptoms, (b) the delta wave or the surface ECG, in patients with ventricular pre-excitation, and (c) the inducibility of SVT with TEAS at least 1 month after the procedure.

Results

Electrophysiologic Characteristics

A total of 45 patients were studied: AVNRT was induced in six patients, while accessory pathways with orthodromic reentrant SVT were found in the remainder, among whom five had experienced clinical episodes of atrial fibrillation. In this group tachycardia desynchronized spontaneously after the induction of SVT.

Among the accessory pathways, either manifest or concealed, 26 were left and 13 were right pathways. In particular, 17 were left lateral, four left posterolateral, four left posteroseptal, one left anterolateral, 12 right posteroseptal, and one right anteroseptal. Among the five patients with atrial fibrillation, three were left lateral, one left posterolateral, and one left anterolateral. In the patient with PJRT the accessory pathway was a right posteroseptal, located near the ostium of the coronary sinus.

Ablation Results

During the period of the study 48 procedures were performed: one patient underwent it three times; a 15-year-old female with a concealed left posteroseptal pathway underwent two unsuccessful attempts using the retrograde transaortic approach and one transseptal successful procedure.

Immediate success was observed in 38 (92.6%) out of 41 procedures for accessory pathways. A transient disappearance of the accessory pathway during one of the RF deliveries was observed in one patient with a right posterolateral pathway in whom the procedure failed.

Mean fluoroscopy time in patients with accessory pathways was 31 ± 18 min. Mean fluoroscopy time in the retrograde transaortic approach was 95% longer than in the transeptal approach (45 ± 10 min versus 23 ± 12 min; $p<0.01$).

In patients with AVNRT, ablation of the slow pathway was successful in 50% of cases (3/6). In the three patients in whom it was impossible to ablate the slow pathway, the procedure was interrupted without attempting to ablate the fast pathway. In one of the three patients treated successfully, ablation of the slow pathway produced a transient complete AV block. The 1:1 conduction recovered as first-degree AV block within a few hours.

In the patient with PJRT, the tachycardia was interrupted by ablating the reentry site of the accessory pathway, but on the day following the procedure a few isolated reentrant beats were recorded.

Follow-up

All patients survived and underwent long-term follow-up (mean 12.9 months, with a range between 5 and 33). Of them, 34 patients were followed up during the first year. All patients in whom treatment was immediately successful remained asymptomatic for tachyarrhythmias. No recurrence of delta waves or episodes of asymptomatic tachycardia were recorded on either the basal ECG or the Holter tape. They were not inducible at TEAS either, with the exception of a 15-year-old female patient with a concealed right anteroseptal pathway. Twenty-five days after the procedure she reported a prolonged episode of palpitations, weakness, and dizziness which recovered spontaneously. After 1 month of follow-up, a reciprocating tachycardia – similar to that she had previously experienced – was induced at TEAS. Propafenone was then given and 1 year after the procedure a new TEAS was performed in pharmacologic washout, inducing tachycardia again. Eighteen months after ablation no arrhythmias were recorded during Holter monitoring, and no tachyarrhythmia was induced at TEAS. Therefore the drug therapy was discontinued and she is now asymptomatic.

At the 1-month and 1-year follow-up examination, the patient with a right posterolateral pathway that was ablated unsuccessfully was asymptomatic: the surface ECG showed no delta wave, and no arrhythmias were recorded during Holter monitoring or were induced at TEAS. Therefore a 100% delayed success was observed in patients with manifest or concealed accessory pathways.

The immediate success of the ablation was later confirmed in only two of the three patients with AVNRT. In one patient, asymptomatic after the procedure, a reciprocating tachycardia was induced at TEAS 1 month after the ablation. Two of the three patients, who were not ablated successfully, experienced symptomatic tachycardia and flecainide was prescribed. The third patient, who was inducible at TEAS, experienced during a 33-month follow-up only one short episode of palpitations, which resolved spontaneously. Therefore a 33% rate of delayed success was observed in patients with AVNRT.

The patient with PJRT, who was ablated with immediate success, experienced the same tachycardia 1 month after the ablation. After 6 months the procedure was repeated and immediate success was obtained. In May 1995, 1 month after the second trial, he is free from tachycardia.

Adverse Events

We reported complications in three patients (6.5%) in whom the transseptal approach was used. One patient had a thrombosis of the femoral vein 6 days after the procedure, which was resolved with medical therapy. The second developed a large hematoma, which disappeared with medical therapy. Holter monitoring showed frequent and monomorphic premature ventricular beats (212 in 24 h) and a short run (7 beats) of monomorphic ventricular tachycardia (150 bpm) with the same morphology of premature ventricular beats in the last patient at the first month of follow-up.

Discussion

SVT due to AV accessory pathways is a congenital cardiac disease with an incidence of about three out of

1000 in the general population. Approximately 85% of the children and adolescents with SVT have a reentry circuit due either to manifest or concealed accessory pathways or to dual AV node physiology .

In 28% of the patients with a manifest AV accessory pathway, electrocardiographic features of pre-excitation disappear during the teenage years and 70% of the 28% have no recurrences during their lives. In contrast, only 40% of patients in whom pre-excitation is still present at ECG do not have recurrences of SVT (1).

About two thirds of the children with reentrant supraventricular tachycardia experience palpitations, chest discomfort, and fatigue. For these reasons they are submitted to long-term antiarrhythmic drug therapy, often requiring strict control which is sometimes difficult to obtain in children and infants. Furthermore, frequent evaluations of therapeutic and side effects should be required.

In the presence of potential side effects of antiarrhythmic drug therapy it is often necessary to take a more aggressive approach in children with SVT. In the past few years, RF transcatheter ablation of overt or concealed accessory pathways and of AVNRT has been increasingly performed in adults (5,6). It is also safe and effective in children and adolescents with symptomatic SVT refractory to antiarrhythmic drug therapy.

Age is an important criteria when considering this procedure as a therapeutic approach: should a SVT occur during the first 4 months of life, it may recur in 22% of patients. A SVT occurring after the first 4 months may recur in 88% of cases. Over a period of 5 years, 80% of patients symptomatic for paroxysmal SVT require long-term drug therapy.

A long-term antiarrhythmic drug therapy may result in the following disadvantages: (a) proarrhythmic or side effects, (b) high economic cost, (c) mild to moderate risk that cardiomegaly develops when supraventricular incessant junctional tachycardia becomes refractory to drug therapy.

The success rate of RF transcatheter ablation in patients suffering from SVT covers a wide range of values, from 50% to 96% in children (7-14,15) and from 82% to 99% in adults (16-18). The lower success rate in pediatric patients might be due to: (a) the frequent association of SVT to congenital heart disease (19), (b) the smaller size of the heart, reducing the maneuvrability of the catheters, (c) fluoroscopy exposure which is too long, suggesting the interruption of the procedure.

In Table 1 the most important studies in infants and adolescents reported in literature have been compared.

An incidence of 4.8% of early and late postablation complications was recently reported by Kugler (18), which is slightly higher when compared to that of catheterization (20). Therefore, pediatric patients should be followed up regularly, even for extracardiac problems, and anticoagulant agents should be used during and after the procedure.

In our patients, the complication rate was similar to that reported by other authors. Evidence of vascular complications after a procedure means that great care should be taken when introducing more than one catheter into the right femoral vein, because of the greater possible risk of trauma occurring in the smaller vascular structures of children. It would be preferable to use smaller catheters than those used up to now.

Although the number of patients in our study is relatively small, our experience confirms the efficacy of

Table 1. Comparison of the results from the most important studies in infants and adolescents

Reference	Year	Patients (n)	Mean age	WPW (n)	Success (%)	AVN reentry	Success (%)	AET	Success (%)	PJRT	Success (%)
(7)	1991	20	12.5 ys	20	74	0	/	0	/	0	/
(8)	1991	17	13.6 ys	12	83	4	100	1	100	0	/
(15)	1992	7	10 mths	6	66	0	/	1	100	0	/
(21)	1992	8	8.2 ys	0	/	0	/	0	/	8	100
(9)	1992	10	10.5 ys	10	100	0	/	0	/	0	/
(20)	1993	71	14 ys	71	93	0	/	0	/	0	/
(10)	1993	17	12.8 ys	17	94	0	/	0	/	0	/
(22)	1993	22	16.5 ys	22	73	0	/	0	/	0	/
(23)	1994	16	15 ys	13	81	0	/	0	/	0	/
(24)	1994	53	9.3 ys	51	96	0	/	0	/	0	/
(25)	1994	652	13.5	508[b]	82	76	82	46	93	0	/
(26)	1994	46	12.6 ys	39	100	6	33	0	/	1	100

WPW, Wolff-Parkinson-White syndrome; AVN, atrioventricular node; AET, atrial ectopic tachycardia; PJRT, permanent junctional reciprocating tachycardia.
[a]Pediatric Electrophysiology Society.
[b]Including patients with PJRT.

RF ablation in the treatment of SVT due to a reentry circuit in the pediatric age. The success rate of the patients with a manifest or concealed accessory pathway is clearly greater than that of the patients with AVNRT. This might be due to the more difficult mapping procedure of the slow pathway, which results in a higher percentage of failure. Thus, RF catheter ablation in patients with AVNRT had a lower success rate, as greater attention has to be paid to avoid an AV block.

K potential recording and careful analysis of the A-K and delta-K intervals have determined a better localization of the ablation site, thus making the procedure easier and shorter (11,12). Fluoroscopy time for the transseptal approach was shorter when compared with the transaortic approach in the ablation of left accessory pathways.

Late disappearance of ventricular pre-excitation in patients in whom the procedure was not immediately successful might be due to the fibrosis which results from the RF deliveries. A progressive extension of the scar might inglobe the accessory pathway not perfectly ablated during the procedure. This can also play a role in new arrhythmias developing as presented by one of our patients during the follow-up. Therefore, postponing ablation to an age when physical maturity assures minimal morphovolumetric change of the heart should be considered mandatory unless severe symptoms occur.

In conclusion, our study confirms the safety and efficacy of RF catheter ablation of SVT in the pediatric age group. The efficacy of RF ablation for the interruption of accessory pathways in children over the age of 6 years has become firmly established.

Thus, at present severe symptoms (syncope and presyncope), resistance to medical treatment, and drug intolerance are primary indications for catheter ablation. The wishes of the patient and their family may sometimes represent an indication for ablation even in patients with mild symptoms. In these cases the family and the patients should be carefully informed about the benefit of the procedure and the risk of complications.

References

1. Klitzner TS, Roberts N (1983) The investigation of an arrhythmia: the invasive approach. In: Roberts N., Gelband H (eds) Cardiac arrhythmias in the neonate, infants and child. Appleton and Lange, East Norwalk, pp 79-103
2. Cox JL, Gallagher JJ, Caim ME (1985) Experience with 118 consecutive patients undergoing operation for the Wolff-Parkinson-White syndrome. J Thorac Cardiovasc Surg 90: 490-501
3. Gillette PC, Garson A, Kugler JD, Cooley DA, Zinner A, McNamara DG (1980) Surgical treatment for SVT in infants and children. Am J Cardiol 46: 281-284
4. Bromberg BI, Dick M, Scott WA, Morady F (1989) Transcatheter electrical ablation of accesssory pathways in children. PACE 12: 1787 1796
5. Borggrefe M, Hindricks G, Haverkamp W, Breithardt G (1990) Catheter ablation using radiofrequency energy. Clin Cardiol 13: 127-131
6. Langberg JJ, Chin MC, Rosenquist M, Cockrell J, Dullett N, Van Hare G, Griffin JC, Scheinman MM (1989) Catheter ablation of the atrioventricular junction with radiofrequency energy. Circulation 80: 1527-1535
7. Dick M, O'Connor BK, Serwer GA, LeRoy S, Armstrong B (1991) Use of radiofrequency current to ablate accessory connections in children. Circulation 84: 2318-2324
8. Van Hare GF, Lesh MD, Scheinman M, Langberg JJ (1991) Percutaneous radiofrequency catheter ablation for supraventricular arrhythmias in children. J Am Coll Cardiol 17: 1613-1620
9. Schluter M, Kuck KH (1992) Radiofrequency current for catheter ablation of accessory atrio-ventricular connections in children and adolescents: emphasis on the single-catheter technique. Pediatrics 89: 930-935
10. Klitzner TS, Wetzel GT, Saxon LA, Stevenson WG (1993) Radiofrequency ablation: a new era in the treatment of pediatrics arrhythmias. Am J Dis Child 147:769-771
11. Montenero AS, Crea F, Bendini MG, Biscione F, Scipione P, Mascellanti M, Cianfrone N, Di Sabato M, De Martino G, Ferro A, Bellocci F, Zecchi P (1993) Radiofrequency catheter ablation of cardiac accessory pathways using the transseptal approach. New Trends Arrhythmias 9: 405
12. Montenero AS, Crea F, Bendini MG, Pelargonio G, Intini A, Finocchiaro ML, Biscione F, Pigozzi F, Bellocci F, Zecchi P. (1995) Electrograms for identification of the atrial ablation site during catheter ablation of accessory pathways. PACE (in press)
13. Jackman WM, Beckman KJ, McClelland JH, et al (1992) Treatment of SVT due to atrio-ventricular nodal reentrant tachycardia by radiofrequency catheter ablation of slow pathway conduction. N Engl J Med 327: 313-318
14. Walsh EP, Saul JP, Hulse JE et al (1992) Transcatheter ablation of ectopic atrial tachycardia in young patients using radiofrequency current. Circulation 86: 1138-1146
15. Case CL, Gillette PC, Oslizlok PC, Knick BJ, Blair HL (1992) Radiofrequency catheter ablation of incessant, medically resistant SVT in infants and small children. J Am Coll Cardiol 20:1405-1410
16. Jackman WM, Wang X, Friday KJ et al (1991) Catheter ablation of accessory atrio-ventricular pathways (Wolff-Parkinson-White syndrome) by radiofrequency current. N Engl J Med 342:1605-1611
17. Calkins H, Sousa J, El-Atassi R, et al (1991) Diagnosis and cure of the Wolff-Parkinson-White syndrome or paroxysmal SVT during a single electrophysiologic test. N Engl J Med 324: 1612-1618
18. Kugler JD, Danford DA, Deal BJ et al for the Pediatric Electrophysiology Society (1994) Radiofrequency catheter ablation for tachyarrhythmias in children and adolescents. N Engl J Med 330: 1481-1487
19. Mullins CE, Latson LA, Neches WH et al (1990) Balloon dilatation of miscellaneous lesions: results of valvuloplasty and angioplasty of congenital anomalies registry. Am J Cardiol 65: 802-803
20. Levine JC, Walsh EP, Saul JP (1993) Radiofrequency ablation of accessory pathways associated with congenital heart disease including heterotaxy syndrome. Am J Cardiol 72: 689-693
21. Ticho BS, Saul JP, Hulse JE, De W, Lulu J, Walsh EP (1992) Variable location of accessory pathways associated with the permanent form of junctional reciprocating tachycardia and confirmation with radiofrequency ablation. Am J Cardiol 70: 1559-1564
22. Sreeram N, Smeets JLRM, Pulles-Heintzberger CFM, Wellens HJJ (1993) Radiofrequency catheter ablation of accessory pathways in children and young adults. Br Heart J 70: 160-165
23. Lemery R, Talajic M, Roy D, Fournier A, Coutu B, TY Hii J, Radzik D, Lavoie L (1994) Cathether ablation using radiofrequency or low-energy direct current in pediatric patients with the Wolff-Parkinson-White syndrome. Am J Cardiol 73: 191-194
24. Hebe J, Schluter M, Kuck KH (1994) Catheter ablation in children with supraventricular tachycardia mediated by accessory pathways: use of radiofrequency current as a first line of therapy. Cardiol Young 4: 28-36
25. Kugler JD, Danford DA, Deal BJ et al for the Pediatric Electrophysiology Society (1994) Radiofrequency catheter ablation for tachyarrhythmias in children and adolescents. N Engl J Med 330: 1481-1487
26. Montenero AS, Drago F, Crea F, Bendini MG, Pelargonio G, Bellocci F, Ragonese P, Zecchi P (1994) Indications and limitations of radiofrequency ablation of supraventricular tachycardia in children. In: Pozzi L (ed) Autoapproach to cardiac arrhythmias in 1994, vol 1, pp 208-213

ATRIAL FIBRILLATION AND
ATRIAL FLUTTER

Lone Atrial Fibrillation: Which Anatomical and Electrophysiologic Substrate?

A. Capucci, M. Biffi*, and G. Boriani*

Ospedale Civile di Piacenza, Italy
*Istituto di Malattie dell'Apparato Cardiovascolare,
Università degli Studi di Bologna, Italy

Introduction

Atrial fibrillation (AF) is the most common arrhythmia seen in clinical practice in all its presentation forms: paroxysmal, recurrent and chronic. Though usually associated with organic heart disease, it is also found in the absence of any structural cardiac abnormality in a substantial number of cases. Its clinical significance, prognosis, and management are largely dependent on underlying or associated heart disease; understanding the electrophysiologic (EP) mechanisms and modulating factors, such as the autonomic nervous system, is of utmost importance in the clinical management of AF patients.

AF Mechanisms: Experimental Models of Atrial Reentry

Mines (1) was first to describe reentry as the EP basis of an arrhythmia. The main findings in Mines' work (1913) are the characteristics required to sustain the reentrant mechanism: unidirectional block and slow conduction.

Slow conduction is the condition by which the area of block can recover excitability for the depolarizing current coming from the opposite direction; this mechanism is enhanced by a short refractory period in the area of block. This experimental model implies that reentry occurs around an anatomical obstacle and implies the existence of a fully excitable gap between the depolarizing wavefront and its own tale of refractoriness.

Lewis et al. (2) confirmed the importance of the reentry mechanism a few years later working on an experimental dog model of atrial flutter. The reentrant loop occurred around the two venae cavae (anatomical obstacles), with an interposed area of functional block determining an excitable gap. Whenever the length of this excitable gap exceeds the circumference of the anatomical obstacle the arrhythmia may collapse and stop, or it may shift to a single-obstacle circuit, thus accelerating to AF.

The concept of a reentry circuit was not subsequently modified until Moe and coworkers reported their observations (3,4). They investigated the role of specialized atrial conduction tissue, such as internodal and Bachman fascicles, as being capable of maintaining atrial flutter without needing anatomical obstacles to sustain reentrant waves.

New insights were brought by Allessie and coworkers in several interesting papers (5-10). The first type of reentrant circuit which they proposed did not necessitate any anatomical obstacle but was defined by pure atrial EP (4) characteristics. The length of the circuit is, in fact, the product of atrial refractoriness and conduction velocity, and is defined as the "wavelength" of the circulating depolarization wavefront. In this model no excitable gap occurs as the reentrant circuit is the shortest allowed by atrial EP characteristics, and the center of the circuit is kept continuously refractory by centripetal wavelets.

Further observations of the presence of areas of slow conduction between anatomical obstacles led to more complex models of atrial reentry. In fact, they described patterns of reentry around an anatomical obstacle (when the wavelength is short enough), either with an anatomical obstacle, an area of slow conduction, or an excitable gap in the normal myocardium (in which the reentry is determined by EP properties only). Thus, reentry may be sustained by coexisting factors, either anatomical or purely functional, and this contributes to the continuously changing shape and characteristics of the depolarizing waves during AF.

Spach and coworkers (11,12) have observed reentry due to purely functional atrial properties, the peculiar spatial arrangement of atrial myocytes. This is responsible for substantial heterogeneity in atrial conduction velocity (greater in longitudinal than in transverse direction) so that areas of slow conduction suitable for reentry are observed at the reflection points. The model of reentry is thus defined by the EP heterogeneity set by the anisotropy of atrial myocytic layers. The geometric shape of the circuit is an ellipsoid with a small gap of excitability at the reflection points.

EP Mechanisms of AF in Humans

Atrial Refractoriness

Although general agreement in the literature has not been achieved, the duration of the atrial refractory period is a critical parameter for the development of clinical AF. In fact, several reports (13-16) have emphasized the significance of markedly shortened atrial refractoriness in patients with clinical AF episodes or with inducible AF at EP study. In the same way, Attuel et al. (17) found a significantly shorter atrial functional and effective refractoriness (evaluated with one up to three extrastimuli) in inducible versus noninducible patients with either AF, atrial flutter and paroxysmal supraventricular tachycardia in various heart diseases. Kumagai et al. (18) evaluated patients with chronic AF the day following transthoracic cardioversion by EP study and found a shorter effective refractory period than in controls.

Michelucci et al. (15) found a significantly greater dispersion of both functional and effective refractoriness either in sinus or during paced rhythm at three atrial sites than in controls.

The same finding was absent in a previous work by Luck and Engel (19), who had evaluated patients with sinus node dysfunction, with and without clinical AF episodes.

In the work of Michelucci, et al. dispersion of atrial refractoriness is also common in patients with sinus node dysfunction without AF, and both atrial refractoriness and its dispersion are related to age in normal subjects (20). Padeletti et al. (21) found that, whereas dispersion of atrial refractoriness (functional and effective) is significantly greater in AF patients, the average value of atrial refractory periods is not significantly different than in controls. Boutjdir et al. (22) made interesting observations at the cellular level, measuring atrial refractory periods in human myocytes on specimens taken during open heart surgery: AF patients exhibited shorter refractoriness at long pacing cycles and greater dispersion than controls.

Other works (23-25) failed to find any significant difference in atrial refractoriness between patients with AF or atrial flutter and controls, though in one study AF patients had shorter refractoriness than atrial flutter patients (23). It is useful to underline that in the work by Simpson (25) atrial refractoriness was measured by pacing at 10 mA, in order to obtain the shortest value of refractoriness, which is different from conventional measurements made by pacing at twice the diastolic threshold.

In their study, Attuel et al. (26) examined the significance of rate adaptation of the refractory periods and found absence of adaptation at high rates of both effective and functional refractoriness in subjects with inducible atrial tachyarrhythmias with or without spontaneous arrhythmias. The lack of rate adaptation was associated with short atrial refractoriness, so that it is not clear whether this phenomenon is primitive or indeed secondary to the presence of short refractoriness at long cycle length.

The observations made by Capucci et al. (27) in patients with lone paroxysmal AF show that atrial functional and effective refractoriness are significantly shorter at both long and short cycle lengths than in control patients, and this correlates with a high degree of vulnerability to fibrillate at long cycle lengths, too (600 ms), with a single extrastimulus.

In a recent study by Ramdat-Misier et al. (28) atrial refractoriness during fibrillation has been evaluated by the analysis of a fibrillation interval as described by Lammers et al. (29) with a multielectrode array during heart surgery. AF patient candidates for the "corridor" procedure showed a significantly shorter mean fibrillation interval and greater dispersion of refractoriness than patients without clinical AF episodes.

Atrial Conduction

An intraatrial conduction delay may be observed on a surface electrocardiogram (ECG), determining a bimodal pattern of the P wave in lead II, and it is associated with the occurrence of atrial arrhythmias (16,18,23) However, in patients with clinical AF episodes the P wave is usually normal (30).

The technique of signal averaging of the P wave has been recently applied (31,32) to improve sensitivity in detecting intraatrial conduction disturbances which may be responsible for the arrhythmogenic substrate in AF patients.

Atrial conduction may be better investigated at EP study. Many parameters have been proposed to define the critical one at AF induction:

S_2-A_2. S_2-A_2 is defined as the atrial activation time measured after a premature stimulus delivered early in diastole, in proximity to the effective atrial refractory period (30).

Concern has been raised as to whether this parameter may reflect actrial activation latency (due to tissue polarization by stimuli falling during absolute refractoriness) rather than true conduction; in this respect, different values have been observed at different atrial sites and during atrial pacing in comparison with sinus rhythm (16,30). These findings are in agreement with the hypothesis that this parameter represents true atrial conduction during relative refractoriness.

In patients with paroxysmal AF a significant delay of S_2-A_2 at the His bundle recording site and in coronary sinus compared to controls has been found by Cosio et al. (16). The same author showed that this parameter was significantly prolonged when the premature beat was delivered at the same site as the paced one (33).

Kumagai et al. (18) found a greater atrial conduction delay (defined as S_2-$A2 > S_1$-$A_1 + 20$ ms) and a wider range of premature beats capable of inducing such a conduction delay in AF patients as compared to controls.

Attuel et al. (17) did not observe significant differences in S_2-A_2 between patients with or without inducible sustained atrial tachyarrhythmias; the difference from other studies (16,18,30,33) lies in the different clinical characteristics of the populations (clinical versus induced arrhythmias; AF or flutter patients versus supraventricular tachycardias).

Patients with lone paroxysmal AF represent a peculiar subset because of the absence of a structural abnormality as compared to patients with organic heart disease; in this subgroup, Capucci et al. (27) did not find any statistically significant difference in S_2-A_2 as compared to subjects without either clinical or inducible atrial arrhytmias.

Intraatrial and Interatrial Conduction Time. Interatrial conduction time is the interval from high right atrium to low right atrium activation during pacing in the high right atrium, and **interatrial conduction time** is the interval from high right atrium to coronary sinus activation during pacing in the high right atrium. Buxton and coworkers (23) found a significant increase in both intraatrial and interatrial conduction times in patients with AF or flutter compared to controls at 600-ms cycle length, but this finding demonstrated specificity only at long paced cycles. The same increase was, in fact, observed also in controls at a 450-ms cycle length.

Simpson et al. (25) also found significantly longer intraatrial and interatrial conduction times than in controls, but the same finding was common to patients with sinus node disease without clinical AF and to patients with atrial arrhythmias other than AF.

Michelucci et al. (34) have reported that a prolongation of interatrial conduction times identifies patients with paroxysmal AF to controls as compared.

A_2 Fragmentation. Ohe et al. (24) first noticed that, in patients with lone AF, the range of premature stimuli determining A_2 fragmentation (widening of $A_2 > 150\%$ of baseline value) in the high right atrium was wider than in control patients. The same phenomenon was also observed in patients with sick sinus syndrome with and without clinical AF, although to a greater extent in those with AF. The fragmented atrial activity was considered analogous to previous observations in the ventricle (35), where it represents an ongoing local electrical activity in response to an extra beat, due to tissue anisotropy determining abnormal and slowed conduction.

Tanigawa et al. (36) confirmed the presence of atrial fragmentation ($A_2 > 100$ ms or with >8 deflections) in 68% of AF patients during atrial mapping. The number of sites showing fragmentation was greater in patients with associated sinus node dysfunction. Konoe et al. (37) studied patients with Wolff-Parkinson-White syndrome: they observed atrial fragmentation in those patients with paroxysmal AF.

Padeletti et al. (21) found significantly longer values in AF patients than in controls simply comparing A_2 values obtained at the refractory period. In their study on patients receiving coronary artery bypass graft (CABG), Capucci et al. (38) found that A_2 fragmentation ($A_2 > 40$ ms with respect to baseline) was more common among those who developed AF in the postoperative period.

In the study by Kumagai et al. (18), AF patients had a wider range of extrastimuli determining fragmentation than controls.

Dispersion of Atrial Conduction Times. The dispersion of atrial conduction times is defined as the difference between A_1-A_2 in the high right atrium and A_1-A_2 in the low right atrium at the same pacing cycle. In patients receiving CABG, Capucci et al. (27) found a greater dispersion of intraatrial conduction in those who developed AF in the postoperative period.

Δ A_1-A_2. The maximal difference of A_1-A_2, Δ A_1-A_2, among each of the three recording sites, high right atrium, low right atrium, and coronary sinus, represents the maximal intra- or interatrial dispersion of conduction. Capucci et al. have recently demonstrated significantly longer A_1-A_2 at all paced cycles than in controls; moreover, a Δ A_1-A_2 greater than 25 ms was never observed in controls.

Association of EP Abnormalities: The Arrhythmogenic Substrate of AF Patients

The most common association of EP abnormalities in patients with paroxysmal AF occurs with short refractoriness and conduction disturbances. It is useful to recall the most significant results:
– Shorter right atrial effective refractory period and a wider range of premature beats capable of prolonging S_2-A_2 either at the His bundle recording site or at the coronary sinus than in controls (16).
– Greater dispersion of both functional and effective atrial refractoriness (measured at five atrial sites) and greater fragmentation of A_2 than in controls (21).
– Longer right atrial conduction time and shorter right atrial effective refractoriness in patients with WPW and AF respect to WPW patients without AF (39). In patients with chronic AF evaluated the day following transthoracic cardioversion, Kumagai et al. (18) demonstrated shorter effective right atrial refractoriness, longer S_2-A_2, and a wider range of extrabeats determining either a delay in intraatrial conduction or A_2 fragmentation than in controls.
– Shorter functional and effective refractoriness at all paced cycles and longer Δ A_1-A_2 in patients with lone paroxysmal AF than in controls were reported in the recent paper by Capucci et al. (27).

In light of the physiopathological background provided by experimental cardiology, the association of short refractoriness and intraatrial or interatrial conduction delay, widely documented in the aforementioned clinical works, is the most likely EP substrate of AF in humans.

References

1. Mines GR (1913) On dynamic equilibrium in the heart. J Physiol 46: 349-383
2. Lewis T, Feil S, Stroud WD (1920) Observations upon flutter and fibrillation. II. The nature of auricolar flutter. Heart 7: 191-246
3. Moe GK, Abildskov JA (1959) Atrial fibrillation as a self-sustaining arrhythmia independent of focal discharge. Am Heart J 58: 59-70
4. Pastelin G, Mendez R, Moe GK (1978) Participation of atrial specialized conduction pathways in atrial flutter. Circ Res 42: 386-393
5. Allessie MA, Bonke FIM, Schopman FJG (1976) Circus movement in rabbit atrial muscle as a mechanism of tachycardia. II. The role of nonuniform recovery of excitability in the occur-

rence of unidirectional block as studied with multiple microelectrodes. Circ Res 39: 168-177

6. Allessie MA, Bonke FIM, Schopman FJG (1977) Circus movement in rabbit atrial muscle as a mechanism of tachycardia. III. The "leading circle" concept: a new model of circus movement in cardiac tissue without the involvement of an anatomical obstacle. Circ Res 41: 9-18

7. Allessie MA, Lammers WJEP, Bonke FIM, Hollen J (1984) Intra-atrial reentry as a mechanism for atrial flutter induced by acetylcholine and rapid pacing in the dog. Circulation 70: 123-135

8. Allessie MA, Lammers WJEP, Rensma PL, Bonke FIM (1987) Flutter and fibrillation in experimental models: what has been learned that can be applied to humans? In: Brugada P, Wellens HJJ (eds) Where to go from here? Futura, Mount Kisco, pp 67-82

9. Allessie MA, Rensma W, Brugada J, Smeets JLRM, Penn O, Kirchhof CJHJ (1990) Models of atrial reentry. In: Touboul P, Waldo AL (eds) Atrial arrhythmias. Current concepts and management. Mosby, St.Louis, pp 112-130

10. Smeets JLRM, Allessie MA, Lammers WJEP, Bonke FIM, Hollen J (1986) The wavelength of the cardiac impulse and reentrant arrhythmias in isolated rabbit atrium. Circ Res 58: 96-108

11. Spach MS, Miller WT, Dolber PC, Kootsey M, Sommer JR, Mosher CE (1982) The functional role of structural complexities in the propagation of depolarisation in the atrium of the dog: cardiac conduction disturbances due to discontinuities of effective axial resistivity. Circ Res 50: 175-191

12. Spach MS Dolber PC (1986) Relating extracellular potentials and their derivatives to anisotropic propagation at a microscopic level in human cardiac muscle. Circ Res 58: 356-371

13. Wyndham CRC, Amat-Y-Lyon F, Wu D, Denes P, Dhingra R,Simpson R, Rosen KM (1977) Effects of cycle length on atrial vulnerability. Circulation 55: 260- 267

14. Michelucci A, Padeletti L, Fradella GA (1982) Atrial refractoriness and spontaneous or induced atrial fibrillation. Acta Cardiol 37:333-344

15. Michelucci A, Padeletti L, Lova RM, Fradella GA, Monizzi D, Franchi F (1982) La refrattarietà atriale e la sua dispersione in differenti condizioni fisiopatologiche. G Ital Cardiol 12: 555- 562

16. Cosio FG, Palacios J, Vidal JM, Cocina EG, Gomez-Sanchez MA, Tamargo L (1983) Electrophysiologic studies in atrial fibrillation. Slow conduction of premature impulses: a possible manifestation of the background for reentry. Am J Cardiol 51:122-136

17. Attuel P, Pellerin D, Gaston J, Seing S, Quatre JM, Mugica J, Coumel P (1989) Latent atrial vulnerability: new means of electrophysiologic investigations in paroxysmal atrial fibrillation. In: Attuel P, Coumel P, Janse M (eds) The atrium in health and disease. Futura, Mount Kisco, pp. 159-200

18. Kumagai K, Akimitsu S, Kawahira K, Kawanami F, Yamanouchi Y, Hiroki T, Arakawa K (1991) EP properties in chronic atrial fibrillation. Circulation 84: 1662- 1668

19. Luck JC, Engel TR (1979) Dispersion of atrial refractoriness in patients with sinus node dysfunction. Circulation 60: 404-412

20. Michelucci A, Padeletti L, Fradella GA, Lova RM, Monizzi D, Giomi A, Fantini F (1984) Ageing and atrial electrophysiologic properties in man. Int J Cardiol 5: 75-81

21. Padeletti L, Michelucci A, Giovannini T, Mezzani A, Monopoli A, Franchi F (1989) Proprietà elettrofisiologiche atriali nella fibrillazione atriale parossistica. Studio effettuato stimolando cinque sedi atriali. G Ital Cardiol 19: 411-416

22. Boutjdir M, LeHeuzey JY, Lavergne T, Chauvaud S, Guize L, Carpentier A, Peronneau P (1986) Inhomogeneity of cellular refractoriness in human atrium: factor of arrhythmia? PACE 9: 1095-1100

23. Buxton AE, Waxman HL, Marchlinski FE, Josephson ME (1984) Atrial conduction : effects of extrastimuli with and without atrial dysrhythmias. Am J Cardiol 54: 755-761

24. Ohe T, Matsuhisa M, Kamakura S, Yamada J, Sato I, Nakajima K, Shimomura K (1983) Relation between the widening of the fragmented atrial activity zone and atrial fibrillation. Am J Cardiol 53: 1219-1222

25. Simpson RJ, Amara I, Foster JR, Woelfel A, Gettes LS (1988) Threshold, refractory periods and conduction times of the normal diseased human atrium. Am Heart J 116: 1080-1090

26. Attuel P, Childers R, Chauchemenez B, Poveda J, Mujica J, Coumel P (1982) Failure in the rate adaptation of atrial refractory period: its relationship to vulnerability. Int J Cardiol 2: 179-197

27. Capucci A, Biffi M, Boriani G, Ravelli F, Nollo G, Sabbatani P, Orsi C, Magnani B (1995) The dynamic electrophysiologic behaviour of human atria during paroxysmal atrial fibrillation. Circulation (in press)

28. Ramdat, Misier AR, Opthof T, van Hemel NM, Defauw JJAM, de Bakker JMT, Janse MJ, van Capelle FJL (1992) Increased dispersion of refractoriness in patients with idiopathic paroxysmal atrial fibrillation. J Am Coll Cardiol 1992; 19: 1531- 1535

29. Lammers WJEP, Allessie MA, Rensma PL, Schalij MJ (1986) The use of fibrillation cycle length to determine spatial dispersion in EP properties and to characterize the underlying mechanism of fibrillation. New Trends Arrhyth 2: 109-112

30. Cosio FG, Arribas F (1989) Role of conduction disturbances in atrial arrhythmias. In: Attuel P, Coumel P, Janse M (eds) The atrium in health and disease. Futura, Mount Kisco, pp 133-157

31. Fukunami M, Yamada T, Ohmori M, Kumagai K, Umemoto K, Sakai A, Kondoh N, Minamino T, Hoki N (1991) Detection of patients at risk for paroxysmal atrial fibrillation during sinus rhythm by p wave-triggered signal-averaged electrocardiogram. Circulation 83: 162-169

32. Opolski G, Stanislawska J, Slomka K, Kraska T (1991) Value of the atrial signal-averaged electrocardiogram in identifying patients with paroxysmal atrial fibrillation. Int J Cardiol 30: 315-319

33. Cosio FG, Paylos J, Requena M, Fernandez-Vanez J (1984) Influence of basic atrial rhythm on intraatrial conduction of extrastimuli. Am J Cardiol 53: 1018-1021

34. Michelucci A, Lagi A, Caneschi A, Giovannini T, Mezzani A, Salvi S, Padeletti L (1990) Importance of left atrial variables in defining atrial arrhythmogenesis. New Trends Arrhyth 6: 795-800

35. Josephson ME, Horowitz LN, Farshidi A (1978) Continous local electrical activity. A mechanism of recurrent ventricular tachycardia. Circulation 57: 659-665

36. Tanigawa M, Fukatani M, Konoe A, Isomoto S, Kadena M, Hashiba K (1991) Prolonged and fractionated right atrial electrograms during sinus rhythm in patients with paroxysmal atrial fibrillation and sick sinus syndrome. J Am Coll Cardiol 17: 403-408

37. Konoe A, Fukatani M, Tanigawa M, Isomoto S, Kadena M, Sakamoto T, Mori M, Shimizu A, Hashiba K (1992) ED abnormalities of the atrial muscle in patients with manifest Wolff-Parkinson-White syndrome associated with paroxysmal atrial fibrillation. PACE 15: 1040-1052

38. Capucci A, Frabetti L, Turinetto B, Pierangeli A, Magnani B (1987) Fibrillazione atriale nei post operati di by-pass aortocoronarico. Correlazione con le proprietà elettrofisiologiche valutate intraoperatoriamente. G Ital Cardiol 17: 575-582

39. Fujimura O, Klein GJ, Yee R, Sharma AD (1990) Mode of on-set of atrial fibrillation in the Wolff-Parkinson-White syndrome: how important is the accessory pathway? J Am Coll Cardiol 15: 1082-1086

Is Mortality in Patients with Atrial Fibrillation Related to the Underlying Heart Disease or to the Arrhythmia?

F. Di Pede and G. Zuin

Divisione di Cardiologia, Ospedale Umberto I,
Mestre-Venice, Italy

Atrial fibrillation (AF) is considered one of the most common clinically relevant cardiac arrhythmias. The prevalence of AF increases with age and is reported to be 0.2%-0.3% at age 25 – 35 years, 3%-4% at age 55 – 64 years, and 5%-9% at age 62 – 90 years (1). AF is usually a consequence of heart disease involving the left atrium, but may also result from extracardiac conditions such as hyperthyroidism, surgery, acute alcohol intoxication, cholinergic drug use, or diagnostic procedures. In a minority of patients, no contributing factors or overt heart disease can be identified (lone AF). In most cases the clinical and hemodynamic consequences of AF are related to the severity of underlying heart disease.

Hemodynamic Consequences of Atrial Fibrillation

The hemodynamic consequences of AF depend on many factors. These include the loss of atrial systole, the irregularity of ventricular rhythm, the heart rate, and the underlying heart disease. It is generally accepted that the loss of atrial contraction may reduce cardiac output by nearly 15%-20% (2). The atrial contribution to cardiac output is greater in patients with reduced diastolic left ventricular compliance (3, 4). The importance of atrial contraction declines in patients with increased end diastolic volume and in those with higher pulmonary artery wedge pressure (5). Moreover, the effect of atrial systole seems to be more relevant at rest than during exercise (3): clinical studies have shown that heart rate is the major determinant of the increase of cardiac output occurring during exercise, and atrial systole produces only a small additional increment (3, 6-9).

Irregularity of ventricular rhythm may produce adverse hemodynamic consequences ascribed to beat-to-beat variations of ventricular filling and emptying characteristics: particularly short ventricular cycles may have a negative direct effect on myocardial contractility and may result in mitral regurgitation leading to a reduction of stroke volume (10). Both animal and clinical studies have shown that irregular ventricular rhythm produces an increase of pulmonary wedge pressure and a reduction of cardiac output (9%-24%) and that the hemodynamic effect is greater in patients with reduced diastolic function (10, 11).

In most cases AF produces an increase of heart rate with a reduction of the diastolic filling period and of stroke volume; this is partially offset by a greater number of beats per minute. The net effect on cardiac output is uncertain and depends on the underlying heart disease. It is well known that chronic tachycardia has a deleterious effect on left ventricular function and may produce congestive heart failure (12, 13). Despite reports of "tachycardia-induced cardiomyopathy" (12, 13), AF in the absence of other heart disease was generally considered a benign entity (14). Only in recent years has AF with a fast ventricular rate (greater than 200/min) been recognized as a cause of severe ventricular dysfunction, which may be reversible after the restoration of sinus rhythm (15).

The extent of the hemodynamic consequences of AF are related to the underlying heart disease (3, 16-25). In patients without heart disease, AF does not affect resting cardiac output and exercise tolerance, but may lead to an increase in atrial pressure (3, 25, 26). The hemodynamic effect of AF is more evident in patients with heart disease, particularly in those with valvular heart disease or hypertrophic cardiomyopathy, as demonstrated by hemodynamic studies on the conversion of AF to normal sinus rhythm (3, 16-25). Hemodynamic benefits of reversion to sinus rhythm increase over time, since the complete recovery of atrial contraction may occur after 3 weeks (27-28).

Echocardiographic studies have shown that the occurrence of AF may increase the left atrial size. Therefore AF has the potential of producing anatomical changes that can be important in the natural history of the disease (28-30).

Stroke in Atrial Fibrillation

AF is now recognized as the most common cardiac disorder leading to systemic emboli and stroke. The increased risk of systemic emboli was first understood in rheumatic AF and only recently in nonrheumatic AF (31, 32). The risk of embolism in rheumatic heart disease is so high (more than 5% per year, risk ratio, 17.56) that anticoagulant therapy is routinely administered to patients with AF and rheumatic heart disease (32, 33). The impact of nonrheumatic AF on stroke incidence has recently been assessed. In an analysis of the Framingham study data including only nonrheumatic AF, the annual incidence of stroke was 3.8%; in comparison with controls matched for multiple risk factors, the relative risk was 4 (34). The consequences of stroke are often devastating: the precentage of strokes that were disabling or fatal in published studies ranges from 44% to 71% (35, 36). The risk of stroke is greater when AF is chronic and when AF develops in patients with heart failure, hypertension, advanced age, and a recent embolic event (34, 37, 38). The risk of stroke is very low only in young patients with paroxysmal lone AF and may not be higher than in a population of comparable age without AF. The risk of stroke in lone AF may be substantial if the patient is elderly and the fibrillation is chronic.

Mortality in Atrial Fibrillation

Available data indicate that mortality in AF patients is mainly related to the underlying disease (39). However, AF might increase the morbidity and mortality rate in some clinical settings. In the Framingham study, during 20 years of follow-up in a cohort of patients initially 30-62 years old, the mortality rate among those who developed AF was about twice that of those who did not; the relative risk for cardiovascular death was higher than that for all-cause mortality (40). Other authors obtained similar results in patient populations similar to the Framingham cohort or in older patients (41, 42). However, the reduced survival with AF is most probably related to the associated heart disease present in about 80% of patients and probably results from the very high rate of stroke (39). Studies on warfarin in chronic nonrheumatic AF showed an increased mortality rate in the placebo group compared with the warfarin group. The study population included patients with lone AF and with heart disease other than rheumatic. In the AFASAK study (43), total and vascular mortality rates were significantly higher in the placebo group than in the warfarin group ($p < 0.02$). Similarly, in the BAATAF study (44) the overall mortality rate was higher in the placebo group (26 deaths) than in the warfarin group (11 deaths; $p = 0.005$); the same effect was seen with death from noncardiac causes (14 versus 4) and from cardiac causes (12 versus 7). In the SPAF study (45), the total mortality rate per year was only slightly higher in the control group than in the treated group (3.1% versus 2.2%; $p =$ NS). However, patients enrolled in the SPAF study were younger than those enrolled in the other two studies. Data from these studies indirectly demonstrate that AF increases the mortality rate mainly in older patients and that mortality can be reduced by warfarin. The effects of specific heart diseases were not analyzed in these studies.

The influence of lone AF on mortality is still poorly defined because of the low incidence of lone AF. AF in absence of organic heart disease comprises only 2% – 6% of all causes of AF (14). Many papers on lone AF mentioned its low mortality (14, 46). However, data from the Framingham study (40) show that patients with AF have nearly twice the annual total mortality rate compared with controls (5% versus 2.8%). In the subgroup of 30 patients with idiopathic AF the yearly mortality rate was lower but still increased at 3.8%. These results seem to conflict with those of Copecky et al. (47), who found a similar mortality rate in patients with idiopathic AF and in controls. However, important differences in patient characteristics exist: Copecky reported on young patients (mean age, 44 years) affected predominantly by paroxysmal AF, while patients in the Framingham study were older (mean age, 70 years); all had chronic AF, and 32% had hypertension, suggesting that some patients in the Framingham study were not truly idiopathic. Data gathered from insurance companies suggest that idiopathic paroxysmal AF does not increase mortality compared with controls, while chronic idiopathic AF produces an eightfold increase in mortality (48). Since cardiovascular abnormalities were ruled out only retrospectively the incidence of heart disease was underestimated. From these data we can argue that the prognosis in lone AF depends on the presence of an occult cardiovascular disease that might not become manifest until follow-up rather than on the arrhythmia itself. Therefore, the prognosis appears to be excellent in young nonhospitalized patients with idiopathic paroxysmal AF, while chronic AF in elderly patients cannot be considered benign (14).

The effects of AF in dilated cardiomyopathy and in congestive heart failure have been studied more extensively. AF is a common rhythm in congestive heart failure and is often believed to be an unfavorable clinical characteristic. However, studies on AF in heart failure offer conflicting results (49, 50). Some authors (51) showed that AF has no effect on survival, while others (52) found a deleterious effect of AF on univariate analysis, but not when multivariate analysis was applied. In a recent study based on patients in NYHA (New York Heart Association) functional class III – IV, AF was associated with a further impairment of survival only in those with lower pulmonary capillary wedge pressure on therapy, but not in those with elevated pulmonary capillary wedge pressure (50). These data may suggest a potential explanation for the conflicting results of previous studies: any additional hemodynamic dysfunction produced by AF is probably relatively insignificant in patients with very severely depressed ventricular function, as indicated by the higher pulmonary capillary wedge pressure; while in patients with low pulmonary capillary wedge pressure, who have a relatively better prognosis, the additional functional impairment may be relevant. This explanation is supported by the study by Greenberg (5), who showed that, in patients with high pulmonary capillary wedge pressure, the loss of atrial contraction does not produce a fall of cardiac output.

The prognostic significance of AF in coronary artery disease has only been poorly analyzed. The frequency of AF in coronary artery disease is less than 2% (53). Coronary Artery Surgery Study (CASS) data established that AF is associated with congestive heart failure or left ventricular dysfunction or mitral regurgitation, but it does not correlate with the extent of coronary artery disease (53). Moreover, AF was identified as an independent predictor of mortality with a relative risk of 1.98 as compared with sinus rhythm (53). Similar results were obtained in the Framingham study: the risk ratio was significantly higher (3:1) in men with coronary artery disease who developed chronic AF (54).

Conclusions

AF is usually a consequence of heart disease, and mortality depends on the underlying structural heart disease. The occurrence of AF, however, may produce systemic embolism and hemodynamic dysfunction, which may aggravate the clinical course of the disease. Available data indicate that the increased mortality rate observed in AF patients is essentially related to embolism. The hemodynamic dysfunction is probably not clinically relevant in lone AF, but may increase mortality in heart failure and in coronary artery disease patients. Moreover, AF with uncontrolled heart rate produces congestive heart failure and probably death even in the absence of structural heart disease.

References

1. Kannel WB, Wolf PA (1992) Epidemiology of atrial fibrillation. In: Falk RH, Podrid PJ (eds) Atrial fibrillation. Mechanisms and management. Raven, New York, pp 81-92
2. Ruskin J, McHale PA, Harley A, Greenfield JC Jr (1970) Pressure-flow studies in man: effects of atrial systole on left ventricular function. J Clin Invest 49: 472-478
3. Atwood JE (1992) Exercise hemodynamics of atrial fibrillation. In: Falk RH, Podrid PJ (eds) Atrial fibrillation. Mechanism and management. Raven, New York, pp 145-163
4. Rahimtoola SH, Ehsani A, Sinno MZ et al (1975) Left atrial transport function in myocardial infarction: importance of its booster function. Am J Med 59: 686-693
5. Greenberg B, Chatterjee K, Parmley WW, Werner JA, Holly AN (1980) The influence of left ventricular filling pressure on atrial contribution to cardiac output. Am Heart J 98: 742-751
6. Pehrsson SK (1983) Influence of heart rate and atrioventricular synchronization on maximal work tolerance in patients treated with artificial pacemaker. Acta Med Scand 214: 311-315
7. Ausubel K, Steingart RM, Shimshi M, Klementowicz P, Furman S (1985) Maintenance of exercise stroke volume during ventricular versus atrial synchronous pacing: role of contractility. Circulation 72: 1037
8. Fananapazir L, Bennet DH, Monks P (1983) Atrial synchronized ventricular pacing: contribution of the chronotropic response to improved exercise performance. Pace 6: 601-605
9. Fananapazir L, Srinivas V, Bennet DH (1983) Comparison of resting hemodynamic indices and exercise performance during atrial synchronized and asynchronous ventricular pacing. Pace 6: 202-206
10. Naito M, David D, Michelson EL, Schaffenburg M, Dreifus LS (1983) The hemodynamic consequences of cardiac arrhythmias: evaluation of the relative roles of abnormal atrioventricular sequencing, irregularity of ventricular rhythm and atrial fibrillation in a canine model. Am Heart J 106: 284-291
11. Piccolo E, Di Pede F, Millosevich P (1993) Ablazione transcatetere della giunzione AV ed impianto di Pace-Maker in pazienti con fibrillazione e flutter atriale: la regolarizzazione dei cicli ventricolari migliora la funzione cardiaca? In: Piccolo E, Raviele A (eds) Third International Workshop on Cardiac Arrythmias, Venice, 21-23 October 1993. Centro Scientifico Editore, Torino, pp 79-92
12. Packer DL, Bardy GH, Worley SJ, Smith MS, Cobb FR, Coleman E, Gallagher JJ, German LD (1986) Tachycardia-induced cardiomyopathy: a reversible form of left ventricular dysfunction. Am J Cardiol 57: 563-570
13. McLaran CJ, Gersh BJ, Sugrue DD, Hammill SC, Seward JB, Holmes DR Jr (1985) Tachycardia induced myocardial dysfunction: a reversible phenomenon? Br Heart J 53: 323-327
14. Leather RA, Kerr CR (1992) Atrial fibrillation in the absence of overt cardiac disease. In: Falk RH, Podrid PJ (eds) Atrial fibrillation: mechanisms and management. Raven, New York, pp 93-108
15. Grogan M, Smith HC, Gersh BJ, Wood DL (1992) Left ventricular dysfunction due to atrial fibrillation in patients initially believed to have idiopathic dilated cardiomyopathy. Am J Cardiol 69: 1570-1573
16. Selzer A (1960) Effects of atrial fibrillation upon the circulation in patients with mitral stenosis. Am Heart J 59: 518-526
17. Graettinger JS, Carleton RA, Muenster JJ (1964) Circulatory consequences of changes in cardiac rhythm produced in patients by transthoracic direct-current shock. J Clin Invest 43: 2290-2295
18. Morris JJ, Entman M, North WC et al (1965) The changes in cardiac output with reversion of atrial fibrillation to sinus rhythm. Circulation 31: 670-678
19. Reale A (1965) Acute effects of countershock conversion of atrial fibrillation upon right and left heart hemodynamics. Circulation 32: 214-222
20. Killip T, Baer R (1965) Hemodynamic effect after reversion from atrial fibrillation to sinus rhythm by precordial shock. J Clin Invest 45: 658-670
21. Shapiro W, Klein G (1968) Alterations in cardiac function immediately following electrical conversion of atrial fibrillation to normal sinus rhythm. Circulation 38: 1074-1078
22. Glancy DL, O'Brein KP, Gold HK et al (1970) Atrial fibrillation in patients with idiopatic hypertrophic subaortic stenosis. Am Heart J 32: 652-658
23. Di Pede F, Raviele A, Zuin G et al (1987) Quando, come e perché riconverire a ritmo una fibrillazione atriale. In: Raviele A, Alboni P (eds) Third International Workshop on Cardiac Arrythmias, Venice, 21-23 October 1993. Il Pensiero Scientifico Editore, Rome, pp 55-62
24. Piccolo E, Delise P, Alboni P et al (1991) Problemi elettrofisiologici e clinici della fibrillazione atriale. G Ital Cardiol 21: 437-459
25. Scarfò S, Papparella N, Fucà G, Yannacopulu P, Alboni P (1993) Perché conquistare a tutti i costi il ritmo sinusale? Quale vantaggio emodinamico per il paziente? G Ital Cardiol 23 [Suppl I]: 98-102
26. Atwood JE, Myers J, Sullivan M et al (1988) Maximal exercise testing and gas exchange in patients with chronic atrial fibrillation. J Am Coll Cardiol 11: 508-513
27. Manning W, Leeman DE, Gotch PJ, Come PC (1989) Pulsed Doppler evaluation of atrial mechanical function after electrical cardioversion of atrial fibrillation. J Am Coll Cardiol 13: 617-623
28. Pollick C (1992) Echocardiography in atrial fibrillation. In: Falk RH, Podrid PJ (eds) Atrial fibrillation: mechamisms and management. Raven, New York, pp 165-180
29. Sanfilippo AJ, Abascal VM, Sheehan M et al (1990) Atrial enlargement has a consecuence of atrial fibrillation. A prospective echocardiographic study. Circulation 82: 791-797
30. Van Gelder IC, Crijns HJ, Van Gilst WH, Hamer HPM, Lie KI (1991) Decrease of right and left atrial size after direct current electrical cardioversion in chronic atrial fibrillation. Am J Cardiol 67: 93-95
31. Hinton RC, Kistler JP, Fallon JT, Friedlich AL, Fisher CM (1977) Influence of etiology of atrial fibrillation on incidence of systemic embolism. Am J Cardiol 40: 509-513
32. Wolf PA, Dawber TR, Thomas HE, Kannel WB (1978) Epidemiologic assessment of chronic atrial fibrillation and risk of stroke: the Framingham study. Neurology 28: 973-977
33. Albers GW, Atwood JE, Hirsh J, Sherman DG, Hughes RA,

Connolly SJ (1991) Stroke prevention in nonvalvular atrial fibrillation. Ann Intern Med 115: 727-736

34. Wolf PA, Abbott RD, Kannel WB (1987) Atrial fibrillation: major contributor to stroke in the elderly. Arch Intern Med 147: 1561-1564
35. Stroke Prevention in Atrial Fibrillation Study Group Investigators (1990) Preliminary report of the Stroke Prevention in Atrial Fibrillation Study. N Engl J Med 322: 863-868
36. Fisher CM (1979) Reducing risk of cerebral embolism. Geriatrics 34: 59-66
37. Stroke Prevention in Atrial Fibrillation Investigators (1992) Predictors of thromboembolism in atrial fibrillation. I. Clinical features of patients at risk. Ann Intern Med 116: 1-5
38. Flegel KM, Hanley J (1989) Risk factors for stroke and other embolic events in patients with nonrheumatic atrial fibrillation. Stroke 20:1000-1004
39. Cairns JA, Connolly SJ (1991) Nonrheumatic atrial fibrillation: risk of stroke and role of antithrombotic theraphy. Circulation 84: 469-481
40. Kannel WB, Abbott RD, Savage DD, McNamara PM (1982) Epidemiologic features of chronic atrial fibrillation: the Framingham study. N Engl J Med 306: 1018-1022
41. Onundarson PT, Thorgeirsson G, Jonmundsson E, Sigfusson N, Hardson T (1987) Chronic atrial fibrillation – epidemiologic features and 14 year follow-up: a case control study. Eur Heart J 3: 521-527
42. Kitchin AH, Milne JS (1977) Longitudinal survey of ischaemic heart disease in randomly selected sample of older population. Br Heart J 39: 889-893
43. Petersen P, Boysen G, Godtfredsen J, Andersen E, Andersen B (1989) Placebo-controlled, randomised trial of warfarin and aspirin for prevention of thromboembolic complications in chronic atrial fibrillation. Lancet 1: 175-178
44. The Boston Area Anticoagulation Trial for Atrial Fibrillation Investigators (1990) The effect of low-dose warfarin on the risk of stroke in patients with nonrheumatic atrial fibrillation. N Engl J Med 323: 1505-1511
45. Stroke Prevention in Atrial Fibrillation Investigators (1991) Stroke prevention in atrial fibrillation study. Final results. Circulation 84: 527-539
46. Evans W, Swann P (1954) Lone auricular fibrillation. Br Heart J 16: 189-194
47. Kopecky SL, Gersh BJ, McGoon MD, Whisnant JP, Holmes DR, Ilstrup DM, Frye RL (1987) The natural history of lone atrial fibrillation. N Engl J Med 317: 669-674
48. Gajewski J, Singer RB (1981) Mortality in an insured population with atrial fibrillation. JAMA 245: 1540-1544
49. Carson PE, Johnson GR, Dunkman WB, Fletcher RD, Farrell L, Cohn JN (1993) The influence of atrial fibrillation on prognosis in mild to moderate heart failure. Circulation 87 [Suppl VI]: 102-110
50. Middlekauff HR, Stevenson WG, Stevenson LW (1991) Prognostic significance of atrial fibrillation in advanced heart failure. A study of 390 patients. Circulation 84: 40-48
51. Keogh AM, Baron DW, Hickie JB (1990) Prognostic guides in patients with idiopathic or ischemic dilated cardiomyopathy assessed for cardiac transplantation. Am J Cardiol 65: 903-908
52. Unverferth DV, Magorien RD, Moescberger ML, Baker PB, Fetters JK, Leier CV (1984) Factors influencing the one-year mortality of dilated cardiomyopathy. Am J Cardiol 54: 147-152
53. Cameron A, Schwartz MJ, Kronmal RA, Kosinski AS (1988) Prevalence and significance of atrial fibrillation in coronary artery disease (CASS Registry). Am J Cardiol 61: 714-717
54. Kannel WB, Abbott RD, Savage DD, McNamara PM (1983) Coronary heart disease and atrial fibrillation: the Framingham study. Am Heart J 106:389-396

Thromboembolic Risk in Patients with Atrial Fibrillation: Can It Be Predicted on the Basis of Clinical Variables?

S. Scardi, C. Mazzone, D. Goldstein, C. Pandullo, and G. Sinagra

Centro Cardiovascolare, Ospedale Maggiore, Trieste, Italy

Introduction

Atrial fibrillation (AF) is a common disorder of cardiac rhythm and its incidence increases with each decade of life (1). In the past, rheumatic mitral valve disease has been the condition most highly associated with AF. However, more recently, other conditions have assumed greater importance, particularly AF which is not associated with rheumatic valvular heart disease (NRAF). The risk of stroke in these patients is estimated to be fivefold greater than that of comparable patients in sinus rhythm (2).

Recent trials demonstrated that prophylactic anticoagulation decreases the rate of stroke significantly with an acceptably low rate of hemorrhagic complications (3-8).

Since the risk of embolism appears to continue indefinitely and the management of anticoagulant therapy is not easy, especially in older patients, it is necessary to identify high and low risk subgroups of subjects; moreover, this classification may influence the decision regarding antithrombotic prophylaxis. The results of subgroup analysis to evaluate embolic risk factors performed in international trials have not been uniform, and the power of the analyses itself has been limited by the relatively small number of embolic events in each study (4).

The TASAF Study

In order to verify the predictive variables of thromboembolic risk in the Italian population, we studied 694 consecutive patients with chronic NRAF who are enrolled in the Trieste Area Study on Nonrheumatic Atrial Fibrillation (TASAF); this was an ongoing prospective community study with a 2-year follow-up.

The study population showed an elevated mean age (71±9 years), a prevalence of males (383/694), a high prevalence of overt or previous heart failure (23%), mitral regurgitation confirmed at echocardiography (30%), and of previous myocardial infarction

Table 1. Characteristics of enrolled population (694 patients)

Characteristic	Number	Percentage
Age (years, mean±s.d.)	71±9	
AF duration (months)	58±66	
Sex (m/f)	383/311	
Smokers	86	12
Hypertension	402	58
Diabetes	63	9
Hyperthyroidism	24	3
Previous myocardial infarction	76	11
Previous heart failure	160	23
Pacemaker	33	5
Mitral regurgitation	210	30
Aortic stenosis	25	4
Aortic regurgitation	54	8
Aortic stenosis and regurgitation	10	2
Lone AF	89	13
No defined cardiopathy	100	14
Coronary heart disease	113	16
Left ventricular hypertrophy	198	28
Congenital heart disease	13	2
Dilated cardiomyopathy	30	4
Degenerative cardiopathy	137	20
Other etiology	14	2

AF, atrial fibrillation.

(11%). Many of the enrolled patients had a history of hypertension (58%; Table 1).

According to the etiology of the underlying heart disease, the following should be emphasized: a high incidence of left ventricle hypertrophy, with or without a history of hypertension (28%), degenerative (20%) or unclassifiable heart disease (14%), and lone AF (13%). Among the echocardiographic findings there were: left ventricular dysfunction (17%), mitral annular calcification (27%), and good mean left ventricular function (ejection fraction, EF, 0.50±0.15); 458 of 694 patients (66%) had a cardiothoracic index > 0.50. (Table 2).

Examining the history of the patients, there were 134 embolic events; 96 were clinically documented in 79 subjects while in 34 patients there were 38 episodes suspected of embolism or transient ischemic attacks. (TIA). Nine patients suffered one recurrence of embolism, three patients suffered two recurrences, one

Table 2. Echocardiographic and chest X-ray findings

Left atrial diameter (cm)	4.6±0.8
Left atrial area (cm²)	27.5±7.8
LVEDD (cm)	5.2±0.8
SF (%)	36±12
EF (%)	58±15
Asynergy (score)	1.4±3.5
Mitral valve prolapse	27 (4%)
Mitral annular calcification	182 (27%)
Left ventricular dysfunction	120 (17%)
CTI > 0.5	458 (66%)

LVEDD, left ventricular end diastolic diameter; SF, ventricular shortening fraction; EF, ejection fraction; CTI, cardiothoracic index.

Table 3. Thromboembolic recurrences and outcome in patients with previous major or suspected embolic event or TIA

	Major event		Suspected event/TIA	
	(n)	%	(n)	%
Single event	66	84.6	29	85.2
First recurrence	7	8.9	2	5.8
Second recurrence	2	2.5	1	2.9
Third recurrence	1	1.2	–	
First suspected recurrence/TIA	2	2.5	2	5.8
Total	78		34	
With disability	16	21		
Without disability	62	79		

TIA, transient ischemic attack.

patient had three recurrences, and four patients had one suspected recurrence of TIA (Table 3). Thirty-five embolic events were clustered around the time of the onset of the arrhythmia, the other 99 thromboembolic complications appeared after the onset of AF: range 1-266 months (Fig. 1). Among the 616 patients without a history of embolism at the time of the first control only 3% were treated with oral anticoagulant agents and 28% with antiplatelet therapy, while among the 78 subjects with documented embolism 28% were receiving anticoagulant therapy and 58% were treated with antiplatelet agents.

Thromboembolic Variables

The group of patients with documented embolic events, as compared with patients without embolism or with suspected embolism or TIA, demonstrated variables predictive of thromboembolic complications: arrhythmia duration (p=0.009) and previous myocar-

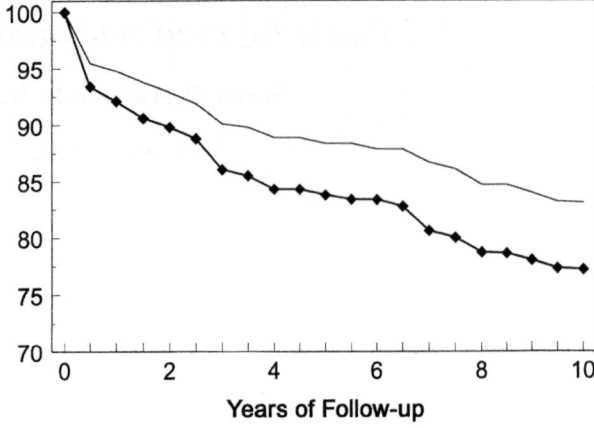

Event free Survival (%)

Fig. 1. Kaplan-Meier curves of event – free survival in patients with major thromboembolism (—) and with total events (major + suspected events/transient ischemic attack; –◆–). Note the clear cluster of thromboembolic events during the first month after the beginning of the atrial fibrillation in both curves

dial infarction (p=0.03). In contrast, mitral annular calcification (p=0.06), history of hypertension (p=0.09) and left ventricular hypertrophy (with or without history of hypertension) (p=0.07) demonstrated only a slight trend towards statistical significance (Table 4). Comparing the clinical characteristics and echocardiographic findings of patients without embolism with those of patients with true embolism or suspected embolism or TIA, the variables predictive of thromboembolic events were arrhythmia duration (p=0.007), history of hypertension (p=0.01), left ventricular hypertrophy, with or without hypertension (p=0.02), and mitral annular calcification (p=0.01). Age showed only a trend towards statistical significance (p=0.06; Table 5).

These data are in agreement with many other reports in the literature. In fact, a previous myocardial infarction is predictive of embolism in the AFASAK (6) and BAATAF (8) studies, while the presence of ischemic heart disease without myocardial infarction or left ventricular dysfunction does not increase the embolic risk.

In our study, the presence of left ventricular hypertrophy, either associated or not with a history of hypertension, was predictive of a thromboembolic event (p=0.02). The same was true for mitral annular calcifications (p=0.01). These last echocardiographic

Table 4. Predictive variables of major embolic events

	Embolic event				
Variable	None or suspected/TIA		Major		p value
	(n)	(%)	(n)	(%)	
Hypertension	350	57	52	67	0.09
Previous MI	62	10	14	18	0.03*
Left ventricular hypertrophy	169	28	29	37	0.07
Mitral annular calcification	155	25	27	35	0.06
Total patients	616		78		
AF duration (months)	56.13±66.08		77.07±62.10		0.009*

AF, atrial fibrillation; MI, acute myocardial infarction.
*= p ≤ 0.05.

Table 5. Predictive variables of all embolic events

Variable	Embolic event					*p* Value
	None			Major or suspected/TIA		
	n	%		*n*	%	
Hypertension	325	56		77	69	0.01*
Left ventricular hypertrophy	156	26		42	37	0.02*
Mitral annular calcification	142	25		40	36	0.01*
Total patients	582			112		
Age (years)	71.2±8.82			72.9±8.3		0.06
AF duration (months)	55.52±66.96			73.89±58.13		0.007*

AF, atrial fibrillation; TIA, transient ischemic attack;
*= $p \leq 0.05$.

findings represent an independent risk factor in the study of Benjamin et al. (9) and in BAATAF (8), but no statistical significance was found in the SPAF (7).

In our study, arrhythmia duration was the most important predictive variable of thromboembolic risk. The Framingham study (10) showed that in 37% of patients with stroke, AF was present for less than a period of 2 years and in most cases the embolism developed a few months after the appearance of the arrhythmia, while Petersen et al. (11) documented an incidence of 13% in the first year and 4% in the following years.

In agreement with other authors (3,5), but contrary to the results of the BAATAF (8) and SPAF (7) studies, left atrial size was not predictive of embolic risk in our patients. It is noteworthy, however, that left atrial geometry is complex, and its echocardiographic evaluation with the M-mode technique may give inadequate results, while a two-dimensional examination is more reliable. Finally, it is not fully understood whether left atrial enlargement is the consequence or the cause of AF (12).

Transesophageal echocardiography

Transthoracic echocardiography (TTE) often fails to disclose an unequivocal cardiac source of embolism; therefore, transesophageal echocardiography (TEE) should be performed (13). TEE is more sensitive in detecting abnormalities than earlier methods and may result in more frequent recognition of cardiogenic embolism, particularly in the left atrial appendage (14). Therefore, the role of TEE in functional evaluation of the left atrial appendage is an important component of the comprehensive evaluation of potential increased risk of thrombus formation (15-18).

For these reasons, TTE and TEE studies were performed in 97 patients (55 males and 42 females, age mean±S.D., 71±9 years at follow-up). The left atrium and appendage were inspected for thrombus and spontaneous echocontrast which was graded from none (0) to severe (4). Outflow velocity profiles were obtained by pulsed wave Doppler at the orifice of the left atrium appendage.

Atrial thrombosis was found in one patient and spontaneous echocontrast in two with TTE. With TEE we found thrombosis in 21 patients (21.6%; in the atrium in two and in the left appendage in 19) and spontaneous echocontrast in 39 patients (40.2%; in both atria

in one; *p*=0.001). Of the 39 patients with spontaneous echocontrast 16 (41%) had left atrial thrombus, compared with five (9%) of the 58 patients without spontaneous echocontrast (*p*=0.0001). Factors related to left atrial thrombus included a history of hypertension (*p*=0.05), larger left atrial area (*p*=0.05), the presence of spontaneous echocontrast (*p*=0.0001), a low ejection fraction (EF%) of the left atrial appendage in horizontal (*p*=0.006) and vertical sections (*p*=0.003), a low peak filling velocity (PFV cm/s; *p*=0.0001) and peak emptying velocity (PEV cm/s; *p*=0.0001) in horizontal and vertical sections (*p*=0.0001 and *p*=0.001, respectively) and a low/absent flow in the left atrial appendage (*p*=0.00001; Table 6).

Variables with statistical significance associated with the presence of spontaneous echocontrast were the left atrial area (*p*=0.03), the presence of thrombosis (*p*=0.0001), a low EF% of the left atrium in horizontal section (*p*=0.01), a low PFV cm/s (*p*= 0.04) and a low PEV cm/s (*p*=0.04) in horizontal section and a low PEV cm/s (*p*=0.02) in vertical section and a low/absent flow in the left appendage (*p*=0.0007); mitral annular calcifications (*p*=0.06) showed only a trend towards statistical significance (Table 7).

It is important to note that the presence of thrombosis and spontaneous echocontrast did not identify

Table 6. Factors related to left atrial/appendage thrombi

Variable	LA thrombus	No LA trhombus	*p* Value
Patients (*n* = 97)	21	76	
Hypertension	13 (62%)	29 (38%)	0.05*
Duration AF (months)	105.6±86	76.2±62	0.08
LA SEC	16 (76%)	23 (30%)	0.0001*
LA AREA (cm²)	30±7	26±7	0.05*
HLAAEF	20.5±11	31±13	0.006*
VLAAEF	22±14	32±12	0.003*
LAA low/absent flow	17%	3%	0.00001*
HPFV (cm/s)	21.7 ± 8	37 ± 11	0.0001*
HPEV (cm/s)	18 ± 4	28.5± 12	0.0001*
VPFV (cm/s)	25.1 ± 13	36.1 ± 11	0.0001*
VPEV (cm/s)	18.7 ± 8	28.4 ± 12	0.001*

LA, left atrium; LAA, left atrial appendage; SEC, spontaneous echocontrast; HLAAEF, left atrial appendage ejection fraction in horizontal section; VLAAEF, left atrial appendage ejection fraction in vertical section; HPFV, horizontal peak filling velocity; HPEV, horizontal peak emptying velocity; VPFV, vertical peak filling velocity; VPEV, vertical peak emptying velocity.
*= $p \leq 0.05$

Table 7. Factors related to left atrial/appendage spontaneous echocontrast

Variable	LA SEC	No LA SEC	p Value
Patients (97)	39	58	
Mitral annular calcification	17 (47%)	15 (28%)	0.06
LAA low/ absent flow	24 (63%)	53 (91%)	0.0007*
LA thrombus	16 (41%)	5 (9%)	0.0001*
LA area	29 ± 6	26 ± 7	0.03*
HLAAEF	24 ± 14	32 ± 12	0.01*
HPFV (cm/s)	30 ± 13	36± 11	0.04*
HPEV(cm/s)	23 ± 11	28 ± 12	0.04*
VPFV (cm/s)	31 ± 14	35.5 ± 10.4	0.08
VPEV (cm/s)	23 ± 12	28.5 ± 12	0.02*

LA, left atrium; LAA, left atrial appendage; SEC, spontaneous echocontrast; HLAAEF, left atrial appendage ejection fraction in horizontal section; VLAAEF, left atrial appendage ejection fraction in vertical section; HPFV, horizontal peak filling velocity; HPEV, horizontal peak emptying velocity, VPFV, vertical peak filling velocity; VPEV, vertical peak emptying velocity.
*= $p \leq 0.05$.

Table 8. Demographic and echocardiographic characteristics in patients with left atrial appendage high (group A) and low (group B) flow profile

Variable	Group A	Group B	p Value
Patients ($n = 89$)	35 (39%)	54 (61%)	
D-dimer (≥ 500 ng/ml)	9	7	0.39
Fibrinogen (>350 mg/dl)	5	6	1.00
Age (years mean±S.D.)	67+/-10	71+/-9	0.06
Previous embolism/TIA	3	6	0.69
Antiaggregant	16 (46%)	19 (35%)	0.32
Anticoagulant	3 (8.6%)	10 (19%)	0.32
Mitral regurgitation	10 (29%)	24 (50%)	0.06
LA SEC	9 (26%)	27 (50%)	0.02*
LA/LAA Thrombus	1 (3%)	18 (33%)	0.001*
LA AREA (cm²)	25 ± 7	29 ± 6	0.004*
HLAAEF (%)	35 ± 11	24 ± 13	0.0001*
VLAEF (%)	35 ± 11	27 ± 13	0.003*
CTI > 0.5	11 (31%)	30 (56%)	0.02*

LA, left atrium; LAA, left atrial appendage; SEC, spontaneous echocontrast; HLAAEF, left atrial appendage ejection fraction in horizontal section; VLAAEF, left atrial appendage ejection fraction in vertical section. TIA, transient ischemic attack.
* = $p \leq 0.05$.

the patients treated with antiplatelet or anticoagulant drugs or those with or without previous thromboembolic complications.

To verify whether there are differences between high and low appendage flow in clinical, demographic, and echocardiographic characteristics, we classified our patients into two groups according to two different left atrial appendage flow patterns: group A with a high flow profile (hf) defined by high peak filling or emptying waves (or ≥ 25 cm/s) and group B with a low flow profile (lf) defined by irregular, very low peak filling or emptying waves (<25 cm/s) associated with almost no visible appendage contractions. In eight patients it was not possible to obtain good Doppler signals (Table 8).

The patients with a low left appendage flow had thrombus and/or spontaneous echocontrast more frequently located in the left atrium/appendage. Low flow was not related to a history of previous thromboembolism, and it was not influenced by anticoagulant and/or antiaggregant drugs or duration of AF. Mitral regurgitation did not seem to protect the left atrium and/or appendage against thrombus formation and /or spontaneous echocontrast.

A low flow pattern was related to a large left atrium ($p=0.004$), with a low left atrial appendage EF% in both sections (in horizontal section $p=0.0001$ and in vertical section $p=0.003$), and with cardiomegaly on chest X-ray ($p=0.02$).

In conclusion, the left atrial appendage function study finds variables with statistical significance associated with the presence of thrombosis and/or spontaneous echocontrast. However, in this first group of patients the findings do not identify those with or without previous thromboembolic complications.

Hematologic Correlates

The onset of NRAF is strictly correlated with an imminent appearance of embolic complications, particularly in the brain. This is probably because the arrhythmia decreases cerebral flow and contributes to the devel-

opment of stroke (4). In fact, in previous studies a higher incidence of embolic episodes was found in the days following the onset of AF (10). This cluster was also confirmed in our study where 26.1% of embolic events occurred in the first month after the appearance of the arrhythmia. However, the embolic risk can be maintained for a long period (266 months). Therefore, it is possible that, besides the cardiac factors, other alterations of coagulation may play an important role in the genesis of thromboembolism (19,20).

Sensitive new biochemical markers for assessing platelet activity (platelet factor 4 and ß-thromboglobulin) and status of thrombin generation (fibrinopeptide A, thrombin-antithrombin III complex) and fibrinolysis (D-dimer, plasma α2 plasmin inhibition complex) have made it possible to evaluate such activities in patients with NRAF (19).

We evaluated two other parameters of the coagulation system to look for a hematologic marker of embolic risk: D-dimer (in 59 patients) and fibrinogen (in 54 patients), considering normal as less than 500 ng/ml and less than or equal to 350 mg/dl, respectively (21). There was no statistically significant relationship between the concentrations of these two parameters and any of the variables tested, either with a history of embolism, the presence of thrombi or spontaneous echocontrast, or the echocardiographic characteristics of left atrial appendage function.

Conclusions

In several studies many risk factors have been identified as being associated with the increased likelihood of thromboembolic events. Although AF is a well-known risk factor for embolic events in patients with conditions of nonrheumatic etiology, it remains unclear whether anticoagulation treatment can prevent embolic stroke. Part of the dilemma is due to the fact that the determinants and predictors of embolic events in patients with NRAF are not clearly defined (Table 9).

Table 9. Clinical and demographic variables and relative risk of embolic events (international studies)

Variable	Relative risk RR 95%	Confidence interval
Previous embolism	3.1	1.9-5.2
Hypertension	1.9	1-2.8
Myocardial infarction	1.7	1.1-2.7
Congestive heart failure	1.7	1.1-2.5
Increasing age	1.4	1.1-1.8

In our study clinical variables with prognostic value included the duration of arrhythmia, left ventricular hypertrophy (with or without a history of hypertension), and previous myocardial infarction. Among the echocardiographic findings mitral annular calcification was significantly related to thromboembolism.

TEE was more sensitive in demonstrating spontaneous echocontrast and/or atrial and auricular thrombus than TTE and was also suitable for measuring other parameters of left atrial appendage function (particularly low flow), which are strictly related to the presence of thrombus and/or spontaneous echocontrast in these cavities. However, the role of alterations of coagulation in the genesis of thromboembolism is unclear.

Patients with NRAF should be treated with low-dose warfarin, especially if high-risk features for thromboembolism are present. In patients in whom anticoagulant therapy is contraindicated and in young patients with lone AF, therapy with 325 mg aspirin per day is preferred. The efficacy of aspirin has not been established in patients with AF who are older than 75 years of age. In the SPAF II study for patients receiving warfarin, a broad anticoagulation target was used: international nomalized ratio (INR) 2.0 to 4.5. In patients ≤ 75 years old, the risk of stroke was 2% in patients treated with either aspirin or warfarin. In those > 75 years old, warfarin was more effective in preventing thromboembolic stroke, but the rate of thrombotic stroke plus intracranial hemorrhage was not significantly different in the two groups (22). Potential bleeding complications with warfarin mandate judicious selection of patients for long-term anticoagulant therapy and they should be monitored strictly for obtaining a reasonable degree of safety.

Acknowledgement. We wish to thank Marie Luise Artero, MD, for her valuable English-language editing of this manuscript.

References

1. Wolf PA, Dawber TR, Thomas HE et al (1978) Epidemiologic assessment of chronic atrial fibrillation and risk of stroke: the Framingham study. Neurology 28: 973-977
2. Chesebro JH, Fuster V, Halperin JL (1990) Atrial fibrillation, risk marker for stroke. N Engl J Med 323: 1556-1558
3. Flegel KM, Shipley MJ, Rose G (1987) Risk of stroke in non-rheumatic atrial fibrillation. Lancet 1: 526-529
4. Scardi S (1993) La profilassi tromboembolica nella fibrillazione atriale non reumatica: quando e come farla? Prim Cardiol 8: 113-121
5. Connoly SJ, Laupacis A, Gent M et al (1991) Canadian Atrial Fibrillation Anticoagulation (CAFA) study. J Am Coll Cardiol 18: 349-355
6. Petersen P, Boysen G, Godtfredsen J et al (1989) Placebo-controlled, randomised trial, of warfarin and aspirin for prevention of thromboembolic complications in chronic atrial fibrillation. Lancet 1: 175-177
7. The Stroke Prevention in Atrial Fibrillation Investigators (1991) Stroke Prevention in Atrial Fibrillation study. Circulation 84: 527-539
8. The Boston Area Anticoagulation Trial in Atrial Fibrillation Investigators (1990) The effect of low-dose warfarin on the risk of stroke in patients with nonrheumatic atrial fibrillation. N Engl J Med 323: 1505-1511
9. Benjamin EJ, Plehn JF, D'Agostino RB et al (1992) Mitral annular calcification and the risk of stroke in an elderly cohort. N Engl J Med 327: 374-379
10. Wolf PA, Kannel WB, Mc Gee DL et al (1983) Duration of atrial fibrillation and imminence of stroke: the Framingham Study. Stroke 14 (5): 664-667
11. Petersen P, Kastrup J, Brinch K et al (1987) Relation between left atrial dimension and duration of atrial fibrillation. Am J Cardiol 60: 382-384
12. Andersen JS, Egelblad H, Abilgaarg J et al (1991) Atrial fibrillation and left atrial enlargement: cause or effect? J Intern Med 229: 253-256
13. Pearson AC, Labowitz AJ, Tatineni S et al (1991) Superiority of transesophageal echocardiography in detecting cardiac source of embolism in patients with cerebral ischemia of uncertain etiology. J Am Coll Cardiol 17: 66-72
14. Black W, Hopkins AP, Lee LCL et al (1991) Left atrial spontaneous echo contrast: a clinical and echocardiographic analysis. J Am Coll Cardiol 18: 398-404
15. Verhorst PMJ, Kamp O, Visser CA et al (1993) Left atrial appendage flow velocity assessment using transesophageal echocardiography in nonrheumatic atrial fibrillation and systemic embolism. Am J Cardiol 71: 192-196
16. Suetsugu M, Matsuzaki M, Toma Y (1988) Detection of mural thrombi and analysis of blood flow velocities in the left atrial appendage using transesophageal two-dimensional echocardiography and pulsed Doppler flowmetry. J Cardiol 18: 385-394
17. Aschenberg W, Schluter M, Kremer P et al (1986) Transesophageal two dimensional echocardiography for the detection of left atrial appendage thrombus. J Am Coll Cardiol 7: 163-166
18. Mugge A, Daniel WG, Hausmann D et al (1990) Diagnosis of left atrial appendage thrombi by transesophageal echocardiography: clinical implication and follow up. Am J Cardiac Imaging 4: 173-179
19. Yamamoto K, Ikeda U, Seino Y et al (1995) Coagulation activity is increased in the left atrium of patients with mitral stenosis. J Am Coll Cardiol 25: 107-112
20. Asakura H, Hifumi S, Jokaji H et al (1992) Prothrombin fragment F1+2 and thrombin-antithrombin III complex are useful markers of the hypercoagulable sate in atrial fibrillation. Blood Coagulation Fibrinolysis 3: 469-473
21. Rylatt DB, Blake AS, Cottis IE et al (1983) An immunoassay for human D-dimer using monoclonal antibodies. Thromb Res 31: 767-778
22. The Stroke Prevention in Atrial Fibrillation Investigators (1994) Warfarin versus aspirin for prevention of thromboembolism in atrial fibrillation: stroke prevention in atrial fibrillation II study. Lancet 343: 687-691

Should All Patients Undergo Transesophageal Echocardiography Before Electrical Cardioversion of Atrial Fibrillation?

B. De Piccoli, F. Rigo, and M. Ragazzo

Divisione di Cardiologia, Ospedale Umberto I,
Mestre-Venice, Italy

Transesophageal Echocardiography and Source of Embolism

Electrical cardioversion may be complicated by cerebral, systemic, and pulmonary embolic events in 0.6%-7% (1-3) of patients undergoing the procedure. Thromboembolism has been attributed to the dislodgment of preformed thrombus from the left atrium (LA) or left atrial appendage (LAA) with the resumption of sinus rhythm and atrial contraction (4).

Recently, spontaneous echocontrast (SEC), that is, an erythrocytic aggregation detectable by ultrasound (5), has also been considered a cause of embolic events (6-8). Thrombus and SEC are on average located in the LA and,above all, in the LAA so their prevalence in patients with atrial fibrillation (AF) may be underestimated by common noninvasive tools such as transthoracic echocardiography (TTE).

We must also outline that abnormalities such as the patent foramen ovale or aneurysm of the interatrial septum, Chiari's network, the mitral or tricuspid strands and the intra-aortic atherosclerotic debris can favour thromboembolism; the diagnostic sensitivity of TTE for these pathologies is poor, ranging from 15% to 19% (9) while transesophageal echocardiography (TEE) exhibits a sensitivity ranging from 57% to 86% (9-12).

The diagnostic sensitivity of TEE for atrial or auricular thrombus and SEC ranges from 83% to 100% (9,13) while the diagnostic sensitivity of TTE ranges from 1.4% to 37% (14-16). Thus TEE is clearly superior to TTE for the detection of potential sources of embolism.

TEE and LAA Dynamics

In the 1990s many papers have emphasized the usefulness of investigating LAA contraction and Doppler flow by TEE. Pollick and Taylor (17) demonstrated that LAA thrombus and SEC were frequent in patients with AF or sinus rhythm when their LAA was enlarged and poorly contracting.

Garcia-Fernandez et al. (18) studied 39 consecutive patients and identified three main patterns of auricular Doppler flow: the first, in subjects with sinus rhythm, was characterized by tall waves of LAA emptying and filling synchronous rhythm with P wave on electrocardiogram (ECG); the second, in subjects with AF, exhibited a sawtooth shape with peak velocities of 49±12 cm/s; the third, also in subjects with AF was characterized by small or unidentifiable waves. Only the last group had evidence of thrombus or SEC.

Verhost and coworkers (19) demonstrated that in patients with nonrheumatic AF auricular Doppler flow waves were lower in subjects with previous embolism. The authors also outlined that in the same patients pulmonary vein flow could not identify subjects with varying embolic risk.

Mügge et al. (20) also observed that in patients with nonrheumatic AF, auricular peaks flow waves lower than 25 cm/s correlated with the presence of thrombus or SEC and with previous embolism.

Thromboembolism After Electrical Cardioversion

Cerebral systemic and pulmonary embolism may occur after direct current countershock (DCC), despite negative results on precardioversion TEE (3,21). In fact, DCC provokes a transient impairment of the dynamics of LAA which, after sinus rhythm, may be worse than during previous AF (22). In such atrial or auricular stunning, SEC may appear or intensify if previously present. In ours and other authors' experience SEC becomes thicker and thicker during the 10 min after DCC and may persist for 72 h. Thus we can hypothesize a de novo formation of thrombus at a variable time interval from DCC (21);the restoration of LA and LAA contraction after DCC takes place at time intervals varying from a few hours to several days and rare cases of 3 month atrial stunning have been reported (23). This problem has been analyzed by serial evaluations of A wave of left and right ventricle Doppler filling curves after DCC (23-25).

Manning et al. (23) outlined that the peak A wave

velocity and percent atrial contribution to total left ventricular filling did not return to normality before 3 weeks after cardioversion in patients who remained in sinus rhythm. Dethy et al. (25) emphasized that an increase of A wave from 4 to 24 h <10% is strongly predictive for recurrence of AF.

These papers allow us to conclude that thromboembolism is not only the consequence of cardiac abnormalities coexisting with AF but it may also be consequent to DCC itself. Doppler echocardiography, above all TEE, constitutes a new window to view the pathophysiology of these ischemic events (2,3,17,18,25).

Thrombus, SEC and Embolic Risk

Previous studies (26,27) have demonstrated a significantly higher prevalence of atrial or auricular thrombosis in subjects who experienced embolic events than in subjects who did not. Thus, thrombus is estimated to be the fundamental cause of embolism. Nevertheless, the prevalence of atrial or auricular thrombosis in patients with AF ranges from 2.5% to 40% (2,3) while the prevalence of embolic events in patients undergoing DCC ranges from 0.6% to 7% (1,2). Thus we cannot establish a direct correlation between intracavitary thrombosis and embolism.

Actually SEC is also considered an independent risk factor for embolism (6-8,12); nevertheless, this conclusion is based upon retrospective studies of patients who previously experienced embolic events, and SEC might be a concomitant phenomenon, not the real cause of embolism.

Fatkin et al. (3) reports four patients who exhibited intensification of SEC and a parallel dynamic impairment of atrial and auricular function after DCC; two of them experienced embolism during follow-up.

We studied 20 cases by TEE during electrical cardioversion; in the only patient who subsequently experienced embolism we noticed a strong thickening of SEC soon after the procedure. This patients was affected by severe mitral stenosis.

In one paper on SEC in enlarged and hypokinetic hearts (28), the authors describe the persistence of the contrast in ventricles in which dynamics did not improve with medical treatment; on the contrary, in the study population studied SEC decreased or dissolved in hearts which improved hemodynamically. Only patients in the former group experienced embolism during the follow up. These reports emphasize that concomitant anatomical or functional pathologies are probably needed to increase the risk of thrombus or SEC.

In previous studies (20,26,29) patients with longstanding AF or more aged as well as patients affected by hypertension, ischemic heart disease, cardiomyopathy, mitral valve disease or mitral prosthesis were considered as high risk subjects for embolism. Other authors (10,12,30), by TEE investigation, often found anatomical and functional cardiac abnormalities favouring embolism in such subjects. Thus, we can clinically identify, at least in part, groups of individuals at higher embolic risk whom we must observe carefully and submit to further investigations if they are undergoing cardioversion.

Thrombus, SEC, and Anticoagulation Treatment

Long-term warfarin treatment can significantly reduce the prevalence of embolic complications in patients with AF who are undergoing DCC (29,31). With this treatment we can also resolve or at least stabilize an intracavitary thrombosis (32). Thus an empiric regimen of anticoagulation for 2-4 weeks before the cardioversion procedure has been recommended (33). There is not yet general agreement on anticoagulation in subjects with echocardiographic detection of "smoke." We know that SEC represents an erythrocytic aggregation conditioned by the interaction with plasma proteins and modulated by the shear rate of the blood flow (3,5). Warfarin treatment does not modify the prevalence and the echocardiographic characteristics of SEC although it also proved effective in preventing thromboembolism in patients with this echocontrast (5,28). We may hypothesize that anticoagulants can prevent "smoke" from transforming into more organized structures such as thrombus. Thus, it seems sensible to extend warfarin or heparin treatment to patients with SEC if they are undergoing cardioversion.

Which Patients Need TEE for cardioversion?

As TEE can give substantial information about abnormalities favouring thromboembolism in patients with AF, it is ethical to propose the diagostic tool to all patients with suspected high risk factors. TEE should be performed several times until the embolic risk is lowered. In this way we can prevent catastrophic and high-cost consequences such as stroke. Furthermore, TEE may obviate the need for several weeks of prophylactic anticoagulant therapy before cardioversion in patients without thrombus or SEC. The treatment is costly and may create problems, depending on the level of education and compliance in these individuals.

A recent analysis (34) of cost-effectiveness of TEE-guided cardioversion with anticoagulation as compared to conventional therapy in patients with AF has considered the following advantages of TEE: decreased embolic risk, guided anticoagulation therapy, convenience, decreased duration of anticoagulant treatment, and earlier DCC. The authors conclude that TEE-guided cardioversion can be expected to reduce costs by 39% compared to conventional therapy.

In low-risk patients TEE would allow us to detect underlying abnormalities that are unlikely but not impossible in this group of subjects with AF (3) and as already mentioned, we could obviate prolonged anticoagulation treatment. Management problems in echocardiographic laboratories do not allow a routine use of TEE in these patients at the present time. Future trends may indicate using this diagnostic tool during cardioversion (3) in order to obtain substantial information about unfavorable anatomical and functional situations before and after DCC. Because these patients are presumed to be free from intracavitary thrombus or intense SEC, the need to perform TEE before the cardioversion is obviated and we can couple TEE with anesthesia induction. The probability of

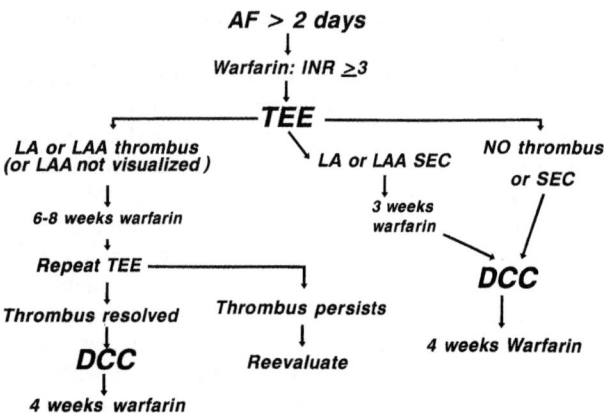

Fig. 1. Algorithm proposed in patients with high embolic risk. *AF*, atrial fibrillation, *INR*, international normalized ratio, *TEE*, transesophogeal echocardiography; *LA*, left atrium; *LAA*, left atrial appendage; *SEC*, spontaneous echocontrast; *DCC*, direct current counterschock. (Modified from [2])

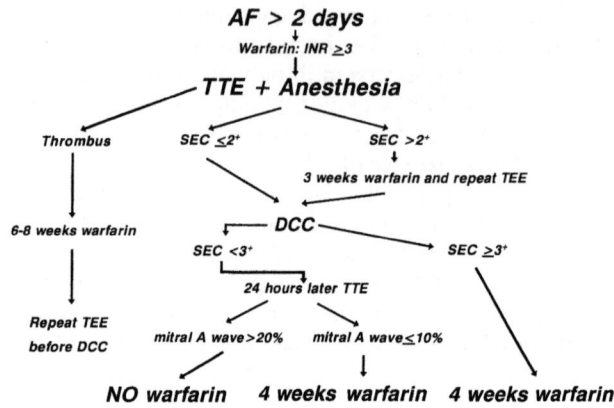

Fig. 2. Future trend in patients with low embolic risk. *TTE*, transthoracic echocardiography. See Fig. 1 legend for other abbreviations.

having to stop the procedure owing to the detection of a clot is remote in such patients. Thus by a single TEE we can obtain useful information before DCC and, by leaving the probe in situ during the delivery of the cardioversion shock, we can analyze LA and LAA function and erythrocytic aggregation after sinus rhythm restoration. If we analyze the A wave of the transmitral and transtricuspidal ventricular filling flow 24 h later by a short transthoracic echo-Doppler investigation, we can completely evaluate the embolic risk of the patients in order to suit subsequent therapy. These advantages surely compensate for the additional 15 min of anesthesia necessary to couple TEE and cardioversion.

Echo-Guided Anticoagulation Therapy

In patients with a high embolic risk TEE should be performed after a short course, 5 days on average, of warfarin treatment which is necessary to reach an optimal therapeutic range (international normalized ratio, INR, close to 3). If no thrombus or SEC is detected, cardioversion can be performed and the coagulation treatment will be maintained for the following 4 weeks in order to prevent postcardioversion thrombosis. If a LA or LAA clot is identified, DCC should be postponed while anticoagulant therapy is maintained for 6-8 weeks. TEE should then be repeated; if the thrombus is resolved, cardioversion and a subsequent 4 weeks treatment by warfarin is indicated. If a clot is still present, then the cost-benefit ratio of cardioversion must be evaluated. Also, if SEC without a clot is detected, DCC should be postponed; the procedure should be performed after 3 weeks of warfarin treatment in order to prevent the "smoke" from transforming into clot. Thereafter, the therapy is maintained for 4 weeks (Fig. 1).

In patients thought to be at low risk, simultaneous TEE and DCC are proposed after an average of 5 days of warfarin treatment. If thrombus and intense SEC are identified, the protocol previously described is followed. If SEC with an intensity degree lower than 2+ (a swirling pattern of smoke that is detectable only transiently during the cardiac cycle in the LAA or LA

cavity) is identified, cardioversion is performed: if thereafter smoke increases to 3+ or to a higher degree of intensity (dense swirling pattern in the LAA and LA cavity detectable constantly throughout the cardiac cycle) subsequent warfarin therapy for 4 weeks is recommended. If SEC does not increase after cardioversion, decisions about therapy are posponed for 24 h after recording the transmitral and transtricuspidal flow by transthoracic doppler echocardiography. At that time, if the atrial contribution to ventricular filling is lower than 10%, patients will be maintained on anticoagulation therapy in the subsequent 4 weeks; if the atrial contribution is greater than 20%, no anticoagulation is prescribed (Fig. 2).

References

1. Lown B (1967) Electrical reversion of cardiac arrhythmias. Br Heart J 29: 469-489
2. Grimm RA, Stewart W, Black IW et al (1994) Should all patients undergo transesophageal echocardiography before electrical cardioversion of atrial fibrillation? J Am Coll Cardiol 23: 533-541
3. Fatkin D, Kuchar DL, Thorburn CW et al (1994) Transesophageal echocardiography before and during direct current cardioversion of atrial fibrillation: evidence for "atrial stunning" as a mechanism of thromboembolic complications. J Am Coll Cardiol 23: 307-316
4. Mancini GBJ, Goldberger AL (1982) Cardioversion of atrial fibrillation: consideration of embolisation, anticoagulation, prophylactic pacemaker, and long-term success. Am Heart J 104: 612-621
5. Merino A, Hamptman P, Badiman L et al (1992) Echocardiographic "smoke" is produced by interaction of erythrocytes and plasma proteins modulated by shear forces. J Am Coll Cardiol 20: 1661-1668
6. Daniel WG, Nellesen V, Schroder E et al (1988) Left atrial spontaneous contrast in mitral valve disease: an indicator for an increase thromboembolic risk. J Am Coll Cardiol 11: 1204-1211
7. Tsai LM, Chen JH, Fang CJ et al (1992) Clinical implication of left atrial spontaneous echocontrast in non-rheumatic atrial fibrillation. Am J Cardiol 70: 327-331
8. Black IW, Chesterman CN, Hopkins AP et al (1993) Hematologic correlates of left atrial spontaneous echo-contrast and thromboembolic in non valvular atrial fibrillation. J Am Coll Cardiol 21: 451-457
9. Pearson AC, Labovitz AJ, Tatinemi S et al (1991) Superiority of transesophageal echocardiography in detecting cardiac

source of embolism in patients with cerebral ischemia of uncertain etiology. J Am Coll Cardiol 17: 66-72

10. Cujec B, Mycyk T, Khovri M (1992) Identification of Chiari's network with transesophageal echocardiography. J Am Soc Echocardiogr 5: 96-99

11. Vandenbogaerde J, De Bleeker J, Decoo D et al (1992) Transesophageal echo-Doppler in patients suspected of a cardiac source of peripheral emboli. Eur Heart J 13: 88-94

12. Derook FA, Comess KA, Albers GV et al (1992) Transesophageal echocardiography in the evaluation of stroke. Ann Intern Med 117: 992-932

13. Acar J, Cormier B, Grimbery D et al (1991) Diagnosis of left atrial thrombi in mitral stenosis, usefulness of ultrasound techniques compared with other methods. Eur Heart J 12 (Suppl B): 70-76

14. Herroy CA, Bass D, Kane M et al (1984) Two dimensional echocardiographic imaging of the left atrial appendage thrombus. J Am Coll Cardiol 1340-1344

15. Daniel WG, Angermann C, Englerding R et al (1989) Transesophageal echocardiography in patients with cerebral ischemic events and arterial embolism. A European multicenter study. Circulation 80 [Suppl 11] II: 473 (abstr)

16. Larandogoitia E, Medina A, Ortega JR et al (1991) Echo-transesofagico en la seleccion de los pacientes para valvuloplastica mitral percutanea. Estudio de 71 pacientes consecutivos. Rev Esp Cardiol 44: 599-604

17. Pollick C, Taylor D (1991) Assessment of left atrial appendage function by transesophageal echocardiography. Implications for the development of thrombus. Circulation 84: 223-231

18. Garcia-Fernander M, Torrecilla EG, San Roman D et al (1992) Left atrial appendage Doppler flow patterns: implications on thrombus formation. Am Heart J 124: 955-961

19. Verhost PMJ, Kemp D, Visser CA et al (1993) Left atrial appendage flow velocity assessment using transesophageal echocardiography in nonrheumatic atrial fibrillation and systemic embolism. Am J Cardiol 71: 192-196

20. Mügge A, Kühn H, Nikutta P et al (1994) Assessment of left atrial appendage function by biplane transesophageal echocardiography in patients with nonrheumatic atrial fibrillation: identification of a subgroup of patients at increased embolic risk. J Am Coll Cardiol 23: 599-607

21. Black IW, Fatkin D, Sagar KB et al (1993) Does exclusion of atrial thrombus by transesophageal echocardiography preclude embolism after cardioversion? A multicenter study. Circulation 88 [Suppl 1] I: 314 (abstr)

22. Grimm RA, Stewart WJ, Maloney JD et al (1993) Impact of electrical cardioversion for atrial fibrillation on left atrial appendage function and spontaneous echo-contrast: characterization by simultaneous transesophageal echocardiography. J Am Coll Cardiol 22: 1359-1360

23. Manning WJ, Leeman DE, Gotch PJ et al (1989) Pulsed Doppler evaluation of atrial mechanical function after electrical cardioversion of atrial fibrillation. J Am Coll Cardiol 13: 617-623

24. Shapiro EP, Effron MB, Lima S et al (1988) Transient atrial dysfunction after conversion of chronic atrial fibrillation to sinus rhythm. Am J Cardiol 1988; 62: 1202-1207

25. Dethy M, Chassat C, Roy D et al (1988) Doppler echocardiographic predictors of recurrence of atrial fibrillation after cardioversion. Am J Cardiol 62: 723-726

26. Pop G, Sutherland GR, Kondstaal PJ et al (1990) Transesophageal echocardiography in the detection of intracardiac embolic sources in patients with ischemic attacks. Stroke 21: 560-561

27. Lee RJ, Bartzokis J, Yeah JK et al (1991) Enhanced detection of intracardiac sources of cerebral emboli by transesophageal echocardiography. Stroke 22: 734-739

28. Doud DN, Jacobs WR, Moran JF et al (1990) The natural history of left ventricular spontaneous contrast. J Am Soc Echocardiogr 3: 465-470

29. Weinberg DM, Mancini J (1989) Anticoagulation for cardioversion of atrial fibrillation. Am J Cardiol 15: 745-746

30. Black IW, Hopkins AP, Lee LCL et al (1991) Left atrial spontaneous echo contrast: a clinical and echocardiographic analysis. J Am Coll Cardiol 18: 398-404

31. Bjerkelund CJ, Orming OM (1969) The efficacy of anticoagulant therapy in preventing embolism related to DC electrical conversion of atrial fibrillation. Am J Cardiol 23: 208-216

32. Tsai LM, Hung JS, Chen JH (1991) Resolution of left atrial appendage thrombus in mitral stenosis after warfarin therapy. Am Heart J 121: 1232-1234

33. Dunn M, Alexander J, de Silva R, Hildner F (1989) Antithrombotic therapy in atrial fibrillation. Chest 95: 118S-127S

34. Klein AL, Grimm RA, Black IW et al (1994) Cost effectiveness of TEE-guided cardioversion with anticoagulation compared to conventional therapy in patients with atrial fibrillation. J Am Coll Cardiol 23: 128A (abstr)

Anticoagulation in Atrial Fibrillation:
Is Aspirin Sufficient?

G. Di Pasquale, S. Urbinati, M.A. Ribani, P. Passarelli, G. Labanti, M.L. Borgatti, and G. Pinelli

Divisione di Cardiologia, Ospedale Bellaria, Bologna, Italy

Introduction

Atrial fibrillation (AF) carries a high risk of systemic embolism, in particular stroke. This is true not only when AF is associated with rheumatic valvular disease, but also in the so-called nonvalvular AF (NVAF) (1-7).

The principal mechanisms for stroke in AF are emboli due to stasis-related left atrial thrombi (associated with enlarged atria and thrombi in the left atrial appendage or atrial septal aneurysm), or stasis-related left ventricular thrombi (associated with left ventricular enlargement). Because of blood flow stasis, activation of the coagulation system with fibrin formation predominates over platelet activation as the principal mechanism in the development of intracavitary thrombi. According to the pathogenetic mechanism anticoagulation seems the most appropriate prophylactic treatment (8).

Alternative mechanisms for stroke in patients with NVAF include structural abnormalities of the mitral valve (including myxomatous or thickened valvular leaflets or mitral annular calcification), coexisting atherosclerotic carotid artery disease (in approximately 25% of AF-associated strokes), or atherosclerotic plaques in the ascending aorta and proximal arch. In these conditions sources of emboli are represented by platelet-fibrin thrombi and therefore platelet inhibition may be effective (9).

Five recent randomized, placebo-controlled, clinical trials (10-14) assessing antithrombotic therapy as primary prevention in NVAF have shown that in patients with NVAF not anticoagulated the annual incidence of ischemic stroke ranges between 3% and 5.8% (mean 5%) with a 2.5% incidence of disabling stroke; also including transient ischemic attacks (TIA) the incidence increases to 7% and to >7% considering silent cerebral infarction detected by computed tomography (CT) scan or magnetic resonance imaging (MRI).

An analysis from the SPAF study (15), subsequently confirmed by meta-analysis of pooled data from the five randomized controlled trials (16), has shown that in the large population of patients with NVAF the risk of stroke is not homogeneous. Stratification of AF patients into those at high and low risk of thromboembolism is possible and warranted in order to plan optimal antithrombotic prophylaxis (17).

Clinical risk factors predictive of stroke include increasing age, history of hypertension, previous TIA or stroke, recent congestive heart failure, and diabetes. Patients younger than 65 years who have none of these predictive factors (15% of all patients in the randomized clinical trials) show a low annual rate of stroke, approximately 1%, in the absence of any antithrombotic prophylaxis (16). These results confirm a previous observation that patients with lone AF (defined also by the absence of hypertension and diabetes) younger than 60 years have a risk for stroke less than 0.5% per year (2,18).

Besides the clinical risk factors, a SPAF analysis has identified echocardiographic predictors of stroke (19). They include left ventricular systolic dysfunction and left atrial enlargement. Transesophageal echocardiography provides further markers of embolic risk, i.e., left atrial thrombi, spontaneous echocontrast, and left atrial appendage dysfunction (20).

Warfarin Therapy

The effectiveness of warfarin therapy for the prevention of ischemic stroke has been definitely assessed by randomized clinical trials (16, 21, 22). Overall, warfarin decreased the frequency of all strokes by 68% (95% confidence interval, CI, 50%-79%), with an absolute annual reduction of 3.1% (p <.001). The incidence of stroke with residual deficit was decreased by 68% (95% CI, 39%-83%) with an absolute annual reduction of 1.4% (p <.001).

The intensity of anticoagulation in the five trials varied consistently, prothrombin time international normalized ratio (INR) ranging between 1.8 and 4.2. No correlation emerges between intensity of anticoagulation and consistency of reduction of stroke. Also low-intensity anticoagulation (INR range 2-3) as adopted in the BAATAF (11) and SPINAF (14) studies confers substantial benefit.

The risk of bleeding in patients receiving warfarin in these studies was quite low. The annual frequency of major bleeding events was 1.3% in warfarin-treated patients (vs 1.0% in patients receiving placebo or controls, and 1.0% in aspirin-treated patients). However, the bleeding risk is likely higher in patients treated in general clinical practice. Patients included in the clinical trials were carefully selected (representing only 7%-39% of the screened patients) and followed up carefully according to strict protocols. This can explain the low bleeding risk during warfarin treatment.

Moreover, the safety and tolerability of long-term anticoagulation to conventional levels has not been completely defined among patients older than 75 years. In the AFASAK (10) study involving AF patients older than those enrolled in every other trial (mean age of 75 years) the withdrawal rate from warfarin was 38% after 1 year. In the SPAF II study (23; INR 2.0-4.5, mean 2.7) the risk of major hemorrhage, mainly cerebral, was substantially higher among AF patients older than 75 years.

Aspirin Therapy

The fears regarding anticoagulation mainly in older AF patients explain the great expectations which have been placed on aspirin among physicians. The efficacy of aspirin for stroke prevention in AF patients is less clear and more controversial. The effect of aspirin in doses between 75 and 325 mg/day has been assessed in three placebo-controlled studies of primary prevention (AFASAK, SPAF I), secondary prevention (EAFT) (24), and in one primary prevention study without placebo arm (SPAF II) (Table 1).

The AFASAK study observed a statistically nonsignificant decrease in the frequency of strokes by 18%

(95% CI, 60%-58%; $p = .57$), while a statistically significant decrease of 44% (95% CI, 7%-66%; $p = .02$) was observed in the SPAF I study. Possible explanations for the different efficacy of aspirin in these two studies include different dosages of aspirin (75 mg in AFASAK and 325 mg in SPAF I) and different age of treated patients (mean age 75 years in AFASAK and 67 in SPAF I).

Other possible explanations for this difference may be the higher prevalence of stasis-related thrombi in the AFASAK study patients than in SPAF as suggested by the higher incidence of congestive heart failure (51% versus 19%). It is conceivable that aspirin does not prevent stasis-related causes of stroke due to left atrial and possibly left ventricular thrombi in patients with enlarged left ventricle.

It is unlikely that different dosages of aspirin could account for different efficacy. Several studies have also demonstrated that dosages of 30 mg/day are equally effective (25). As far as the age is concerned it is important to consider that a further analysis of SPAF has demonstrated that aspirin was ineffective in the subgroup of AF patients older than 75 years. The differential effect of aspirin associated with age could be accounted for by differences in the effect of aspirin on platelets, different stroke mechanisms, or age-related patient characteristics (e.g., intrinsic fibrinolytic activity or intra-atrial stasis of blood due to congestive heart failure) which might render the antithrombotic effect of aspirin inadequate.

The third trial in which aspirin was tested is the EAFT study (24). In this trial 1007 NVAF patients with a recent TIA or minor ischemic stroke were randomized to open anticoagulation or double-blind treatment with either 300 mg aspirin per day or placebo; patients with contraindications to anticoagulation were randomized to receive aspirin or placebo. In

Table 1. Efficacy of aspirin for the prevention of stroke in patients with nonvalvular atrial fibrillation

Study	Patients Total (n)	ASA treatment (n)	Dose of ASA (mg)	Treatment	Stroke reduction with ASA
AFASAK (10)	1007	336	75	W, ASA, PL	- 18% (ns)
SPAF I (11)	1330	552	325	Group 1 AC candidates W, ASA, PL	- 95% Groups 1+2 combined[a] All strokes -44% (p<0.02)
				Group 2 non AC candidates ASA, PL	- 8% Moderately - severely disabling strokes -24%
EAFT b (24)	1007	545	300	Group 1 AC eligible W, ASA, PL	
				Group 2 AC not eligible ASA, PL	- 14% (ns)
SPAF II (23)	1100		325	W, ASA	<75 years: absolute event rate (stroke + SE) 0.7% per year higher with ASA vs W >75 years: absolute event rate (stroke + SE) 1.2% per year higher with ASA vs W

W, warfarin; ASA, aspirin; PL, placebo; AC, anticoagulation; SE, systemic embolism; ns, not significant.
[a] In patients >75 years nonsignificant stroke reduction.
[b] Secondary prevention trial.

these high-risk patients warfarin was very effective, reducing the risk of stroke from 12% per year to 4% per year, while aspirin showed only a modest efficacy, reducing that risk from 12% to 10% per year.

Finally, more data on aspirin can be derived from the BAATAF study, in which control patients could choose to take aspirin on a nonrandomized basis, and approximately half did. A "treatment received" analysis provides no support for the efficacy of aspirin in preventing stroke in AF (26).

Combining the three placebo-controlled studies (AFASAK, SPAF, EAFT), the overall risk reduction with aspirin was statistically significant, 25% (range 14%-44%). In AFASAK and SPAF combined analysis the reduction of stroke was significantly higher in men, 44% (95% CI, 3%-68%; $p = .04$) than in women, 23% (95% CI, 40%-58%; $p = .38$).

A direct comparison of aspirin with warfarin has been made in three studies (AFASAK, SPAF II, EAFT). Aspirin was significantly less effective (combined risk reduction was 47% by warfarin relative to aspirin) but associated with a substantially lower risk of bleeding.

An analysis performed combining data sets from aspirin-assigned patients in both SPAF I and II has identified a number of aspirin-resistant patients who experienced a thromboembolic event during aspirin therapy (27). AF patients with a high rate of stroke during aspirin therapy are women older than 75 years and patients with impaired left ventricular function, congestive heart failure, systolic hypertension, and previous thromboembolism. In the presence of any of these conditions the annual risk of stroke was 8%; if none of these risk factors were present the risk was only 1%. The results of this analysis confirm that in high-risk NVAF patients, as those in the EAFT, aspirin is less efficacious.

A correlation of each of these variables with an increased risk of thromboembolism had already been found in other primary prevention studies in patients with AF (16). Moreover, the EAFT has shown that aspirin has only a modest efficacy in preventing recurrences of thromboembolism in patients with AF and recent TIA or stroke.

Finally, in a case-control study Bornstein et al. (28) found that ischemic heart disease is a risk factor for stroke recurrence despite aspirin treatment.

In other words, in high-risk AF patients aspirin has limited efficacy, providing inadequate thromboembolic prophylaxis.

Only speculative explanations can be provided regarding the modest efficacy of aspirin in certain patients.

Impaired left ventricular function, defined by the presence of clinical congestive heart failure or subclinical echocardiographic abnormalities, increases stasis in the left atrium, potentially rendering the effect of aspirin inadequate. The scarce efficacy of aspirin in the AFASAK study has been partially attributed to the high prevalence of congestive heart failure in treated patients.

Female gender is another independent predictor of thromboembolism only in older patients over the age of 75 years, while younger women had rates similar to

men. A difference in response to aspirin by gender has long been controversial. Less efficacy of aspirin in women has been reported in some trials (29, 30) involving patients with a history of TIA or stroke. An overview of randomized trials of prolonged aspirin therapy in various categories of patients does not show any difference in response for aspirin by gender (31). It is likely that the high risk of thromboembolism during aspirin therapy in elderly women could be due to other clinical risk factors associated with gender and advanced age (e.g. congestive heart failure, systolic hypertension).

The association of *high systolic blood pressure* with stroke and embolic events in patients with NVAF has been demonstrated in several studies (32, 33). In patients with paroxysmal NVAF a history of hypertension has also resulted in a significant independent risk factor for systemic embolism (34). Systolic hypertension does not imply only a vascular risk, but interacts specifically with AF to greatly increase the absolute risk of stroke. In the presence of hypertension, possibly associated with left ventricular hypertrophy, myocardial compliance is decreased, which results in an increased left atrial work load and distention. This favors stasis and thrombi formation in the left atrium, rendering the effect of aspirin inadequate. The importance of left ventricular hypertrophy is confirmed by the high embolic risk of AF in patients with hypertrophic cardiomyopathy (35).

Finally, *previous thromboembolism* is a high-risk condition for embolic recurrences. Patients with NVAF and prior stroke, TIA, or systemic arterial embolism should be treated with warfarin because of the excessive recurrence rate of thromboembolism during aspirin therapy.

In contrast, in the SPAF analysis aspirin proved to be a sufficient therapy for younger AF patients (<75 years) identified as at low risk based on clinical criteria: in this subgroup the risk of thromboembolism during aspirin therapy is extremely low, averaging 0.5% per year (95% CI, 0.1% per year to 1.9% per year).

In AF patients older than 75 years, especially women, aspirin is ineffective and warfarin should be the treatment of choice, irrespective of the presence or absence of risk factors. However, warfarin in these older patients carries a high risk of bleeding complications. Possible alternative options, under evaluation in the SPAF III and AFASAK II studies, include warfarin at less intense levels and fixed warfarin doses (1-3 mg) plus aspirin (36).

A differential effect of aspirin according to stroke mechanism is another important issue. Platelet inhibitors and anticoagulants may influence cardioembolic and noncardioembolic sources of stroke differently. Aspirin may have a greater prophylactic impact on noncardioembolic mechanisms than on strokes of presumed cardioembolic origin in AF patients. In a SPAF secondary analysis strokes were categorized as cardioembolic or noncardioembolic according to clinical and neuroradiologic criteria (37). The preventive effect of aspirin therapy was different for cardioembolic relative to noncardioembolic ischemic strokes ($p = 0.001$). Aspirin was associated with a risk reduction in noncardioembolic strokes of 100% (95% CI, 60%-

100%; p=0.001), but with a risk reduction of only 31% for cardioembolic strokes (95% CI, -35%-65%; p=0.31).

Another intriguing issue concerning aspirin treatment is the evidence that among patients taking aspirin about one third are nonresponders. This has been demonstrated by the platelet reactivity test in stroke patients under aspirin treatment (38). The clinical relevance of these laboratory findings has to be assessed, looking at the clinical outcomes in a long-term follow-up of aspirin treatment nonresponders and aspirin responders.

Antiplatelet agents other than aspirin might have a different efficacy for stroke prevention in NVAF (39). In the Italian study SIFA (Studio Italiano Fibrillazione Atriale) the efficacy and safety of the antiplatelet drug indobufen, a reversible cyclooxygenase inhibitor (100-200 mg bid) has been compared with warfarin (INR 2.0-3.5) in patients with NVAF and a recent (≤ 14 days) TIA or stroke (40).

In this multicenter, open trial 950 NVAF patients were randomized to anticoagulation or indobufen. Preliminary results after 1 year follow-up show a comparable incidence (approximately 10%) of primary outcome events (nonfatal stroke, systemic embolism, nonfatal myocardial infarction or vascular death) in the two groups. In comparison with the EAFT study, the efficacy of antiplatelet treatment was substantially higher.

Finally, coagulation abnormalities have been demonstrated in patients with AF. Significantly higher concentrations of von Willebrand factor, factor VIII: c, fibrinogen, D-dimer, thromboglobulin, and platelet factor 4 have been found in NVAF patients than in healthy controls (41-43). Recently, Yamamoto et al. (44) have demonstrated an increased coagulation activity in the left atrium of patients with mitral stenosis and AF, even during anticoagulation. Thus, alterations in hemostatic function may contribute to the increased risk of stroke in patients with AF.

Conclusions

In conclusion, according to current knowledge from the literature the following guidelines can be suggested (45) (Table 2):

1. In patients <75 years with NVAF and without risk factors aspirin is a sufficient prophylaxis, pending confirmation from the ongoing SPAF III prophylaxis study; in younger patients <60 years and without risk factors probably no treatment is required.

2. Elderly patients >75 years still represent a therapeutic dilemma, because aspirin may not be sufficient, especially in women, and conventional anticoagulation may carry substantial toxicity. In this latter group of patients the choice of treatment should be based on the evaluation of the risk/benefit ratio in the individual case. It appears reasonable to consider aspirin for those who are poor candidates for anticoagulation, patients with extracardiac causes of embolism (i.e., carotid artery disease, aortic plaques), and patients without gross echocardiographic abnormalities (i.e., left atrial and left ventricle enlargement) favoring thrombi formation.

Table 2. Guidelines for antithrombotic prophylaxis in patients with nonvalvular atrial fibrillation

Primary prevention
< 60 years
  No risk factors → no treatment
  Yes risk factors → warfarin (INR 2.0 - 3.0)
60-75 years
  No risk factors → aspirin
  Yes risk factors → warfarin (INR 2.0 - 3.0)
> 75 years
  Warfarin (INR 1.5 - 2.0)
  Warfarin fixed dose (1 - 3 mg) + aspirin 325 mg
  Aspirin 325 mg

Secondary prevention
  Warfarin (INR 2.5 - 4.0)
  Aspirin 325 mg in poor candidates for
  anticoagulation

INR, international normalized ratio.
a As optimal antithrombotic therapy is not established, possible treatment options are proposed.

Further studies, some already ongoing, are necessary to establish:

1. Efficacy of lower intensity regimens of anticoagulation, and combinations of fixed-dose warfarin (1-3 mg/day) possibly associated with aspirin;

2. Elucidation of stroke mechanisms in AF;

3. Better characterization of the role of aspirin and confirmation of its efficacy in low-risk patients;

4. Role of transesophageal echocardiography (intra-atrial thrombi, spontaneous echocontrast, left atrial appendage filling and emptying velocities) for risk stratification;

5. Role of hemostatic variables (prothrombotic states) as contributing factors for intracardiac thrombosis and stroke in patients with AF.

References

1. Halperin JL, Hart RG (1988) Atrial fibrillation and stroke: new ideas, persisting dilemmas (editorial). Stroke 19: 937-941
2. Cerebral Embolism Task Force (1989) Cardiogenic brain embolism: the second report of the Cerebral Embolism Task Force. Arch Neurol 46: 727-743
3. Petersen P (1990) Thromboembolic complications in atrial fibrillation. Stroke 21: 4-13
4. Cairns JA, Connolly SJ (1991) Nonrheumatic atrial fibrillation. Risk of stroke and role of antithrombotic therapy. Circulation 84: 469-481
5. Hart RG (1992) Thromboembolism in nonrheumatic atrial fibrillation: what have we learned? In: Di Pasquale G, Pinelli G (eds) Heart-brain interactions. Springer, Berlin Heidelberg New York, pp 83-86
6. The National Heart, Lung and Blood Institute Working Group on Atrial Fibrillation (1993) Atrial fibrillation: current understandings and research imperatives. J Am Coll Cardiol 32: 1830-1834
7. Hart RG, Halperin JL (1994) Atrial fibrillation and stroke: revisiting the dilemmas. Stroke 25: 1337-1341
8. Stein B, Fuster V, Halperin JL, Chesebro JH (1989) Antithrombotic therapy in cardiac disease. An emerging approach based on pathogenesis and risk. Circulation 80: 1501-1513
9. Chesebro JH, Fuster V, Halperin JL (1991) Atrial fibrillation: risk marker for stroke. N Engl J Med 323: 1556- 1558
10. Petersen P, Boysen G, Godtfredsen J, Andersen ED, Andersen B (1989) Placebo-controlled, randomised trial of warfarin and aspirin for prevention of thromboembolic complications in

chronic atrial fibrillation. The Copenhagen AFASAK Study. Lancet 1: 175-179

11. The Stroke Prevention in Atrial Fibrillation Investigators (1991) The Stroke Prevention in Atrial Fibrillation trial: final results. Circulation 84: 527-539

12. The Boston Area Anticoagulation Trial for Atrial Fibrillation Investigators (1990) The effect of low-dose warfarin on the risk of stroke in patients with nonrheumatic atrial fibrillation. N Engl J Med 325: 1505-1511

13. Connolly SJ , Laupacis A, Gent M, Roberts RS, Cairns JA, Joyner C, for the CAFA study coinvestigators (1991) Canadian Atrial Fibrillation Anticoagulation (CAFA) study. J Am Coll Cardiol 18: 349-355

14. Ezeckowitz MD, Bridgers SL, James KE, Carliner NH, Colling CL, Gornick CC, Krause-Steinrauf H, Kurtzke JF, Nazarian SM, Radford MJ, Rickles FR, Shabetai R, Deykin D, for the Veterans Affairs Stroke Prevention in Nonrheumatic Atrial Fibrillation Investigators (1992) Warfarin in the prevention of stroke associated with nonrheumatic atrial fibrillation. N Engl J Med 327: 1406-1412

15. The Stroke Prevention in Atrial Fibrillation Investigators (1992) Predictors of thromboembolism in atrial fibrillation: I. clinical features of patients at risk. Ann Intern Med 116: 1-5

16. Atrial Fibrillation Investigators (1994) Risk factors for stroke and efficacy of antithrombotic therapy in atrial fibrillation: analysis of pooled data from five randomized controlled trials. Arch Intern Med 154: 1449-1457

17. Di Pasquale G, Urbinati S, Ribani MA, Passarelli P, Pinelli G (1994) Clinical markers of embolic risk in patients with atrial fibrillation. G Ital Cardiol 24: 315-324

18. Kopecky Sl, Gersh BJ, Mc Goon MD, Whisnant JP, Holmes DR Jr, Ilstrup DM, Frye RL (1987) The natural history of lone atrial fibrillation: a population-based study over three decades. N Engl J Med 327: 1406-1412

19. The Stroke Prevention in Atrial Fibrillation Investigators (1992) Predictors of thromboembolism in atrial fibrillation: II. echocardiographic features of patients at risk. Ann Intern Med 116: 6-12

20. Di Pasquale G, Urbinati S, Pinelli G (1995) New echocardiographic markers of embolic risk in atrial fibrillation. Cerebrovasc Dis (in press)

21. Albers G, Atwood JE, Hirsch J, Sherman DG, Hughes RA, Connolly SJ (1991) Stroke prevention in nonvalvular atrial fibrillation. Ann Intern Med 115: 727-736

22. Laupacis A, Albers G, Dunn M, Feinberg W (1992) Antithrombotic therapy in atrial fibrillation. Chest 102 [Suppl]: 426S-433S

23. Stroke Prevention in Atrial Fibrillation Investigators (1994) Warfarin versus aspirin for prevention of thromboembolism in atrial fibrilllation: Stroke Prevention in Atrial Fibrillation II Study. Lancet 346: 687-691

24. EAFT (European Atrial Fibrillation Trial) Study Group (1993) Secondary prevention in non-rheumatic atrial fibrillation after transient ischaemic attack or minor stroke. Lancet 342: 1255-1262

25. Patrono C (1994) Aspirin as an antiplatelet drug. N Engl J Med 330: 1287-1294

26. Singer DE, Hughes RA, Gress DR, Sheehan MA, Oertel LB, Maraventano SW, Blewett DR, Rosner B, Kistler JP for the BAATAF Investigators (1992) The effect of aspirin on the risk of stroke in patients with nonrheumatic atrial fibrillation: the BAATAF Study. Am Heart J 124: 1567-1573

27. Mc Anulty JH, Hart RG, Pearce RA for the SPAF Investigators (1993) Atrial fibrillation and thromboembolism: predictors

of high risk during aspirin therapy. Circulation 88 [suppl]: I-222 (abstr)

28. Bornstein NM, Karepov VG, Aronovich BD, Gorbulev AY, Treves TA, Korczyn AD (1994) Failure of aspirin treatment after stroke. Stroke 25: 275-277

29. Canadian Cooperative Study Group (1978) A randomized trial of aspirin and sulfinpyrazone in threatened stroke. N Engl J Med 299: 53-59

30. UK-TIA Study Group (1988) United Kingdom transient ischaemic attack (UK-TIA) aspirin trial: interim results. Br Med J 296: 316-320

31. Antiplatelet Trialists' Collaboration (1994) Collaborative overview of randomized trials of antiplatelet therapy - I: prevention of death, myocardial infarction, and stroke by prolonged antiplatelet therapy in various categories of patients. Br Med J 306: 81-106

32. Flegel KM, Hanley J (1989) Risk factors for stroke and other embolic events in patients with nonrheumatic atrial fibrillation. Stroke 20: 1000-1004

33. Moulton AW, Singer DE, Haas JS (1991) Risk factors for stroke in patients with nonrheumatic atrial fibrillation: a case-control study. Am J Med 91: 156-161

34. Corbalan R, Arriagada D, Braun S, Tapia J, Huete I, Kramer A, Chavez A (1992) Risk factors for systemic embolism in patients with paroxysmal atrial fibrillation. Am Heart J 124: 149-153

35. Di Pasquale G, Andreoli A, Lusa AM, Urbinati S, Grazi P, Carini GC, Ruffini M, Pinelli G (1990) Cerebral embolic risk in hypertrophic cardiomyopathy. In: Baroldi G, Camerini F, Goodwin JF (eds) Advances in cardiomyopathies. Springer, Berlin Heidelberg New York, pp 90- 96

36. Major Ongoing Stroke Trials (1995) Stroke 26: 349-353

37. Miller VT, Rothrock JF, Pearce LA, Feinberg WM, Hart RG, Anderson DC (1993) Ischemic stroke in patients with atrial fibrillation: clinical characteristics and the effect of aspirin. Neurology 43: 32-36

38. Grotemeyer KH (1991) Effect of acetylsalicylic acid in stroke patients. Evidence of nonresponders in a subpopulation of treated patients. Thromb Res 63: 587-593

39. Fornaro GL, Rossi P, Mantica P, Caccia ME, Aralda D, Lavezzari M, Pamparana F, Milanesi G (1993) Indobufen in the prevention of thromboembolic complications in patients with heart disease. A randomized, placebo-controlled, double-blind study. Circulation 87: 162-164

40. Cataldo G, SIFA Study Group (1995) Secondary prevention of stroke in non-valvular atrial fibrillation: results of the SIFA (Studio Italiano Fibrillazione Atriale). J Am Coll Cardiol 25 [Suppl] 144A (abstr)

41. Gustafsson C, Blombäck M, Britton M, Hamsten A, Svensson J (1990) Coagulation factors and the increased risk of stroke in nonvalvular atrial fibrillation. Stroke 21: 47-51

42. Kumagai K, Fukunami M, Ohmori M, Kitabatake A, Kamada T, Hoki N (1990) Increased intracardiovascular clotting in patients with chronic atrial fibrillation. J Am Coll Cardiol 16: 377-380

43. Boysen G, Petersen P, Felding P (1991) Coagulation and fibrinolysis in patients with chronic atrial fibrillation. Cerebrovasc Dis 1: 235-238

44. Yamamoto K, Ikeda V, Seino Y, Mito H, Fujikawa H, Sekiguchi H, Shimada K (1995) Coagulation activity is increased in the left atrium of patients with mitral stenosis. J Am Coll Cardiol 25: 1107-1112

45. Di Pasquale G, Ribani MA, Urbinati S, Passarelli P, Pinelli G (1995) Come si deve trattare oggi la fibrillazione atriale. In: Prati PL (ed) Conoscere e curare il cuore '95. CIBA Edizioni, Milan, pp 285-299

Pharmacologic Cardioversion of Atrial Fibrillation: Always the Same Algorithm or Different Drugs for Different Patients?

N. Baldi, V.A. Russo, G. Marasco, G. Polimeni, and V. Morrone

Divisione di Cardiologia, Ospedale SS. Annunziata, Taranto, Italy

The clinical use of class IC antiarrhythmic drugs and amiodarone during the last 10 years has represented a great achievement in the restoration of the sinus rhythm during atrial fibrillation (AF) of recent onset. In fact, the advantages of the pharmacologic treatment depend not only on the effectiveness of these drugs (quinidine, a very old drug, has also shown an effectiveness in the range of 30% – 91%), but much more on the velocity of the sinus rhythm restoration, often during the intravenous infusion of the drug. This avoids patient hospitalization. The drugs mainly employed in the treatment of AF are 1A and 1C antiarrhythmic agents, amiodarone, and sometimes verapamil, beta-blocking agents, and digoxin. Clinical practice suggests that the appropriate drug be chosen in each individual situation. However, before discussing the different clinical situations in which AF may occur, we must emphasize that to our knowledge no homogeneous, controlled, and randomized studies in large groups of patients that suggest the correct way of treating this arrhythmia have been performed. In fact, in all the studies patients the group were heterogenous as far as the etiology of heart disease and the duration of AF were different. In our opinion, however, it is possible to suggest some guidelines about the clinical use of different drugs in different patients using our knowledge of the electrophysiologic and hemodynamic properties of drugs, their effectiveness, and side effects occurring in clinical practice. Regarding cardioversion, if we take into account anticoagulant prophylaxis, it is useful to divide AF in-to AF of recent onset (less than 3 days) and prolonged AF (more than 3 days). In fact, according to the College of Chest Physicians (1), AF with a duration longer than 3 days needs to be treated with anticoagulant drugs for at least 3 weeks before cardioversion. Therefore, this practice identifies two groups of patients with AF: the first group can be treated within 3 days, and the second cannot be treated before 3 weeks. It is well known that AF duration is the main factor conditioning the probability of sinus rhythm restoration (2). As we now have several drugs whose effectiveness may be different according to AF duration, it follows that AF duration is one of the main factors determining the choice of drug.

Pharmacologic Cardioversion of Atrial Fibrillation in Different Clinical Situations

Lone Atrial Fibrillation

Lone or idiopathic AF in the absence of known heart disease accounts for less than 10% of all cases of AF and often affects young people. This is the clinical situation in which class 1C antiarrhythmic agents may be most useful. Different studies in which intravenous flecainide (3 – 7) and propafenone (7 – 11) have proved to be effective investigated groups of patients affected by both lone AF and AF in the presence of different underlying heart diseases. It is not possible, however, to evaluate separately the effectiveness of drugs in the subgroup of patients, but in some studies in which the subgroup of patients affected by lone AF is dominant or can be easily distinguished from the remaining cases, the percentage of success ranges between 85% and 93% for flecainide (4, 5, 7) and between 57% and 87.5% for propaferone (5, 7, 10). The actual use of these drugs depends not only on their effectiveness, but also on the time until sinus rhythm restoration (generally within 1 h and often during the drug infusion). Although, for example, amiodarone is a drug which shows a percentage of success ranging between 25% and 80.8% (10, 12, 13), the average times of sinus rhythm restoration are usually longer. Recently, a dose of propafenone and flecainide per os has been proposed in two groups of patients in whom idiopathic AF accounted for 50% of all cases (14). The conversion rate of AF into sinus rhythm 3 h after administration was 59% for flecainide and 52% for propafenone. If this treatment is confirmed by other studies we will be able to considerably reduce the duration of the AF, thus avoiding patient hospitalization.

Wolff-Parkinson-White Syndrome

The incidence of AF in Wolff-Parkinson-White (WPW) syndrome patients is higher than in the normal population, and ventricular fibrillation may develop during an attack of AF if conduction through the accessory pathway is rapid (15). Drugs such as digoxin, verapamil, and amiodarone are contraindicated because of their depressive action on nodal conduction, which may speed up the ventricular response during AF and increase the risk of degeneration to ventricular fibrillation (15-19). Flecainide and propafenone can be considered as the drugs of choice in the treatment of AF; in these patients, many studies have shown that both drugs determine the prolongation of the anterograde and retrograde refractory period of the accessory pathway – both in patients with a long and those with a short refractory period – as well as the complete block of conduction, via the accessory pathway (20-27). Thus, these drugs considerably slow down the ventricular response during AF with pre-excited ventricular response (20, 22, 25, 28, 29). Thus, their effects are twofold: (1) restoration of sinus rhythm and (2) prolongation of pre-excited beat intervals or block of conduction, via the accessory pathway with slowing down of the ventricular rate. Other class 1A antiarrhythmic agents, such as procainamide, are also clinically useful in the immediate treatment of AF associated with the WPW syndrome (30). However, in comparison with class 1C antiarrhythmic drugs, procainamide shows two disadvantages: (1) it prolongs the anterograde refractory period of the atrioventricular pathway with relatively long refractory periods (31); (2) it is inferior in immediately slowing down the ventricular response during AF (30). Recently, some authors have proposed the use of disopyramide or sotalol as the drugs of choice in this kind of arrhythmia (32). Disopyramide, like 1C drugs, is also effective in patients in whom the shortest R-R interval was initially less than 200 ms (33). Sotalol has a balanced action in prolonging refractoriness and conduction velocity in the atrioventricular node and the atrioventricular accessory pathway, and it also slows down the ventricular response during AF (34, 35), but no conduction block in the accessory pathway either in the anterograde or retrograde direction was observed (35). However, disopyramide has only been tested in small groups of patients, and the effect of sotalol in patients with WPW syndrome and documented AF has yet to be established.

Sick Sinus Syndrome

Presently, no data are available about the pharmacologic conversion of AF in patients with sick sinus syndrome, because the presence of the syndrome has been an exclusion criteria in most studies. We suggest several forms of treatment based on the electrophysiologic action of certain drugs on the sinus node. Intravenous administration of flecainide in these patients showed a clear prolongation of the maximal sinus node recovery time and the corrected sinus node recovery time (36). Amiodarone can sometimes produce sinus bradycardia and other types of sinus node dysfunctions (37). Some observations about propafenone (38) also suggest that

caution needs to be applied in using it in these patients, even if the few clinical observations carried out have not shown any relevant side effect (9). Considering this uncertainty, the use of compounds with vagolytic properties has been suggested for these patients, and disopyramide is therefore primarily recommended (32). Nevertheless, before pharmacologic treatment, the best thing to do seems to be to use a temporary, preferably transthoracic pacemaker to avoid the introduction of an electrode catheter.

Bundle Branch Block or Multifascicular Block

There is a potential risk in patients with bundle branch block or multifascicular block of a complete paroxysmal atrioventricular block due to drugs which hardly depress the conduction through the His-Purkinje system. The H-V interval is actually prolonged by 1A class drugs, such as procainamide (39), and 1C class drugs, such as flecainide and propafenone (40, 41), whereas amiodarone does not slow down conduction through the His-Purkinje system (42). Thus, in such patients the drug of choice is amiodarone to avoid the risk of a complete paroxysmal atrioventricular block.

Left Ventricular Dysfunction Without Heart Failure

In patients with left ventricular dysfunction without heart failure we suggest the use of amiodarone, a drug with a very slight negative inotropic effect (43), instead of 1A class drugs, such as disopyramide (44) and procainamide (45) and 1C class drugs such as flecainide (46) and propafenone (47), drugs with a clearly negative inotropic effect.

Acute Myocardial Infarction in a Steady Hemodynamic State

AF occurs in 10%–15% of patients with acute myocardial infarction; it is usually transient and tends to occur in patients with left ventricular failure, but it is also observed in patients with pericarditis and ischemic injury to the atria. Digoxin is commonly administered to those patients not requiring immediate direct current (DC) cardioversion (48), but amiodarone is the only drug that has shown a certain effectiveness in restoring the sinus rhythm in a randomized open study. In fact, in a comparative study with digoxin, amiodarone showed a rate of conversion into sinus rhythm of 75%, compared to 10% using digoxin ($p < 0.05$), without clinically relevant side effects (49). Thus, amiodarone must be considered the drug of choice in such conditions.

Atrial Fibrillation Lasting Longer than 3 Days

It is generally accepted that AF lasting longer than 3 days requires anticoagulant treatment for at least 3 weeks before any attempt at conversion into sinus rhythm is made. In these case DC shocks is the treatment of choice. As far as pharmacologic treatment is concerned, the percentage of success for different drugs employed decreases as the duration of AF increases. The treatment currently still suggested is quinidine with beta-blocking agents, a combination which has proved to be able to restore the sinus rhythm even during AF lasting several months in patients with different underlying heart disease (50).

Conclusion

In conclusion, we believe that knowledge of both the physiopathology of the different clinical conditions in which AF can occur and the electrophysiologic and hemodynamic effects of the antiarrhythmic drugs must be used to indicate the most appropriate drug to restore the sinus rhythm in AF.

References

1. Dunn M, Alexander J, de Silva R, Hildner F (1989) Antithrombotic therapy in atrial fibrillation. Chest 95: 118S-124S
2. Baldi N, Lenti V, Marasco G, Russo VA, Montervino C (1991) Riconversione della fibrillazione atriale: quando e perché. In Piccolo E, Raviele A (eds) Aritmie cardiache, Centro Scientifico Editore, Torino, pp 293-300
3. Goy JJ, Gbric M, Hurni M, Finci L, Maendly R, Duc J, Sigwart U (1985) Conversion of supraventricular arrhythmias to sinus rhythm using flecainide. Eur Heart J 6: 518-524
4. Borgeat A, Goy JJ, Maendly R, Kaufman U, Grbic M, Sigwart U (1986) Flecainide versus quinidine for conversion of atrial fibrillation to sinus rhythm. Am J Cardiol 58: 496-498
5. Suttorp MJ, Kingma JH, Jessuron ER, Lie-A-Huen L, Van Hemel NM, Lie KI (1990) The value of class 1C antiarrhythmic drugs for acute conversion of paroxysmal atrial fibrillation or flutter to sinus rhythm. J Am Coll Cardiol 16: 1722-1727
6. Donovan KD, Dobb GJ, Coombs LJ, Kok-Yeng Lee, Weekes JN, Murdock CJ, Clarke GM (1992) Efficacy of flecainide for the reversion of acute onset atrial fibrillation. Am J Cardiol 70: 50A-55A
7. Baldi N, Lenti V, Marasco G, Russo VA, Montervino C (1992) Propafenone vs flecainide in the acute treatment of atrial fibrillation of recent onset: a randomized study. New Trends Arrhith 8: 499-505
8. Capucci A, Gubelli S, Carini G, Frabetti L, Magnani B (1987) Cardioversione farmacologica con propafenone di fibrillazione atriale di recente insorgenza. G Ital Cardiol 17: 975-982
9. Bianconi L, Boccadamo R, Pappalardo A, Gentili C, Pistolese M (1989) Effectiveness of intravenous propafenone for conversion of atrial fibrillation and flutter of recent onset. Am J Cardiol 64: 335-338
10. Bertini G, Conti A, Fradella G, Francardelli L, Giglioli G, Mangialavori G, Margheri M, Moschi G (1990) Propafenone versus amiodarone in field treatment of primary atrial tachydysrhythmias. J Emerg Med 8: 15-20
11. Bracchetti D, Palmieri M (1992) Sicurezza ed efficacia del propafenone e.v. nella cardioversione della fibrillazione atriale parossistica di recente insorgenza. G Ital Cardiol 23: 186 (abstr)
12. Faniel R, Schönfeld PG (1983) Efficacy of i.v. amiodarone in converting rapid atrial fibrillation and flutter to sinus rhythm in intensive care patients. Eur Heart J 4: 180-185
13. Noc M, Stajer D, Horvat M (1990) Intravenous amiodarone versus verapamil for acute conversion of paroxysmal atrial fibrillation to sinus rhythm. Am J Cardiol 65: 679-680
14. Capucci A, Boriani G, Botto GL, Lenzi T, Rubino I, Falcone C, Trisolino G, Della Casa S, Binetti N, Cavazza M, Sanguinetti M, Magnani B (1994) Conversion of recent-onset atrial fibrillation by a single oral loading dose of propafenone or flecainide. Am J Cardiol 74; 503-505
15. Klein GJ, Bashore TM, Sellers TD, Pritchett ELC, Smith WM, Gallagher JJ (1979) Ventricular fibrillation in the Wolff-Parkinson-White syndrome. N Engl J Med 301: 1080-1085
16. Wellens HJ, Durrer D (1973) Effect of digitalis on atrioventricular conduction and circus-movement tachycardias in patients with Wolff-Parkinson-White syndrome. Circulation 47: 1229-1233
17. Harper RW, Whitford E, Middlebrook K, Federman J, Anderson S, Pitt A (1982) Effect of verapamil on the electrophysiologic properties of the accessory pathway in patients with the Wolff-Parkinson-White syndrome. Am J Cardiol 50: 1323-1330
18. Michel B, Goy JJ, Kappenberger L (1989) Syndrome de Wolff-Parkinson-White et verapamil: à propos d'un cas de fibrillation auricolaire. Schweiz Med Wochenschr 13/119 (19): 630-634
19. Vitale P, De Stefano R, Auricchio A (1986) Possibile pericolosità dell'amiodarone per via endovenosa rapida nel corso di tachicardia da rientro in soggetti con Wolff-Parkinson-White. G Ital Cardiol 16: 969-974
20. Neuss H, Buss J, Schlepper M, Berthold R, Mitrovic V, Kramer A, Musial WJ (1983) Effects of flecainide on electrophysiological properties of accessory pathways in the Wolff-Parkinson-White syndrome. Eur Heart J 4: 347-353
21. Hellestrand KJ, Nathan AW, Bexton RS, Camm AJ (1984) Electrophysiologic effects of flectainide acetate on sinus node function anomalous atrioventricular connections and pacemaker threshold. Am J Cardiol 53 [Suppl B]: 30-38
22. Breithardt G, Borggrefe M, Wiebringhaus E, Seipel L (1984) Effect of propafenone in the Wolff-Parkinson-White syndrome: electrophysiological findings and long-term follow-up. Am J Cardiol 54: 29D-39D
23. Kim SS, Lal R, Ruffy R (1986) Treatment of paroxysmal supraventricular tachycardia with flecainide acetate. Am J Cardiol 58: 80-85
24. Shen EN, Keung E, Huycke E, Dohrmann ML, Nguyenn N, Morady F, Sung RJ (1986) Intravenous propafenone for termination of reentrant supraventricular tachycardia. A placebo-controlled, randomized, double-blind, crossover study. Ann Intern Med 105: 655-659
25. Hammil SC, McLaran CJ, Wood DL, Osborne MJ, Gersh BJ, Holmes DR (1987) Double blind study of intravenous propafenone for paroxysmal supraventricular reentrant tachycardia. J Am Coll Cardiol 9: 1364-1368
26. Ludmer PL, McCowan NE, Antman EM, Friedman PL (1987) Efficacy of propafenone in Wolff-Parkinson-White syndrome: electrophysiologic findings and long-term follow-up. J Am Coll Cardiol 9: 1357-1363
27. Dubuc M, Kus T, Campa MA, Lambert C, Rosengarten M, Shenasa M (1989) Electrophysiologic effects of intravenous propafenone in Wolff-Parkinson-White syndrome. Am Heart J 117: 370-376
28. Kappenberger LJ, Fromer MA, Shenasa M, Gloor HO (1985) Evaluation of flecainide acetate in rapid atrial fibrillation complicating Wolff-Parkinson-White syndrome. Clin Cardiol 8: 321-326
29. Manolis AS, Salen DN, Estes NAm (1989) Electrophysiologic effects, efficacy and tolerance of class 1C antiarrhythmic agents in Wolff-Parkinson-White syndrome. Am J Cardiol 63: 746-750
30. Boahene KA, Klein GJ, Yee R, Sharma AD, Fujimura O (1990) Termination of acute atrial fibrillation in the Wolff-Parkinson-White syndrome by procainamide and propafenone: importance of atrial fibrillatory cycle length. J Am Coll Cardiol 16: 1408-1414
31. Wellens HJ, Bar FW, Dassen WRM, Brugada P, Vanagt EG, Farre J (1980) Effect of drugs in the Wolff-Parkinson-White syndrome. Am J Cardiol 46: 665-669
32. Asplund K, Beerman B, Bergfeld L, Blomstrom P, Blomstrom Lundqvist C, Boman K, Britton M, Dale J, Edvarsson N, Forfang K, Godtfredsen J, Gustafsson C, Juul-Moller S, Norrving B, Olsson SB, Rehnqvist N, Ronvall J (1993) Treatment of atrial fibrillation. Eur Heart J 14: 1427-1433
33. Kerr CR, Prystowsky EN, Smith WM, Cook L, Gallagher JJ (1982) Electrophysiologic effects of disopyramide-phosphate in patients with Wolff-Parkinson-White syndrome. Circulation 65: 869-878
34. Mitchell LB, Wyse DC, Duff HJ (1987) Electropharmacology of sotalol in patients with Wolff-Parkinson-White syndrome. Circulation 76: 810-818
35. Kunze KP, Schluter M, Kulk KH (1987) Sotalol in patients with Wolff-Parkinson-White syndrome. Circulation 75: 1050-1057
36. Vik-Mo H, Ohm O-J, Lund-Johansen I (1982) Electrophysiologic effects of flecainide acetate in patients with sinus nodal dysfunction. Am J Cardiol 50: 1090-1094

37. Reifel JA, Estes NAM, Waldo AL, Pristowsky EN, Di Bianco R (1994) A consensus report on antiarrhythmic drugs use. Clin Cardiol 17: 103-116
38. Alboni P, Filippi L, Pirani R, Preziosi S, Paparella N (1984) Effetti elettrofisiologici del propafenone in pazienti con disfunzione del nodo del seno. G Ital Cardiol 14: 297-303
39. Ogunkelu JB, Damato AN, Akhtar M, Reddy CP, Caracta AR, Lau SH (1976) Electrophysiologic effects of procainamide in subtherapeutic to therapeutic doses on human atrioventricular conduction system. Am J Cardiol 37: 724-731
40. Hellenstrand KJ, Bexton RS, Nathan AW, Spurrel RA, Camm AJ (1982) Acute electrophysiological effects of flecainide acetate on cardiac conduction and refractoriness in man. Br Heart J 48: 140-148
41. Pristowsky EN, Heger JJ, Chilson DA, Miles WM, Hubbard J, Zipes DP (1984) Antiarrhythmic and electrophysiologic effects of oral propafenone. Am J Cardiol 54: 26D-28D
42. Finerman WB Jr, Peter TB, Mandel WJ (1980) Studies on the electrophysiologic effects of amiodarone in man. Circulation 62 [Suppl III]: 152
43. Schwartz A, Shen E, Morady F, Gillespie K, Scheinman M, Chatterjee K (1983) Hemodynamic effects of intravenous amiodarone in patients with depressed left ventricular function and recurrent ventricular tachycardia. Am Heart J 106: 848-852
44. Leach AJ, Brown JE, Armstrong PW (1980) Cardiac depression by intravenous disopyramide in patients with left ventricular dysfunction. Am J Med 68: 839-844
45. Burton JR, Mathew MT, Armstrong PW (1976) Comparative effects of lidocaine and procainamide on acutely impaired hemodynamics. Am J Med 61: 215-220
46. Legrand V, Vandormael M, Collgnon P, Kulbertus HE (1983) Hemodynamic effects of a new antiarrhythmic agent, flecainide (R-818) in coronary heart disease. Am J Cardiol 51: 422-426
47. Podrid PJ, Cytryn R, Lown B (1984) Propafenone: non-invasive evaluation of efficacy. Am J Cardiol 54: 53D-59D
48. Pentecost BI (1983) Myocardial infarction. In: Weatherall DJ, Ledingham JGG, Warrel DA (eds) Oxford Textbook of Medicine. Oxford University Press, Oxford, pp 174-188
49. Cowan JC, Gardiner P, Reid DS, Newell DJ, Campbell RWF (1986) A comparison of amiodarone and digoxin in the treatment of atrial fibrillation complicating suspected acute myocardial infarction. J Cardiovasc Pharmacol 8: 252-256
50. Levi F, Proto C (1972) Combined treatment of atrial fibrillation with quinidine and beta-blockers. Br Heart J 34: 911-914

Prophylaxis of Atrial Fibrillation: What are the Benefits and Risks of the Different Antiarrhythmic Drugs?

M. Chimienti[1] and S. Barbieri[2]

[1]Sezione di Cardiologia, Istituto di Medicina Interna,
Università di Pavia, Pavia, Italy
[2]Centro Cardiovascolare "E. Malan", Ospedale Universitario di S. Donato,
S. Donato Milanese, Italy

Introduction

The role of antiarrhythmic drugs in the prevention of chronic recurrences or paroxysmal episodes of atrial fibrillation (AF) has recently come into question after some observations showing the risks that treated patients may face in terms of morbidity or mortality (1-5). On the other hand, AF may be strongly symptomatic, particularly in the paroxysmal form, and is not without risks in terms of complications secondary to thromboembolism (6-8) and left ventricular dysfunction (9-11). For these reasons the decision to treat a patient is not easy and the risks/benefits balance of such a therapeutic intervention should first always be considered.

Risks of Treatment

The main risk in administering an antiarrhythmic agent to a patient is the so-called proarrhythmic effect: any drug given to reduce, suppress, or prevent an arrhythmia may, under particular and often unforeseeable circumstances, increase the incidence or severity of the arrhythmia itself and even favor the occurrence of new and possibly life-threatening arrhythmias. The proarrhythmic effect has been reported with different incidence for any antiarrhythmic agent and is often increased by the presence of structural heart disease (myocardial infarction, valvular heart disease, cardiomyopathy, etc.), cardiac failure, acute ischemia, and electrolyte imbalance (12-15).

A second point to be taken into account before starting an antiarrhythmic treatment is the potential for hemodynamic worsening: almost all antiarrhythmic drugs have a negative inotropic effect which may cause or contribute to the aggravation of a cardiac failure (16).

Finally, possible interactions with the metabolism of other drugs (for instance, quinidine and digitalis, amiodarone and digitalis, amiodarone and flecainide, etc.) may cause unpredictable and potentially dangerous changes in plasma concentrations (16).

Benefits of Treatment

The main benefits of preventing recurrences of AF derive from the suppression of related symptoms (palpitations, dyspnea, dizziness, syncope, and angina). Most importantly, suppression of AF may also eliminate the risk of thromboembolism as well as the need for anticoagulant therapy, with its potential hemorrhagic complications. Moreover, the presence of sinus rhythm has strong hemodynamic consequences, due both to the regulating of rhythm at rest and on effort and maintaining of atrial contribution to the stroke volume, which is particularly important in the presence of heart disease (17-21).

Studies of Antiarrhythmic Agents

Many drugs of different classes have been demonstrated to be effective in preventing recurrences of both chronic AF after cardioversion and paroxysmal attacks of AF (16-21). Any drug has been more or less extensively studied with different protocols, most of which compare an active drug with a corresponding placebo. Unfortunately, enormous differences are reported in the selection of patients, who may not only have clinically different symptom characteristics, but also different physiologic and/or anatomical substrates. Drugs are often given at different dosages (e.g., at the *maximum tolerated* dose or at the *minimum effective* dose); the endpoints and the effectiveness criteria (e.g., subjective symptoms, ECG, documentation of recurrences, total or partial suppression of arrhythmias, etc.) are not always the same; safety criteria (e.g., relationship of adverse medical experiences to study drug) are difficult to ascertain; the incidence of patients with atrial flutter is different, and this arrhythmia is notoriously less responsive to drugs. Finally, there are few protocols directly comparing two or more drugs and the dosages utilized are often criticizable. For all these reasons, the analysis of the risk/benefit ratio of antiarrhythmic treatment in the prevention of AF appears extremely difficult. We will try to examine this ratio for each of the most commonly given antiarrhythmic agents for the prevention of paroxysmal and chronic AF.

Quinidine

Quinidine is the archetype of class IA antiarrhyhmic agents and is the oldest drug still available for the prevention of AF. For many years now it has been the most common treatment of AF all over the world and still has a predominant role, at least in the United States.

Quinidine exerts a direct depressant effect on all cardiac tissues and slows impulse conduction (22). It also possesses mild anticholinergic activity, which may be important in enhancing conduction through the atrioventricular (AV) node; if the latter exceeds the direct depressant effect of the drug on AV conduction the final result may be sometimes a paradoxical acceleration of the ventricular response. Moreover, it is not infrequent that quinidine, given during AF, may slow the atrial rate and result in organization of the fibrillatory impulses, changing the latter into flutter waves; also in this situation a paradoxical ventricular acceleration may occur. To prevent this, it is standard clinical practice to administer a drug capable of reducing AV conduction (digitalis, ß-blockers, or calcium antagonists) before giving quinidine.

The efficacy of quinidine salts in preventing recurrences of both chronic and paroxysmal AF has been widely proven in many clinical trials (23-26). In a recently published meta-analysis of six controlled trials in which a total of 373 patients received quinidine treatment and 354 received placebo or no therapy, Coplen et al. (2) found that quinidine-treated patients were about twice as likely to remain in sinus rhythm as the untreated patients 1 year after cardioversion; however, there were six deaths (three of which were sudden) of cardiovascular causes in the quinidine group as compared with two in the control group. Even if the small number of patients does not permit any clinically significant comparison, the risk that quinidine may contribute to improve symptoms but not survival in patients with AF (if not to favor cardiovascular death) should always be taken into account.

The beneficial effects of quinidine are unfortunately counterbalanced by a high incidence of adverse effects, particularly QT prolongation, which may favor the appearance of ventricular arrhythmias such as torsade de pointes (27-31). That is why quinidine treatment should always be started with the patient in the hospital under careful ECG monitoring.

In our experience, dihydroquinidine (which is neither a quinidine salt, nor a quinidine metabolite, but simply a quinidine derivative usually contaminating the quinidine preparations) offers some advantages as compared to quinidine. The drug, commercially available in most European countries but not in the United States, has demonstrated a greater effectiveness than quinidine salts in both ventricular and supraventricular tachyarrhythmias at lower dosages, with more stable plasma concentrations and a low incidence of side effects (32,33). Dihydroquinidine has been used clinically for many years, especially in the pharmacologic con-

version of chronic AF, but it is still utilized today in many cardiological institutions as a first-choice drug also in the prevention of AF recurrences.

Disopyramide

Disopyramide, a class IA antiarrhythmic drug, exerts electrophysiologic activity similar to that of quinidine (34); its use has thus been suggested to maintain sinus rhythm after cardioversion. Hartel et al. (35) compared the efficacy of this drug to placebo in a randomized, double-blind study involving 38 patients with chronic AF. Three months after cardioversion, 72% of the patients given disopyramide remained in sinus rhythm, as compared to 30% of patients given placebo ($p<0.05$). Karlson et al. (36) studied 90 patients randomized to disopyramide or placebo after cardioversion for AF. After 1 year of treatment, sinus rhythm was present in 54% of the patients on disopyramide and 30% of those on placebo ($p<0.01$).

Unfortunately, the high incidence of side effects observed during disopyramide treatment (particularly of the anticholinergic type, including urinary retention, dry eyes and mouth, constipation, and visual disturbances) reduces the possibility of its safe and widespread use (37). A sizeable negative inotropic action also has to be taken into account before making any therapeutic decision for disopyramide (38).

Flecainide

Flecainide, a class IC agent, exerts substantial depressive activity on impulse conduction in all myocardial tissues. This strong effect on atrial tissues is the mechanism by which the drug prevents recurrences of AF, while the slow conduction through the AV node permits some reduction of ventricular response rate during AF (39).

The efficacy of this drug in preventing AF recurrences has been demonstrated in a number of clinical trials (40-46). Van Gelder et al. (40) studied the efficacy and safety of flecainide in the maintenance of sinus rhythm after electrical cardioversion for chronic AF or atrial flutter. Eighty-one patients were randomized to receive flecainide (at an average dose of 199 mg daily) or no treatment. After 1, 3, 6, and 12 months 69%, 64%, 58%, and 49% in the group of patients treated with flecainide maintained sinus rhythm, versus 54%, 49%, 49%, and 36% in the untreated group. Multiple regression analysis showed that NYHA class for exercise tolerance and flecainide treatment were the only significant predicting factors, while left atrial size and AF duration had no influence in increasing the arrhythmia-free interval. Adverse cardiac events occurred in 9% of a total of 58 patients treated with flecainide. Recently, Anderson and the Flecainide Supraventricular Tachycardia Study Group (41) reported the results of a multicenter, double-blind, crossover study of flecainide and placebo in 64 patients with frequent (at least two episodes in a month) symptomatic recurrences of paroxysmal AF. The efficacy of the drug was assessed by suppression of symptoms as well as by the use of transtelephonic ECG monitoring. The flecainide dosage was 200 to 400 mg/day and was based on the presence of side effects and patient tolerance. During the trial the period of time to the first recurrence of AF lengthened from a median of 3 days on placebo to 14.5 days on flecainide ($p<0.001$). Treatment with flecainide also significantly increased the average time interval between attacks of AF from a median of 6.2 days (on placebo) to 27 days ($p<0.001$) and increased the percentage of patients who remained free of arrhythmias during the follow-up period (from 9% on placebo to 31% on flecainide). Adverse cardiac events occurred in 11% of patients treated with flecainide. Pietersen and the Danish-Norwegian Flecainide Multicenter Study Group (42) reported the efficacy of flecainide in 43 patients with paroxysmal AF and atrial flutter using a randomized, double-blind, crossover protocol. Patients were given either placebo or flecainide 150 mg twice daily for consecutive periods of 3 months. If intolerable symptoms developed, the protocol allowed patients to cross over between treatments before the end of the first 3-month period. Complete suppression with flecainide was seen in 35% of the patients treated for 1 week with both regimens, in 46% treated for 1 month, and in 50% completing all 3 months. Leclercq et al. (43) studied the effects of flecainide (100 mg twice daily) in 52 patients with frequent symptomatic AF attacks who were resistant or intolerant to quinidine. Vagally induced paroxysmal AF was clinically documented in 35 patients. Amiodarone, previously used and ineffective, was combined with flecainide in 33 patients. Complete disappearance of paroxysmal AF was observed in 73% of patients after a follow-up of 1-5.8 years. Extracardiac side effects necessitated withdrawal in only three cases. Two patients, with previously documented atrial flutter, experienced presyncopal episodes of atrial flutter with a 1:1 AV conduction and a wide QRS complex. No death occurred during the observation period. Recently Hohnloser and Zabel (44) analyzed the efficacy and safety data for flecainide in the treatment of supraventricular arrhythmias from 60 original articles. In spite of the different definitions of efficacy criteria, they were able to assess a long-term efficacy of the drug in 49% of the patients, with similar efficacy rates in 11 comparative trials and in 16 uncontrolled studies.

While the efficacy of flecainide in the prevention of AF has been widely proven, the safety of the drug was put up for debate again after the report of the CAST data (3), showing a nearly threefold increase in mortality in patients treated with antiarrhythmic agents for asymptomatic ventricular arrhythmias and recent myocardial infarction compared to placebo-treated patients. In order to reassess long-term safety of this drug in a large group of patients, a multicenter study was recently carried out in Italy by the Flecainide and Propafenone Italian Study (FAPIS) Group (45-46). Two-hundred patients with paroxysmal AF and no history of heart disease were enrolled in a randomized, open label, parallel group trial comparing the relative safety of flecainide to propafenone. The initial daily doses were 200 mg flecainide or 450 mg propafenone; dose escalations up to a maximum of 300 mg flecainide or 900 mg propafenone daily were permitted after at least two attacks of AF. The patients were assessed for safety and drug tolerance at designated intervals over a 12-month period, unless discontinued because of adverse events or inadequate response. Ten patients on flecainide reported 14 cardiac adverse events; four of them discontinued treatment. Seven patients receiving propafenone reported eight cardiac adverse experiences; five of them discontinued treatment. Three proarrhythmic events occurred: one patient on propafenone developed ventricular tachycardia and two patients on flecainide experienced AF with rapid ventricular response. An intention-to-treat analysis showed that the probability of safe and effective treatment after 12 months was 77% for flecainide-treated patients and 75% for propafenone-treated patients. No drug-related death occurred during the 1-year follow-up. Thus, the study demonstrated an acceptable risk/benefit profile in patients with paroxysmal AF and no evidence of clinically significant heart disease who were treated with flecainide and propafenone for 12 months.

Propafenone

Propafenone, a class IC antiarrhythmic agent, has effects on cardiac tissues similar to those produced by flecainide (47). By means of its electrophysiologic activity decreasing impulse conduction through the atrial tissue, propafenone is effective in preventing AF. Moreover, the drug may be useful in reducing the ventricular response to AF as a result of its action on the AV node. The drug has a negative inotropic effect, which is dose dependent but may occur even when low doses are administered (48).

In addition to the above-mentioned multicenter trial by the FAPIS Group (45-46), many other studies have been published showing efficacy and safety of propafenone in patients with paroxysmal or chronic AF. Antman et al. (49) studied the efficacy of long-term oral propafenone (mean total dose: 795 mg daily) for preventing frequent paroxysmal episodes of symptomatic AF or atrial flutter, or both, in 60 patients. After a 1-month follow-up, 54% of patients were free of recurrent AF, after 3 months 44% were without arrhythmia, and at 6 months 40% of patients were free of recurrent episodes of AF. Drug-related adverse reactions were reported in 22% of patients and were severe enough to require early discontinuation of the drug in 5% of the patients. Connolly and Hoffert (50) studied the efficacy of propafenone for suppression of recurrent paroxysmal symptomatic AF in 18 patients by means of a cross-over protocol: the patients were subsequently randomized to alternate between propafenone and placebo every month for 4 months. The mean dose of propafenone at the end of the initial dose-ranging, open label phase, was 644 mg/day. During the cross-over study the percentage of days with an attack of AF was significantly reduced from 51% on placebo to 27% on propafenone. The rate of early cross-over or withdrawal from the study was 14% with propafenone and 45% with placebo. There were 29 minor side effects reported with the active drug and 11 with placebo. Reimold et al. (51) compared the efficacy of propafenone (at a mean maintenance dose of 737 mg/day) and sotalol (mean dose of 335 mg/day) in preventing recurrences of chronic (53 patients) or paroxysmal (43 patients) AF. For patients randomized to propafenone, 46%, 41%, and 30% remained in sinus rhythm at 3, 6, and 12 months, respectively; a similar proportion of patients treated with sotalol remained in sinus rhythm at follow-up (49%, 46%, and 37% at 3, 6, and 12 months, respectively); the difference between the two treatments was not significant. Proarrhythmic effects, defined as the new onset of sustained ventricular tachycardia, ventricular fibrillation, or torsades de pointes, occurred in one patient treated with propafenone and in three treated with sotalol; new, nonsustained ventricular tachycardia also occurred in one patient receiving propafenone.

Amiodarone

Amiodarone is the prototype of class III antiarrhythmic agents. Its main electrophysiologic action consists in a prolongation of action potential duration. It also demonstrates some sodium channel blocking activity, as well as mild noncompetitive ß-blocking and calcium channel-blocking activity (52). Moreover, because the drug contains substantial amounts of iodine, it has been postulated that some of the drug antiarrhythmic activity may be due to its interaction with thyroxine metabolism. Amiodarone has been widely used for AF, particularly in European countries (it is not yet approved for this indication in the United States). A major limitation to the use of amiodarone is the high incidence of toxicity, which may affect many organs (hypo- or hyperthyroidism, pulmonary fibrosis, gastrointestinal and neurological complaints, photodermatitis, corneal microdeposits, etc.). Adverse cardiac events are not infrequent and include sinus bradycardia, atrioventricular block, and QT prolongation, even if torsades de pointes are very rare (53).

Most of the clinical studies carried out with amiodarone have been uncontrolled (54-57), owing to its self-evident side effects and its peculiar pharmacokinetics, which make a blind comparison with placebo or other drugs particularly difficult. Graboys et al. (54) reported their experience in 95 patients with chronic or paroxysmal AF of long duration treated with amiodarone. Complete prevention of AF was achieved in 78% of the patients, whereas in an additional 6% there was a partial effect, defined as a reduction in the frequency or duration of the AF episodes. Gold et al. (55) treated 68 patients with paroxysmal or chronic AF for a mean period of 21 months. They found that treatment at a maintenance dose of 200 to 400 mg/day was effective in preventing recurrent AF in 79% of the patients; the presence of chronic AF for longer than 1 year was the only predictor of drug failure. However, 35% of the patients had side effects, requiring discontinuation of the drug in 10%. Brodsky et al. (56) demonstrated the efficacy of the drug in 28 patients with a dilated left atrium (>45 mm). Amiodarone treatment was considered successful in ten patients who remained in sinus rhythm 1 year after cardioversion and partially successful in an additional 11 patients who maintained sinus rhythm for at least 6 months. The outcome of treatment was related to left atrium dimension, as the drug was completely effective in nine of 18 patients with a left atrium size < 60 mm, but in only one of ten with a left atrium size > 60 mm. More recently, Gosselink et al. (57) studied the efficacy and safety of low-dose amiodarone (mean daily maintenance dose of 204 mg) in 80 patients with chronic AF; the mean follow-up was 20.7 months. The cumulative percentages of patients remaining in sinus rhythm during 1, 2, and 3 years after cardioversion were 61%, 56%, and 53%, respectively. Serious side effects occurred in 4% of the patients, whereas minor side effects were observed in 13% of the patients.

It should be pointed out that the reduction and regularization of ventricular rate observed during AF in patients treated with amiodarone make it difficult to judge the real suppression of AF recurrences in the absence of any objective documentation of the maintenance of sinus rhythm; the use of random ECG recording obtained with a transtelephonic system has partially contributed to obviate this bias (58). For this reason the success rates observed during amiodarone treatment are probably overestimated, particularly in patients with paroxysmal AF.

Sotalol

Sotalol exerts both class II ß-blocking activity as well as class III properties; it is available as a racemic mixture of its l- and d- stereoisomers: the l-isomer is primarily responsible for the ß-blocking activity while the d-isomer has the class-III properties (59).

Recently, Juul-Moller et al. (60) reported on a multicenter study comparing sotalol (98 patients) with quinidine (85 patients) for maintenance of sinus rhythm after cardioversion of chronic AF. After 6 months, 52% of the patients in the sotalol group and 48% of the patients in the quinidine group remained in sinus rhythm. It is noteworthy that, thanks to sotalol ß-blocking activity, the heart rate after relapsing into AF was much lower in the patients treated with sotalol (78 beats/min) than in the patients treated with quinidine (109 beats/min, $p<0.001$). In terms of safety, more patients were withdrawn from quinidine than from sotalol treatment (26% versus 11%, $p<0.05$) and sotalol was generally better tolerated than quinidine. Twenty-eight percent of the patients on sotalol and 50% of the patients on quinidine reported side effects ($p<0.01$). Unfortunately, one of the problems of sotalol treatment in patients with ventricular arrhythmias is the potential for QT prolongation and ventricular arrhythmia aggravation, which may lead to the occurrence of torsades de pointes (61). The actual incidence of this life-threatening side effect in a large population affected by AF, with or without organic heart disease, has not yet been established.

Clinical Considerations

The ideal antiarrhythmic drug for the prevention of recurrences of both chronic AF after cardioversion and paroxysmal AF is unfortunately not yet available. The characteristics of this ideal drug are: good efficacy, no proarrhythmic effect, no negative hemodynamic activity, good tolerance, and favorable pharmacokinetic profile.

So far, the available drugs demonstrate many disadvantages. On the other hand, the presence of AF has many clinical consequences, not only due to troublesome subjective symptoms, but also to an increased risk of thromboembolism and a potential aggravation of heart failure.

From the experiences of all the published clinical trials the clinician has to learn the importance of keeping the *patient* and not the *arrhythmia* in the center of his clinical judgment: the actual clinical conditions, in terms of heart disease, ischemia, hypertrophy, electrolyte imbalance, concomitant therapy, etc., are far more important in the prognosis of the arrhythmia than the arrhythmia itself. In other words, the decision to treat a patient must take all these variables into consideration, whereas the choice of the drug is usually less important.

References

1. IMPACT Research Group (1984) International mexiletine and placebo antiarrhythmic coronary trial: I. Report on arrhythmia and other findings. J Am Coll Cardiol 4:1148-1163
2. Coplen SE, Antman EM, Berlin JA et al (1990) Efficacy and safety of quinidine therapy for maintenance of sinus rhythm after cardioversion: a meta-analysis of randomized control trials. Circulation 82:1106-1116
3. Echt DS, Liebson PR, Mitchell LB et al (1991) Mortality and morbidity in patients receiving encainide, flecainide, or placebo: the Cardiac Arrhythmia Suppression Trial. N Engl J Med 324:781-788
4. The Cardiac Arrhythmia Suppression Trial II Investigators (1991) Effect of the antiarrhythmic agent moricizine on survival after myocardial infarction. N Engl J Med 327:227-233
5. Flaker GC, Blackshear JL, McBride R (1992) Antiarrhythmic drug therapy and cardiac mortality in atrial fibrillation. J Am Coll Cardiol 20:527-532
6. Stroke Prevention in Atrial Fibrillation Investigators (1991) Stroke prevention in atrial fibrillation study: final results. Circulation 84:527-539
7. Wolf PA, Abbott R, Kannel W (1991) Atrial fibrillation as an independent risk factor for stroke: the Framingham study. Stroke 22:938-988
8. Cheng TO (1994) Atrial fibrillation, stroke, and antithrombotic treatment. Am Heart J 127:961-968
9. Grogan M, Smith HC, Gersh BJ, Wood DL (1992) Left ventricular dysfunction due to atrial fibrillation in patients initially believed to have idiopathic dilated cardiomyopathy. Am J Cardiol 69:1570-1573
10. Shite J, Yokoyama M (1993) Heterogeneity and time course of improvement in cardiac function after conversion of chronic atrial fibrillation: assessment of serial echocardiographic indices. Br Heart J 70:154-159
11. Van Gelder IC, Crijns HJGM, Blanksman PK et al (1993) Time course of hemodynamic changes and improvement of exercise tolerance after cardioversion of chronic atrial fibrillation unassociated with cardiac valve disease. Am J Cardiol 72:560-566
12. Velebit V, Podrid P, Lown B et al (1982) Aggravation and provocation of ventricular arrhythmias by antiarrhythmic drugs. Circulation 65:886-894
13. Ruskin JN, McGovern B, Garan H et al (1983) Antiarrhythmic drugs: a possible cause of out-of-hospital cardiac arrest. N Engl J Med 309:1302-1306
14. Morganroth J (1987) Risk factors for the development of proarrhythmic events. Am J Cardiol 59:32E-37E
15. Kerin NZ, Somberg J (1994) Proarrhythmia: definition, risk factors, causes, treatment, and controversies. Am Heart J 128:575-585
16. Podrid PJ (1992) Oral antiarrhythmic drugs used for atrial fibrillation: clinical pharmacology. In: Falk RH, Podrid PJ (eds) Atrial fibrillation: mechanisms and management. Raven, New York, pp 197-231
17. Feld GK (1990) Atrial fibrillation: is there a safe and highly effective pharmacological treatment? Circulation 82:2248-2250
18. Pritchett ELC (1992) Management of atrial fibrillation. N Engl J Med 326:1264-1271
19. Mandel WJ (1994) Should every patient with atrial fibrillation have the rhythm converted to sinus rhythm? Clin Cardiol 17:II 16-II 20
20. Roden DM (1994) Risks and benefits of antiarrhythmic therapy. N Engl J Med 331:785-791
21. Crijns HJGM, Van Gelder IC, Lie KI (1994) Benefits and risks of antiarrhythmic drug therapy after DC electrical cardioversion of atrial fibrillation or flutter. Eur Heart J 15 [Suppl A]:17-21
22. Weld FM, Coromilas J, Rottman JN, Bigger JT (1982) Mechanism of quinidine induced depression of maximum upstroke velocity in ovine cardiac Purkinje fibers. Circ Res 50:369-376
23. Hartel G, Vouhija A, Konttinen A et al (1970) Value of quinidine in maintenance of sinus rhythm after electric conversion of atrial fibrillation. Br Heart J 32:57-60
24. Sodermark T, Jonsson B, Olsson A et al (1975) Effect of quinidine on maintaining sinus rhythm after conversion of atrial fibrillation or flutter: a multicentre study from Stockholm. Br Heart J 37:486-492
25. Normand JP, Legendre M, Kahn JC et al (1976) Comparative efficacy of short-acting and long-acting quinidine for maintenance of sinus rhythm after electrical conversion of atrial fibrillation. Br Heart J 38:381-386
26. Boissel JP, Wolf E, Gillet J et al (1981) Controlled trial of a long-acting quinidine for maintenance of sinus rhythm after conversion of sustained atrial fibrillation. Eur Heart J 2:49-55
27. Selzer A, Wray HW (1964) Quinidine syncope: paroxysmal ventricular fibrillation occurring during treatment of chronic atrial arrhythmias. Circulation 30:17-26
28. Jenzer HR, Hagemeijer F (1976) Quinidine syncope: torsade de pointes with low quinidine plasma concentrations. Eur J Cardiol 4:447-451
29. Bauman JL, Bauerfeind RA, Hoff JV et al (1984) Torsade de pointes due to quinidine: observations in 31 patients. Am Heart J 107:425-430
30. Morganroth J, Horowitz LN (1985) Incidence of proarrhythmic effects from quinidine in the outpatient treatment of benign or potentially lethal ventricular arrhythmias. Am J Cardiol 56:585-587
31. Roden DM, Woosley RL, Primm RK (1986) Incidence and clinical features of the quinidine-associated long QT syndrome: implications for patient care. Am Heart J 111.1088-1093
32. Chimienti M, Panciroli C, Salerno JA et al (1984) Dihydroquinidine versus disopyramide: efficacy in patients with chronic stable ventricular ectopy. Clin Cardiol 7:538-546
33. Chimienti M, Regazzi BM, La Rovere MT et al (1988) Comparison of the effectiveness of dihydroquinidine and quinidine on ventricular ectopy after acute and chronic administration. Cardiovasc Drugs Ther 2:679-686
34. Kus T, Sasyniuk BI (1975) Electrophysiologic actions of disopyramide phosphate on canine ventricular muscle and Purkinje fibers. Cir Res 37:844-854
35. Hartel G, Louhija A, Konttinen A (1974) Disopyramide in the prevention of recurrence atrial fibrillation after electroversion. Clin Pharmacol Ther 15:551-555
36. Karlson BW, Torstensson I, Abjorn C et al (1988) Disopyramide in the maintenance of sinus rhythm after electroconversion of atrial fibrillation. A placebo-controlled one-year follow-up study. Eur Heart J 9:284-290
37. Wald RW, Waxman MB, Colman JM (1981) Torsade de pointes ventricular tachycardia: a complication of disopyramide shared with quinidine. J Electrocardiol 14:301-307
38. Podrid PJ, Schoeneberger A, Lown B (1980) Congestive heart failure caused by oral disopyramide. N Engl J Med 302:614-620
39. Hodess AB, Follansbee WP, Spear JF, Moore EM (1979) Electrophysiologic effects of a new antiarrhythmic drug, flecainide, on the intact canine heart. J Cardiovasc Pharmacol 1:427-439

40. Van Gelder IC, Crijns HJGM, Van Gilst WH et al (1989) Efficacy and safety of flecainide acetate in the maintenance of sinus rhythm after electrical conversion of chronic atrial fibrillation or atrial flutter. Am J Cardiol 64:1317-1321

41. Anderson JL, Gilbert EM, Alpert BL et al (1989) Prevention of symptomatic recurrences of paroxysmal atrial fibrillation in patients initially tolerating antiarrhythmic therapy: a multicenter, double-blind, crossover study of flecainide and placebo with transtelephonic monitoring. Circulation 80:1557-1569

42. Pietersen AH, Hellemann H, for the Danish-Norwegian Flecainide Multicenter Study Group (1991) Usefulness of flecainide for prevention of paroxysmal atrial fibrillation and flutter. Am J Cardiol 67:713-717

43. Leclercq JF, Chouty F, Denjoy I et al (1992) Flecainide in quinidine-resistant atrial fibrillation. Am J Cardiol 70:62A-65A

44. Hohnloser SH, Zabel M (1992) Short- and long-term efficacy and safety of flecainide acetate for supraventricular arrhythmias. Am J Cardiol 70:3A-10A

45. Chimienti M, Cullen MT, Casadei G (1995) Safety of long-term flecainide and propafenone in the management of patients with symptomatic paroxysmal atrial fibrillation: report from the Flecainide and Propafenone Italian Study (FAPIS) investigators. Am J Cardiol (in press)

46. Chimienti M, Cullen MT, Casadei G (1995) Safety of flecainide versus propafenone for the long-term management of symptomatic paroxysmal supraventricular tachyarrhythmias. Eur Heart J (in press)

47. Kohlhardt M (1984) Block of sodium currents by antiarrhythmic agents: analysis of the electrophysiologic effects of propafenone in heart muscle. Am J Cardiol 54:13D-19D

48. Baker BJ, Dinh H, Kroskey D et al (1984) Effect of propafenone on left ventricular ejection fraction. Am J Cardiol 54:20D-22D

49. Antman EM, Beamer AD, Cantillon CO et al (1988) Long-term oral propafenone therapy for suppression of refractory symptomatic atrial fibrillation and atrial flutter. J Am Coll Cardiol 12:1005-1011

50. Connolly SJ, Hoffert DL (1989) Usefulness of propafenone for recurrent paroxysmal atrial fibrillation. Am J Cardiol 63:817-819

51. Reimold SC, Cantillon CO, Friedman PL, Antman EM (1993) Propafenone versus sotalol for suppression of recurrent symptomatic atrial fibrillation. Am J Cardiol 71:558-563

52. Mason JW (1987) Drug therapy: amiodarone. N Engl J Med 316:455-466

53. Sclarovsky S, Lewin RF, Krakoff O et al (1983) Amiodarone-induced polymorphous ventricular tachycardia. Am Heart J 105:6-12

54. Graboys TB, Podrid PJ, Lown B (1983) Efficacy of amiodarone for refractory supraventricular arrhythmias. Am Heart J 106:870-876

55. Gold RL, Haffajee CL, Charos G et al (1986) Amiodarone for refractory atrial fibrillation. Am J Cardiol 57:124-127

56. Brodsky MA, Allen BJ, Waler CJ et al (1987) Amiodarone for maintenance of sinus rhythm after conversion of atrial fibrillation in the setting of a dilated left atrium. Am J Cardiol 60:572-575

57. Gosselink ATM, Crijns HJGM, Van Gelder IC et al (1992) Low-dose amiodarone for maintenance of sinus rhythm after cardioversion of atrial fibrillation or flutter. JAMA 267:3289-3293

58. Bhandari AK, Anderson JL, Gilbert EM et al (1992) Correlation of symptoms with occurrence of paroxysmal supraventricular tachycardia or atrial fibrillation: a transtelephonic monitoring study. Am Heart J 124:381-386

59. Singh BN, Deedwania P, Nademanee K et al (1987) Sotalol: a review of its pharmacodynamic and pharmacokinetic properties and therapeutic use. Drugs 34:311-349

60. Juul-Moller S, Edvardsson N, Rehnqvist-Ahlberg (1990) Sotalol versus quinidine for the maintenance of sinus rhythm after direct current conversion of atrial fibrillation. Circulation 82:1932-1939

61. McKibbin JK, Pocock WA, Barlow JB et al (1984) Sotalol, hypokalemia, syncope and torsade de pointes. Br Heart J 51:157-162.

Atrial Fibrillation with a Slow Ventricular Response: Is Theophylline a Good Alternative to a Pacemaker?

N. Paparella, R. Pirani, and P. Alboni

Divisione di Cardiologia, Ospedale Civile, Cento (Fe), Italy

There is no agreement on the definition of atrial fibrillation (AF) with a slow ventricular response: the condition may be characterized as an AF with slow resting heart rate or as an AF with normal resting heart rate but with prolonged ventricular pauses. Symptoms such as asthenia, easy fatigue, and dyspnea may be attributable to low cardiac output due to a low heart rate, and cardiac pauses may be responsible for neurologic symptoms such as presyncope or syncope.

Our knowledge on the clinical and prognostic significance of AF with a slow ventricular response is very limited. In fact, we do not know whether the clinical course and the prognosis of patients with this bradyarrhythmia, in particular the incidence of sudden death, is similar to that of patients with AF and normal heart rate.

Recently, some light has been shed on the significance of ventricular pauses in patients with AF and normal heart rate:
1. Pauses lasting 3 s or more are frequent, being present in Holter recordings not only at night but also during the day in a high precentage of subjects (24%) (1).
2. The cardiac pauses do not correlate with the neurologic symptoms (2).
3. The prevalence of ventricular pauses longer than 2 s is similar in patients with and without syncope (3).

These data suggest that asymptomatic cardiac pauses in subjects with AF require no treatment. In contrast, in the presence of neurologic symptoms such as syncope or symptoms due to a low cardiac output, patients with AF and slow ventricular response or cardiac pauses must be treated.

It is obviously difficult to evaluate the real benefit of a treatment without knowing the natural history of the arrhythmia. The currently most commonly used therapy for symptomatic slow-response AF is permanent ventricular stimulation. Based on previously published data and on general knowledge, a few statements can be made about this kind of treatment:
– VVI pacemaker implantation shows the advantage of a regular cardiac rhythm, but it induces an abnormal ventricular activation and consequently an abnormal contraction, which leads to a more or less marked reduction in cardiac function. It is unknown whether, after pacemaker implantation in patients with AF, the advantage of the regularization of cardiac rhythm outweighs the disadvantage of the asynchronous contraction. In dogs, the latter seems to be dominant (4).
– A higher incidence of embolic complications in patients with AF treated with electrical treatment has been reported compared with untreated patients (5).
– A very high incidence of spontaneous remission of syncope (about 80%) in patients with chronic AF and cardiac pauses during Holter monitoring has recently been reported by Saxon et al. (3) Neurological symptoms disappeared as frequently in patients with as in those without a pacemaker.

These data seem to suggest that the cause of neurologic symptoms in subjects with AF is different from patient to patient, with frequent spontaneous remissions. The syncope may be the result of an abnormal neural reflex, as demonstrated in patients with sick sinus syndrome and syncope (6, 7). Moreover, pacemaker implantation seems not to play an important part in the treatment of syncope in patients with AF. Since electrical therapy does not appear to be an ideal treatment in patients with AF with a slow ventricular response, the question arises as to whether pharmacologic therapy is a good alternative. So far only theophylline has been systematically evaluated in long-term treatment.

Theophylline Treatment

There have been a number of reports substantiating a positive chronotropic and dromotropic effect of theophylline. Electrophysiological investigations showed that the drug enhances atrioventricular (AV) nodal conduction; it shortens both the A-H interval and the cycle length of the fastest 1:1 AV conduction (8, 9). These reports indicate that oral theophylline is a probable candidate for effective therapy of symptomatic AF with a slow ventricular response.

We selected 17 consecutive patients with chronic

AF and a slow ventricular response not induced by drugs. The criteria for inclusion were the following: mean resting heart of less than 60 beats/min constantly present for some days in several resting standard electrocardiograms (ECG) recorded during daytime hours; symptoms attributable to slow heart rate; absence of bundle branch block of advanced degree (QRS less than 120 ms). The exclusion criteria were the following: recent myocardial infarction, acute disease of any type, significant renal or hepatic disease, and congestive heart failure (New York Heart Association class IV).

The mean age was 78±9 years (range, 52-92 years); eight patients were men and nine women. Fourteen patients had organic heart disease: eight had hypertensive cardiovascular disease, four had ischemic heart disease, and two had mitral valve disease. Sixteen patients had New York Heart Association class I-II and one class III heart failure. Twelve patients complained of syncope or presyncope before hospitalization; four complained of marked asthenia and easy fatigue, and one complained of dyspnea after slight effort. Two patients were smokers at the time of entry into the study. None of the patients engaged in an exercise program. Electrolytes and thyroid hormones were within the normal range. None of the patients was taking cardioactive medication or drugs known to interfere significantly with the autonomic system or with adenosine metabolism (dipyridamole or diazepam). Diuretics, converting enzyme inhibitors, and nitrates were administered if the patient needed them; in this case, the control evaluation was done during administration of these drugs, which were then maintained during the follow-up period.

Each patient gave informed consent. The steady state evaluation was performed during hospitalization. Chest X-ray examination, echocardiogram, and standard laboratory tests for hematologic, renal, and hepatic function were performed. The resting heart rate was measured from a 10-s standard ECG strip after a 15-min rest period. Patients underwent a 24-h Holter monitoring for 2 consecutive days using a two-channel recorder. The data were analyzed to obtain the mean 24-h heart rate, the minimum 24-h heart rate, the maximum 24-h heart rate, the number of cardiac pauses longer than 2500 ms, the longest R-R interval, the number of wide QRS complexes and the number of episodes of two and three or more than three consecu-

tive wide QRS complexes. Oral theophylline therapy was then initiated at a dosage of 700 mg daily in two divided doses using a slow-release tablet. Five to 6 days later, standard ECG and Holter recording were repeated with the same methods. Both before and after theophylline treatment, the parameters were reported as the mean of two consecutive 24-h Holter recordings in order to reduce spontaneous variability and therefore to better evaluate the effects of the drug. The serum theophylline level was determined on the same day as the second 24-h Holter recording, 3 h after the intake of the morning dose.

The patients were then enrolled in a long-term study, and were seen at the outpatient clinic 1 month later and every 3 months thereafter. A clinical history, physical examination, resting ECG, 24-h Holter recording, and serum theophylline level were obtained during each visit. Dosage modifications were made as necessary to eliminate symptoms and cardiac pauses and to limit drug-related side effects. If any episode of syncope recurred or if side effects persisted despite dosage reduction, theophylline therapy was discontinued.

Statistical evaluations were performed using the Wilcoxon test. Results are given as mean ± standard deviation.

Results

Steady State

The effects of the drug on heart rate are reported in Table 1 and Fig. 1. The mean resting heart rate, the mean 24-h heart rate, the minimum 24-h heart rate, and the maximum 24-h heart rate increased significantly after drug administration by 42%, 31%, 34%, and 14% respectively. The percentage increases in daytime heart rate and sleep heart rate were very similar: +31.4% and +31.6%, respectively. The daily number of cardiac pauses longer than 2500 ms decreased after administration from 806 ± 2472 to 31 ± 118 ($p < 0.01$). The longest R-R interval decreased in all subjects from 3030 ± 771 to 2195 ± 468 ms ($p < 0.01$). The daily number of couplets and triplets did not change significantly (21 ± 78 versus 29 ± 108). In no patients were episodes of ventricular tachycardia observed either before of after drug administration.

Table 1. Effects of oral theophylline on the electrocardiographic parameters during long-term treatment

	Basal evaluation (n = 17)	Steady state (n = 17)	Theophylline treatment follow-up (months)			
			1 (n = 15)	12 (n = 10)	24 (n = 7)	36 (n = 5)
Daily theophylline dosage (mg)		700	485±80	421±163	429±170	480±164
Serum theophylline level (ng/ml)		13±4	10±3	8±4	9±4	10±3
Resting HR (beats/min)	47±5	67±10	66±12	64±11	62±8	61±3
Mean 24-h HR (beats/min)	51±6	67±12	65±14	60±8	60±6	60±3
Minim. 24-h HR (beats/min)	32±5	43±10	42±10	37±5	36±4	37±3
Maxim. 24-h HR (beats/min)	96±18	109±20	105±25	111±12	109±13	112±12
Daily no. of pauses > 2500 ms	806±2472	31±119	7±16	11±27	15±24	8±8
Daily no. of wide QRS complexes	530±769	1076±1652	1459±3324	530±411	560±541	466±157

HR, Heart rate

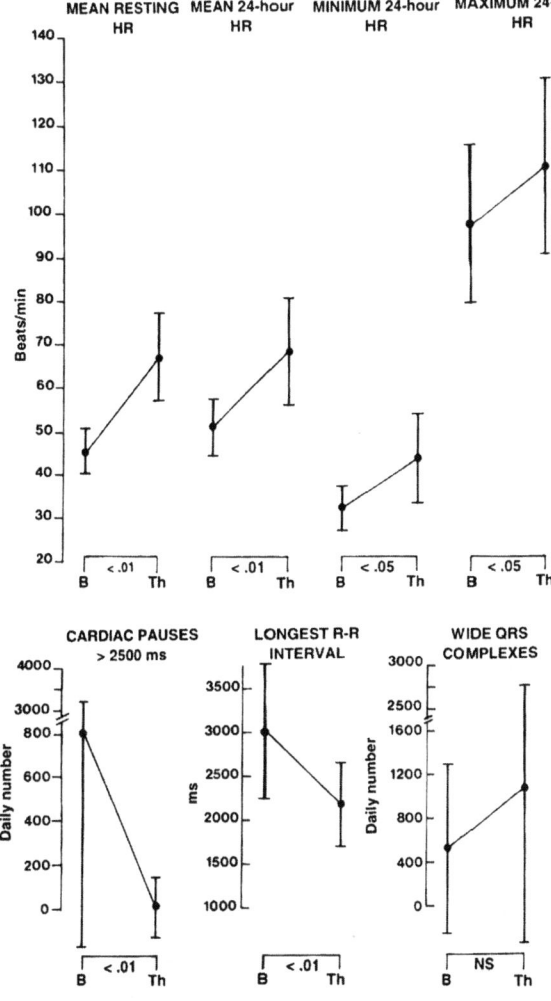

Fig. 1. Effects of oral theophylline on the electrocardiographic parameters at the steady state evaluation. *B*, basal evaluation; *Th*, after theophylline; *HR*, heart rate

Theophylline did not significantly change systolic and diastolic blood pressure. The serum theophylline level was 13 ± 4 ng/ml (range, 5-21 ng/ml). The correlation between the serum theophylline level and the percentage change in the resting heart rate, the mean 24-h heart rate, and the minimum 24-h heart rate was poor.

Follow-up

The mean follow-up period was 20 ± 18 months (range, 1-55 months). Long-term therapy was initiated at a dosage of 400 – 600 mg daily.

During the follow-up, seven patients died after 15 ± 14 months of treatment. One patient died of heart failure, two of arterial embolism, and four of noncardiovascular disease (pneumonia, pulmonary neoplasm, rectal neoplasm, and pulmonary complications after prostatectomy). None of these patients died suddenly.

These seven patients were followed in the hospital for their terminal illness; they continued to take theophylline, and in all cases, the resting heart rate was similar to that observed at the steady state evaluation.

One patient complained of syncope; he refused pacemaker implantation, continued theophylline treatment, and remained asymptomatic in the subsequent 21 months. In the other patients, syncope or presyncope did not occur during the follow-up period. The

drug markedly reduced asthenia and fatigue in the patients complaining of these symptoms. Three patients complained of palpitations, despite the reduction in the daily dosage of the drug to 200-300 mg; the resting heart rate was 90, 95, and 110 beats/min, respectively. The drug was discontinued after 20 ± 11 months of treatment, and in the subsequent visits the resting heart rate was between 80 and 100 beast/min for a mean period of 8 ± 3 months. In these three patients, thyroid hormones were within the normal range, signs of heart failure were absent, and there were no obvious causes for the increase in heart rate.

In two patients, theophylline had to be discontinued at about 1 month because of nausea. During the follow-up period, other patients complained of slight gastric disturbances, which disappeared after a temporary or permanent reduction of the dosage.

The values of the ECG parameters during the follow-up period are presented in Table 1 and in Fig. 2. In the latter, the ECG parameters of the seven patients followed for at least 24 months are shown graphically; this is an intrapatient comparison that allows us to better evaluate the effects of the drug on heart rate. The values of the resting heart rate, the mean 24-h heart rate, and the minimum 24-h heart rate during the fol-

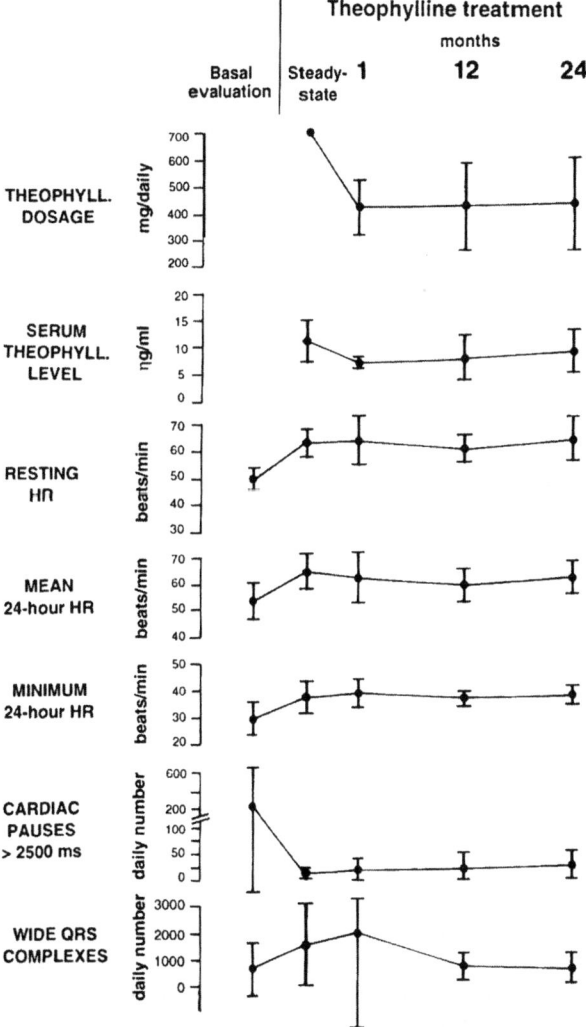

Fig. 2. Long-term effects of oral theophylline. The parameters of the seven patients followed for at least 24 months are shown. *HR*, heart rate

lowing period were similar to those observed at the steady-state evaluation, though the mean dosage of theophylline had been reduced. The daily number of cardiac pauses during the follow-up was similar to that observed at the steady state. In two patients, the follow-up heart rate decreased to control values at one visit; in both patients the serum theophylline level was less than 5 ng/ml and it is possible that they were noncompliant with their medication schedule for a period of time.

Comments

The mean age of our patients with AF and a slow ventricular response was high (about 80 years). This may partially explain the high mortality rate observed during the follow-up period. However, in no patients was death attributable to the AV conduction disturbance, since none died suddenly. We did not include patients with bundle branch block, in which the slow ventricular response might be an expression of a conduction disturbance within the His-Purkinje system, where theophylline does not appear effective. At the steady state evaluation, the drug significantly increased the resting heart rate, the mean 24-h heart rate and the minimum 24-h heart rate and abolished or markedly decreased the number of cardiac pauses. We previously reported an increase in exercise heart rate by 26% (10). These data confirm that theophylline improves AV nodal conduction, resulting in a faster response rate.

Theophylline has several possible mechanisms that might explain the positive chronotropic and dromotropic action: inhibition of phosphodiesterase, activation of the sympathetic nervous system, and antagonism of cardiac effects of adenosine; however, several observations suggest that the primary action of theophylline at therapeutic concentrations is the blockade of adenosine receptors (11, 12). Adenosine has been shown to slow down the sinus rate and depress AV nodal conduction in laboratory animals and in clinical patients (13, 14).

During long-term therapy, the heart rate was similar to that observed at the steady state evaluation despite the reduction in the daily dosage. This suggests that the positive dromotropic action of the drug does not decrease in time.

During the follow-up period, only one patient complained of syncope; the remaining patients remained free of neurologic symptoms. Our results, therefore, suggest a reduction in bradycardia-related symptoms in patients with AF and a slow ventricular response treated with theophylline; this observation seems to be supported by the marked reduction in the frequency of cardiac pauses. However, the natural history of AF with a slow ventricular response is unknown; in particular, we do not know whether the course of neurologic symptoms in this type of arrhythmia is variable from patient to patient, with frequent spontanous remissions as in sick sinus syndrome, or whether the clinical course is constantly changing (15-17).

It has been recently demonstrated that, at least in the majority of cases, a patient with sick sinus syndrome is symptomatic with syncope only if he or she has an abnormal neural reflex in addition to the sinus node dysfunction (6, 7).

At present, we do not know whether an AF with a slow ventricular response syncope is an expression of exhaustion of AV nodal conduction or of an abnormal neural reflex. However, theophylline seems effective in both these circumstances, since it markedly decreases cardiac pauses and prevents tilt-induced neuromediated syncope (18). The reduction in asthenia and fatigue during long-term treatment is interesting; it can be related both to the increase in heart rate and to a stimulant effect on the central nervous system (19).

At the steady state evaluation, oral theophylline, as well as increasing the heart rate, increased the number of wide QRS complexes, albeit not significantly. An arrhythmogenic effect of the drug has been reported in previous investigations conducted in patients with normal sinus rhythm or sinus bradycardia (20-24). In the present study, however, it is not possible to define with certainty in the Holter recording whether the wide QRS complexes were ventricular beats or aberrantly conducted supraventricular beats related to the increase of the heart rate induced by theophylline.

After a mean period of treatment of $1\frac{1}{2}$ years, three patients (17%) complained of severe palpitations; their heart rate had increased spontaneously and the drug was discontinued. Thus we observed spontaeous recovery of the AV conduction disturbance of uncertain origin, something which has not been described before.

In two patients, theophylline had to be discontinued because of nausea; it has already been reported that in about 15% of subjects the drug has to be discontinued because of gastric intolerance (19). It was recently reported that in patients with AF and a normal resting heart rate, oral theophylline significantly increases the exercise heart rate, but only slightly increases the resting heart rate (+3%) (25). Moreover, the drug induces a more marked increase of the resting sinus rate in subjects with sinus bradycardia (+34%) than in those with normal sinus rate (+5%) (20, 26, 27). The reason for a more marked effect of the drug when the heart rate is slow is unclear. Adenosine, which is antagonized by theophylline, may play an important role in the pathophysiology of the sick sinus syndrome and of the AV nodal block (28).

Our data indicate oral theophylline as an effective therapy in most patients with AF and a slow ventricular response and suggest that the initial dosage of the drug should be 500 – 600 mg daily; it can be then slightly decreased or increased according to the clinical course. Serum theophylline levels should be 5 ng/ml or more; with lower values, the effects of the drug on heart rate are unreliable. Furthermore, to prevent side effects of the drug, the serum concentration should not be greater than 15 ng/ml.

At present, there are no data to help define whether electrical therapy or oral theophylline treatment in patients with AF and slow ventricular response is preferable. In the absence of clear data, the following guidelines seem reasonable:
1. Patients with AF, slow ventricular response, and

narrow QRS complex: oral theophylline; if the drug fails to bring therapeutic benefit or causes undesirable side effects, we can proceed to pacemaker implantation.

2. Patients with AF with slow ventricular response and wide QRS complex: pacemaker implantation.

3. Patients with "brady-tachy AF": pacemaker implantation and concomitant antiarrhythmic therapy.

References

1. Pitcher D (1986) Twenty-four hour ambulatory electrocardiography in patients with chronic atrial fibrillation. Br Med J 292: 594
2. Hilgard J, Ezri M, Denes P (1985) Significance of ventricular pauses of three seconds or more detected on twenty-four-hour Holter recordings. Am J Cardiol 55: 1005-1008
3. Saxon LA, Albert BH, Uretz EF et al (1990) Permanent pacemaker placement in chronic atrial fibrillation with intermittent AV block and cerebral symptoms. PACE 13: 724-729
4. Lee MA, Dae MW, Langberg JJ et al (1994) Effects of long-term right ventricular apical pacing on left ventricular perfusion, innervation, function and histology. J Am Coll Cardiol 24: 225-232
5. Mitrovic V, Thormann J, Schelepper M, Neuss H (1983) Thrombotic complications with pacemakers. Int J Cardiol 2: 363-374
6. Brignole M, Menozzi C, Gianfranchi L et al (1991) Neurally mediated syncope detected by carotid sinus message and head-up tilt test in sick sinus syndrome. Am J Cardiol 68: 1032-1036
7. Alboni P, Menozzi C, Brignole M et al (1993) An abnormal neural reflex plays a role in causing syncope in sinus bradycardia. J Am Coll Cardiol 22 (4): 1130-1134
8. Benditt DG, Benson W Jr, Kreitt J et al (1983) Electrophysiologic effects of theophylline in young patients with recurrent symptomatic bradyarrhythmias. Am J Cardiol 52: 1223-1229
9. Eiriksson CE, Writer SL, Vestal RE (1987) Theophylline-induced alterations in cardiac electrophysiology in patients with chronic obstructive pulmonary disease. Am Rev Respir Dis 135: 322-326
10. Alboni P, Ratto B, Scarfò S et al (1991) Dromotropic effects of oral theophylline in patients with atrial fibrillation and a slow ventricular response. Eur Heart J 12: 630-634
11. Belardinelli L, Fenton RA, West A et al (1982) Extracellular action of adenosine and the antagonism by aminophylline on the atrioventricular conduction of isolated perfused guinea pig and rat hearts. Circ Res 51: 569-579
12. Rall TW (1982) Evaluation of the mechanism of action of methylxanthines from calcium mobilizers to antagonist of adenosine receptors. Pharmacologist 24: 277-287
13. James TN, Bear ES, Frink RJ, Urthaler F (1971) Pharmacologic production of atrioventricular block with and without initial bundle branch block. J Pharmacol Exp Ther 179: 346-388
14. Favale S, Di Biase M, Rizzo U, Belardinelli L, Rizzon P (1985) Effects of adenosine and adenosine-5-triphosphate on atrioventricular conduction in patients. J Am Coll Cardiol 5: 1212-1219
15. Baldi N, Castelli M, Alberti E et al (1979) La sindrome del seno malato: storia naturale. In: Consolo F, Arrigo F, Oreto G (eds) La sindrome del seno malato. Piccin, Padova, p 133
16. Gann D, Tolentino A, Samet P (1979) Electrophysiologic evaluation of elderly patients with sinus bradycardia; a long-term follow-up study. Ann Intern Med 90: 24-29
17. Sasaki Y, Shimotori M, Akahane K et al (1988) Long-term follow-up of patients with sick sinus syndrome: a comparison of clinical aspects among unpaced, ventricular inhibited paced and physiologically paced group. PACE 11: 1575-1583
18. Nelson SD, Stanley M, Love CJ et al (1991) The autonomic and hemodynamic effects of oral theophylline in patients with vasodepressor syncope. Arch Intern Med 151: 2425-2429
19. Rall TW (1985) The methylanthines. In: Gilman AG, Goodman LS (eds) MacMillan Publishing Co, New York, p 589
20. Alboni P, Ratto B, Cappato R et al (1991) Clinical effects of oral theophylline in sick sinus syndrome. Am Heart J 122: 1361-1367
21. Banner AS, Sunderrajan EV, Agarval MK et al (1979) Arrhythmogenic effects of orall administered bronchodilators. Arch Intern Med 139: 434-437
22. Patel AK, Skatrud B, Thomsen JH (1981) Cardiac arrhythmias due to orally aminophylline in patients with chronic obstructive pulmonary disease. Chest 80: 661-665
23. Dutt AK, De Soyza ND, Au WY et al (1983) The effects of aminophylline on cardiac rhythm in advanced chronic obstructive pulmonary disease: correlation with serum thephylline levels. Eur J Respir Dis 64: 264-270
24. Conradson T, Eklundh G, Olofsson B et al (1987) Arrhythmogenicity from combined bronchodilator therapy in patients with obstructive lung disease and concomitant ischemic heart disease. Chest 91: 5-9
25. Dattilo Gl, Eiriksson CE Jr, Vestal RE (1992) Increased ventricular response rate during exercise in patients with atrial fibrillation treated with theophylline. Arch Intern Med 152: 797-803
26. Blinks JR, Olson CB, Jewell BR et al (1972) Influence of caffeine and other methylxanthines on mechanical properties of isolated mammalian heart muscle. Circ Res 30: 367-392
27. Vestal RE, Eiriksson CE Jr, Musser B et al (1983) Effect of intravenous aminophylline on plasma levels of catecholamines and related cardiovascular and metabolic responses in man. Circulation 67: 162-171
28. Watt AH (1985) Sick sinus syndrome: and adenosine-mediated disease. Lancet 1: 786-788

Control of Rapid Heart Rate in Patients with Atrial Fibrillation: Drugs or Ablation?

M. Brignole[1], C. Menozzi[2], and L. Gianfranchi[1]

[1]Ospedali Riuniti, Sezione di Aritmologia, Lavagna, Genoa, Italy
[2]Ospedale S. Maria Nuova, Sezione di Aritmologia, Reggio Emilia, Italy

Epidemiology

Atrial fibrillation is by far the most frequent arrhythmia. It is particularly frequent in the elderly, in males, and in patients with heart disease. The prevalence of atrial fibrillation is 9.1% in men and women with cardiovascular disease (1). Data from the Framingham study (2) indicate that the overall incidence of developing atrial fibrillation was 529 new cases per year per 100 000 inhabitants aged 50-79 years (250 and 279 for paroxysmal and chronic forms, respectively). Given this high incidence, even if catheter ablation therapy were prescribed for a minority of drug-refractory patients, the total number of potential candidates for this treatment would be high. For example, during 1994 in our institutions radiofrequency catheter ablation of the atrioventricular junction and subsequent pacemaker implantation were performed in 6.4 patients per 100.000 inhabitants; that was only 1.2% of the patients with a new atrial fibrillation, but 18% of the total number of pacemakers implanted during the same period in that population. For comparison, it should be noted that the annual incidence of a new case of Wolff-Parkinson-White syndrome is 4 persons per 100 000 inhabitants (3), about one third of whom may perhaps benefit from radiofrequency therapy.

Reasons for Converting Atrial Fibrillation to Sinus Rhythm

Sinus rhythm is preferable to atrial fibrillation. The major reasons for converting atrial fibrillation to sinus rhythm are ventricular rate control, hemodynamic improvement, a sense of well-being and, possibly, the avoidance of embolism (4). The question of ventricular rate control is generally straigthforward, as the vast majority of patients clearly are not confortable at ventricular rates >100 bpm, while rapid ventricular rates for prolonged periods lead to ventricular dilatation, congestive heart failure, and a rate-related cardiomyopathy (5-8). Generally, restoration of sinus rhythm produces prompt improvement of cardiovascular per-formance. Therefore, the principle that sinus rhythm must be maintained whenever possible is generally accepted (4). However, failure to maintain stable sinus rhythm occurs in 35%-50% of patients with paroxysmal atrial fibrillation or chronic atrial fibrillation of recent onset within 1 or 2 years even if serial antiarrhythmic drug treatments are used (9-12). Causes of failure are: long-lasting atrial fibrillation, unsuccessful cardioversion, frequent recurrences despite multiple drug trials (including amiodarone), the risk of proarrhythmia (especially in patients with heart failure), and poor compliance with prolonged pharmacological treatment.

In patients with chronic atrial fibrillation and in those with paroxysmal atrial fibrillation in whom recurrences are frequent or poorly tolerated, it is important to provide therapy to control ventricular response. In such cases, therapy is prescribed on the assumption that ventricular rate control provides greater comfort for the patients and may ameliorate their cardiac performance. This assumption has largely been undemonstrated even though it is widely accepted. Ventricular rate during atrial fibrillation can be successfully controlled by means of drugs or ablative techniques.

Pharmacological Control of Heart Rate

In many patients with atrial fibrillation and a rapid ventricular rate, the current pharmacological approach is largely unsatisfactory.

Digoxin

Monotherapy with digoxin has been shown to slow resting heart rate in comparison with placebo in most patients, but because digoxin's predominant effect on the resting heart rate is mediated by an enhanced vagal tone, the beneficial effects frequently may not be maintained during exertion, when vagal influences are withdrawn. Indeed, in one study (13), mean decrease in heart rate was 13% at rest (from 93±5 bpm during the placebo phase to 81±5 bpm during the digoxin phase) with an average decrease of 11% during 24-h monitoring (from 102±5 bpm to 91±4 bpm), whereas it remained unchanged during exercise (from 175±3 bpm to 177±2). Two other studies (14,15) showed that, with increasing digoxin concentration, the heart rate decreased significantly both at rest and during exercise, with a maximum decrease of 24% at rest and 8%-14% during exercise. In contrast, long-term digoxin therapy does not seem to be effective in reducing the ventricular response in patients with paroxysmal atrial fibrillation, despite adequate therapeutic levels (16,17). Digoxin proved unable to increase exercise tolerance (13,18,19) and, in about 50% of cases, loss of control of heart rate occurs during such therapy (20). Digoxin's advantages as a once-daily, inexpensive, and relatively safe choice with no contraindications still make it the first line of therapy. When ineffective, digoxin can be combined with either calcium channel antagonists or ß-blockers to produce greater decreases in heart rate than either digoxin or the added agent alone. This suggests that this combination may be the optimal therapy for the control of exertional rate increases. However, the side effects produced by calcium antagonists and ß-blockers necessitate drug discontinuation in a considerable number of patients.

Calcium Channel Antagonists (Verapamil, Diltiazem)

Verapamil and diltiazem have similar effects on rate slowing. Medium doses of verapamil and diltiazem are comparable to therapeutic doses of digoxin at rest, but superior during exercise (15,21,23). Symptom control is also similar with the two drugs (22). Therapy with a combination of digoxin and verapamil or diltiazem enhances the effects of digoxin alone and results in significantly better control of heart rate at rest and during exercise (Table 1) (15,21,23-30). Indeed, the decrease in heart rate ranges from 15% to 26% at rest, from 11% to 29% during peak exercise, and from 9% to 21% during an average of 24 h of ambulatory electrocardiographic monitoring. The ventricular rate control achieved with the calcium channel antagonists has disparate effects on exercise tolerance, with improvement varying from 2% to 33%.

ß-Adrenergic Blocking Agents

Like calcium-antagonists, ß-blockers used as an adjuvant to digoxin, are significantly more effective than digoxin alone in controlling rapid ventricular rates at rest and during exercise (Table 2) (13,19,31-33). The magnitude of the decrease in heart rate is similar to that observed with calcium antagonists at rest (range from 9% to 25%), during exercise (range from 13% to 31%), and during 24-h electrocardiographic monitoring (range from 1% to 22%). Owing to their negative inotropic effect, ß-blockers generally impair exercise capacity (31,32), but not always. For example, in one study (13) labelalol, owing to its unique property of combined α- and ß-blockade, increased exercise tolerance by 13%. In another study (33), sotalol did not affect exercise capacity; this was probably because the adverse effect of ß-adrenergic blockade was counterbalanced by the favorable class III drug effect of prolongation of repolariza-

Table 1. Effects of combined therapy with calcium channel antagonists and digitalis in comparison with digitalis alone according to data from some available randomized, placebo-controlled studies

Author	Drug	Dose (mg/day)	Patients (n)	Rest heart rate (bpm)			Exercise heart rate (bmp)			Exercise tolerance (sec*; watts†; mets')			Average 24-h heart rate (bpm)		
				Placebo	Active	Δ%	Placebo	Active	Δ%	Placebo	Active	Δ%	Placebo	Active	Δ%
Schwartz et al. (26)	V	320	10	-	-	-	151±26	106±22	-29%	-	-	-	87±9	72±6	-17%
Lang et al. (15)	V	240	52	88±24	75±20	-15%	147±29	114±19	-22%	-	-	-	-	-	-
Panidis et al. (25)	V	240-480	27	87±20	69±13	-21%	136±23	104±14	-24%	-	-	-	-	-	-
Lang et al. (24)	V	240-320	20	90±22	70±16	-22%	165±28	136±29	-18%	219±77*	292±71*	+33%	-	-	-
Roth et al. (21)	D	240	12	86±12	67±16	-22%	170±20	132±32	-23%	-	-	-	-	-	-
Roth et al. (21)	D	320	12	86±12	65±15	-24%	170±20	121±24	-29%	-	-	-	-	-	-
Steinberg et al. (27)	D	240-360	16	96±17	69±10	-26%	163±14	133±26	-18%	7.0±2.3'	7.3±2.4'	+4%	87±13	69±10	-21%
Maragno et al. (28)	D	180-240	16	96±19	79±16	-18%	150±22	120±24	-20%	-	-	-	83±15	69±10	-16%
Atwood et al. (30)	D	240	9	91±17	68±13	-23%	171±30	142±27	-29%	672*	684*	+2%	-	-	-
Lewis et al. (23)	D	180	14	100±17	83±12	-17%	152±23	128±28	-16%	-	-	-	87±20	70±10	-20%
Lundstrom et al. (29)	D	270	18	-	-	-	179±13	159±21	-11%	127±39'	136±42'	+7%	88±14	76±13	-14%
Lundstrom et al. (29)	V	240	18	-	-	-	179±13	158±23	-12%	127±39'	137±39'	+8%	88±14	80±11	-9%

V, verapamil; D, diltiazem.

237

Table 2. Effects of combined therapy with ß-blocking agents and digitalis in comparison with digitalis alone according to data from some available, randomized, placebo-controlled studies

Author	Drug	Dose (mg/day)	Patients (n)	Rest heart rate (bpm)			Exercise heart rate (bmp)			Exercise tolerance (min)			Average 24-h heart rate (bpm)		
				Placebo	Active	Δ%	Placebo	Active	Δ%	Placebo	Active	Δ%	Placebo	Active	Δ%
DiBianco et al. (31)	N	90	20	92±19	73±16	-21%	153±26	111±24	-27%	7.8±2.4	6.3±2.4	-19%	94±18	73±14	-22%
Atwood et al. (32)	C	600	9	91±17	77±15	-15%	171±30	118±20	-31%	11.3	10.3	-9%	-	-	-
Zoble et al. (19)	N	20-120	32	-	-	-	162	120	-26%	9.1	9.6	+5%	-	-	-
Wong et al. (13)	L	100-400	10	81±5	74±4	-9%	177±5	154±4	-13%	14.2±1.5	16.1±1.1	+13%	91±4	90±4	-1%
Brodsky et al. (33)	S	80	20	95±4	79±3	-17%	173±6	150±6	-20%	-	-	-	-	-	-20%
	S	160	19	97±4	79±3	-18%	179±5	153±6	-16%	-	-	-	-	-	-13%

N, Nadolol; C, Celiprolol; L, Labetalol; S, Sotalol.

tion and by its vasodilatatory effect. However, the rate control achieved with sotalol was unassociated with a significant improvement in symptoms.

Amiodarone

The effect of amiodarone in controlling rapid ventricular rates has only seldom been evaluated. In one study (10) heart rate decreased at rest from a mean of 89 bpm to 67 bpm (25% decrease).

Unresolved Issues Concerning Pharmacologic Control of Heart Rate

It is generally accepted that control of heart rate to values <90 bpm makes most patients more comfortable, but controlled studies are lacking (4). Channer et al. (34) found that both high-dose digoxin and verapamil significantly reduced symptom scores for palpitation, but both treatments were unable to improve dyspnea or walking distance. Lewis et al (23) found no evidence that the further reduction in ventricular rate seen with the combination of digoxin and diltiazem was associated with improved exercise tolerance; they concluded that the use of diltiazem does not appear to be of benefit in the majority of patients. Moreover, very little is to be found in the literature about an improvement in cardiac performance and/or survival as a result of heart rate control. Only few case reports exist which show the reversible effect of successful control of rapid heart rate on tachycardia-induced cardiomyopathy (6,35). On the other hand, an increased ventricular rate partially compensates for the reduction in stroke volume due to the loss of atrial contraction. Thus, within certain ranges, tachycardia can be a beneficial phenomenon, partially counteracting an even greater fall in cardiac output than would otherwise occur; the optimal heart rate varies from patient to patient (4). This could explain why exercise tolerance is only slightly increased, if at all, by reducing ventricular rate. Furthermore, pharmacologic therapy is always unable to suppress rhythm irregularity. It is well known that rhythm irregularity greatly affects cardiac contractility and decreases cardiac output (4).

The role and safety of standard doses of calcium-channel antagonists and ß-blockers in patients with congestive heart failure remain controversial. Verapamil and diltiazem have negative inotropic effects that may cause hemodynamic deterioration, particularly in patients with marked left ventricular dysfunction. ß-adrenergic blockers, which also exert negative inotropic effects, not only may precipitate congestive heart failure but also may be contraindicated in patients with underlying bronchospasm caused by asthma or chronic obstructive pulmonary disease. It is not clear whether either class of drugs can be safely recommended for patients with underlying cardiac or pulmonary disease, particularly when relatively high doses are needed for rate control (19,21,25,29,31). Amiodarone, too, which could be a valid alternative to calcium antagonists and to ß-blockers, may cause many side effects involving all organ systems; side effects are considered clinically significant in about 20% of cases and require discontinuation of therapy in 8% of cases (36).

In conclusion, although sufficient heart rate control can probably be achieved in most cases with pharmacologic therapy, its clinical benefits still remain unclear.

Radiofrequency Catheter Ablation

Benefits

Catheter ablation of the atrioventricular junction is an excellent alternative for those patients with atrial fibrillation in whom arrhythmia is refractory or who cannot tolerate the drugs needed. The success rate of inducing complete atrioventricular block by using radiofrequency energy is close to 100%, especially if a sequential right- and left-sided approach is used (37-43). It must be noted that atrioventricular junction ablation is not curative, since these patients require chronic cardiac pacing. However, radiofrequency ablation plus pacemaker-guided rhythm allows a virtually optimal rate control to be achieved, which is undoubtedly superior to that obtainable with drugs.

This better heart rate control, together with the absence of the adverse effects of drugs, also seems to be able to determine better clinical results. Ablation therapy has proved to be particularly efficacious in controlling palpitations, which virtually disappeared in all patients with both paroxysmal and chronic forms (43-45). In a controlled, prospective study by our group (44), ablation greatly increased the functional capacity of patients with severe symptoms; the symptom scores for palpitations, rest dyspnea, effort dyspnea, exercise tolerance, asthenia, and NYHA class improved by 13%-96% after ablation. The beneficial effects were nearly twice as great as those seen in the control group. It is likely that cardiac performance can also be improved by ablation in comparison with conventional therapy. Indeed, in studies by various authors, exercise tolerance increased by 17%-54% after ablation (39,44,46) and a reduction in left ventricular diameters resulting in an improvement of fractional shortening of 34%-44% was observed in the patients with originally depressed function (39,40,44,47). Benefits are maintained during long-term follow-up in many cases (45). In our own series, 90 patients (mean age 70±10 years) underwent radiofrequency ablation for drug-refractory paroxysmal (n=30) or chronic (n=60) atrial fibrillation. Heart failure was present in 47%. After ablation, they were followed for up to 24 months (mean 14 months): compared with the pre-ablation value, NYHA class improved at the end of

follow-up in 46%, worsened only in 1%, and remained unchanged in 53% of cases. There were only 9 hospitalizations for cardiac problems after ablation, in comparison with 215 hospitalizations before ablation.

Risk

There are several disadvantages to catheter ablation, other than the need for pacemaker implant. These include serious procedure-related complications and the risk of sudden death. Complications of atrioventricular junction ablation with radiofrequency energy in 1643 patients from the available patient series (42,43,48-51) have been pooled together and reported in table 3. These include a mortality rate from the procedure of 0.3%, ventricular tachycardia/fibrillation in 0.4%, and an incidence of early life-threatening complications, such as pulmonary embolism and cardiac tamponade, of 0.4%. However, complications are fairly rare and their incidence is significantly lower than that observed in the historical series of patients treated with direct current (DC) shock energy (52-56). The high rate of complications observed with DC energy has probably led to some overestimation of the risks of radiofrequency therapy. Although no clear proarrhythmic effects have been established, ablation of cardiac tissue is potentially arrhythmogenic. This mechanism is not completely known; in some cases improper cardiac electrostimulation was the cause (38). Basically, the observed risk was very low (0.4%), being five times lower than that incurred with DC shock energy (Table 3). Since ventricular tachycardia/fibrillation occur in the first 24-48 h after ablation, this potentially lethal complication can be corrected by monitoring the patient in the intensive care unit during this period. Most of the patients who die in the periablation observation period are reported to have severely depressed left ventricular function with very low ejection fraction values (53).

There is no evidence of an increased risk of death during long-term follow-up in patients treated with radiofrequency ablation. Indeed, during a follow-up duration ranging from 5 to 24 months, a pooled group of 438 patients including our own series and two studied by other authors (43,50) showed a 4.8% total death rate and a 1.6% sudden death rate. In our own series consisting of 90 patients, actuarial mortality rates were 5% and 12% after 1 and 2 years, respectively (Fig 1). Overall, there were eight deaths, five of which were due to heart failure, one to sudden death and two to noncardiac causes. The observed survival curve was

Table 3. Procedure-related complications of atrioventricular junction ablation with radiofrequency energy (1643 patients) [a] and with DC shock energy (903 patients) [b] from the available patient series

Complication	RF group (n=1643)		DC group (n=903)		p value	Odds ratio (±95% confidence limit)
	(n)	(%)	(n)	(%)		
Procedure-related deaths	4	0.3	13	1.4	0.0001	0.2 (0.05-0.5)
Non-fatal VT-VF	6	0.4	13	1.4	0.005	0.2 (0.08-0.7)
Early life-threatening events (embolisms, tamponade)	8	0.5	11	1.2	0.07	0.4 (0.1-1.1)
Other minor events	40	2.4	40	4.4	0.008	0.5 (0.3-0.9)

DC, direct current.
[a] Radiofrequency series (42,43,48-51).
[b] DC series (52-56)

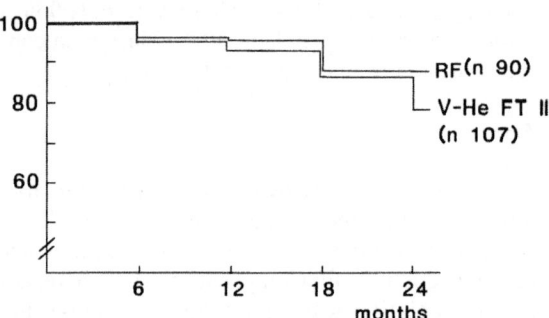

% SURVIVAL

RF (n 90)

V-He FT II (n 107)

Fig 1. Actuarial estimate of death rate in our own series of 90 patients affected by drug-refractory atrial fibrillation who had received radiofrequency ablation of atrioventricular junction and subsequent pacemaker implant (RF). The survival curve of a large series of medically treated patients affected by atrial fibrillation enrolled in the V-HeFT II study (54), whose clinical characteristics seem to be similar to those of our population, is superimposed

Table 4. Advantages and disadvantages of catheter ablation of the atrioventricular junction versus drug therapy for the control of rapid ventricular rate in patients with atrial fibrillation

Advantages	Disadvantages
Better ventricular rate control	Need for pacemaker implant
Improved symptom control	Procedure-related complications
Improved myocardial function for some	Long-term outcome not well known
No need for antiarrhythmic drugs (drug toxicity and proarrhythmia)	
Lesser need for hospitalization for refractory cases	

closely similar to that of the large group of patients enrolled in the V-HeFT II study (57) whose clinical characteristics seem to be similar to those of our population (Fig 1).

Conclusion

The potential benefits and disadvantages of catheter ablation versus pharmacologic therapy for the control of rapid ventricular rate are listed in Table 4. The timing of ablative therapy is a matter of clinical judgment. It is not appropriate to exhaust every possible combination of antiarrhythmic drug therapy before proceeding with ablation. The benefits of improved myocardial function and obviating the need for hospitalization have been demonstrated for ablation therapy. The risk of procedure-related complications, though fairly rare, remains a concern. Catheter ablation technique is sufficiently refined, safe, and efficacious that randomized trials comparing catheter ablation and drug therapy should be considered.

References

1. Furberg C, Psaty B, Manolio T, Gardin J, Smith V, Rautaharju P (1994) Prevalence of atrial fibrillation in elderly subjects (the Cardiovascular Heart Study). Am J Cardiol 74: 236-241
2. Kannel W, Abbott R, Savage D, McNamara P (1983) Coronary heart disease and atrial fibrillation: the Framingham study. Am Heart J 106: 389-396
3. Munger T, Packer D, Hammill S, Feldman B, Bailey K, Ballard D, Holmes D, Gersh B (1993) A population study of the natural history of Wolff-Parkinson-White syndrome in Olmsted County, Minnesota, 1953-1989. Circulation 87: 866-873
4. Brignole M, Menozzi C, Bottoni N, Bertulla A (1992) Comportamento della performance cardiaca nella fibrillazione atriale di diverse patogenesi. In: Rovelli F, De Vita C, Moreo A (eds) Cardiologia 1992. Librex, Milan, pp 443-451
5. Phillips E, Levine SA (1949) Auricular fibrillation without other evidence of heart disease: a cause of reversible heart failure. Am J Med 7: 479-489
6. Grogan M, Smith H, Gersh B, Wood D (1992) Left ventricular dysfunction due to atrial fibrillation in patients initially believed to have idiopathic dilated cardiomyopathy. Am J Cardiol 69: 1570-1573
7. Lemery R, Brugada P, Cheriex E, Wellens H (1987) Reversibility of tachycardia-induced left ventricular dysfunction after closed-chest catheter ablation of the atrioventricular junction for intractable atrial fibrillation. Am J Cardiol 60: 1406-1408
8. Peters KG, Kienzle MG (1988) Severe cardiomyopathy due to chronic rapidly conducted atrial fibrillation: complete recovery after restoration of sinus rhythm. Am J Med 85: 242-244
9. Crijns H, Van gelder I, Van Gilst W, Hillege H, Gosselink M, Lie K (1991) Serial antiarrhythmic drug treatment to maintain sinus rhythm after electrical cardioversion for chronic atrial fibrillation or atrial flutter. Am J Cardiol 68: 335-341
10. Zehender M, Hohnloser S, Muller B, Meinertz T, Jost H (1992) Effects of amiodarone versus quinidine and verapamil in patients with chronic atrial fibrillation: results of a comparative study and a 2-year follow-up. J Am Coll Cardiol 19: 1054-1059
11. Hohnloser S (1994) Indications and limitations of class II and III antiarrhythmic drugs in atrial fibrillation. PACE 17: 1019-1025
12. Antman E, Beamer A, Cantillon C, McGowan N, Friedman P (1990) Therapy of refractory symptomatic atrial fibrillation and atrial flutter: a staged care approach with new antiarrhythmic drugs. J Am Coll Cardiol 15: 698-707
13. Wong C, Lau C, Leung W, Cheng C (1990) Usefulness of labetalol in chronic atrial fibrillation. Am J Cardiol 66: 1212-1215
14. Beasley R, Smith D, McHaffie D (1985) Exercise heart rates at different serum digoxin concentrations in patients with atrial fibrillation. Br Med J 290: 9-11
15. Lang R, Klein H, Weiss E, David D, Sareli P, Levy A, Guerrero J, Di Segni E, Kaplinsky E (1983) Superiority of oral verapamil therapy to digoxin in treatment of chronic atrial fibrillation. Chest 83: 491-499
16. Rawles J, Metcalfe M, Jennings K (1990) Time of occurrence, duration, and ventricular rate of paroxysmal atrial fibrillation: the effect of digoxin. Br Heart J 63: 225-227
17. Galun E, Flugelman M, Glikson M, Eliakim M (1991) Failure of long-term digitalization to prevent rapid ventricular response in patients with paroxysmal atrial fibrillation. Chest 99: 1038-1040
18. Zarowitz B, Gheorghiade M (1992) Optimal heart rate control for patients with chronic atrial fibrillation: are pharmacologic choices truly changing? Am Heart J 123: 1401-1403
19. Zoble R, Brewington J, Olukotun A, Gore R (1987) Comparative effects of nadolol-digoxin combination therapy and digoxin monotherapy for chronic atrial fibrillation. Am J Cardiol 60: 39D-45D
20. Roberts S, Diaz C, Nolan P, Salerno D, Stapczynski S, Zbrozek A, Ritz E, Bauman J, Vlasses P (1993) Effectiveness and costs of digoxin treatment for atrial fibrillation and flutter. Am J Cardiol 72: 567-573
21. Roth A, Harrison E, Mitani G, Cohen J, Rahimtoola S, Elkayam U (1986) Efficacy and safety of medium- and high-dose diltiazem alone and in combination with digoxin for control of heart rate at rest and during exercise in patients with chronic atrial fibrillation. Circulation 73: 316-324
22. Lewis R, Lakhani M, Moreland A, McDevitt D (1987) A comparison of verapamil and digoxin in the treatment of atrial fibrillation. Eur Heart J 8: 148-153
23. Lewis R, Laing E, Moreland T, Service E, McDevitt D (1988) A comparison of digoxin, diltiazem and their combination in the treatment of atrial fibrillation. Eur Heart J 9: 279-283
24. Lang R, Klein H, Di Segni E, Gefen J, Sareli P, Libhaber C, David D, Weiss E, Guerrero J, Kaplinsky E (1983) Verapamil

improves exercise capacity in chronic atrial fibrillation: double-blind crossover study. Am Heart J 105: 820-824

25. Panidis I, Monganroth J, Baessler C (1983) Effectiveness and safety of oral verapamil to control exercise-induced tachycardia in patients with atrial fibrillation receiving digitalis. Am J Cardiol 52: 1197-1201

26. Schwartz J, Keefe D, Kates D, Kirsten E, Harrison D (1982) Acute and chronic pharmacodynamic interaction of verapamil and digoxin in atrial fibrillation. Circulation 65: 1163-1170

27. Steinberg J, Katz R, Bren G, Buff L, Varghese J (1987) Efficacy of oral diltiazem to control ventricular response in chronic atrial fibrillation at rest and during exercise. J Am Coll Cardiol 9: 405-411

28. Maragno E, Santostasi G, Gaion R, Trento M, Grion A, Miraglia G, Dalla Volta S (1988) Low- and medium-dose diltiazem in chronic atrial fibrillation: comparison with digoxin and correlation with drug plasma levels. Am Heart J 116: 385-392

29. Lundstrom T, Ryden L (1990) Ventricular rate control and exercise performance in chronic atrial fibrillation: effects of diltiazem and verapamil. J Am Coll Cardiol 16: 86-90

30. Atwood E, Myers J, Sullivan M, Forbes S, Pewen W, Froelicher V (1988) Diltiazem and exercise performance in patients with chronic atrial fibrillation. Chest 92: 20-25

31. DiBianco R, Monganroth J, Freitag J, Ronan J, Lindgren K, Donohue D, Larca L, Chadda K, Olukotun A (1984) Effects of nadolol on the spontaneous and exercise-provoked heart rate of patients with chronic atrial fibrillation receiving stable dosages of digoxin. Am Heart J 108: 1121-1127

32. Atwood E, Sullivan M, Forbes S, Myers J, Pewen W, Olson H, Froelicher V (1987) Effect of beta-adrenergic blockade on exercise performance in patients with chronic atrial fibrillation. J Am Coll Cardiol 10: 314-320

33. Brodsky M, Saini R, Bellinger R, Zoble R, Weiss R, Powers L (1994) Comparative effects of the combination of digoxin and dl-sotalol therapy versus digoxin monotherapy for control of ventricular response in chronic atrial fibrillation. Am Heart J 127: 572-577

34. Channer K, Papouchado M, James M, Pitcher D, Russell Rees J (1987) Towards improved control of atrial fibrillation. Eur Heart J 8: 141-147

35. Packer DL, Bardy GH, Worley SJ, Smith MS, Cabb FR, Coleman E, Gallagher JJ, German LD (1986) Tachycardia-induced cardiomyopathy: a reversible form of left ventricular dysfunction. Am J Cardiol 57: 563-570

36. Raeder E, Podrid P, Lown B (1985) Side effects and complications of amiodarone therapy. Am Heart J 109: 975-983

37. Souza O, Gursoy S, Simonis F, Steurer G, Andries E, Brugada P (1992) Right-sided versus left-sided radiofrequency ablation of the His bundle. PACE 15: 1454-1459

38. Trohman R, Simmons T, Moore S, Firstenberg M, Williams D, Maloney J (1992) Catheter ablation of the atrioventricular junction using radiofrequency energy and a bilateral cardiac approach. Am J Cardiol 70: 1438-1443

39. Twidale N, Sutton K, Bartlett L, Dooley A, Winstanley S, Heddle W, Hassam R, Koutsounis H (1993) Effects on cardiac performance of atrioventricular node catheter ablation using radiofrequency current for drug-refractory atrial arrhythmias. PACE 16: 1275-1284

40. Heinz G, Siostrzonek P, Kreiner G, Gossinger H (1992) Improvement in left ventricular systolic function after successful radiofrequency His bundle ablation for drug-refractory, chronic atrial fibrillation and recurrent atrial flutter. Am J Cardiol 69: 489-492

41. Kalbfleisch S, Williamson B, Man C, Volperian V, Hummel J, Calkins H, Strickberger A, Langberg J, Morady F (1993) A randomized comparison of the right- and left-sided approaches to ablation of the atrioventricular junction. Am J Cardiol 72: 1406-1410

42. Menozzi C, Brignole M, Gianfranchi L, Lolli G, Oddone D, Gaggioli G, Bottoni N (1994) Radiofrequency catheter ablation and modulation of atrioventricular conduction in patients with atrial fibrillation. PACE 17: 2143-2149

43. Kay N, Epstein A, Dailey S, Plumb V (1993) Role of radiofrequency ablation in the management of supraventricular arrhythmias: experience in 760 consecutive patients. J Cardiovasc Electrophysiol 4: 371-389

44. Brignole M, Gianfranchi L, Menozzi C, Bottoni N, Bollini R, Lolli G, Oddone D, Gaggioli G (1994) Influence of atrio-ventricular junction radiofrequency ablation in patients with chronic atrial fibrillation and flutter on quality of life and cardiac performance. Am J Cardiol 74: 242-246

45. Rosenquist M, Lee M, Moulinier L, Springer M, Abbott J, Wu J, Langberg J, Griffin J, Scheinman M (1990) Long-term follow-up of patients after transcatheter direct current ablation of the atrioventricular junction. J Am Coll Cardiol 16: 1467-1474

46. Kay N, Bubien R, Epstein A, Plumb V (1988) Effect of catheter ablation of the atrioventricular junction on quality of life and exercise tolerance in paroxysmal atrial fibrillation. Am J Cardiol 62: 741-744

47. Rodriguez LM, Smeets J, Xie B, de Chillou C, Cheriex E, Pieters F, metzger J, den Dulk K, Wellens H (1993) Improvement in left ventricular function by ablation of atrioventricular nodal conduction in selected patients with lone atrial fibrillation. Am J Cardiol 72: 1137-1141

48. Hindricks G (1993) The Multicentre European Radiofrequency Survey (MERFS): complications of radiofrequency catheter ablation of arrhythmias. Eur Heart J 14: 1644-1653

49. Scheinman M (1994) Patterns of catheter ablation practice in the United States: results of the 1992 NASPE survey. PACE 17: 873-875

50. Raviele A, Delise P, Themistoclakis S, Coluccia S (1994) Complicanze dell'ablazione transcatetere. G Ital Cardiol 24: 132-147

51. Olgin J, Scheinman M (1995) Catheter ablation of the atrioventricular node for treatment of supraventricular tachyarrhythmias. In: Zipes D and Jalife J (eds) Cardiac electrophysiology. From cell to bedside. Saunders, Philadelphia, pp 1453-1460

52. Evans T, Scheinman M, Zipes D, Benditt D, Breithardt G, Camm J, El-Sherif N, Fisher J, Fontaine G, Levy S, Pristosky E, Josephson M, Morady F, Ruskin J (1988) The percutaneous cardiac mapping and ablation registry: final summary of results. PACE 11: 1621-1626

53. Evans T (1991) Predictors of in-hospital mortality after DC catheter ablation of atrioventricular junction. Results of a prospective, international, multicenter study. Circulation 84: 1924-1937

54. Olgin J, Scheinman M (1993) Comparison of high energy direct current and radiofrequency catheter ablation of the atrioventricular junction. J Am Coll Cardiol 21: 557-564

55. Levy S, Bru P, Aliot E, Attuel P, Barnay C, Clementy J, Ebagosti A, Fauchier JP, Fontaine G, Leclercq JF (1988) Long-term follow-up of atrioventricular junctional transcatheter electrical ablation. PACE 11: 1149-1153

56. Sadoul N, de Chillou C, Lamouri F, Simon JP, Reeb T, Pescariou S, Dodinot B, Aliot E (1994) Results, complications and long-term outcome of percutaneous ablation of atrioventricular conduction: a series of 85 cases. Arch Mal Coeur 87: 1453-1458

57. Carson P, Jonhson G, Dunkman B, Fletcher R, Farrell L, Cohn J (1993) The influence of atrial fibrillation on prognosis in mild to moderate heart failure. The V-HeFT studies. Circulation 87: VI102-VI110

How Effective and Safe Is Internal Direct Current Shock for Atrial Fibrillation Refractory to External Cardioversion?

M. Santini, C. Pandozi, S. Toscano, G. Altamura,
A. Castro, S. Tonioni, and B. Magris

Dipartimento delle Malattie del Cuore, Ospedale S Filippo Neri,
Rome, Italy

In a group of patients (6%-50% in different series) with atrial fibrillation (AF) external cardioversion and pharmacological therapy failed to restore sinus rhythm. AF is not a benign arrhythmia; it causes disabling symptoms and hemodynamic disturbances related to the rapid ventricular response and/or to the loss of the atrial kick. Moreover, patients with AF are at a higher risk of systemic embolism and stroke as assessed by the Framingham study (1, 2). In patients with AF resistant to pharmacologic and transthoracic electrical cardioversion the following therapeutic options are available:
– Drugs acting on the atrioventricular (AV) node conduction (verapamil, beta-blocking agents)
– AV node or His bundle ablation with subsequent pacemaker insertion
– High energy internal cardioversion (HEIC)
– Low energy internal cardioversion (LEIC)

The first two treatments improve symptoms and hemodynamics with no effect on the embolic risk, which is reduced only by the latter procedures when successful. The purpose of the present study was to assess the short and long-term efficacy and the safety of internal cardioversion (IC) with both high and low energy in such patients.

Methods

From March 1992 to February 1995, 34 patients with AF underwent IC; 23 were men and 11 women, with a mean age of 56.6 years (±10). An underlying heart disease was present in 26 patients (76%): ten patients had coronary heart disease, nine a dilated and one a hypertrofic cardiomyopathy, four had mitral valve disease, and two congestive heart failure. AF duration ranged from 1 day to 30 months (mean, 7.7 months).

The mean body weight was 85.1 kg (±17,8), and the mean left atrial size 45,2 mm (±7.4). All patients had failed at least one pharmacologic and one transthoracic electrical cardioversion attempt. All but two patients had chronic AF (lasting more than 1 month)

External cardioversion consisted of synchronized direct current (DC) shocks delivered at increasing energy levels: 100, 200, and 300 J, the latter repeated twice. The need for and type of anticoagulation were decided according to our protocol. In brief, patients with arrhythmia duration less than 3 days were not generally anticoagulated. Those with AF lasting more than 3 days were fully anticoagulated in the presence of atrial or auricular thrombi discovered by transesophageal echocardiography or in the presence of mitral stenosis, heart failure, or previous embolism. If smoke effect without atrial thrombi was detected, subcutaneous heparin was administered for 2 days before the procedure. If AF lasted more than 3 days but there was no evidence of atrial thrombi or smoke effect, no treatment was given. Full anticoagulation was performed in all the patients after successful cardioversion for at least 1 week.

The first 29 patients underwent HEIC, the last five LEIC; the latter procedure was started in our Institution in May 1994.

All the patients undergoing HEIC were treated with antiarrhythmic drugs before the procedure (750 mg propafenone die in 18 patients and 200 mg amiodarone die in the remaining 11 with left ventricular dysfunction); these were usually discontinued if IC failed. Patients treated with LEIC started antiarrhythmic drugs immediately after sinus rhythm was restored (generally 2 mg propafenone/kg i.v. followed by 750 mg propafenone per os die) to avoid defibrillation threshold increase.

HEIC was performed in the fasting state during anaesthesia induced with 100-150 mg propofol i.v., while patients undergoing LEIC were only slightly sedated with diazepam (5 mg i.v.). In patients undergoing HEIC, two quadripolar unused catheters were inserted in the right cavities through the femoral or subclavian vein. One was left in the right ventricular apex for emergency pacing. The other was positioned in the right atrium to administer shock. In the first five patients, the tip of the atrial lead was in contact with the tricuspidal annulus and the most proximal electrode was in the cavity of right atrium, as suggested by Levy

(3); in the following 24 patients the catheter was floating in the middle of the atrium, far from the atrial walls as assessed by left (LAO) and right anterior oblique view (RAO) projections. Unipolar synchronized shocks were delivered between a back plate (anode) and the proximal (first five patients) or one of the middle (following 24 patients) electrodes of the atrial lead (cathode). The following energy values were used in sequence: 100, 200, and 300 J.

The procedure was ended after restoration of the sinus rhythm or after the 300 J shock discharge.

In patients undergoing LEIC, two unused decapolar catheters were advanced from the femoral vein up to the distal coronary sinus and the lateral right free wall, respectively. A quadripolar catheter was placed in the right ventricular apex to enable ventricular synchronization. The electrodes of each decapolar catheter were electrically coupled to create two electrodes. Using the right atrial catheter as the anode and the coronary sinus catheter as the cathode, R wave synchronized shocks were delivered at increasing energy levels of 0.2, 0.6, 1.4, 2.5, 4.0, 5.7, 7.7, and 10 J. Shocks were biphasic, truncated and exponential. All the catheters were generally inserted via the right femoral vein.

An electrocardiographic (ECG) recording was obtained during the cardioversion procedure and for the following 15 min; data were analyzed using the chi-square analysis. A p value of 0.005 or less was considered significant.

Results

High-Energy Internal Cardioversion

Sinus rhythm was restored in 23 patients (79%): in seven (30%) with one, in nine (39%) with two and in seven (30%) with three shocks. Transient complete AV block, treated with prophylactic ventricular pacing, occurred in two patients (7%) – in two of the first five patients (40%) and in none of the following 24 (p=0.0049). First degree AV block occurred in two of 21 patients (10%) without transient complete AV block in which sinus rhythm was restored – in two of three in the first five patients and in none of the following. In total, four of the first five patients (80%) showed transient AV conduction disturbances compared with none in the remaining 24 (p=0.0001.)

Transient bradycardia appeared in one patient. No other complication was noted after IC, as assessed by echocardiography performed at the end of the procedure and 24 h later.

No correlation was found between sinus rhythm restoration and left atrial size, body weight, or AF duration.

At a mean follow-up of 15 months, AF recurred in only nine patients (39%). A second IC attempt was not performed in patients with AF recurrence. A total of 14 patients (48%) of the whole patient population that underwent IC were in sinus rhythm at 12 months follow-up. No patient that underwent IC died during the follow-up, and no correlation was found between AF recurrence and left atrial size, body weight, or AF duration.

Low-Energy Internal Cardioversion

In the five patients undergoing LEIC, sinus rhythm was restored in all with energy levels ranging from 1 to 10 J. Two patients with paroxysmal AF had the lowest defibrillation threshold (0.6 and 1.4, respectively). Patients complained of increasing levels of discomfort with increasing energy levels. No complication was noted in any patient as assessed by echocardiography performed at the end of the procedure and 24 h later.

At a mean follow-up of 6 months (range, 2-11 months), AF recurred in one patient. The small number of the patients treated with LEIC does not permit any correlation between sinus rhythm restoration or AF recurrences and left atrial size, AF duration or body weight.

Discussion

AF was considered a benign arrhythmia until the late 1970s, when several studies demonstrated a higher incidence of stroke in patients with AF without rheumatic valvular disease and even in those without heart disease compared to normal population matched for age and blood pressure (1, 2, 4).

The pathogenesis of stroke in such patients is probably multifactorial but the most important factor is embolization of left atrial thrombi whose formation is closely related to the presence of AF (5).

These new insights had two important effects:
– A more aggressive management of AF in order to restore sinus rhythm even in patients with AF of long duration
– The widespread use of antithrombotic medication in patients in whom sinus rhythm restoration attempatients failed

Patients in whom pharmacologic or electrical transthoracic cardioversion were unsuccessful were usually treated with drugs acting on AV node conduction such as verapamil or beta blockers. More recently, AV node or His bundle transcatheter ablation, with subsequent implantation of a permanent pacemaker, has been employed in such patients (6, 7).

The above therapeutic options ameliorate symptoms and hemodynamics but have no impact on embolic risk because the atria remain in AF.

A third and new approach is IC that can be performed using high (8-10) or low energy (11, 12). In external cardioversion, a large part of the energy does not reach the heart because of transthoracic impedance (13), while during IC the energy is delivered directly to the atrium. This accounts for the success of IC in patients in whom external cardioversion failed to restore sinus rhythm. In fact, in all patients undergoing IC in this study, one or more attempts with transthoracic DC shock had been unsuccessful.

High-Energy Internal Cardioversion

The immediate success (sinus rhythm restoration) was very high (79%) and comparable with that reported by other authors in patients with AF resistant to external cardioversion (3, 8, 9).

In accordance with other studies (3, 8-10) we had a low rate of complications during and after IC. No patients had pericardial effusion, ventricular arrhythmias, or permanent complete AV block.

In contrast to the data reported by Levy (8), we noted a lower incidence of transient AV block (8%); in our series, it appeared to be related to the position of the atrial lead delivering the shock.

When the catheter was positioned in the tricuspidal area, as in the first five patients, we observed transient complete AV block in two patients (40%); moreover transient prolongation of AV conduction was noted in two of the remaining three. Levy reported a 37% incidence of transient complete AV block after shock delivered through a catheter positioned in the tricuspid area (8); the incidence of transient AV conduction prolongation in patients with restored sinus rhythm and without transient complete AV block was not reported.

When the shock was delivered through a lead floating in the middle of the atrial cavity, as in the following 24 patients, no AV conduction disturbance was noted in our patients.

The difference between our two groups in developing any kind of transient AV conduction disturbance or specifically transient AV block is statistically significant ($p=0.0001$ and $p=0.049$, respectively). Mechanical trauma of the AV junction during the shock accounts for the high incidence of AV conduction disturbances observed when the atrial lead was left in contact with the tricuspid annulus.

During 1 year of follow-up, 39% patients had AF recurrence. The incidence of AF recurrence in our study seems to be lower than that reported by Levy (8) and Levy and Morady (10); the only difference between our and Levy's studies was the extensive use of propafenone for AF recurrence prophylaxis in our patients. The low AF recurrence rate in our study does not imply a superior efficacy of IC in the prevention of AF recurrence. Animal and clinical studies (8, 9) have suggested that stretching of atrial fibers and a long-lasting alteration in transmembrane ion flux might lead to a better efficacy of HEIC respect to transthoracic cardioversion in preventing AF recurrence (8, 9). However, the recent study by Levy and Morady (10) has shown that the recurrence rate of AF is not different in patients in whom sinus rhythm was restored with HEIC or external cardioversion.

No correlation was found in our study between sinus rhythm restoration or AF recurrence and body weight, atrial size, or AF duration.

Levy and Morady (10) reported that body weight was the only variable associated with the outcome of cardioversion; their study population consisted of 112 patients randomized to undergo external cardioversion or IC. An inverse correlation between body weight and successful cardioversion applies to the whole population, with no distinction being made between patients undergoing external cardioversion and those undergoing HEIC.

Body weight correlates with chest diameter and consequently with transthoracic impedance which is inversely related to the current flow traversing the heart during external cardioversion (14 – 16). Consequently a correlation between body weight and suc-

cessful cardioversion is expected in external cardioversion but not in HEIC.

The results reported by Levy and Morady probably reflect only the effect of body weight on external cardioversion. In our study, no correlation was found between body weight and sinus rhythm restoration in patients who underwent HEIC. The inverse relation between body weight and the transthoracic cardioversion success rate is indirectly confirmed by the fact that, not surprisingly, the mean body weight of our patients (in all of whom at least one external cardioversion attempt had failed) was very high.

Some investigators have reported a relation between atrial size or AF duration and cardioversion success rates (17-20), others between atrial size or AF duration and AF recurrence (19, 21).

Our and other recent studies using both HEIC and transthoracic cardioversion have not found any of the above correlations (8-10, 22). These differences probably reflect the fact that the prevalence of the underlying heart diseases is now different.

Low-Energy Internal Cardioversion

Recent animal (23, 24) studies showed that conversion of AF to sinus rhythm is feasible by intracardiac application of low energy shocks. Our and other studies (11, 12) demonstrate that the procedure is safe and effective in humans too. Moreover, in our patients previous attempts with external shock had failed; this fact suggests that LEIC may be used in other groups of patients achieving a lower defibrillation threshold. In our study, sinus rhythm was successfully restored with about 5% of the energy normally used during transthoracic cardioversion, which explains the absence of any kind of complication. Our preliminary results in patients with AF refractory to external DC shock suggest that LEIC may be used in the future as the treatment of first choice in patients with paroxysmal or chronic AF because of its safety, efficacy, and the low energy required; moreover general anesthesia is unnecessary.

Conclusions

IC with both high and low energy is a safe and effective procedure to restore sinus rhythm in patients with AF in whom one or more attempts at external cardioversion had failed. In HEIC, shocks delivered through a catheter floating in the right atrial cavity, far from the AV ring and His bundle, reduce the risk of transient complete AV block and other AV conduction disturbances. In our and other studies, ventricular tachyarrhytmias have been never induced with either HEIC or LEIC.

In our institution LEIC is actually the treatment of choice for patients in whom transthoracic defibrillation was unsuccessful, because it does not require general anesthesia; moreover, LEIC requires a significantly lower energy level, thus avoiding the uncommon side effects of HEIC; if LEIC is not effective, HEIC represents the last therapeutic option in these patients. IC is an additional important tool in the treatment of patients with AF. In our study, at 15 months follow-up, 46% of the whole patients population that underwent IC remained in sinus rhythm. These patients would be in AF if a non aggressive approach had not included IC, with either high or low energy, after the failure of external DC shock.

References

1. Wolf PA, Dawber TR, Thomas HE Jr (1978) Epidemiologic assessment of chronic atrial fibrillation and risk of stroke: the Framingham study. Neurology 28: 973-977
2. Wolf PA, Abbott RD, Kannel WB (1987) Atrial fibrillation: a major contributor to stroke in the elderly. The Framingham study. Arch Intern Med 147: 1561-1564
3. Levy S, Lacombe P, Cointe R, Bru P (1988) High energy transcatheter cardioversion of chronic atrial fibrillation. J Am Coll Cardiol 12: 514-518
4. Hinton RC, Kistler P, Fallon JR, Friedlich AL, Fisher CM (1977) Influence of etiology of atrial fibrillation on incidence of systemic embolism. Am J Cardiol 40: 509-513
5. Aberg H (1969) Atrial fibrillation: a study of atrial thrombosis and sistemic embolism in a necropsy material. Acta Med Scand 185: 373-379
6. Jackman WM, Xunzhang W, Friday KJ, Fitzgerald DM; Roman C et al (1991) Catheter ablation of atrioventricular junction using radiofrequency current in 17 patients. Circulation 83: 1562-1576
7. Yeung-Lai-Wah AJ, Alison JF, Lonergan L, Mohama R, Leather R, Kerr CR (1991) High success rate of atrioventricular node ablation with radiofrequency energy. J Am Coll Cardiol 18: 1753-1758
8. Levy S, Dolla E, Ebagosti A, Bru P (1990) Internal cardioversion for chronic atrial fibrillation. In: Touboul P, Waldo AL (eds) Atrial arrythmias. Mosby, St. Louis, pp 411-418
9. Kumagay K, Yamanouchi Y, Tadayuki H, Arakawa K (1991) Effects of transcatheter cardioversion on chronic lone atrial fibrillation. PACE 14: 1571-1575
10. Levy S, Philippe Lauribe, Dolla E, Kou W, Kadish A, Kalkins H et al (1992) A randomized comparison of external and internal cardioversion of chronic atrial fibrillation. Circulation 86: 1415-1420
11. Alt E, Schmitt C, Ammer R et al (1994) Initial experience with intracardiac atrial defibrillation in patients with chronic atrial fibrillation. PACE 17: 1067-1078
12. Baker B M, Botteron GW, Smith JM (1995) Low-energy internal cardioversion for atrial fibrillation resistant to external cardioversion. J Cardiovasc Electrophysiol 6: 44-47
13. Hoyt R, Grayzel J, Kerber RE (1981) Determinants of intracardiac current in defibrillation: experimental studies in dogs. Circulation 64: 818-823
14. Geddes LA, Tacker WA, Rosborough JP, Moore AG, Cabler PS (1974) Electrical dose for ventricular defibrillation of large and small animals using precordial electrodes. J Clin Invest 53: 310-319
15. Connell PN, Ewy GA, Dahl CF, Ewy MD (1973) Transthoracic impedance to defibrillator discharge: effect of electrode size and chest wall interface. J Electrocardiogr 6: 313-317
16. Ewy GA (1980) Direct current shock and trancardiac impedance. Am J Cardiol 45: 909-913
17. Flugelman MY, Hasin Y, Katznelson N (1984) Restoration and maintenance of sinus rhythm after mitral valve surgery for mitral stenosis. Am J Cardiol 54: 617-619
18. Henry WL, Morganroth J, Pearlman AS (1976) Relation between echocardiographically determined left atrial size and atrial fibrillation. Circulation 53: 273-279
19. Ewy G, Ulfers L, Hager WD (1980) Response of atrial fibrillation to therapy: role of etiology and left atrial diameter. J Electrocardiol 13: 119-124
20. Waris E, Kreus KE, Salokannel J (1971) Factors influencing persistence of sinus rhythm after DC shock treatment of atrial fibrillation. Acta Med Scand 189: 161-166
21. Mancini GBJ, Goldberger LA (1982) Cardioversion of atrial fibrillation: considerations of embolization, anticoagulation, prophylactic pacemaker, and long-term success. Am Heart J 104: 617-621
22. Dittrich HC, Erickson JS, Schneiderman T, Blacky R, Savides T, Nicod PH (1989) Echocardiographic and clinical predictors for outcome of elective cardioversion of atrial fibrillation. Am J Cardiol 63: 193-197
23. Cooper R, Alferness C, Smith W et al (1993) Internal cardioversion of atrial defibrillation in sheep. Circulation 87: 1673-1686
24. Powell AC, Garan H, McGovern BA et al (1992) Low energy conversion of atrial fibrillation in the sheep. J Am Coll Cardiol 20: 707-711

Automatic Implantable Atrial Defibrillator: A Dream or a Real Prospect?

S. Lévy

University of Marseille, School of Medicine, Division of Cardiology,
Hôpital Nord, Marseille, France

Introduction

A few years ago, John Camm and I wrote an editorial (1) presenting the conditions necessary to make the dream of an atrial defribillator come true. These conditions include feasibility, safety, and tolerability. The atrial defibrillator should be able to reliably detect and terminate atrial fibrillation (AF). The feasibility and safety of such a device must be discussed together with the possible need for an implantable atrial defibrillator (IAD) and its role among the therapeutic strategies for AF.

Is There a Need for an Automatic Implantable Atrial Defibrillator?

AF is an extremely common arrhythmia seen in clinical practice, as shown by a number of epidemiologic studies. Pharmacologic therapy represents a first-line treatment, and a number of patients respond favorably, at least for a given period of time. However, a significant number of patients have recurrent attacks of AF despite pharmacologic therapy; others are controlled, but the drug is discontinued as the patient develops intolerable side effects. Symptoms related to the arrhythmia may be due to the rapid ventricular response and/or irregular rhythm. Other symptoms or complications include a deleterious effect on cardiac function, reduced cardiac output, and peripheral emboli. The embolic risk averages 3%–5% per year and depends on the age of the patient, the presence and type of underlying heart disease, and ventricular function. The clinical presentation of AF is quite heterogenous, and a classification system has recently been proposed (Table 1). Obviously, symptomatic patients in class III, i.e., patients who experience symptomatic episodes of AF despite the use of antiarrhythmic agents (sodium channel blockers and potassium channel blockers), represent potential candidates. The number and duration of episodes should be taken into account in the indications. Patients with frequent episodes (several episodes per day) must be excluded,

Table 1. Proposed clinical classification of atrial fibrillation (AF)

Class	Symptoms
I	First attack of AF
A	Spontaneous termination
B	Pharmacologic or electrical cardioversion
II	Recurrent attacks of AF (untreated)
A	Asymptomatic
B	Less than one attack in 3 months
C	More than one attack in 3 months
III	Recurrent attacks of AF (treated)
A	Asymptomatic
B	Less than one attack in 3 months
C	More than ,one attack in 3 months

as IAD implantation may result in too frequent discharges, patient discomfort, and rapid battery depletion. Similarly, patients with episodes of short duration and spontaneous termination may not be good candidates.

The severity of patient symptom(s) and arrhythmia tolerance must be taken into account. Selected patients with infrequent attacks, fewer than one episode per 3-month period, may benefit from an IAD, particularly those patients with long-lasting episodes of AF that require pharmacologic or electrical reversion. It is not known whether there is an indication for an IAD in patients with asymptomatic AF and a history of embolic complications. In selected AF patients resistant to antiarrhythmic therapy aimed at preventing recurrences and assessed with ambulatory electrocardiogram (ECG) monitoring, an IAD may be considered.

Other therapeutic options in patients with recurrent AF resistant to pharmacologic therapy include controlling the ventricular rate with agents such as verapamil, diltiazem, beta-blocking agents, and digitalis. Such therapeutic options have not been systematically tested. When control of ventricular rate and symptoms cannot be achieved with pharmacologic treatment, atrioventricular (AV) node ablation with pacemaker implantation may be an alternative. Recently, AV node modification was proposed, which may obviate the need for pacemaker implantation in a large number of patients (6). Preliminary results are encouraging. There are no data indicating that the control of ventricular rate reduces embolic risk.

Unlike other forms of supraventricular tachycardias, catheter ablation of AF is not yet possible. Surgery for AF prevention includes the "corridor" (7) and the "maze" operations (8). Although the results reported are impressive, this major surgery carries a significant risk of operative mortality, and long-term results of morbidity in a large series are not yet available (9).

Therefore, we believe that there are indications for an IAD, provided it is technically feasible, reliable in terms of arrhythmia detection and termination, and safe.

Can Atrial Fibrillation Be Reliably Detected?

An IAD should be able to reliably detect AF. Detection of AF obviously requires an electrode in the right atrium. Atrial electrograms are more difficult to detect than ventricular electrograms, as the signal amplitude is less and it may be mistaken for a distant ventricular signal or interference withe other electromagnetic signals. However, recent studies (10, 11) have shown that AF may be recognized using atrial electrograms on the basis of atrial rate, amplitude, probability density function, and spectral analysis with a sensitivity greater than 88% and a specificity of 100%. The detection algorithm may include irregular ventricular cycles detected using a ventricular electrode, which is required for R wave synchronization. The detection algorithms may be further refined, as there is no urgency to terminate AF as opposed to ventricular fibrillation.

Atrial Defibrillation

Atrial defibrillation is feasible in humans using high-energy shocks (12, 13). However, as the shock for AF is delivered to an awake patient, the energy used should be low enough to avoid shock-related discomfort. Initial studies by Mower et al. (14) using two catheters, one in the right atrium and the other in the superior vena cava, have shown successful defibrillation in 125 episodes in acetylcholine-induced AF in dogs with energies ranging from 0.05 to 3 J. Dunbar et al. (15) were able to terminate only 26% of AF episodes induced by talc-induced pericarditis in dog. The electrode used included both anode and cathode on the same catheter. Using a similar catheter in humans, Nathan et al. (16) were not successful in terminating AF and obtained better results with atrial flutter. In contrast, using the technique of Lévy et al. (12), Kumagai et al. (17) were able to terminate 81 episodes of AF in dogs with talc-induced pericarditis using shocks of 5 J or less. In 57 attempts (70%), shocks of 1 J or less resulted in successful cardioversion. Recently, Cooper et al. (18) studied different electrode configurations and found that delivering a shock between one catheter in the right atrium and the other in the coronary sinus and using a biphasic waveform in a sheep model of AF resulted in successful defibrillation with energies ranging from 1 to 7 J. In 50% of the episodes, successful cardioversion was obtained, with energies of 1.3 ± 0.4 J. The question arises as to whether these results can be extrapolated to AF in humans with areas of atrial fibrosis and underlying heart disease in 80% of cases. In 16 patients with flutter fibrillation, Kean et al. (19) reported successful cardioversion in 15 patients with energies less than 7 J. In two patients, termination of atrial flutter was obtained with an energy level less than 1 J. In six patients with inducible sustained AF, Johnson et al. (20) compared a 6-ms monophasic with a 3/3-ms biphasic truncated waveform. Biphasic shocks resulted in lower defibrillation thresholds (2.5 ± 1.4 versus 4.7 ± 3.1 J). Murgatroyd et al. (21) attempted cardioversion with two electrodes (coronary sinus and right atrium) in eight patients with sustained AF and were successful using a mean energy of 2.2 J (range, 0.7 – 3.4 J). Furthermore, they found that shocks of less than 1 J were well tolerated. This is important, since discomfort due to shock is acceptable for a malignant ventricular arrhythmia often associated with hypotension and syncope, but may not be tolerated for a supraventricular arrhythmia, which is usually not life-threatening. Alt et al. (22) compared 14 patients with chronic AF and dilated left atrium and were able to successfully cardiovert using a mean energy of 3.7 ± 1.7 J. The XAD study on internal cardioversion of atrial fibrillation using an external atrial defibrillator in a multicenter trial with 123 patients showed that is it possible to successfully defibrillate the atria with an energy level of less than 2.5 J in 75% or more of cases. Not surprisingly, the energy needed for paroxysmal spontaneous or induced atrial fibrillation was significantly lower than that required for chronic atrial defibrillation.

Safety of an Automatic Implantable Atrial Defibrillator

A major concern with an IAD is safety, i.e., the potential risk of inducing ventricular tachycardia or fibrillation when delivering a shock to convert AF. Obviously, the shock delivered to the right atrium should be synchronized to the ventricular electrogram recorded through an electrode positioned in the right ventricle. Such an electrode catheter may also be useful for pacing the ventricles in the case of shock-related bradycardia (asystole or AV block). Dunbar et al. (15) reported an incidence of ventricular fibrillation ranging from 2% – 6.5% in dogs following shocks (0.1 – 5 J) delivered in the right atrium. As already mentioned, this may be due to the electrode configuration they used, as Kumagai et al. (17) did not observe such a complication. Ayers et al. (23) addressed this issue in an elegant study in sheep. They observed 11 episodes of ventricular fibrillation in a total of 1870 shocks delivered and evaluated the conditions favoring such ventricular proarrhythmic effects. They found that the cycle length preceding R wave-synchronized shock delivery played a role, because no episodes of ventricular fibrillation occurred after a cycle length of more than 300 ms. Such a study may contribute toward reducing the risk of ventricular proarrhythmia. One way to treat such a potential risk would be to combine the IAD with an implantable cardioverter defibrillator (ICD), the latter delivering a shock to the ventricles in the case of ventricular fibrillation following an attempt to convert AF. Ongoing studies on atrial defibrillation in a large number of patients with AF, with or without underlying heart disease, will determine the incidence of ventricular proarrhythmia. Preliminary results in humans so far have not shown any ventricular proarrhythmic events. To be acceptable, the risk should certainly be very low (less than 0.1%). However, it should also be taken into account that the use of antiarrhythmic agents is associated with ventricular proarrhythmia. A useful step in the develpment of an IAD and in the evaluation of its safety and efficacy might be a physician-activated device.

A further issue relates to the tolerance of shocks. Our experience in nonsedated patients showed a wide individual variability in the tolerance of shocks. This issue remains to be studied in a systematic fashion. Pain may turn out to be less of a problem in real life than in the laboratory, where the patient is very anxious.

An automatic atrial defibrillator is already available (Metrix system), and clinical trials are about to start. The first step should be to study the detection and the termination of AF using such an implanted device activated by the physician. Such a trial is essential to define the safety of atrial defibrillation before using the automatic mode. Thus atrial defibrillator is no longer merely a dream, but is now a real prospect, and clinical trials are needed.

References

1. Lévy S, Camm AJ (1993) An implantable atrial defibrillator: an impossible dream? Circulation 87: 1769-1772
2. Kannel WB, Abbott RD, Savage DD et al (1992) Epidemiologic features of chronic atrial fibrillation: the Framingham study. N Engl J Med 306: 1018-1022
3. Bialy D, Lehmann MH, Schumacher DM et al (1992) Hospitalization of arrhythmias in the United States: importance of atrial fibrillation. J Am Coll Cardiol 19: 41A
4. Pritchett ELC (1992) Management of atrial fibrillation. N Engl J Med 326: 1264-1271
5. Lévy S, Novella P, Richard P et al (1995) Paroxysmal atrial fibrillation: a need for classification. J Cardiovasc Electrophysiol 6: 69-74
6. Williamson BD, Ching Man K, Daoud E et al (1994) Radiofrequency catheter modification of atrioventricular conduction to control the ventricular rate during atrial fibrillation. N Engl J Med 331: 910-917
7. Leitch JW, Klein G, Yee R et al (1991) Sinus node-atrioventricular node isolation: long-term results with the "corridor" operation for atrial fibrillation. J Am Coll Cardiol 17: 970-975
8. Cox JL, Shnessler RB, D'Agostino HJ et al (1991) The surgical treatment of atrial fibrillation. III. Development of a definitive surgical procedure. J Thorac Cardiovasc Surg 101: 509-583
9. McCarthy PM, Castle LW, Maloney JD et al (1993) Initial experience with the maze procedure for atrial fibrillation. J Thorac Cardiovasc Surg 105: 1077-1087
10. Slocum J, Sahakian KH, Swiryn S (1988) Computer discrimination of atrial fibrillation and regular atrial rhythms from intraatrial electrograms. Pace 11: 610-621
11. Jenkins J, Noth KH, Guezennec A et al (1988) Diagnosis of atrial fibrillation using electrograms from chronic leads: evaluation of computer algorithms. Pace 11: 622-631
12. Lévy S, Lacombe P, Coint R et al (1988) High energy transcatheter cardioversion of chronic atrial fibrillation. J Am Coll Cardiol 12: 514-518
13. Lévy S, Lauribe P, Dolla E et al (1992) A randomized comparison of external and internal cardioversion of chronic atrial fibrillation. Circulation 86: 1415-1420
14. Mower MM, Mirowski M, Denniston RH (1972) Assessment of various models of acetylcholine induced atrial fibrillation for study of intra-atrial cardioversion. Clin Res 20: 388 (abstr)
15. Dunbar DN, Tobler HG, Fetter J et al (1986) Intracavitary electrode catheter cardioversion of atrial tachyarrhythmias in the dog. J Am Coll Cardiol 7: 1015-1027
16. Nathan AW, Bexton RS, Spurrell RA et al (1984) Internal transvenous low energy cardioversion for the treatment of cardiac arrhythmias. Br Heart J 52: 377-384
17. Kumagai K, Yamanouchi Y, Tashiro N et al (1990) Low energy synchronous transcatheter cardioversion of atrial flutter/fibrillation in the dog. J Am Coll Cardiol 16: 467-501
18. Cooper RAS, ALferness CA, Smith WM et al (1993) Internal cardioversion of atrial fibrillation in sheep. Circulation 87: 1673-1686
19. Keane D, Sulke N, Cooke R et al (1993) Endocardial cardioversion of atrial flutter and fibrillation. Pace 16: 928
20. Johnson E, Smith W, Yarger M et al (1994) Clinical predictors of low energy defibrillation thresholds in patients undergoing internal cardioversion of atrial fibrillation. Pace 17: 742 (abstr)
21. Murgatroyd FD, Slade AKB, O'Farrell DM et al (1994) Low energy internal atrioversion in man. Cardiostimulation, Nice, 1994 (abstr 662)
22. Alt E, Schmitt C, Ammer R et al (1992) Initial experience with intracardiac atrial defibrillation in patients with chronic atrial fibrillation. Pace 17: 1067-1078
23. Ayers GM, Alferness CA, Ilina M et al (1994) Ventricular proarrhythmic effects of ventricular cycle length and shock strength in a sheep model of transvenous atrial defibrillaion. Circulation 89: 413-422

Paroxysmal Atrial Flutter: Which Mechanism and Treatment in the Era of Catheter Ablation?

F. Ambrosini, M. Arlotti, and A. Lotto

Divisione di Cardiologia, Ospedale Maggiore, IRCCS, Milan, Italy

Atrial flutter (AF), a common rhythm disturbance, was first described several decades ago (1). Despite extensive investigation, several important issues remain unresolved concerning its mechanism and its management. Indeed, for greater clarity, it should be recalled that this term mainly covers the common form (still called type I flutter), defined as an atrial tachycardia with a constant rate, polarity, and morphology of locally recorded electrograms. A "saw tooth" pattern (inverted P waves) is present in the inferior leads on the electrocardiogram. The morphological criterion is actually prevalent, the diagnosis of flutter being compatible with atrial frequencies higher than 300/min, or lower between 200 and 250/min. Type II AF is characterized by a similar uniformity of the atrial electrogram appearance, but the rate is faster. While both are likely due to a reentrant mechanism, type I AF can often be stopped by rapid atrial pacing or can be transformed to type II AF (2-5).

Present therapeutic strategies often appear effective in preventing and terminating AF; however, controlled trials and definitive studies comparing the various treatment options are surprisingly scarce. While antiarrhythmic drugs continue to be used to prevent recurrent AF, little data prove the efficacy of these drugs, their mechanism of action, or their safety.

Experimental and clinical approaches to this arrhythmia have brought about evidence for a macro-reentrant mechanism in the right atrium (3, 5-16). This has led to the use of catheter ablation as a mode of treatment for drug refractory AF (17-19).

Basic Concepts

The Circular Activation of the Right Atrium

Experimental models of AF can have an anatomical or functional basis, or a combination of both. In Rosenblueth's "tricuspid ring" model, dependent on a large, purely anatomical obstacle in the posterior right atrial wall, another lesion ablating all myocardium between the central obstacle and the tricuspid ring would make reentry impossible (20). However, in Allessie's model, under vagal stimulation, reentry is based mainly on functional changes and can appear almost anywhere in either atrium; therefore no simple ablative intervention can prevent it.

A third AF model is based on a combination of an anatomical obstacle (typically the superior vena cava or inferior vena cava) and adjacent areas of slow conduction and/or functional block. This type of reentry best resembles common human AF circuits, and it may be amenable to ablative interruption if there is a strong enough anatomical dependence (8-11, 13-16).

Puech in 1970 (2) and Chauvin in 1983 (8) used endocardial mapping to localize most human AF circuits to the right atrium. Most recently, Cosio has confirmed these findings and defined in more detailed the anatomical and functional bases of AF circuits (4-6, 17, 21-23). By sequential endocardial mapping, the author found circular activation patterns in the right atrium (RA) in all cases of common AF and in some AF with positive or low voltage waves. In common AF, the septum is activated caudocranially, the anterolateral RA craniocaudally (counterclockwise rotation in the frontal plane), and the circuit is closed through the relatively narrow isthmus between inferior vena cava (IVC) and the tricuspid valve (T). This isthmus is located on the anterior (ventral) side of the RA caudal end. The coronary sinus is activated from right to left, suggesting passive activation from the RA (Fig. 1).

Abnormal electrograms, suggestive of abnormal conduction, are recorded from different areas of the RA during AF, and some of them, located within the circuit, may be important in the reentry mechanism. Double-spike electrograms are constantly recorded along a line in the posterolateral RA; a likely explanation of these findings is that anisotropic conduction in the posterior internodal pathway (crista terminalis) creates a functional barrier between the posterior and lateral RA walls which, added to the IVC opening, constitutes a large enough central obstacle to sustain reentrant activation (5, 17, 22, 24-26).

Fragmented or double-spike electrograms are also recorded reproducibly from the low and midpos-

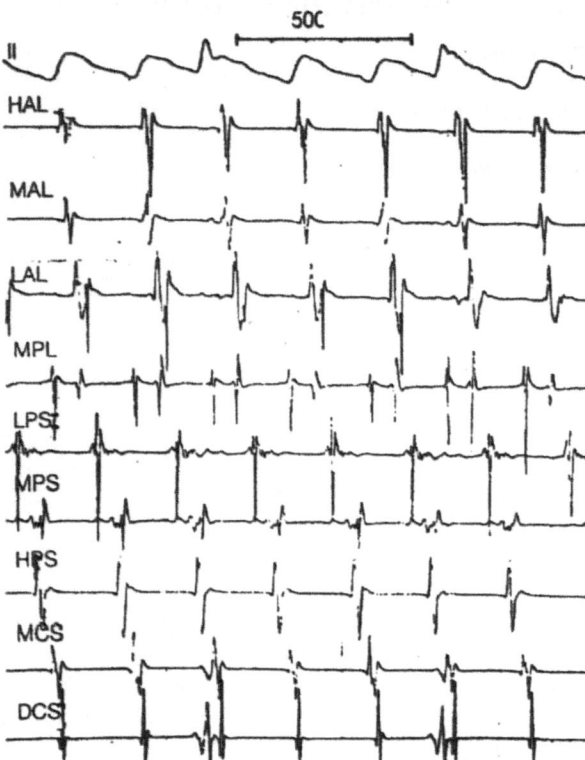

Fig. 1. Multiple simultaneous recordings in common flutter. From top to bottom: lead II, right atrial electrograms from high anterolateral (*HAL*), midanterolateral (*MAL*), low anterolateral (*MPL*), low posteroseptal (*LPS*), midposteroseptal (*MPS*), and high posteroseptal (*HPS*) areas, midcoronary sinus (*MCS*), and distal coronary sinus (*DCS*). Note the general trend of craniocaudal activation on the anterolateral right atrial wall and caudocranial activation on the posteroseptal wall. The MPL electrogram inscribes two spikes, one of which is close in time to the LAL electrogram, while the other is close to the MPS electrogram. Wide fragmented electrograms are recorded at LPS and MPS, suggesting local conduction delay (54)

teroseptal RA in the area of Kock's triangle. Fragmentation in this area is more likely a marker of local slow conduction, because electrogram duration fills the gap between activation of the more medial part of the IVC – TV isthmus and the activation of the midseptum.

This may be the location of the slow conduction zone; detailed intraoperative mapping of this area has shown very slow conduction from the IVC-TV isthmus toward the dorsal and cranial RA on both sides of the coronary sinus ostium (7, 27, 28). This local slow conduction would tend to support reentry by enlarging the excitable gap in the circuit. The cause of conduction slowing is unclear, but again it may be related to anisotropy, as internodal pathways converge in this area from several directions (29-33).

In fact, it is most probable that AF is related to the architecture of the RA. This cavity includes the orifices of the superior and inferior venae cavae as well as the fossa ovalis, which constitute obstacles to the progression of the excitation wave. Conduction within the RA is confined to three muscular columns linking the sinus node to the atrioventricular node: the crista terminalis and two internodal patways in the septum separated by the fossa ovalis. The endocardial depolarization splits into three main currents converging around the atrioventricular node. There is the potential anatomical basis for the creation of a circus movement.

However, the presence of a slow conduction area must be postulated in any structure able to develop a reentrant activity (Fig. 2) (16).

AF of the common type thus seems dependent on an abnormal excitation process of the RA, the participation of the left atrium only being contingent. The data concerning type II flutter are still a subject of debate. They tend, however, to support a circus movement of clockwise rotation in the RA, with descending depolarization of the atrial septum as a possible mechanism (4-6, 23).

Entrainment and Reset

The studies by Waldo et al. (34-36) in postoperative AF introduced the concept of entrainment of a reentrant circuit and provided evidence that reentry is the basic mechanism of human AF. Pacing from the high RA increased the atrial rate to the pacing rate, but the F waves remained negative in the inferior ECG leads despite the "high" pacing site. After pacing interruption, the basic F rate was resumed immediately. As pacing rate increased progressively, the F wave morphology changed, becoming less negative. In some cases, when a critical rate was reached, F waves became positive, and pacing interruption led to the restoration of sinus rhythm. These observations were interpreted as the result of penetration of the paced activation front "orthodromically" and "antidromically" in the AF circuit. In each paced cycle, collision would occur between the antidromically directed activation and the orthodromic penetration of the previous stimulus. As the pacing rate shortened, more antidromic penetration occurred, and progressive "fusion" between the orthodromic and the antidromic fronts changed the F morphology. Every time pacing was discontinued, the last orthodromic penetration would restart the AF circuit. A change to a positive P wave would mean that the AF cicuit was broken, atri-

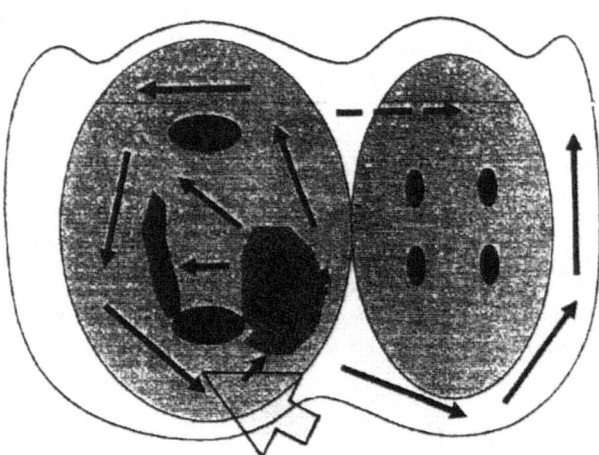

Fig. 2. Typical activation map in common atrial flutter (AF). Both atria are shown in a schematic anterior wave from the atrioventricular rings. *Shaded areas* represent endocardium and *white areas* epicardium. The location of the venae cavae, coronary sinus, and pulmonary veins are shown. The septal, posterior, and lateral right atrium (RA) walls are represented on the endocardial side. The activation proceeds "down" the anterior wall and "up" the septum. An area of slow conduction is present in the low posteroseptal RA. The *arrow* shows the region of the inferior vena cava (IVC) – tricuspid valve (T) isthmus. From (54)

al activation then starting at the high RA pacing site (37-42).

The actual events during entrainment have been documented in atrioventricular accessory pathway tachycardia and in AF in dog models. Orthodromic and antidromic penetration as well as progressive fusion have been confirmed, with collision at a different point for each entrainment rate. The increased rate during entrainment modifies the properties of the circuit, mainly in terms of conduction velocity. Slow conduction may develop in different parts of the AF circuit due to a faster driving rate and may progress to block of both the antidromic and orthodromic fronts, resulting in AF interruption. Entrainment can be conceived as a continuous resetting of the AF cycle by regularly spaced stimuli. Resetting by a single stimulus produces the same sequence changes as entrainment, supporting the presence of a large circular activation pathway, although without precisely defining its limits (40).

Clinical Approach to the Patient

Despite the interest in the mechanism of AF and the relative frequency of its occurrence, surprisingly few definitive long-term, controlled trials have addressed management of those patients with only AF while excluding patients with atrial fibrillation.

AF is usually symptomatic. The most common symptoms are palpitations, but AF can also cause hypotension, angina, or heart failure. The symptoms depend on the underlying heart disease and on the ventricular rate.

Treatment of AF is not mandatory in the asymptomatic patient with a controlled ventricular response rate, as it is unlikely to alter the long-term prognosis. Unfortunately, an asymtomatic patient is rare to find. In contrast, treatment with IC antiarrhythmic drugs may accelerate the ventricular rate during AF, while paradoxically slowing the atrial rate, ultimately worsening symptoms. Other adverse effects of antiarrhythmic drug therapy must be considered. Several clinical issues in the management of patients with AF are worth addressing. These includes the following:
1. Etiology and types of AF
2. Ventricular rate control during AF
3. Long-term pharmacologic management in patients with AF
4. Nonpharmacologic therapy

Pharmacological Management

Although generally not life-threatening, AF is usually associated with symptoms that can be severe. AF can cause hemodynamic impairment in some patients, especially in those with impaired ventricular function. In the pediatric age-group, AF can be life-threatening if concomitant congenital heart disease is present. In such patients, the atrial contribution to cardiac output may be critical. Compared to atrial fibrillation, few randomized, prospective studies demonstrate the utility of antiarrhythmic drug therapy to terminate and to prevent AF. There is not a drug presently available that will terminate human AF reliably (an important

difference between the animal models of AF and man). The most effective approach to stop human AF is a nonpharmacologic approach (endocardial or transesophageal rapid atrial pacing and/or synchronized cardioversion) (43). In certain patients subgroups, such as those with postoperative AF, it appears worthwhile to use β-adrenergic blockers to stop and prevent AF or class I antiarrhythmic drugs (44).

β-Adrenergic blockers are particularly useful in patients with AF following cardiac surgery (45). Amiodarone has also been used in patients postoperatively, but it is not clear whether it is more effective than other drugs for AF. Antiarrhythmic drugs can help aid termination of AF by atrial pacing (46).

However, few data show that patients benefit long-term from antiarrhythmic drug therapy for AF (most data combine AF with fibrillation), and few data are available to indicate how long antiarrhythmic therapy is necessary or effective. While antiarrhythmic drugs may be effective, adverse drug effects worse than the AF itself are common. In addition, these drugs may trigger other more life-threatening arrhythmias and increase the risk of sudden death. Encainide and flecainide have been shown to do this in patients with coronary artery disease and asymptomatic ventricular ectopy. In addition, there may be a higher death rate in patients with atrial fibrillation who take quinidine, although the data are not conclusive.

Nevertheless, for patients with recurrent AF, especially when symptomatic, chronic antiarrhythmic drug therapy is effective to prevent arrhythmia recurrence and may be recommended. Several drugs are available, but their comparative efficacy is unknown. β-Adrenergic blockers – especially sotalol – are particularly useful in preventing paroxysmal AF. Amiodarone is also an effective drug, but several important side effects preclude its use as a first-line drug. Not only can amiodarone terminate and prevent AF, but it can also maintain a slower ventricular response rate to AF due to its atrioventricular nodal blocking effect.

Direct Radiofrequency Catheter Ablation of the AF Circuit

As previously described, the reproducible configuration of common flutter circuits in patients with and without different types of cardiac disease suggests a strong dependence on RA anatomy. This would refer to the "holes" made by the veins and to the myocardial arrangement in bundles (internodal tracts) with its important effects on conduction. This anatomical arrangement might be the reason for the tendency to develop the same type of reentry circuit in many different disease processes.

The IVC – T isthmus closes the caudal end of circuit. Thus this narrow isthmus appears to be an optimal target for ablation to interrupt common AF (17). The apparent anatomical dependence of the AF circuit also suggests that ablation of this area could also prevent recurrences. Technically speaking, the IVC – T isthmus is easily accessible, of small width, and located far from the atrioventricular node.

To interrupt the circuit permanently, the difficult

aim would be the production of a continuous line of necrosis cutting across the IVC-T isthmus, from the T ring to the IVC.

It is possible to interrupt the circuit permanently, delivering radiofrequency (RF) energy to other anatomical sites (isthmus between the IVC and the coronary sinus and isthmus between T and the coronary sinus)(anatomical criterion, see Table 1) (47-52).

In 1992, Feld et al. (53) reported that RF energy applied to a discrete area in the low posteroseptal RA can terminate AF and prevent its immediate reinduction by programmed stimulation. RF ablation was successful at sites demonstrating earliest activation with a discrete electrogram and an exact entrainment pace map with a relatively short stimulus-to-P wave interval of 20-40 ms, suggesting that these sites were at the exit from the area of slow conduction (electrophysiological criterion; see Table 1).

Our Experience (51, 52)

Sixteen patients (mean age, 59±13 years) with symptomatic, recurrent type I AF (mean cycle, 238±39 ms, resistant to 2-4 antiarrhythmic drugs, underwent endocardial mapping of RA and RF catheter ablation. The underlying heart disease was: mitral valve prolapse (n = 3), valvular heart disease (n = 3), dilated cardiomyopathy (n = 2), ischemic heart disease (n = 1) and restrictive cardiomyopathy (n = 1). Six patients had a normal heart. Target sites for RF energy delivery were identified by recording fragmented atriograms, by activation time, and by entrainment pace mapping in 10 patients (group 1); in 6 patients RF was applied to the IVC – T isthmus (group 2).

We applied a mean of 18±7 RF impulses (10-30 W for 5-20 s) by means of the distal electrode of a four-polar lead with a thermocouple for temperature recording, used in unipolar configuration. In group 1, sinus rhythm was restored in 4/10 patients (40%), in group 2, in 5/6 patients (83%) (Fig. 3). Modulation of atrioventricular nodal conduction was performed in six patients. The long-term results (follow-up, 4-58 months; mean, 19±9 months) are shown in Table 2.

Table 2. Follow-up (19±9 months)

	Patients	Sinus rhythm restored		AF (paroxysmal)		Atrial fibrillation	
	(n)	(n)	(%)	(n)	(%)	(n)	(%)
Group 1	10	4	40	4	40	2	20
Group 2	6	5	83	2	33	1	16

AF, atrial flutter

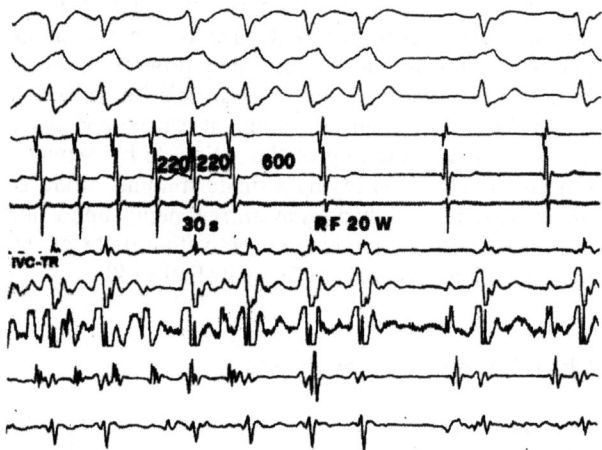

Fig. 3. Interruption of atrial flutter (AF) 20 s after radiofrequency (*RF*) application at the inferior vena cava – tricuspid valve (*IVC – T*) isthmus.

Conclusions

These few studies have shown that RF catheter ablation may have a role in the treatment of drug-resistant AF without the need for nodal ablation and a permanent pacemaker. However, RF ablation still puts the following problems. The success of this approach is related to atrial mapping and careful identification of the critical slow conduction area by well-trained staff. Clearly, there are many questions that remain to be answered about the nature of the reentrant circuit in AF. While it seems clear that most flutter involves reentry in the RA, we are still only beginning to clearly understand the nature of AF. Although the careful studies, such as those by Cosio et al. (54), are extremely helpful, improvements in recording techniques and the ability to study AF intraoperatively in patients us-

Table 1. Radiofrequency ablation studies

Reference	Patients (n)	Target	Recurrences (n)	Follow-up (months)
(51) (52)	16	IVC–T / EPS	9/16	5-48
(53)	12	EPS	10/12	5 weeks
(17)	9	IVC–T	3/9	3-18
(49)	9	IVC–T	4/9	1-10
(55)	8	IVC–T / T–CS	6/8	12
(56)	6	IVC–T / T–CS	3/6	7.5
(57)	16	EPS	9/16	4-10
(50)	70	IVC–T / T–CS / IVC–CS	37/70	1-24
(58)	40	IVC–T / T–CS	25/40	9.8
(59)	20	NR	16/20	5.3
(60)	14	T–CS / CS–LRA	9/14	1-17

IVC–T, isthmus between inferior vena cava (IVC) and tricuspid valve; T–CS, isthmus between tricuspid valve and coronary sinus; IVC–CS, isthmus between inferior vena cava and coronary sinus; EPS, electrophysiologic criterion; NR, not reported

ing simultaneous multisite mapping tecnhiques are still needed to provide more accurate data on the nature of AF reentrant circuits. Hopefully, we will then be able to answer the many questions that remain: where is the precise location of the reentrant circuit of AF in patients? Does it always involve reentrant excitation in part or in full around an anatomical obstacle? Can the obstacle be entirely functional? Is there a relationship between the so-called slow pathway of atrioventricular nodal reentrant tachycardia and an area of slow conduction posteroinferior in the RA in AF?

Finally, a longer follow-up period will clearly be required to confirm that this form of therapy is an effective alternative to currently available treatment, because late recurrence of new AF morphologies or atrial fibrillation may limit its usefulness.

References

1. Lewis T, Feil S, Stroud WD (1920) Observations upon flutter and fibrillation. II. The nature of auricular flutter. Heart 7/ 191-233
2. Puech P, Latour H, Grolleau R (1970) Le flutter et ses limites. Arch Mal Coeur 63: 116-144
3. Disertori M, Inama G, Vergara G, Guarnerio M, Del Favero A, Furlanello F (1983) Evidence of a reentry circuit in the common type of atrial flutter in man. Circulation 67: 434-440
4. Cosio FG (1992) Atrial vulnerability. Clin Cardiol 15: 198-202
5. · Cosio FG, Lopez-Gil M, Goicolea A, Arribas F (1992) Electrophysiologic studies in atrial flutter. Clin Cardiol 15: 667-673
6. Cosio FG, Palacios J, Vidal JM, Cocina EG, Gomez-Sanches MA, Tamargo L (1983) Electrophysiologic studies in atrial fibrillation. Slow conduction of premature impulse: a possible manifestation of the background for reentry. Am J Cardiol 51: 122-130
7. Klein GJ, Guiraudon GM, Sharma AD, Milstein S (1986) Demonstration of macroreentry and feasibility of operative therapy in the common type of atrial flutter. Am J Cardiol 57: 587-591
8. Frame LH, Page RL, Hoffman BF (1986) Atrial reentry around an anatomic barrier with a partially refractory execitable gap. A canine model of atrial flutter. Circ Res 58: 495-511
9. Frame LH, Page RL, Boyden PA, Fenoglio JJ, Hoffman BF (1987) Circus movement in the canine atrium around the tricuspid ring during experimental atrial flutter and during reentry in vitro. Circ Res 76: 1155-1175
10. Boyden PA, Frame LH, Hoffman BF (1989) Activation mapping of reentry around an anatomic barrier in the canine atrium. Observation during entrainment and termination. Circ 79: 406-416
11. Boyden PA (1988) Activation sequence during atrial flutter in dogs with surgically induced right atrial enlargement I: observation during sustained rhythms. Circ Res 62: 596-608
12. Page PL, Plumb VJ, Okumura K, Waldo AL (1986) A new animal model of atrial flutter. J Am Coll Cardiol 8: 872-879
13. Shoels W, Gough WB, Restivo M, El-Sherif N (1990) Circus movement atrial flutter in the canine sterile pericarditis model. Activation patterns during initiation, termination, and sustained reentry in vivo. Circ Res 67: 35-50
14. Schoels W, Kuebler W, Yang H, Gough WB, El-Sherif N (1993) A unified functional/anatomic substrate for circus movement atrial flutter: activation and refractory patterns in the canine right atrial enlargement model. J Am Coll Cardiol 1: 73-84
15. Isber N, Restivo M, Gough WB, Yang H, El-Sherif N (1993) Circus movement atrial flutter in the canine sterile pericarditis model. Cryothermal termination from the epicardial site of the slow zone of the reentrant circuit. Circulation 87: 1649-1660
16. Gough WB, Restivo M, Yang H, El-Sherif N (1991) The slow zone in circus movement atrial flutter: the critical epicardial substrate. Circulation 84 [Suppl II]: 503 (abstr)
17. Cosio FG, Lopez-Gil M, Goicolea A, Arribas F, Barroso JL (1993) Radiofrequency ablation of the inferior vena cava – tricuspid valve isthmus in common atrial flutter. Am J Cardiol 71: 705-709
18. Chauvin M, Brechenmacher C, Voegtlin JR (1983) Application de la cartographie endocavitare a l'étude du flutter auriculaire. Arch Mal Coeur 76: 1020-1030
19. Chauvin M, Brechenmacher C (1989) A clinical study of application of endocardial fulguration in the treatment of recurrent atrial flutter. Pace 12: 219-224
20. Rosenblueth S, Garcia Ramos I (1947) Studies of flutter and fibrillation. II. The influence of artificial obstacles on experimental auricular flutter. Am Heart J 33: 677-684
21. Cosio FG, Arribas F, Palacios G, Tascon J, Lopez-Gil M (1986) Fragmented electrograms and continuous electrical activity in atrial flutter. Am J Cardiol 57: 1309-1314
22. Cosio FG, Arribas F, Barbero JM, Kellmeyer C, Goicolea A (1988) Validation of double spike electrograms as markers of conduction delay or block in atrial flutter. Am J Cardiol 61: 775-780
23. Cosio FG, Lopez-Gil M, Arribas F, Palacios J, Goicolea A, Nu͂nez A (1994) Mechanisms of entrainment of human common flutter studied with multiple endocardial recordings. Circulation 89: 2117-2125
24. Gravilescu S, Luca C (1975) Right atrium monophasic action potentials during atrial flutter and fibrillation in man. Am Heart J 90: 199-205
25. Boineau JP, Schuessler RB, Cain ME, Corr PB, Cox JL (1990) Activation mapping during normal atrial rhythms and atrial flutter. In: Zipes DP, Jalife J (eds) Cardiac electrophysiology. From cell to bedside. Saunders, Philadelphia, pp 537-548
26. Scherf L, James TN (1979) Fine structures of cells and their histologic organization within internodal pathways of the heart: clinical and electrocardiographic implications. Am J Cardiol 44: 345-369
27. Wells JL, MacLean WAH, James TN, Waldo AL (1979) Characterization of atrial flutter. Studies in man after open heart surgery using fixed atrial electrodes. Circulation 60: 665-673
28. Saumarez RC, Parker J, Camm J (1992) Geometrically accurate mapping of the atrioventricular node region during surgery. J Am Coll Cardiol 19: 601-606
29. Boineau JP, Schuessler RB, Mooney CR, Miller CB, Wylds AC, Hudson RD, Borremans JM, Brockus CW (1980) Natural and evoked atrial flutter due to circus movement in dogs. Role of abnormal atrial pathways, slow conduction, nonuniform refractory period distribution and premature beats. Am J Cardiol 45: 1167-1181
30. Dillon S, Allessie MA, Ursell PC, Wit Al (1988) Influence of anisotropic tissue structure on reentrant circuits in the epicardial border zone of subacute canine infarcts. Circ Res 63: 182-206
31. Spach MS, Dolber PC (1986) Relating extracellular potentials and their derivatives to anisotropic propagation at a microscopic level in human cardiac muscle: evidence for electrical uncoupling of side-to-side fiber connections with increasing age. Circ Res 58: 356-371
32. Spach MS, Miller WT, Dolber PC, Kootsey JM, Sommer JR, Mosher CE (1982) The functional role of structural complexities in the propagation of depolarization in the atrium of the dog: cardiac conduction disturbances due to discontinuities of effective axial resistivity. Circ Res 50: 175-191
33. Spach MS, Dolber PC, Heidlage JF (1988) Influence of the passive anisotropic properties on directional differences in propagation following modification of the sodium conductance in human atrial muscle: a model of reentry based on anisotropic discontinous propagation. Circ Res 62: 811-832
34. Waldo AL, McLean WAH, Karp RB, Kouchoukos NT, James TN (1977) Entrainment and interruption of atrial flutter with atrial pacing: studies in man following open heart surgery. Circulation 56: 737-745
35. Waldo AL, Plumb VJ, Arciniegas JG, McLean WAH, Coopert Tb, Priest MF, James TN (1982) Transient entrainment and interruption of A-V bypass pathway type paroxysmal atrial tachycardia: a model for understanding and identifying reentrant arrhythmias in man. Circulation 67: 73-83
36. Waldo AL, Henthorn RW, Plumb VJ, McLean WAH (1984) Demonstration of the mechanism of transient entrainment and interruption of ventricular tachycardia with rapid atrial pacing. J Am Coll Cardiol 3: 422-430

37. Okumura K, Henkthorn RW, Epstein AED, Plumb VJ, Waldo AL (1985) Further observations on transient entrainment: importance of pacing site and properties of the components of the reentry circuit. Circulation 72: 1293-1307

38. Beckman K, Huang TL, Frafchek J, Wyndham CRC (1986) Classic and concealed entrainment of typical and atypical atrial flutter. Pace 9: 826-835

39. Okumura K, Plumb VJ, Page PL (1991) Atrial activation sequence during atrial flutter in the canine pericarditis model and its correlation with the polarity of the flutter wave in the electrocardiogram. J Am Cardiol 17: 338-345

40. Arenal A, Almendral J, San Roman D, Delcan JL, Josephson ME (1992) Frequency and implications of resetting and entrainment with right atrial stimulation in atrial flutter. Am J Cardiol 70: 1292-1298

41. Henthorn RW, Okumura K, Olshansky B, Plumb VJ, Waldo AL (1988) A fourth criterion for transient entrainment: the electrogram equivalent of progressive fusion. Circulation 77: 1003-1012

42. Olshansky B, Okumura K, Henthorn RW, Waldo AL (1990) Characterization of double potentials in human atrial flutter: studies during transient entrainment. J Am Coll Cardiol 86: 833-841

43. Guarnerio M, Furlanello F, Del Greo M (1989) Transesophageal atrial pacing: a first choice technique in atrial flutter therapy. Am Heart J 117: 1241-1252

44. Olshansky B, Kleinman B, Wilber D (1991) Management of arrhythmias and conduction disturbances in the perioperative settings. In: Naccarelli GV (ed) Clinical cardiovascular therapeutics: cardiac arrhythmias: a pratical approach. Futura, Mount Kisco, pp 325-358

45. Leone L, Silverman A, Siouffi S (1987) Efficacy of nadolol in preventing supraventricular tachycardia after coronary artery bypass grafting. Am J Cardiol 60: 51D-58D

46. McAlister HF, Luke RA, Whitlock RM (1990) Intravenous amiodarone bolus versus oral quinidine for atrial flutter and fibrillation after cardiac operations. J Thorac Cardiovasc Surg 99: 911-918

47. Saoudi N, Atallah G, Kirkorian G, Touboul P (1990) Catheter ablation of the atrial myoicardium in human type I atrial flutter. Circulation 81: 762-771

48. Saoudi N, Derumeaux G, Cribier A (1991) The role of catheter ablation techniques in the treatment of classic (type I) atrial flutter. Pace 14: 2022-2027

49. Kirkorian G, Canu G, Moncada E, Atallah G, Chevalier P, Claudel JP, Touboul P (1993) Efficacy of radiofrequency ablation of atrial tissue in common atrial flutter. Pace 16/4: 851

50. Fisher B, Haissaguerre M, Le Metayer P, Egloff P, Warin JF (1993) Radiofrequency catheter ablation of common atrial flutter in 42 patients. Pace 16/5: 1099

51. Ambrosini F, Arlotti M, Landolina M, Manfredini R, Broglia P, Sernesi L, Lotto A (1992) Treatment and conversion of drug-resistant atrial flutter with radiofrequency energy. New Trends Arrhythm VII 1/2: 481-486

52. Arlotti M, Landolina M, Ambrosini F, Sernesi L, Mantica M, Lotto A (1993) Radiofrequency catheter ablation of drug-resistant atrial flutter: short and long term results. Pace 16/5: 1099

53. Feld GK, Fleck RP, Chen PS, Boyce K, Bahson TD, Stein JB, Calisi CM, Ibarra M (1992) Radiofrequency catheter ablation for the treatment of human type I atrial flutter. Identification of a critical zone in the reentrant circuit by endocardial mapping techniques. Circulation 86/4: 1233-1240

54. Cosio FG, Arribas F, Lopez-Gil M, Goicolea A (1993) Endocardial catheter mapping of atrial arrhythmias. In: Shenasa, Borggrefe, Breithardt (eds) Cardiac mapping. Futura, New York, pp 443-459

55. Nakagawa H, McClelland J, Beckman K, Wang X, Lazzara R, Hazlitt A, Santoro I, Aruda M, Abdalla I, Singh A, Sweidan R, Gossinger H, Hirao K, Wjdman L, Jackman W (1993) Radiofrequency catheter ablation of common type atrial flutter. PACE 16,4, Part II: 850 (Abstr)

56. Lesh M, Van Hare GF, Kwasman MA, Scheinman MM, Grogin HR, Lee RJ, Epstein LM, Gonzales R, Griffin JC (1993) Curative radiofrequency (RF) catheter ablation of atrial tachycardia and flutter. J Am Coll Cardiol 21: 374A (Abstr)

57. Calkins H, Leon AR, Deam AG, Kalbfleisch SJ, Langberg JJ, Morady F (1994) Catheter ablation of atrial flutter using radiofrequency energy. Am J Cardiol 73, 5: 353-356

58. Philippon F, Epstein AE, Plumb VJ, Douglas AW, Baker JH, Kay GN (1994) Predictors of atrial fibrillation following catheter ablation of atrial flutter. PACE 17,4, Part II: 758 (Abstr)

59. Mounsey JP, Nath S, Haines DE, DiMarco JP (1994) Normal right atrial size is required for success in radiofrequency ablation of atrial flutter. PACE 17,4, Part II: 757 (Abstr)

60. Ricard P, Mansouri C, Lauribe P, Gueunoun M, Paganelli F, Levy S (1994) Radiofrequency ablation of atrial flutter: a new anatomical approach. PACE 17,4, Part II: 758 (Abstr)

Author Index

GPSR Compliance

The European Union's (EU) General Product Safety Regulation (GPSR)
is a set of rules that requires consumer products to be safe and our
obligations to ensure this.

If you have any concerns about our products, you can contact us on
ProductSafety@springernature.com

In case Publisher is established outside the EU, the EU authorized
representative is:

Springer Nature Customer Service Center GmbH
Europaplatz 3
69115 Heidelberg, Germany

Batch number: 09635764

Printed by Printforce, the Netherlands